ALLE ZEIT WACH
1842

Kazuo Tabuchi (Ed.)

Biological Aspects of Brain Tumors

Proceedings of the 8th Nikko Brain Tumor Conference, Karatsu (Saga) 1990

With 214 Figures Including 13 in Color

Springer-Verlag
Tokyo Berlin Heidelberg
New York London Paris
Hong Kong Barcelona

Kazuo Tabuchi, m.d.
Professor and Chairman, Department of Neurosurgery, Saga Medical School,
Nabeshima, Saga, 849 Japan

ISBN 978-4-431-70078-4 Springer-Verlag Tokyo Berlin Heidelberg New York
ISBN 978-3-540-70078-4 Springer-Verlag Berlin Heidelberg New York Tokyo
ISBN 978-0-387-70078-6 Springer-Verlag New York Berlin Heidelberg Tokyo

Library of Congress Cataloging-in-Publication Data
Nikko Brain Tumor Conference (8th: 1990: Karatsu-shi, Japan) Biological aspects of brain tumors: proceedings of the 8th Nikko Brain Tumor Conference, Karatsu (Saga) 1990/K. Tabuchi (ed.). p. cm. Includes bibliographical references and index.ISBN 978-4-431-70078-4 -ISBN 978-3-540-70078-4. — ISBN 978-0-387-70078-6 1. Brain—Cancer—Congresses. 2. Gliomas—Congresses. I. Tabuchi, K. (Kazuo), 1940- . II. Title. [DNLM: 1. Brain Neoplasms—congresses. 2. Drug Resistance—congresses. 3. Glioma—congresses. 4. Oncogenes—physiology—congresses. WL 358 N692b 1990], RC280.B7N55 1990, 616.99′481—dc20, DNLM/DLC, for Library of Congress. 91-4993

Preface

Biological Aspects of Brain Tumors comprises the proceedings of the 8th Nikko Brain Tumor Conference held on November 6–8, 1990, in Karatsu (Saga Prefecture), Japan. The intention of the meeting was to bring together basic and clinical neuroscientists in order to exchange new ideas and information relevant to brain tumor research. The main theme of the 1990 Conference was "Recent Progress in Brain Tumor Biology." Several major topics related to the main theme were discussed, such as: growth activity of brain tumor, metabolism of brain tumor, brain tumor and cytokines, drug resistance of brain tumor, oncogene and anti-oncogene of brain tumor, and basic studies in brain tumor biology and therapy.

Glioma, particularly malignant glioma which is still one of the most challenging form of tumor, frustrating the efforts in current cancer treatment, is the major target of research in neuro-oncology and was therefore the primary focus of this meeting. The aim of this volume is to provide new concepts concerning our understanding of malignant glioma as well as an up-to-date summary of significant and potentially valuable works for the purposes of further investigation in the field of brain tumor biology. It is my hope that this volume may serve as a milestone for research into the 21st century at which time malignant glioma should be amenable to treatment.

A total of 64 papers have been selected from the oral and poster presentations at the Conference. The volume is divided into two parts: Part I is devoted to the seven special lectures which were given by the invited speakers and Part II includes the selected papers and consists of six sections dealing with the major topics mentioned above.

The Conference was fruitful not only from the point of view of the scientific material presented, but also with regard to the exchange of ideas and information during formal and informal discussions. All the authors submitted their manuscripts on time which allowed the prompt publication of this volume, and I gratefully acknowledge their endeavors. In the preparation of these proceedings, I have been helped greatly by the staff of Springer-Verlag, who have cooperated efficiently with the English copy-editing of this book. Finally, I am also much indebted to all the participants and sponsors who actively contributed to the success of this meeting.

Saga, Japan KAZUO TABUCHI

Contents

Section 4. Drug Resistance of Brain Tumor

Section 5. Oncogene and Anti-Oncogene of Brain Tumor

List of Contributors

Biological Aspects of Brain Tumors

Part I. Special Lectures

An Introduction to Molecular Biology for the Neuro-Oncologist

MARK A. ISRAEL[1]

There is now overwhelming evidence that cancer is a genetic disease resulting from alterations in DNA. Over the past decade, advances in molecular biology and recombinant DNA technology have permitted us to make great strides in the understanding of cancer. The powerful genetic tools provided by these experimental approaches have made it possible to identify chemical and biological alterations that occur during the transformation of normal cells to malignant ones, and to catalogue the cellular changes resulting from these alterations. Molecular approaches to the pathologic classification of tumors should soon provide a rational basis upon which novel therapeutic possibilities can be examined.

Such progress in recombinant DNA technology and molecular genetics can be expected to have a major impact on the clinical practice of oncology in the near future, and clinicians will need to develop a familiarity with the concepts and experimental techniques of this discipline. This paper briefly outlines techniques frequently referred to in the molecular biology literature and highlights selected topics in molecular biology, summarizing current themes important for understanding tumors of the central nervous system (CNS).

Glial Tumorigenesis: Molecular Approaches

The key laboratory techniques of molecular biology, including nucleic acid hybridization and gene cloning, are based on the complementary nature of the nucleic acid base that characterizes the primary structure of the DNA molecule [1]. The recognition of one strand of nucleic acid by a second, complementary strand, and the ability of one strand to act as a template for the second strand are fundamental to each of the techniques used by molecular geneticists to study tumorigenesis.

[1]Preuss Laboratory for Molecular Neuro-Oncology, Brain Tumor Research Center, Department of Neurological Surgery, School of Medicine, University of California, San Francisco, CA 94122, USA

Molecular Hybridization

Among molecular genetic techniques, the most important for the clinician is *DNA hybridization analysis*. Hybridization is the process by which two complementary strands of nucleic acid anneal to form a double-stranded molecule. To analyze DNA from tumor specimens for any particular gene, a molecular probe consisting of radionuclide-labeled DNA corresponding to the gene of interest is prepared. The individual strands of the probe DNA and specimen DNA preparations can be separated (denatured) and annealed to form specimen DNA-probe DNA hybrids. The presence of such hybrids indicates that DNA nucleotide sequences present in the probe were also present in the specimen. Experimental procedures used to detect such hybrid double-stranded molecules are now performed routinely and form the basis of all hybridization analyses (Table 1).

Hybridization analysis of clinical specimens was greatly enhanced by the discovery of restriction endonucleases, enzymes that catalyze the cleavage of both strands of DNA at sequence-specific locations [2]. Most cells contain only two DNA copies of each gene per cell, and the distribution of various restriction enzyme recognition sites in each gene are unique to that stretch of DNA. The digestion of cellular DNA by restriction enzymes, therefore, results in DNA fragments of characteristic sizes that mark every gene. Southern blot analysis takes advantage of these findings and allows a quantitative evaluation of gene copy number as well as an evaluation of gene structure [3] (Fig. 1). In this type of analysis, gel electrophoresis is used to separate DNA restriction fragments by size and the DNA is transferred *in situ* from the gel onto a solid matrix, typically a sheet of nitrocellulose or nylon. This matrix binds and immobilizes the DNA fragments at their exact migration position in the gel.

Table 1. Types of DNA hybridization analysis useful in the evaluation of human tumor specimens

Southern blotting analysis—a technique for characterizing DNA. A DNA sample digested with restriction enzymes is fractionated by size in agarose gels, transferred to a nitrocellulose membrane, and hybridized to a isotopically labeled nucleic acid probe.

Northern blotting analysis—a technique for evaluating gene expression by characterizing mRNA sequences. RNA is purified from cells, fractioned by size on agarose gels, transferred to a nitrocellulose membrane, and analyzed by hybridization as described for Southern analysis.

***In situ* hybridization to histologic tissue specimens**—isotopically labeled nucleic acid probes are hybridized to tissue sections mounted for microscopic evaluation. After the reaction is complete, the tissue is covered with a photographic emulsion in which silver grains mark to sites of probe reactivity following development. With emulsion in place, slides can be stained for routine histologic evaluation.

***In situ* hybridization to chromosomal spreads**—isotopically labeled nucleic acid probes are hybridized to metaphase chromosome preparations on a microscope slide. After the reaction is complete, the specimen is analyzed and stained for G-banding in a manner analogous to that described above for tissue specimens.

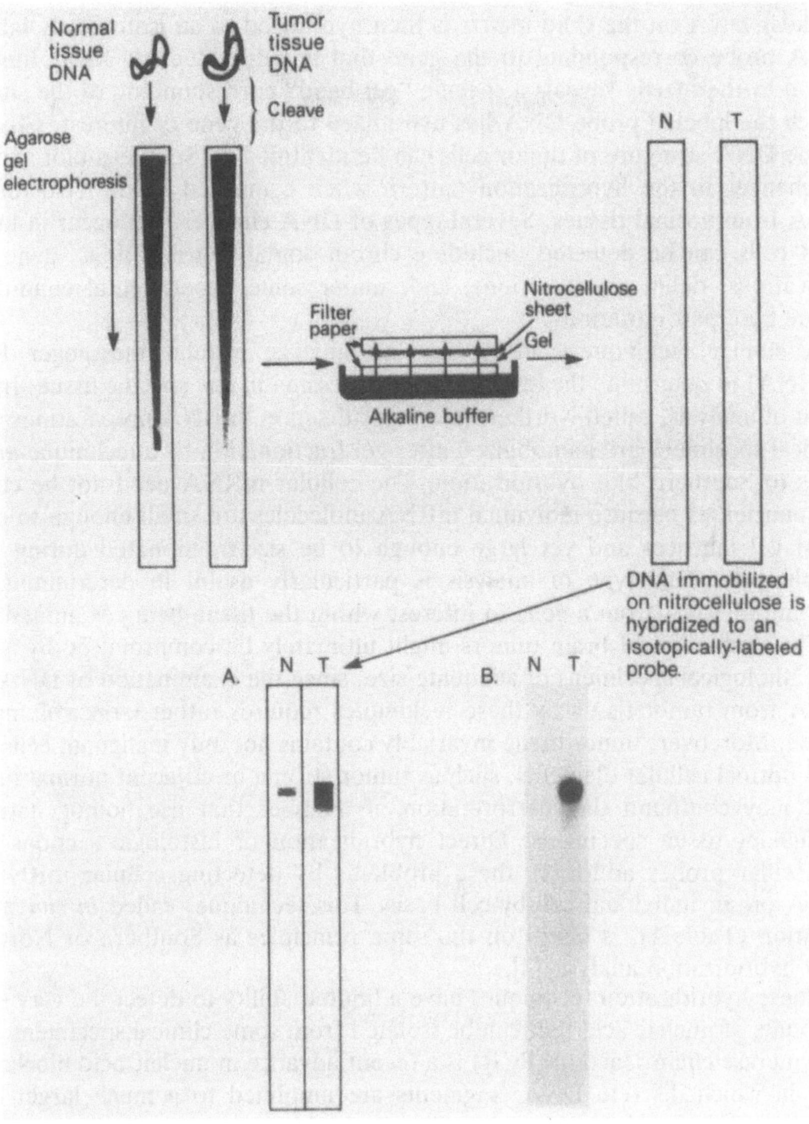

Fig. 1. Southern blot hybridization analysis of tumor cell DNA. This cartoon depicts the hypothetical pattern one might expect to observe in the analysis of DNA which is amplified during the development of a particular malignancy. Cleavage of DNA from both a normal cell and a tumor cell results in innumerable different-sized fragments that can be distributed along a migration path during gel electrophoresis. Transfer of this DNA and hybridization analysis using a molecular probe corresponding to the amplified gene leads to an increased amount of radioactivity at a location in the migration path where the DNA fragment containing the gene of interest has migrated. The location and intensity of this DNA fragment can be identified by autoradiography revealing both the structure and copy number of DNA fragments containing the gene of interest. This is indicated figuratively in panel A. In panel B, an autoradiogram from such an experiment demonstrates an intense signal in tumor specimen [T] compared with a barely visible signal in the normal specimen [N]

Cellular DNA on the solid matrix is then hybridized to an isotopically labeled DNA probe corresponding to the gene that is being studied. X-ray film exposed to the matrix reveals a specific "gel band" corresponding to the sites at which the labeled probe DNA has hybridized to the gene of interest. Changes in the DNA structure of tumor cells can be identified by Southern blot analysis as changes in the hybridization pattern when compared to the structure of DNA from normal tissues. Several types of DNA changes that occur in malignant cells can be detected, including chromosomal translocations, gene amplifications, deletions, insertions, and, under some experimental conditions, single base pair mutations.

A similar technique can be used to analyze cellular messenger RNA (mRNA) to determine the level of gene expression in any specific tissue. In this form of analysis, called Northern blot hybridization, mRNA preparations from clinical specimens are immobilized after gel fractionation by a technique analogous to Southern blot hybridization. The cellular mRNA need not be cut by endonucleases because individual mRNA molecules are small enough to enter most gel matrices and yet large enough to be size-fractionated during electrophoresis. This type of analysis is particularly useful in determining the amount of RNA from a gene of interest within the tissue being examined.

The evaluation of brain tumors might ultimately be compromised by a lack of pathological specimens of adequate size, since the examination of DNA and RNA from tumor tissue by these techniques requires rather large volumes of tissue. Moreover, tumor tissue invariably contains not only malignant cells, but also normal cellular elements, such as tumor stroma or adjacent normal tissue, that may confound the interpretation of analyses that use homogenates of malignant tissue specimens. Direct hybridization of histologic sections with molecular probes addresses these problems by detecting cellular mRNA or DNA on an individual cell-by-cell basis. This technique, called *in situ* hybridization (Table 1), is based on the same principles as Southern or Northern blot hybridization analysis [4].

These hybridization techniques have a limited ability to detect the very small amounts of nucleic acid that can be isolated from some clinical specimens. The polymerase chain reaction (PCR) is a recent advance in nucleic acid biochemistry, in which discrete DNA fragments are amplified to a much larger copy number and thereby become readily detectable using standard probes and hybridization techniques [5] (Fig. 2). When using PCR to amplify DNA, the double-stranded DNA of interest is heat-denatured and annealed to a pair of oligonucleotide primers that are complementary to the opposite strands of the DNA. DNA synthesis extending from these primers is mediated by a DNA polymerase that is thermostable, thereby facilitating the repeated denaturation-renaturation cycles necessary to achieve high levels of amplification. Each cycle of PCR doubles the number of DNA copies. With polymerases that are now available, these cycles can be repeated up to 25 times in rapid succession without the need for additional enzyme, resulting in up to a 10^5-fold increase in the amount of the DNA available for analysis.

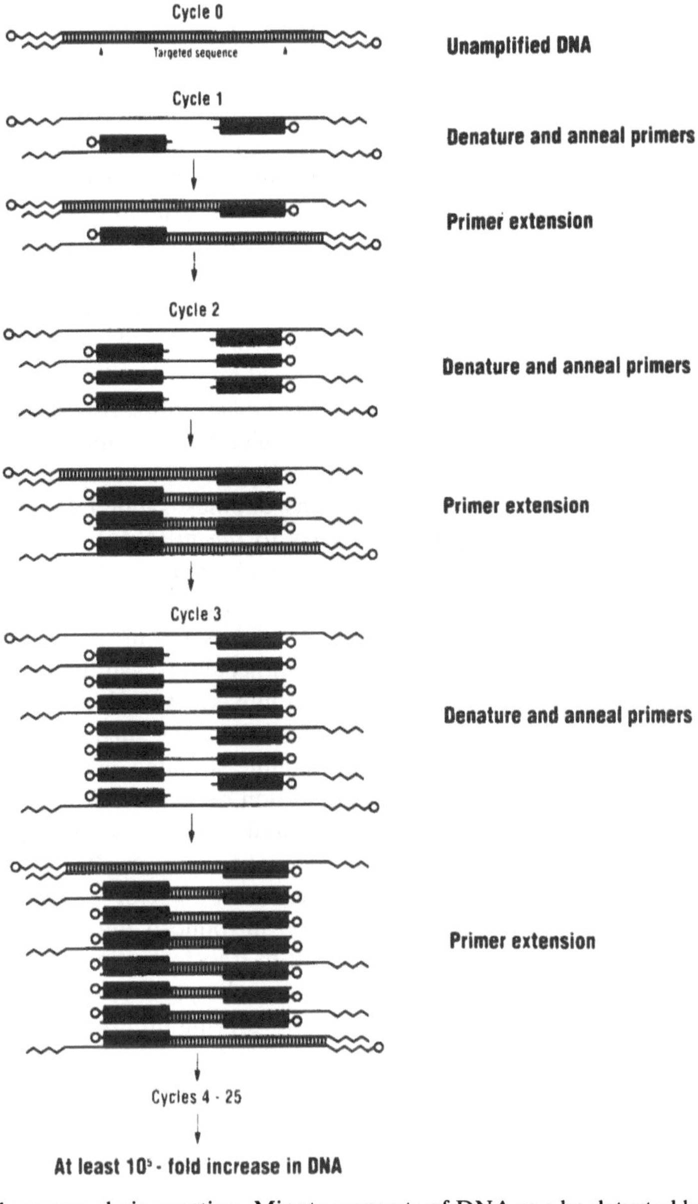

Fig. 2. Polymerase chain reaction. Minute amounts of DNA can be detected by increasing the number of copies of the specific DNA segment. The DNA sequence of interest is heat denatured, annealed to DNA primers homologous to the 5′ and 3′ ends of the sequence by heat renaturation, and undergoes primer extension. This process results in producing a new DNA copy for every DNA sequence of interest present. This cycle of heat denaturation and primer extension can be repeated multiple times to yield at least a 100,000-fold increase in copy number of the DNA sequence of interest

Gene Cloning

Since the hybridization techniques outlined above depend upon the availability of molecular probes, the means to clone genes that can serve as such probes is another critical technique in the molecular genetic arsenal. Genes for which probes might be of interest to the clinician include: (a) oncogenes, (b) tissue-specific genes, which are effective indicators of the tissue in which a tumor may arise, (c) genes involved in the regulation of growth and differentiation, (d) genes encoding therapeutic resistance, and (e) genes encoding proteins involved in metastases and other clinically important features of malignancy.

Gene cloning requires the identification and selection of a DNA segment of interest from a library of numerous nucleic acid molecules. Recombinant DNA libraries can be a collection of DNA from the cell's entire genetic constitution, i.e., genomic library, or only the DNA molecules corresponding to those genes that are actually expressed in any given cell type, i.e., a complementary DNA (cDNA) library. A cDNA library contains double-stranded DNA molecules with a nucleotide sequence complementary to the mRNA from a cell line or tissue. For the preparation of such a recombinant DNA library, purified mRNA is extracted from a cell line or tissue of interest and a poly-T DNA primer molecule is annealed to the poly-A mRNA tail in the presence of the enzyme reverse transcriptase. A cDNA molecule is synthesized from the mRNA template. This template is then removed by RNAse and a second complementary strand of DNA is synthesized from the single-stranded cDNA molecule using DNA polymerase. This double-stranded cDNA is then prepared for insertion into a vector by the addition of artificial restriction enzyme sites (linkers) to its ends or by adding homopolymeric deoxynucleotide tails to the 5′ ends of each DNA strand using terminal transferase. These stretches of double-stranded DNA can now be combined with a vector, resulting in a new "recombinant DNA molecule" that can be introduced into host bacteria, a process called "transformation". As a result of transformation, each bacterium in a culture acquires a different DNA corresponding to a different cloned gene segment. The collection of different bacteria carrying different cloned genes is called a "library".

Genes can be cloned in many types of vectors, including plasmids, bacteriophage, and cosmids. Plasmids, which are the most frequently used vectors, consist of double-stranded DNA molecules that replicate independently of the host chromosome within bacteria. Bacteriophage, which are bacterial viruses, have two distinct advantages over plasmids when used for cloning. First, recombinant phages are more efficient than plasmids in their ability to be transferred into host bacteria. Second, phages can hold larger DNA inserts than plasmids can. Cosmid vectors can hold even larger pieces of DNA than can bacteriophage and can be used to clone very long stretches of genomic DNA.

To screen the recombinant DNA library for a gene of interest, bacterial colonies containing recombinant plasmids are plated onto agar. Using a solid matrix, such as nylon, a replica of the bacterial colonies is made. Most commonly, this large collection of bacterial clones is screened by a nucleic acid hybridization assay for the presence of nucleic acid that bears homology to a probe of interest. DNA from these clones is prepared on the replica in situ and hybridized to a radio-labeled probe in a manner similar to Southern blotting. The filter paper is then exposed to X-ray film revealing a "hot" spot corresponding to the bacterial colony on the original agar plate that contains the cDNA of interest. The DNA from the identified bacterial colony can be extracted and purified. This screening method is useful if a molecular probe corresponding to DNA closely related to the gene of interest already exists. Alternatively, if no probe exists but the protein sequence of the gene is known, oligonucleotide probes whose DNA sequence is based on the known protein sequence can be constructed and used for hybridization.

Glial Tumorigenesis: Genetic Alterations

Cytogenetic Changes

The identification of disease-associated, nonrandom cytogenetic rearrangements in a wide variety of tumours, including brain tumors, has been of fundamental importance in establishing the genetic basis for cancer, directing researchers towards the identification of tumor-specific genetic alterations, and providing a novel basis for the development of a tumor classification schema. Glial tumors of the CNS frequently have a diploid stemline [6]. Although, occasionally, no chromosomal abnormalities are found, more typically chromosomal alterations, which are now recognized to occur rather frequently, have been detected in these tumors [6–9]. Additional copies of chromosome 7 and losses of chromosome 10 seem to be associated with the most malignant gliomas. Losses of chromosomes 22, 9p, and the sex chromosome have also been reported. Structural abnormalities have been most frequently detected in 9p and 19q, whereas 1, 6p, 7q, 8p, 9p, 11, 3q, 15q, and 19q have been implicated less frequently [6–8]. In these same tumors, double minute chromosomes are also frequently found [6]. Cytogenetic examination of glial tumors of different grades suggests that high-grade tumors are more likely to have detectable genetic alterations than are lower grade tumors [7], although the observed spectrum of cytogenetic changes is very similar [10].

Pediatric glial tumors of the CNS have also been examined for the presence of clonal cytogenetic alterations, although the number of tumors examined to date has been small [6]. Interestingly, the limited spectrum of alterations recognized to date for these (glial) tumors is indistinguishable from the changes identified in more commonly occurring undifferentiated CNS tumors of children such as medulloblastomas [6,11]. The most common changes seen in both types of tumors are numerical: i (17q) was found in six out of seven pediatric tumors examined in one study [11] and in two out of ten such tumors in another [12]. Deletions, duplications, and translocations of chromosome 1 with breakpoints on 1p, sometimes resulting in trisomy of lp, lq, or both arms, were also frequently observed in both pediatric glial tumors and medulloblastomas [11,12].

An additional cytogenetic alteration in both pediatric and adult glial tumors is double minute chromosomes [6]. These are among the changes thought to occur early during glial tumorigenesis [13] and are of particular interest because the double minute chromosomes contain amplified gene segments, presumably selected for their encoding of some pathologic feature of the tumor that provides it with a biologic advantage. To date, most interest in amplified genes in glial tumors has focused on the epidermal growth factor receptor (EGFR) in adult, high-grade glial tumors (discussed below) [14,15]. The amplified genes of pediatric, undifferentiated CNS tumors seem to occur most frequently in genes other than the EGFR, although only a few childhood glioblastoma multiforme tumors have been examined to date [16].

Many chromosomal alterations in glial tumors, including changes in ploidy, structural alterations, and the presence of double minutes are maintained during the passage of tumor cells as xenografts in nude mice [17]. The stability of these genetic changes during passage makes this laboratory model particularly valuable for examining specific pathological changes that are mediated by such genetic alterations. In tissue culture, many biological features of cell lines from malignant tumors also remain stable for a very prolonged period. However, cell lines carried in vitro may have somewhat less genetic stability, especially in regard to the ploidy of such lines [9].

Based upon experience in the hematopoietic malignancies, it is thought that cytogenetically detected chromosomal rearrangements mark sites of alterations in oncogenes and other genes that are of potential pathological importance. Presumably, specific rearrangements orchestrate a specific cellular phenotype. We now know that some of the cytogenetic alterations recognized as occuring in association with brain tumors involve genes that can contribute to the disordered growth that characterizes these tumors. In other cases, specific genes known to be important for tumors induced in the laboratory are found at the sites of cytegenetic alterations in glial tumors, although their precise function in these tumors is not yet understood. These genes include several known oncogenes.

Molecular Genetic Alterations: Oncogenes

Cellular oncogenes (proto-oncogenes) are present in the genome of every cell and can be activated to cause malignant transformation of a cell [18,19]. The activated form of a proto-oncogene is known as an oncogene. Although

Table 2. Proto-oncogenes expressed in glioma tumor cell lines

erb-B1	N-*myc*	c-*mil*/*raf*
c-*ros*	c-*myc*	*neu*
c-*myb*	c-*abl*	c-*fos*
c-*raf*-1	N-*ras*	c-*sis*

oncogenes were first recognized during the characterization of retroviruses, proto-oncogenes are now known to be components of the normal genetic constitution of every animal cell. When incorporated into a viral genome, they sometimes become mutated, leading to the production of an altered protein product. In other cases, they come under the control of viral regulatory elements and are expressed at inappropriately high levels, thereby contributing to the malignant transformation of infected animal cells. In spontaneous human tumors, it is thought that the "random" mutation or overexpression of these genes similarly contributes to tumor development.

Every mammalian cell genome is now thought to contain at least 60 proto-oncogenes [18]. Although the functions of the proteins encoded by most protooncogenes are not precisely known, biochemical activities of several protooncogene products have been identified. Some of the gene products are identical to, or related to, proteins known to be important in growth regulation. Table 2 lists oncogenes that have been implicated in the pathogenesis of brain tumors.

The best characterized of the oncogenes thought to be important in the development of glial tumors in the erb-B1 gene. This gene encodes the EGFR, a transmembrane protein that catalyzes the phosphorylation of tyrosine re-

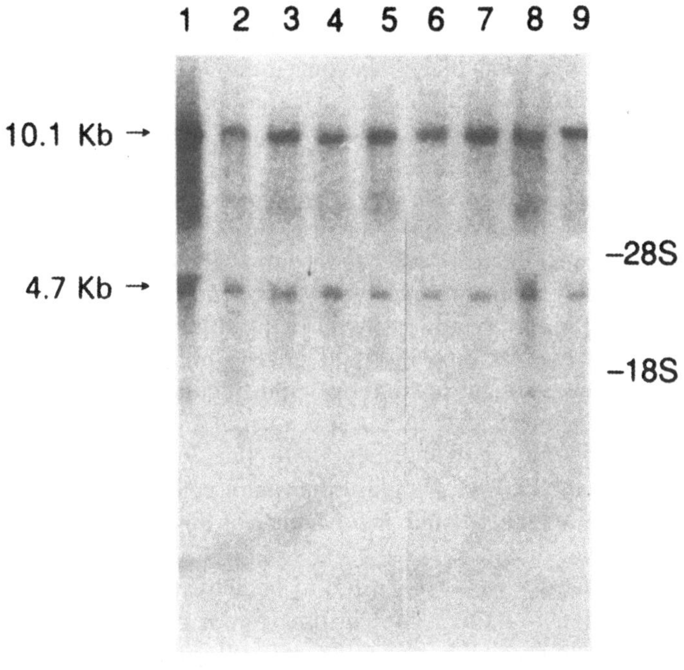

Fig. 3. C-*erb* B mRNA expression in human glioma cell lines. Northern blot hybridization analysis of 30 μg of total RNA isolated from glioma cell lines was hybridized with a 32p-labeled EGF-R DNA probe. *Lane 1*, U-343 MGA c12:6; *lane 2*, U-87 MG; *lane 3*, U-1796 MG; *lane 4*, U-118 MG; *lane 5*, U-178 MG; *lane 6*, U-251 MG sp; *lane 7*, U-343 MG; *lane 8*, U-138 MG; *lane 9*, U-410 MG

sidues in cellular proteins following the binding of its extracellular domain to the epidermal growth factor. This receptor has been found to be amplified in tissue from 50% to 70% of glioblastoma multiforme tumors [14,15,20,21], although it may be amplified somewhat less frequently in glial tumors presenting during childhood [16]. In such tumors, it is frequently rearranged to encode a truncated EGFR that also contains point mutations [20,22]. The amplification of this gene grequently corresponds to the presence of double minute chromosomes in glioma tumor specimens [23], and increased expression of EGFR in gliomas seems to be invariably associated with gene amplification [24]. Since EGFR amplification is retained during the passage of xenografts in athymic mice [25], but is found only infrequently in glioblastoma tumor cell lines [26] (Fig. 3), it seems likely that expression of this gene confers some sort of biologic advantage upon these tumor cells that is particularly important for growth in vivo.

EGF induces a mitogenic response in both normal glial and some glioblastoma-derived tumor cell lines [27], although antibodies directed against EGFR do not typically inhibit glioma tumor cell growth. In at least one glioblastoma tumor cell line, EGFR-associated tyrosine kinase is not stimulated in association with the binding of EGF by tumor cells [28]. Also, the level of EGFR expression in early passage primary cultures of glioma tumors does not correlate with either the growth of these cells in soft agar or as athymic mouse xenografts [29]. These findings and the observation that amplification and high-level EGFR expression in glioblastoma tumors has not been associated with any particular histologic or pathologic feature of these tumors [30] make it difficult at the present time, confidently to assign a precise biologic activity to the amplified EGFR in glial tumors.

Another tyrosine kinase encoding oncogene of interest in the study of glial tumors is the *ros* oncogene. This gene was originally detected in a human glioblastoma tumor cell line [31] and has recently been characterized to encode a 280 kilodalton (d) transmembrane tyrosine-specific protein kinase that possesses *in vitro* autophosphorylating activity [32]. Although most gliomal tumor cell lines examined express high levels of mRNA encoded by the *ros* proto-oncogene, it has not yet been possible to identify either amplification of high levels of ros expression in glial tumor specimens [33]. Truncation of the *ros* gene as the result of a rearrangement with the 5′ end of the gene has, however, been detected in one glioblastoma tumor cell line [34], providing yet additional evidence for the possible involvement of this gene in the pathogenesis of high grade glial tumors.

Other genes that have been recognized to be activated by either rearrangement or amplification in human glioblastoma tumor cell lines include: c-*myb* [35], N-*myc* 30,36], c-*myc* [30], *gli* [37], c-*abl* [38], and c-*raf*-1 [39]. In some cases, more than one tumor or cell line has been recognized to contain alterations in one of these genes, but evidence for the involvement of any one of these in a particular type of glial tumor or in glial tumors in general is lacking. Similarly, the expression of a large number of different proto-oncogenes in glioblastoma tumors [20,36,37,40] and tumor cell lines [26–45] has been documented. These include c-*erb*-B1 [20,26,41,44], N-*ras* [37], c-*sis* [26,40,42-44], *fos* [40], N-*myc* [36,40], c-*mil*/*raf*-1 [26], *neu* [26], and c-*myb* [26]. In contrast to the presumption that proto-oncogenes activated by amplification or gene rearrangement are of etiologic importance, we do not know the significance of prot-oncogene expression in glioblastoma tumors. Such expression may mark genetic programs activated during the course of oncogenesis. Alternatively, these genes might also be expressed simply as a reflection of the cell type in which a particular malignancy arose.

Tumors arise in immature precursor cells of fully mature tissues that we can recognize in the adult organism. The finding of slightly different patterns of proto-oncogene expression in tumor cell lines with different degrees of differentiation along the glial lineage [26,45] has raised the possibility that these cell lines may correspond to glial precursors that are present at sequential stages of normal glial development. The finding that the expression of a variety of different proto-oncogenes can be regulated in glial tumor cell lines by agents such as cyclic AMP [46], phorbol esters [47], and transforming growth factor β [48], which have been recognized to induce the differentiation of other cell types, is consistent with this possibility.

Observations made during the study of familial retinoblastoma led to the hypothesis that recessive genes might be found that are important for the development of this tumor [49–51]. The association of a loss of genetic material with the development of cancer is consistent with the idea that the normal allele protecting against the formation of retinoblastoma must be dominant and, therefore, must be inactivated or deleted before the mutant, recessive retinoblastoma allele can be expressed, giving rise to a tumor [49–51]. Such recessive cancer genes have also been called anti-oncogenes.

Researchers sought the specific allele associated with retinoblastoma tumor development by the analysis of DNA from members of families in which this tumor was hereditary. Using probes recognizing restriction fragment-length polymorphisms (RFLPs), stretches of DNA from normal tissues in which at least two different-sized restriction fragments can result following enzymatic digestion, investigators can study the association of an unknown allele with a specific, inherited trait. DNA can be homozygous at a locus recognized by an RFLP probe, showing only one size band on a Southern blot hybridization, or it can be heterozygous at this locus and yield two different-sized gel bands after hybridization with the RFLP. These different DNA fragments correspond to the maternally and paternally derived alleles. The finding of a single allele in tumor DNA from an individual in which similarly examined normal tissue DNA contains two identifiable alleles indicates that tumor cells have lost DNA from one of the two chromosomes containing this genomic region.

Using RFLP probes to examine glial tumors, losses of genetic material from chromosomes 10, 13, 17, and 22 have been identified [52]. Among these chromosomal regions, the only one in which a specific locus likely to be of importance in the development of glial tumors has been recognized is chromosome 17p11.2-pter [53]. The p53 gene is located within this region and in at least some glial tumor cell lines in which homozygosity of 17p can be demonstrated, mutation of the remaining p53 allele has been identified [54]. This finding and the experimental demonstration that wild type p53 can suppress the *in vitro* growth of a glial tumor cell line provide strong evidence for a role for p53 in the pathogenesis of glial tumors [55]. The identification of recessive oncogenes located within chromosomal regions that are converted to homozygosity during the course of glial tumor development is an active area of research that should contribute important information regarding the pathology of these tumors.

Conclusion

Although there have been many advances in the understanding of carcinogenesis, and many genes have been identified that are known to be involved in the development of the malignant phenotype, our understanding of the sequence of events that transform a normal cell to a malignant one remains incomplete. Numerous pieces of evidence, however, suggest that more than one genetic change is usually necessary for the development of malignancy. Also, the variety of different cell types present in individual tumors suggests that malignant cells retain considerable plasticity to differentiate along multiple lineages in association with the oncogenic process. The identification of cells with different morphologies within the same tumor that contain the same genetic alteration [14] provides evidence that the cytologic heterogeneity of tumor cells so obvious to the neuropathologist may reflect underlying genetic events and be important for progression of the malignant process.

References

1. Bonner TI, Brenner DJ, Neufeld Br, Britten RJ (1973) Reduction in the rate of DNA reassociation by sequence divergence. J Mol Biol 81:123–135
2. Smith HO, Wilcox KW (1970) A restriction enzyme from *Hemophilus influenzae*. II. Base sequence of the recognition site. J Mol Biol 51:393–409
3. Southern EM (1975) Detection of specific seqences among DNA fragments separated by gel electrophoresis. J Mol Biol 98:503–517
4. Haase AT, Gantz D, Blum H, Stowring L, Ventura P, Geballe, A (1985) Combined macroscopic and microscopic detection of viral genes in tissues. Virology 140:201–206
5. Mullis KB, Faloona FA (1987) Specific synthesis of DNA *in vitro* via a polymerase catalysed chain reaction. Methods Enzymol 1155:335–350
6. Bigner SH, Mark J, Burger PC, Mahaley MS Jr, Bullard DE, Muhlbaier LH, Bigner DD (1988) Specific chromosomal abnormalities in malignant human gliomas. Cancer Res 48:405–411
7. Jenkins RB, Kimmel DW, Moertel CA, Schultz CG, Scheithauer BW, Kelly PJ, Dewald GW (1989) A cytogenetic study of 53 human gliomas. Cancer Genet Cytogenet 39:253–279
8. Rey JA, Bello MJ, de Campos JM, Kusak ME, Ramos C, Benitez J (1987) Chromosomal patterns in human malignant astrocytomas. Cancer Genet Cytogenet 29:201–221

9. Rey JA, Bello MJ, de Campos JM, Kusak ME, Moreno S (1989) Cytogenetic follow-up from direct preparation to advanced *in vitro* passage of a human malignant glioma. Cancer Genet Cytogenet 41:175–183
10. Rey JA, Bello MJ, de Campos JM, Kusak ME, Moreno S (1987) Chromosomal composition of a series of 22 human low-grade gliomas. Cancer Genet Cytogenet 29:223–237
11. Bigner SH, Mark J, Friedman HS, Biegel JA, Bigner DD (1988) Structural chromosomal abnormalities in human medulloblastoma. Cancer Genet Cytogenet 30:91–101
12. Griffin CA, Hawkins AL, Packer RJ, Rorke LB, Emanuel BS (1988) Chromosome abnormalities in pediatric brain tumors. Cancer Res 48:175–180
13. Bigner SH, Mark J, Bullard De, Mahaley MS Jr, Bigner DD (1986) Chromosomal evolution in malignant human gliomas starts with specific and usually numerical deviations. Cancer Genet Cytogenet 22:121–135
14. Libermann TA, Nusbaum HR, Razon N, Kris R, Lax I, Soreq H, Whittle N, Waterfield MD, Ullrich A, Schlessinger J (1985) Amplification, enhanced expression and possible rearrangement of EGF receptor gene in primary human brain tumours of glial origin. Nature 313:144–147
15. Libermann TA, Razon N, Bartal AD, Yarden Y, Schlessinger J, Soreq H (1984) Expression of epidermal growth factor receptors in human brain tumors. Cancer Res 44:753–760
16. Wasson JC, Saylors RL, Zeltzer P, Friedman HS, Bigner SH, Burger PC, Bigner DD, Look AT, Douglass EC, Brodeur GM (1990) Oncogene amplification in pediatric brain tumors. Cancer Res 50:2987–2990
17. Bigner SH, Schold SC, Friedman HS, Mark J, Bigner DD (1989) Chromosomal composition of malignant human gliomas through serial subcutaneous transplantation in athymic mice. Cancer Genet Cytogenet 40:111–120
18. Bishop JM (1985) Viral oncogenes. Cell 42:23–38
19. Bishop JM (1987) The molecular genetics of cancer. Science 235:305–311
20. Yamazaki H, Fukui Y, Ueyama Y, Tamaoki N, Kawamoto T, Taniguchi S, Shibuya M (1988) Amplification of the structurally and functionally altered epidermal growth factor receptor gene (c-*erb*B) in human brain tumors. Mol Cell Biol 8:1816–1820
21. Helseth E, Unsgaard G, Dalen A, Fure H, Skandsen T, Odegaard A, Vik R (1988) Amplification of the epidermal growth factor receptor gene in biopsy specimens from human intracranial tumours. Br J Neurosurg 2:217–255
22. Humphrey PA, Wong AJ, Vogelstein B, Zalutsky MR, Fuller GN, Archer GE, Friedman HS, Kwatra MM, Bigner SH, Bigner DD (1990) Anti-synthetic peptide antibody reacting at the fusion junction of deletion-mutant epidermal growth factor receptors in human glioblastoma. Proc Natl Acad Sci USA 87:4207–4211
23. Bigner SH, Wong AJ, Mark J, Muhlbaier LH, Kinzler KW, Vogelstein B, Bigner DD (1987) Relationship between gene amplification and chromosomal deviations in malignant human gliomas. Cancer Genet Cytogenet 29:165–170
24. Wong AJ, Bigner SH, Bigner DD, Kinzler KW, Hamilton SR, Vogelstein B (1987) Increased expression of the epidermal growth factor receptor gene in malignant gliomas is invariably associated with gene amplification. Proc Natl Acad Sci USA 84:6899–6903
25. Humphrey PA, Wong AJ, Vogelstein B, Friedman HS, Werner MH, Bigner DD, Bigner SH (1988) Amplification and expression of the epidermal growth factor receptor gene in human glioma xenografts. Cancer Res 48:2231–2238

26. LaRocca RV, Roseblum M, Westermark B, Israel MA (1989) Patterns of proto-oncogene expression in human glioma cell lines. J Neurosci Res 24:97–106.
27. Pollack IF, Randall MS, Kristofik MP, Kelly RH, Selker RG, Vertosick FT (1990) Response of malignant glioma cell lines to epidermal growth factor and platelet-derived growth factor in a serum-free medium. J Neurosurg 73:106–112
28. Wells A, Bishop JM. Helmeste D (1988) Amplified gene for the epidermal growth factor receptor in a human glioblastoma cell line encodes an enzymatically inactive protein. Mol Cell Biol 8:4561–4565
29. U HS, Kelley PY, Hatton JD, Shew JY (1989) Proto-oncogene abnormalities and their relationship to tumorigenicity in some human glioblastomas. J Neurosurg 71:83-90
30. Bigner SH, Burger PC, Wong AJ, Werner MH, Hamilton SR, Muhlbaier LH, Vogelstein B, Bigner DD (1988) Gene amplification in malignant human gliomas: Clinical and histopathologic aspects. J Neuropathol Exp Neurol 47:191–205
31. Birchmeier C, Birnbaum D, Waitches G, Fasano O, Wigler M (1986) Characterization of an activated human *ros* gene. Mol Cell Biol 6:3109–3116
32. Sharma S, Birchmeier C, Nikawa J, O'Neill K, Rodgers L, Wigler M (1989) Characterization of the *ros*1-gene products expressed in human glioblastoma cell lines. Oncogene Res 5:91–100
33. Wu JK, Chikaraishi DM (1990) Differential expression of *ros* oncogene in primary human astrocytomas and astrocytoma cell lines. Cancer Res 50:3032-3035
34. Birchmeier C, O'Neill K, Riggs M, Wigler M (1990) Characterization of *ROS*1 cDNA from a human glioblastoma cell line. Proc Natl Acad Sci USA 87:4799–4803
35. Welter C, Henn W, Theisinger B, Fischer H, Zang KD, Blin N (1990) The cellular *myb* oncogene is amplified, rearranged and activated in human glioblastoma cell lines. Cancer Lett 52:57–62
36. Fujimoto M, Sheridan PJ, Sharp ZD, Weaker FJ, Kagan-Hallet S, Story JL (1989) Proto-oncogene analyses in brain tumors. J Neurosurg 70:910–915
37. Kinzler KW, Bigner SH, Bigner DD, Trent JM, Law ML, O'Brien SJ, Wong AJ, Vogelstein B (1987) Identification of an amplified, highly expressed gene in a human glioma. Science 236:70–73
38. Heisterkamp N, Morris C, Sender L, Knoppel E, Uribe L, Cui MY, Groffen J (1990) Rearrangement of the human *ABL* oncogene in a glioblastoma. Cancer Res 50:3429–3434
39. Fukui M, Yamamoto T, Kawai S, Mitsunobu F, Toyoshima K (1987) Molecular cloning and characterization of an activated human c-*raf*-1 gene. Mol Cell Biol 7:1776–1781
40. Fujimoto M, Weaker FJ, Herbert DC, Sharp ZD, Sheridan PJ, Story JL (1988) Expression of three viral oncogenes (v-*sis*, v-*myc*, v-*fos*) in primary human brain tumors of neuroectodermal origin. Neurology 38:289–293
41. Steck PA, Gallick GE, Maxwell SA, Kloetzer WS, Arlinghaus RB, Moser RP, Gutterman JU, Yung WK (1986) Expression of epidermal growth factor receptor and associated glycoprotein on cultured human brain tumor cells. J Cell Biochem 32:1–10
42. Shapiro JR (1986) Biology of gliomas: Heterogeneity, oncogenes, growth factors. Semin Oncol 13:4–15
43. Westermark B, Nister M, Heldin CH (1985) Growth factors and oncogenes in human malignant glioma. Neurol Clin 3:785–799
44. Harsh GR 4th, Rosenblum ML, Williams LT (1989) Oncogene-related growth factors and growth factor receptors in human malignant glioma-derived cell lines. J Neurooncol 7:47–56

45. Blin N, Muller-Brechlin R, Carstens C, Meese E, Zang KD (1987) Enhanced expression of four cellular oncogenes in a human glioblastoma cell line. Cancer Genet Cytogenet 25:285–292
46. Harsh GR, Kavanaugh WM, Starksen NF, Williams LT (1989) Cyclic AMP blocks expression of the c-*sis* gene in tumor cells. Oncogene Res 4:65–73
47. Press RD, Misra A, Gillaspy G, Samols D, Goldthwait DA (1989) Control of the expression of c-*sis* mRNA in human glioblastoma cells by phorbol ester and transforming growth factor beta 1. Cancer Res 49:2914–2920
48. Helseth E, Unsgaard G, Dalen A, Vik R (1988) The effects of type beta transforming growth factor on proliferation and epidermal growth factor receptor expression in a human glioblastoma cell line. J Neurooncol 6:269–276
49. Knudson AG (1971) Mutation and cancer. Statistical study of retinoblastoma. Proc Nat Acad Sci USA 68:820–823
50. Cavenee WK, Dryja TP, Phillips RA, Benedict WF, Godbout R, Gallie BL, Murphree AL, Strong LC, White RL (1983) Expression of recessive alleles by chromosomal mechanisms in retinoblastoma. Nature 305:779–784
51. Murphree AL, Benedict WF (1984) Retinoblastoma: Clues to human oncogenesis. Science 223:1028–1033
52. James CD, Carlbom E, Dumanski JP, Hansen M, Nordenskjold M, Collins VP, Cavenee WK (1988) Clonal genomic alterations in glioma malignancy stages. Cancer Res 48:5546–5551
53. James CD, Carlbom E, Nordenskjold M, Collins VP, Cavenee WK (1989) Mitotic recombination of chromosome 17 in astrocytomas. Proc Natl Acad Sci USA 86:2858–2862
54. Nigro JM, Baker SJ, Preisinger AC, Jessup JM, Hostetter R, Cleary K, Bigner SH, Davidson N, Baylin S, Devilee P (1989) Mutations in the p53 gene occur in diverse human tumour types. Nature 342:705–708
55. Mercer WE, Shields MT, Amin M, Sauve GJ, Appella E, Romano JW, Ullrich SJ (1990) Negative growth regulation in a glioblastoma tumor cell line that conditionally expresses human wild-type p53. Proc Natl Acad Sci USA 87:6166–6170

Genetic Alterations of Nervous System Tumors

Robert L. Martuza[1]

Introduction

The last decade has witnessed revolutionary advances in our understanding of the basic molecular changes associated with carcinogenesis in general and with nervous system tumorigenesis in particular. This report discusses the genetic alterations in nervous system tumors from two viewpoints. The first represents a summary of the descriptive changes that have been documented in various nervous system tumors. Here, the molecular and chromosomal changes associated with schwannomas, meningiomas, gliomas, and other nervous system tumors are described. These represent the naturally occurring genetic alterations associated with tumorigenesis and tumor progression. The second discusses alterations in tumor cells that may be purposefully induced in order to study their cellular biology or to test novel therapeutic approaches. This section represents a new era in tumor studies which is still in its elemental stages, but its impact could result in the development of new therapies for some tumors which are invariably fatal despite maximal conventional therapy.

Molecular Genetic Studies of Neurofibromatosis-2, Acoustic Neuroma, and Meningioma

Among the first central nervous system tumors to be studied using molecular genetic techniques was the acoustic neuroma. My colleagues and I initially chose this tumor for a variety of reasons: (1) we were interested in localizing and understanding the gene for neurofibromatosis-2 (NF2) [1], (2) we postulated that the gene associated with acoustic neuroma formation in NF2 would probably be the same gene associated with the much more common acoustic neuromas occurring unilaterally and sporadically in the general population, (3) meningiomas occur in NF2 and have been shown to have a loss of one copy of chromosome 22 in many instances [2] and thus became a candidate area for

---

[1] Molecular Neurogenetics Laboratory, Massachusetts General Hospital, Charlestown, MA 02129, USA

study (4) acoustic neuromas have such a low mitotic rate that they do not lend themselves to other approaches such as karyotypes which require cell division in culture, making direct molecular techniques essential, (5) acoustic neuromas are the most common Schwann cell tumors in humans (we operate on approximately one per week at the Massachusetts General Hospital), and (6) acoustic neuromas are histologically relatively pure masses of Schwann cells, thus contaminating cell populations present in some other tumors, such as neurofibromas or astrocytomas, are less likely to confound the results.

NF2 is a serious, debilitating autosomal dominant genetic disorder associated with bilateral acoustic neuromas (eighth cranial nerve schwannomas) in almost all cases as well as with other nervous system tumors such as meningiomas, spinal root schwannomas, and ependymomas in a variable number of cases [1]. Studies of DNA extracted from acoustic neuromas in the general population as well as from patients with NF2 tumors had demonstrated loss of genetic material on chromosome 22 but no losses on other chromosomes studied [3]. Similar results were obtained with other tumors in patients with NF2 tumors including spinal schwannomas [4]. This suggested that the locus associated with tumorigenesis in NF2 is on chromosome 22. Further linkage analysis study of a large kindred with NF2 demonstrated that the inherited locus of the NF2 gene is on the long arm of chromosome 22 [5,6]. Taken together, these studies have localized the NF2 gene (and the gene for acoustic neuromas in the general population) to the long arm of chromosome 22, with the mechanism appearing to be similar to that described for retinoblastoma. Thus, it is currently thought that the long arm of chromosome 22 contains a gene, NF2, which is involved with the growth suppression of Schwann cells (and others). Loss of function of both copies of this gene leads to tumor formation.

Meningiomas were next studied by this approach and also demonstrated loss of genetic material on the long arm of chromosome 22 [7]. However, other areas of genetic change have also been noted, most commonly on chromosome 14 and on the Y-chromosome in males [8]. This suggests the possibility that there may be an initiator locus for meningiomas on chromosome 22 as well as other progressor loci on other chromosomes. This also fits with the clinical data that indicate that whereas acoustic neuromas virtually never progress to become malignant, meningiomas may progress to become aggressive or even frankly malignant. Thus, further study of these progressor loci may have clinical relevance. Additionally, the chromosome 22 locus for meningiomas may not be identical with that for acoustic neuromas [9]. Once both are cloned, this issue will be finally resolved and the interactions of these two putative loci will be available for study.

Gliomas, Neurofibromas, Neurofibrosarcomas, and Neurofibromatosis-1

Gliomas are of even greater complexity and interest. Karyotype studies have demonstrated that the most common chromosomal abnormalities in human malignant gliomas are losses of chromosomes 10 and 22 and gains of chromosome 7 [10,11]. The earliest molecular studies focused on the gain of function were thought to be related to dominantly acting oncogenes. The gain on chromosome 7 was shown to be related to amplification of the epidermal growth factor receptor gene, and alterations in the gene and its product have been described in many but not all glioblastomas [12–14]. Other less common examples of increased oncogene expression (e.g., c-myc [15], sis [16,17], and ROS1 [18]) or of novel oncogenes (e.g., gli [19]) have also been demonstrated in glioblastomas. However, the role of some of these less common abnormalities is uncertain at present, and it is not clear if all play a frequent and key role in tumorigenesis or if the changes are induced in some cases by the process of tumorigenesis itself.

Recently, interest in gliomas has also focused on losses of genetic function at putative tumor suppressor loci. Loss of genetic material has been identified on chromosome 17 and on chromosome 10 [20–22]. In most instances, losses on 17 have been associated with early events in astrocytoma formation, and losses on chromosome 10 with progression to a more malignant phenotype. Both of these probably precede the amplification at the epidermal growth factor receptor (EGFR) locus on chromosome 7 noted above. Thus, the development of gliomas demonstrates multiple progressive genetic events, a concept which is consistent with clinical observations of histologic progression that is often seen in tumors of the astrocytic series.

At present, the gene or genes involved in glioma formation on chromosome 10 are not defined, but the gene or one of the genes involved on chromosome 17 may be the p53 gene (R.Y. Chung and B.R. Seizinger 1990, personal communication and [23]) [23]. This is of special interest since the p53 gene has been implicated in the development of other human tumors such as colon carcinoma [24] and sarcomas [25]. Further, the p53 gene has been cloned and its protein product is available for study [26]. It is likely that research in the next few years will allow elucidation of the mechanisms of interaction of these genes that play a role in the initiation and progression of gliomas in the general population.

Gliomas also occur in certain genetic syndromes such as neurofibromatosis, tuberous sclerosis, and Turcot's syndrome. The most common of these is neurofibromatosis-1 (NF1) also known as von Recklinghausen's disease [27]. Gliomas occur in at least 10% of patients with NF1 [28]. However, the study of tumorigenesis in NF1 is important not only for the understanding of glioma formation. More common in patients with NF1 are tumors of Schwann cells, such as benign neurofibromas and the malignant counterpart, neurofibrosarcoma.

Linkage analysis of large NF1 kindreds localized the NF1 gene to the long arm of chromosome 17 [29,30]. Recently, large portions of the NF1 gene have been cloned and appear to code for a GTPase activating protein (GAP) [31,34]. This is of great interest since GAPs have been studied in other systems and play a critical role in modulating the function of the ras oncogene [36]. Whether the primary effect of the NF1 protein is on the ras oncogene or on another gene is yet unknown. However, this major breakthrough will probably lead to an improved understanding of tumorigenesis not only in NF1 but also in histologically similar tumors occurring in the general population. The exact mechanism of neurofibroma formation by the NF1 gene is not yet known. It is hoped that this will be elucidated very shortly. However, it appears that the histologic progression of a neurofibroma to a malignant neurofibrosarcoma probably involves an additional mutation, not at the NF1 locus on the long arm of chromosome 17, but rather at a locus on the short arm of chromosome 17 [36]. Some evidence indicates that this progressor locus may be the p53 gene.

Can Molecular Genetic Techniques be Used to Develop New Strategies of Tumor Therapy?

The search for genetic abnormalities associated with tumorigenesis has proceeded in a straightforward manner over the last decade. In many instances, the work involved was intense and competetive, but the outcome of gene localization and the ultimate cloning of tumor-associated genes was virtually certain, with only the time frame being unpredictable. The search for the Rb gene and the NF1 gene are examples of this. In contrast, the use of current molecular genetic data and techniques to design strategies for tumor therapy are not so sharply defined at present. A clear-cut framework for experimental design has not been evident and multiple strategies may need to be pursued in order for a few to work.

Two general approaches are worthy of investigation: systemic therapy and local therapy. Each may be complementary and both may ultimately prove useful. Systemic approaches include the use of pharmaceuticals which block the effects of growth factors on tumor cells. Since glioblastoma cells have been shown to contain receptors for the epidermal growth factor, platelet-derived growth factor, and others, agents which block the induction of cell growth by these routes are currently being explored in several laboratories [37]. However, multiple problems exist. These include the observations that cells within a gilioblastoma can be heterogeneous. Thus, an agent may affect some but not all tumor cells. Additionally, the epidermal growth factor receptor in a glioblastoma may be an altered form of the normal receptor molecule, thus it may lack an extracellular determinant needed for pharmaceutical binding. Therapy may therefore be designed toward altering a later step in cell control such as EGF kinase. One group has created multiple agents capable of such action [38]. However, with all such systemic approaches, one must be careful of induced alterations in growth factor systems that are also performing an essential function in normal cells throughout the body. Systemic toxicity is a concern.

For these reasons, we have explored the possibilities of locally administered therapy. One novel approach is the use of viral vectors to genetically alter or to destroy tumor cells without causing harm to normal brain cells. We are currently exploring two such strategies. In one, a retrovirus is used to deliver a gene to alter cell function or to sensitize a cell to an exogenous agent, thereby permitting selective cell modulation or destruction. In the second strategy, a herpes virus is used to alter or to kill tumor cells while sparing normal brain cells.

Several studies have demonstrated that tumors associated with loss of function of a tumor suppressor gene can revert to a more normal phenotype following insertion and expression of a normal copy of the tumor suppressor gene. This was first demonstrated for the Rb gene [39]. Huang and co-workers created a construct containing the normal Rb gene under a strong promoter (the retrovirus long terminal repeat sequence, LTR) and transfected Rb-deficient retinoblatoma cells in culture. The cells taking up and expressing the new copy of the Rb gene reverted to a more normal phenotype in culture and were no longer tumorigenic in animals. In contrast, insertion under a strong promoter of an unrelated gene, luciferase, caused no phenotypic change. Similar results were obtained with osteogenic sarcoma. More recently, insertion and expression of the p53 gene into p53-defective colon carcinoma cells has been demonstrated to cause reversion to a normalized phenotype [40]. Further, some evidence now exists that p53 may play a role in the formation of gliomas (R.Y. Chung and B.R. Seizinger 1990, personal communication and [20–22]). Using a construct in which p53 is driven by a dexamethasone-inducible promoter, one group has now shown that insertion of this p53 construct into glioblastoma cells followed by induced expression of the p53 product is associated with growth suppression of the cells in culture [23]. Thus, in several systems, it now appears that re-introduction of a missing or non-functional tumor suppressor gene has the ability to normalize the cell phenotype. However, these studies have all been done in a cell culture environment where, even if the technique of gene transfer is relatively inefficient, the transfected cell population can be expanded for further testing. Therefore, while such strategies are very worthwhile in order to study tumor cell biology and gene function and regulation, it is not immediately apparent that such techniques can be readily adapted to an in vivo situation.

The major hindrance to developing a strategy of tumor treatment using gene transfer techniques in vivo appears to be the inefficiency of the technique of transfer. Techniques such as calcium-phosphate overlay, plasmid transfection, electroporation, and lipofection are convenient for cell culture studies, but not for in vivo gene transfer. The only relatively efficient method of in vivo gene transfer currently available is the use of viruses. Replication-defective retroviruses are particulary appealing for initial study because they can be engineered to contain the gene of interest but can not replicate to pose a systemic threat or an environmental problem [41,42]. Further, brain tumors represent a dividing cell population within an organ containing cells that are post-mitotic, and retroviruses contain a built-in selectivity for tumor cells in the nervous system since they will only incorporate into dividing cells. Therefore, my colleagues and I have begun to explore the efficiency of such vectors to effect gene transfer in the adult rodent brain.

We used a replication-defective retroviral construct ("BAG") which contained the bacterial beta-galactosidase gene driven by the strong LTR promoter. This viral vector has been shown to be able to incorporate into dividing cells in the fetal brain and has been particularly useful for studying cell lineages in embryologic neural development [43]. However, in the adult rat brain, we found virtually no expression of the beta-galactosidase gene in normal brain cells after stereotactic innoculation of the BAG vector into the right frontal lobe [44]. We next grew a C6 rat glioma in the brain and innoculated it with the BAG vector. Despite the fact that these tumor cells divide, the BAG vector was very inefficient at effecting gene transfer into the tumor cells. Only rare tumor cells and rare endothelial cells were noted to express the beta-galactosidase gene product. We suspect that this represents a relatively short half-life of the BAG vector in vivo and that many tumor cells are not in a state of active division during that short time period. To improve the efficiency, the next set of experiments involved grafting of the virus-producing cells (psi-2-BAG) into the brain. In normal brain, these cells survived less than 5 days and no endogenous cells were noted to take up and express the foreign gene. In contrast, when this packaging line was grafted into a tumor bed in the adult rat brain, improved efficiency of gene transfer and expression were noted. Nonetheless, this efficiency was still 10% or less under the conditions studied. While this may not be adequate for therapeutic studies, it opens avenues for further improvement of efficiency by using syngeneic packaging cells that would not be subject to immune rejection or by using motile packaging cells that are more likely to release virus over a wider area of the tumor. Such a system could be used to deliver tumor suppressor genes to modulate tumor cell growth or to cause tumor cell killing [45].

The use of a replication-defective virus system may always be hampered by the physical constraint that each tumor cell must be contacted by at least one viral particle in order for this strategy to work. Thus, we have considered that it may be worthwhile to use replication-competent viruses in some cases. The use of replication-competent retroviruses is worthy of experimental study but could be associated with systemic complications such as a hematopoetic neoplasia. We have thus begun to explore replication-competent herpes viruses, initially using a strategy aimed at relatively selective glioma cell killing. The advantage of a replication competent virus is that a small innoculum can multiply in the tumor cells and sequentially release virus to additional tumor cells where it can multiply further. However, to prevent neurologic toxicity, some selectivity must be engineered into the virus. Herpes viruses were chosen for initial study because they have been shown to have the ability to grow in the brain and because various mutants have been developed that have reduced neuropathogenicity. Additionally, systemic herpes infections are uncommon and drugs exist to inhibit systemic spread should it occur.

Our initial studies have been with a thymidine kinase mutant of the wild-type KOS strain of herpes simplex-1 (HSV-1). Thymidine kinase deficient strains of HSV-1 have been shown to have reduced neurovirulence [46–48]. The genetically engineered strain that we have tested (dlsptk) [48] contains a large deletion in the thymidine kianase gene so that thymidine kinase activity is virtually undetectable and the chance of reverting to wild-type is nil. We have shown that this virus is capable of a productive infection in two human glioma cell lines and in three human gliomas in culture at the second passage. We have further shown that intraneoplastic innoculation of this virus can kill human glioma cells grafted into a nude mouse [49]. This virus represents a starting point for further studies. Other mutants with compromised neurovirulence are worthy of testing and the construction of viruses containing several mutations may further decrease neurovirulence while retaining the desired properties of glioma cell killing. Other mechanisms of cell selectivity may also be explored, including the use of cell-specific promoters for genes essential for viral replication. Additionally, the herpes virus has a much larger genome than retroviruses, thus the ability to use the herpes system not only for cell killing but also for gene transfer and cell modulation should also be considered.

Summary

In this brief review, I have outlined some of the uses of molecular genetic techniques to define the molecular abnormalities associated with tumorigenesis and with tumor progression. I have also suggested that we are at a point where novel techniques may be contemplated for the study of tumor biology and tumor therapy, and have given two recent examples studied by my colleagues and myself using genetically engineered viruses in experimental settings. This is but a beginning. As more of the tumor-associated genes are cloned and their function is determined, more creative strategies will undoubtedly develop. Many of these will fail but the few which succeed are likely to change the way we think about and treat tumors of the nervous system.

Acknowledgment. This work was supported in part by grants from the National Institutes of Health (NS 24279) and from Neurofibromatosis, Inc. (Mass. Bay area).

References

1. Martuza RL, Eldridge, R (1988) Neurofibromatosis 2 (bilateral acoustic neurofibromatosis). N Engl J Med 318:684–688
2. Zankl H, Zang KD (1972) Cytological and cytogenetical studies on brain tumors. IV. Identification of the missing G chromosome in human meningiomas as no. 22 by fluorescence technique. Hum Genet 14:167–169
3. Seizinger BR, Martuza RL, Gusella JF (1986) Loss of genes on chromosome 22 in tumorigenesis of acoustic neuroma. Nature 322:644–647
4. Seizinger BR, Rouleau G, Ozelius LJ, Lane AH, St. George-Hyslop P, Huson S. Gusella JF, Martuza RL (1987). Common pathogenetic mechanism for three tumor types in bilateral acoustic neurofibromatosis. Science 236:317–319
5. Rouleau GA, Wertelecki W, Haines JL, Hobbs WJ, Trofatter JA, Seizinger BR, Martuza RL, Superneau DW, Conneally PM, Gusella JF (1987) Genetic linkage of bilateral acoustic neurofibromatosis to a DNA marker on chromosome 22. Nature 329:246–248

6. Rouleau GA, Seizinger BR, Wertelecki W, Haines JL, Superneau DW, Martuza RL, Gusella JF (1990) Flanking markers bracket the neurofibromatosis type 2 (NF2) gene on chromosome 22. Am J Hum Genet 46:323–328
7. Seizinger BR, de la Monte S, Atkins L, Gusella JF, Martuza RL (1987) Molecular genetic approach to human meningioma: Loss of genes on chromosome 22. Proc Natl Acad Sci USA 84: 5419–5423
8. Logan JA, Seizinger BR, Atkins L, Martuza RL (1990) Loss of the Y chromosome in meningiomas: A molecular genetic approach. Cancer Genet Cytogenet 45:41–47
9. Dumanski JP, Rouleau GA, Nordenskjold M, Collins VP (1990) Molecular genetic analysis of chromosome 22 in 81 cases of meningioma. Cancer Res 50:5863–5867
10. Bigner SH, Mark J, Mahaley MS Jr, Bigner DD (1984) Patterns of the early, gross chromosomal changes in malignant human gliomas. Hereditas 101:103–113
11. Bigner SH, Mark J, Burger PC, Mahaley MS Jr, Bullard DE, Muhlbaier LH, Bigner DD (1988) Specific chromosomal abnormalities in malignant human gliomas. Cancer Res 88:405–411
12. Libermann TA, Nusbaum HR, Razon N, Kris R, Lax I, Soreq H, Whittle N, Waterfield MD, Ullrich A, Schlessinger J (1985) Amplification, enhanced expression and possible rearrangement of EGF receptor gene in primary human brain tumors of glial origin. Nature 313:144–147
13. Wong AJ, Bigner SH, Kinzler KW, Hamilton SR, Vogelstein B (1987) Increased expression of the epidermal growth factor receptor gene in malignant gliomas is invariably associated with gene amplification. Proc Natl Acad Sci USA 84:6899–6903
14. Malden LT, Novak U, Kaye AH, Burgess AW (1988) Selective amplification of the cytoplasmic domain of the epidermal growth factor receptor gene in glioblastoma multiforme. Cancer Res 48:2711–2714
15. Trent J, Meltzer P, Rosenblum M, Harsh G, Kinzler K, Mashal R, Feinberg A, Vogelstein B (1986) Evidence for rearrangement, amplification, and expression of c-myc in a human glioblastoma. Proc Natl Acad Sci USA 83:470–473
16. Hermansson M, Nister M, Betsholtz C, Heldin C-H, Westermark B, Funa K (1988) Endothelial cell hyperplasia in human glioblastoma: Coexpression of mRNA for platelet-derived growth factor (PDGF) B chain and PDGF receptor suggests autocrine growth stimulation. Proc Natl Acad Sci USA 85:7748–7752
17. Maxwell M, Naber SP, Wolfe HJ, Galanopoulos T, Hedley-Whyte ET, Black P McL, Antoniades HN (1990) Coexpression of platelet-derived growth factor (PDGF) and PDGF-receptor genes by primary human astrocytomas may contribute to their development and maintenance. J Clin Invest 86:131–140
18. Birchmeier C, Sharma S, Wigler M (1987) Expression and rearrangement of the ROS1 gene in human glioblastoma cells. Proc Natl Acad Sci USA 84:9270–9274
19. Kinzler KW, Bigner SH, Bigner DD, Trent JM, Law ML, O'Brien SJ, Wong AJ, Vogelstein B (1987) Identification of and amplified, highly expressed gene in a human glioma. Science 236:70–73
20. James CD, Carlbom E, Dumanski JP, Hansen M, Nordenskjold M, Collins VP, Cavenee WK (1988) Clonal genomic alterations in glioma malignancy stages. Cancer Res 48:5546–5551
21. El-Azouzi M, Chung R, Farmer GE, Martuza RL, Black PMcL, Rouleau GA, Hettlich C, Hedley-Whyte ET, Zervas NT, Panagopoulos K, Nakamura Y, Gusella JF, Seizinger BR (1989). Loss of distinct regions on the short arm of chromosome 17 associated with tumorigenesis of human astrocytomas. Proc Natl Acad Sci USA 86:7186–7190

22. James CD, Carlbom E, Nordenskjold M, Collins VP, Cavenee WK (1989) Mitotic recombination of chromosome 17 in astrocytomas. Proc Natl Acad Sci USA 86:2858–2862
23. Mercer WE, Shields MT, AMin M, Sauve GJ, Appella E, Romano JW, Ullrich SJ (1990) Negative growth regulation in a glioblastoma tumor cell line that conditionally expresses human wild-type p53. Proc Natl Acad Sci USA 87:6166–6170
24. Vogelstein B, Fearon ER, Hamilton SR, Kern SE, Preisinger AC, Leppert M, Nakamura Y, White R, Smits AMM, Bos JL (1988) Genetic alterations during colorectal-tumor development. N Engl J Med 319:525–532
25. Mulligan LM, Matlashewski GJ, Scrable HJ, Cavenee WK (1990) Mechanisms of p53 loss in human sarcomas. Proc Natl Acad Sci USA 87:5863–5867
26. Levine AL, Momand J (1990) Tumor suppressor genes: The p53 gene and the retinoblastoma sensitivity gene and gene products. Biochim Biophys Acta 1032: 119–136
27. Rubenstein AE, Bunge BP, Housman DE (eds) (1986) Neurofibromatosis. Ann NY Acad Sci 486:1–414
28. Blatt J, Jaffe R, Deutsch M, Adkins JC (1986) Neurofibromatosis and childhood tumors. Cancer 57:1225–1229
29. Barker D, Wright E, Nguyen K, Cannon L, Fain P, Goldgar D, Bishop DT, Carey J, Baty B, Kivlin J, Willard H, Waye JS, Greig G, Leinwand L, Nakamura Y, O'Connell P, Leppert M, Lalouel J-M, White R, Skolnick M (1987) Science 236:1100–1102
30. Seizinger BR, Rouleau GA, Ozelius LJ, Lane AH, Fayniarz AG, Chao MV, Huson S, Korf BR, Parry DM, Pericak-Vance MA, Collins FS, Hobbs WJ, Falcone BG, Iannazzi JA, Roy JC, St George-Hyslop PH, Tanzi RE, Bothwell MA, Upadhyaya M, Harper P, Goldstein AE, Hoover DL, Bader JL, Spence MA, Mulvihill JJ, Ayslworth AS, Vance JM, Rosenwasser GOD, Gaskell PC, Roses AD, Martuza RL, Breakefield XO, Gusella JF (1987) Genetic linkage of von Recklinghausen neurofibromatosis to the nerve growth factor receptor gene. Cell 49:589–594
31. Wallace MR, Marchuk DA, Andersen LB, Letcher R, Odeh HM, Saulino AM, Fountain JW, Brereton A, Nicholson J, Mitchell AL, Brownstein BH, Collins FS (1990) Type 1 neurofibromatosis gene: Identification of a large transcript disrupted in three NF1 patients. Science 249:181–186
32. Viskochil D, Buchberg AM, Xu G, Cawthon RM, Stevens J, Wolff RK, Culver M, Carey JC, Copeland NG, Jenkins NA, White R, O'Connell P (1990) Deletions and a translocation interrupt a cloned gene at the neurofibromatosis type 1 locus. Cell 62:187–192
33. Cawthon RM, Weiss R, Xu G, Viskochil D, Culver M, Stevens J, Robertson M, Dunn D, Gesteland R, O'Connell P, White R (1990) A major segment of the neurofibromatosis type 1 gene: cDNA sequence, genomic structure, and point mutations. Cell 62:193–201
34. Xu G, O'Connell P, Viskochil D, Cawthon RM, Robertson M, Culver M, Dunn D, Stevens J, Gesteland R, White R, Weiss R (1990) The neurofibromatosis type 1 gene encodes a protein related to GAP. Cell 62:599–608
35. Hall A (1990) ras and GAP Who's controlling whom? Cell 61:921–923
36. Menon AG, Anderson KM, Riccardi VM, Chung RY, Whaley JM, Yandell DW, Farmer GE, Freiman RN, Lee JK, Li FP, Barker DF, Ledbetter DH, Kleider A, Martuza RL, Gusella JF, Seizinger BR (1990) Chromosome 17p deletions and p53

gene mutations associated with the formation of malignant neurofibrosarcomas in von Recklinghausen neurofibromatosis. Proc Natl Acad Sci USA 87:5435–5439
37. Humphrey PA, Wong AJ, Vogelstein B, Zalutsky MR, Fuller GN, Archer GE, Friedman HS, Kwatra MM, Bigner SH, Bigner DD (1990) Anti-synthetic peptide antibody reacting at the fusion junction of deletion-mutant epidermal growth factor receptors in human glioblastom. Proc Natl Acad Sci USA 87:4207–4211
38. Yaish P, Gazit A, Gilon C, Levitzki A (1988) Blocking of EGF-dependent cell proliferation by EGF receptor kinase inhibitors. Science 242:933–935
39. Huang H-J S, Yee J-K, Shew J-Y, Chen P-L, Bookstein R, Friedmann T, Lee EY-H P, Lee W-H (1988) Suppression of the neoplastic phenotype by replacement of the RB gene in human cancer cells. Science 242:1563–1566
40. Baker SJ, Markowitz S, Fearnon ER, Willson JKV, Vogelstein B (1990) Suppression of human colorectal carcinoma cell growth by wild-type p53. Science 249:912–915
41. Cone Rd, Mulligan RC (1984) High-efficiency gene transfer into mammalian cells: Generation of helper-free recombinant retrovirus with broad mammalian host range. Proc Natl Acad Sci USA 81:6349–6353
42. Cepko C (1989) Immortalization of neural cells via retrovirus-mediated oncogene transduction. Annu Rev Neurosci 12:47–65
43. Price J, Turner D, Cepko C (1987) Lineage analysis in the vertebrate nervous system by retrovirus-mediated gene transfer. Proc Natl Acad Sci USA 84:156–160
44. Short MP, Choi B, Lee J-K, Malick A, Breakefield XO, Martuza RL (to be published) Gene delivery to glioma cells in rat brain by grafting of a retrovirus packaging cell line. J Neurosci Res
45. Moolten F (1986) Tumor chemosensitivity conferred by inserted herpes thymidine kinase genes: Paradigm for a prospective cancer control strategy. Cancer Res 46:5276–5281
46. Chiocca EA, Choi BB, Cai W, DeLuca NA, Schaffer PA, DiFiglia M, Breakefield XO, Martuza RL (1990) Transfer and expression of the lacZ gene in rat brain neurons mediated by herpes simplex virus mutants. The New Biologist 2:739–746
47. Field HJ and Wildy P (1978) The pathogenicity of thymidine kinase-deficient mutants of herpes simplex virus in mice. J Hyg (Camb) 81:267–277
48. Coen DM, Kosz-Vnenchak M, Jacobson JG, Leib DA, Bogard CL, Schaffer PA, Tyler KL, Knipe DM (1989) Thymidine kinase-negative herpes simplex mutants establish latency in mouse trigeminal ganglia but do not reactivate. Proc Natl Acad Sci USA 86:4736–4740
49. Martuza RL, Malick A, Markert JM, Ruffner KL, Coen DM (1991) Experimental therapy of human glioma by means of a genetically engineered virus mutant. Science 252:854–856

Activation of Proto-Oncogenes in Human Brain Tumors

MASABUMI SHIBUYA[1], HITOSHI YAMAZAKI[1,2], YOSHITO OHBA[1,3], YASUHISA FUKUI[1], YOSHITO UEYAMA[2], and NORIKAZU TAMAOKI[2]

Introduction

Recent studies on carcinogenesis have revealed that genetic alteration, including both activation of proto-oncogenes and inactivation of anti-oncogenes, are crucial for initiation and progression of human malignant lesions. Glioblastoma multiforme (astrocytoma grades III and IV) is recognized as the major malignant type of tumor of the human brain. Several proto-oncogenes were found to be activated in glioblastoma. The epidermal growth factor (EGF) receptor gene (c-*erbB* gene) was amplified in about one-third of these tumors [1,2]. Other oncogenes or possible oncogenes, c-*myc* [3], N-*myc* [4], *gli* [5] and *ros*-1 [6] genes were also observed to be amplified or rearranged. However. the presence of activation of the latter four genes in glioblastoma is thought to be rare. Thus, the activation of proto-oncogenes in the DNA level, in about one-half of the glioblastoma multiforme in humans is still unclear. Furthermore, although the EGF receptor gene was found to be frequently amplified in these tumors, it has not been fully determined whether or not these amplified genes are changed structurally and functionally.

In this report, we describe two cases of human glioblastoma multiforme which carried amplification of structurally altered EGF receptor genes [7]. The alteration of the EGF receptor gene was found to be due to a single deletion mutation within the ligand-binding domain, and the mutated EGF receptor gene had an intermediate but ligand-independent transforming activity on the NIH/3T3 cells [8]. Humphrey et al. have also reported a few cases of human glioblastoma carrying amplification of a structurally altered EGF receptor gene [9,10].

[1] Institute of Medical Science, University of Tokyo, Minato-ku, Tokyo, 108 Japan
[2] Department of Pathology, Tokai University, Isehara, Kanagawa, 259-11 Japan
[3] Institute of Clinical Endocrinology, Tokyo Women's Medical College, Shinjuku-ku, Tokyo, 162 Japan

Materials and Methods

In vitro Phosphorylation Reaction Using GL-3 and GL-5 Cells

Fresh-frozen tissues of GL-3, GL-5, and placenta were homogenized and centrifuged at 600 × g for 3 min. The supernatants were recentrifuged at 100,000 × g for 30 min. The pellet was suspended in a buffer to prepare the membrane fraction which was preincubated with or without the EGF at 21°C for 30 min. Phosphorylation was initiated by the addition of [γ-^{32}P]ATP, performed at 0°C for 1 min, and stopped by the addition of modified RIPA buffer. After the phosphorylation reaction was observed, portions of samples and the immunoprecipitates were electrophoresed on a 7.5% polyacrylamide slab gel in the presence of 0.4% sodium dodecyl sulfate (SDS).

Screening of the cDNA Library

GL-5 cells were maintained in athymic nude mice by transplantation of a tumor piece. Total RNA was isolated from fresh-frozen GL-5 cells, and poly(A)$^+$ RNA was purified by affinity chromatography using oligo-d(T) cellulose. A complementary DNA library was constructed in λgt11 via a unique *Eco*RI site and screened by plaque hybridization with a cloned EGF receptor cDNA, pE7, as a probe.

DNA Transfection Assay

DNA transfer into NIH3T3 cells was carried out by a method using polycation and dimethyl sulfoxide as described elsewhere [11]. The transfected cells were grown in Dulbecco's modified Eagle's medium (DMEM) supplemented with 6% fetal or newborn calf serum in the presence or absence of 400 µg/ml of G418.

Results and Discussion

Amplification of Rearranged EGF Receptor Genes in Human Glioblastoma

In our initial screening, we surveyed 8 cases of transplantable human brain tumors (6 glioblastomas and 2 ependymomas) for the presence of abnormal proto-oncogenes using Southern blot analysis. Among 19 oncogene-probes employed, no amplification or rearrangement was detected except for those by the v-*erbB* probe: two glioblastomas, GL-3 and GL-5, carried an amplified EGF receptor gene. These tumors were obtained from two male patients, aged 47 and 50 years, with glioblastoma multiforme and maintained in athymic nude mice. The histological characteristics of these tumors were not drastically changed during serial passages.

We used a human EGF receptor cDNA as a probe (kindly provided by I. Pastan, National Cancer Institute, Bethesda, Md.) in order to examine the fine structure of the amplified c-*erbB* gene in glioblastomas. *Eco*RI-digested DNAs of GL-3 and GL-5 cells carry a high copy number (20–30 copies) of the EGF receptor gene. Additionally possible rearranged DNA fragments were detected in both GL-3 and GL-5 among 5–7 kilobases (kb) DNA fragments (Fig. 1).

For localizing the rearranged DNA fragments in the EGF receptor gene, various portions of the EGF receptor cDNA were purified and used as probes. No abnormal bands were detected in the region downstream from the middle portion of the extracellular domain to the carboxy terminus. However, using 0.7-kb probe corresponding to the central portion of the extracellular domain, rearranged fragments of 25-kb and 11-kb long were detected in *Hin*dIII-digested GL-3 and GL-3 DNA, respectively (data not shown).

A portion of the extracellular domain was found to be lost in these two tumors. A 0.2-kb probe lying upstream of the 0.7-kb fragment in EGF receptor cDNA could not detect amplified bands in either GL-3 or GL-5, although this probe showed gene amplification in A431 cells. Interestingly, a synthetic 40-mer oligonucleotide, corresponding to the 5′-terminus of the coding region in the EGF receptor gene, clearly detected amplified DNA fragments both in GL-3 and GL-5. These results strongly suggest that GL-3 and GL-5 have similar, but not identical, short deletions within the extracellular domain of this gene.

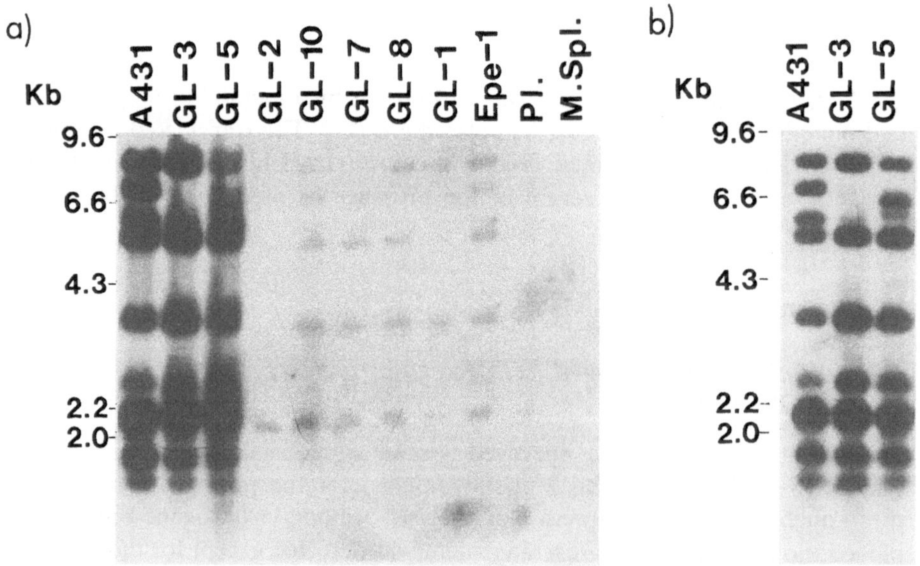

Fig. 1. Southern blot analysis of EGF receptor gene in human brain tumors. **a** Total cellular DNA (10 μg) of human brain tumors, *A431* human epidermoid carcinoma cell line, human placenta (*Pl.*), and nude mouse spleen (*M. Spl.*) were digested with restriction endonuclease *Eco*RI and examined by the Southern blotting method. The probe used was the ^{32}P-labeled 2.3-kb DNA fragment of pE7 human EGF receptor cDNA. **b** *A431* and glioblastoma *GL-3* and *GL-5* cellular DNAs (2 μg each) were analyzed essentially as described above

In further screening studies on 43 cases of glioblastoma multiforme, we found another case with a structurally altered and amplified EGF receptor gene, and 6 cases with amplification of the normal type EGF receptor gene in the DNA level.

Functional Alteration of Amplified EGF Receptor Genes in GL-3 and GL-5

In order to examine the features of the gene products translated from these rearranged EGF receptor genes, [^{35}S] methionine labeling of GL-5 cells and immunoprecipitation with anti-human EGF receptor monoclonal antibody (528 IgG, kindly provided by T. Kawamoto and S. Taniguchi, Okayama University, Japan) were carried out. In the GL-5 cells, the normal EGF receptor of 170 kDa was not detected, while an abnormal molecule of about 140 kDa was observed.

Membrane fractions of GL-3 and GL-5 or placental tissue (which is well known to express a considerable amount of normal EGF receptor) were used for in vitro phosphorylation reactions with or without ligand in order to analyze the tyrosine kinase activity of the 140 kd (kilodalton)-mutated EGF receptor.

Figure 2 shows the result of SDS-polyacrylamide gel electrophoresis of the total membrane fraction after phosphorylation, and of the immunoprecipitates from the same phosphorylated membrane fraction by using #528 IgG monoc-

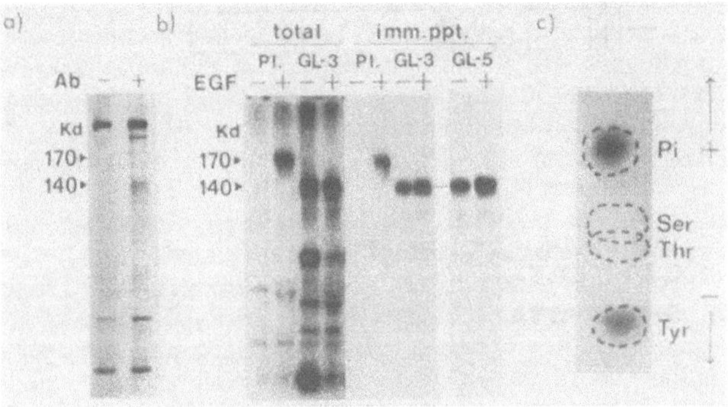

Fig. 2. [^{35}S]methionine labeling and ligand-independent phosphorylation of mutated EGF receptors. **a** A fresh *GL-5* tumor was cut into tiny pieces and labeled with [^{35}S]methionine for 10 h. Samples of cell lysate were mixed with protein A or with protein A plus #528 IgG, and precipitates were analyzed by SDS-polyacrylamide gel electrophoresis. **b** Total membrane fractions of *GL-3*, *GL-5*, and placenta (*Pl.*) were preincubated with or without *EGF* and phosphorylated with [γ-^{32}P]ATP. The samples were immunoprecipitated (*lanes imm. ppt.*) with #528 IgG and electrophoresed on a polyacrylamide gel. **c** Identification of phosphoamino acid in the 140-kd phosphoprotein of the GL-5 membrane fraction. The *band* of *140-kd protein*, phosphorylated without EGF as shown in *panel b*, was cut and analyzed. Authentic phosphoamino acids were added to the radioactive sample before electrophoresis

lonal antibody. As expected, the normal EGF receptor in the placenta was strongly phosphorylated only in the presence of EGF. On the other hand, abnormal EGF receptors of 140 kd in both GL-3 and GL-5 were found to be heavily phosphorylated even without the addition of EGF. In the cell lysates of GL-5, EGF or EGF-like activity was not detected, indicating that the presence of an autocrine-type model is not supported. The amino acid residue in the 140 kDa protein which phosphorylated in vitro in the absence of ligand was exclusively tyrosine.

Structure of EGF Receptor cDNA Obtained from Glioblastoma GL-5

Southern blotting analysis of GL-3 and GL-5 strongly suggested a large deletion mutation(s) within the ligand-binding domain in the level of genomic DNA [7]. The primary structure of the GL-5 EGF receptor cDNA was compared with that reported by Ullrich et al. [12]. Consistent with the results of Southern blotting, GL-5 cDNA carried a large deletion within the extracellular domain of 801-base pair (bp) long (nucleotide residue 275 to 1075 in the published EGF receptor sequence [12]) (Fig. 3). The starting site for this

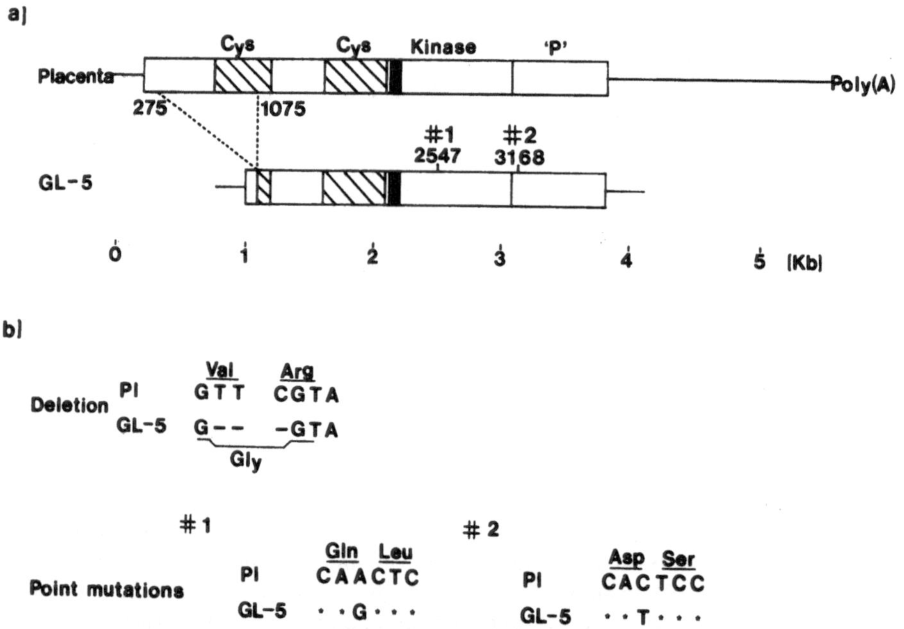

Fig. 3. Deletion mutation within the ligand binding domain of EGF receptor gene in glioblastoma multiforme GL-5. **a** Schematic representation of the EGF receptor cDNA cloned from GL-5 glioblastoma cells. The nucleotide numbers, *2547* and *3168* indicate silent point mutations. Cysteine-rich regions, tyrosine kinase domain, and autophosphorylation region are designated as *Cys*, *Kinase* and '*P*', respectively. **b** An amino acid change at the junction of deletion mutation and silent base changes in the GL-5 EGF receptor cDNA

deletion in the cDNA molecule was essentially the same as the 3′-end of the 1st exon of the EGF receptor gene in the genomic DNA [13]. Furthermore, the terminal site for this deletion in the cDNA was the 5′-terminus of the 7th exon of the EGF receptor gene, based on the nucleotide sequencing analysis of placental genomic DNA and on the physical map of the human EGF receptor gene reported by Haley et al. [14]. These results strongly suggest that the lack of 801 bp stretch in the GL-5 EGF receptor cDNA is due to a deletion mutation starting from a site within the 1st intron to another site in the 6th intron.

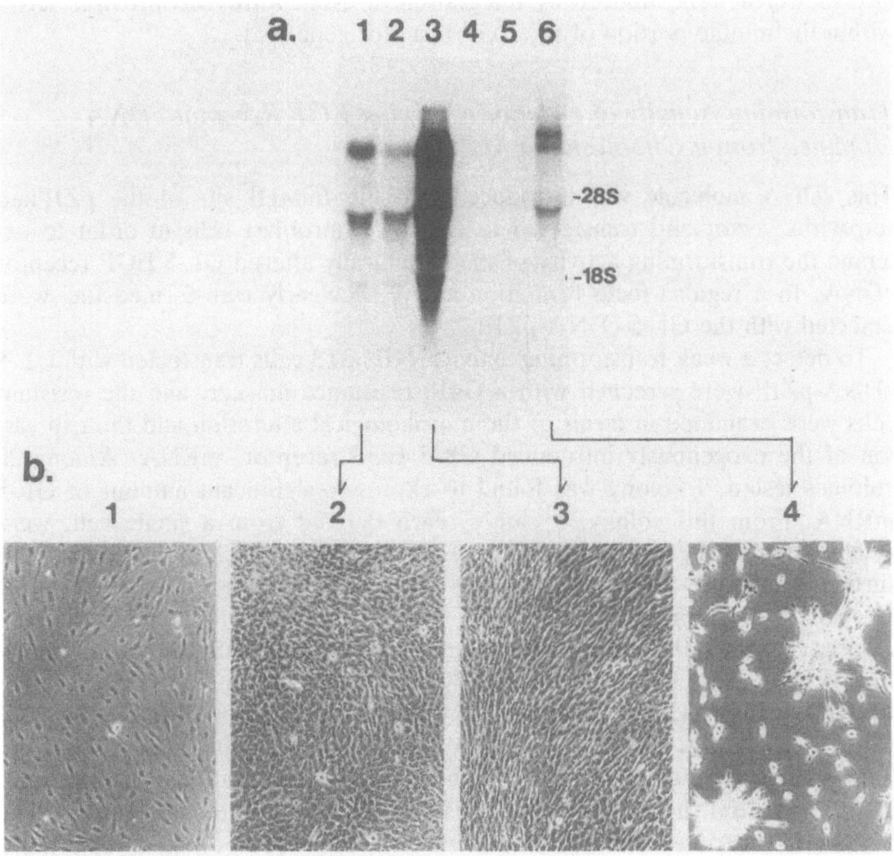

Fig. 4. Transforming activity of the mutated EGF receptor cDNA obtained from GL-5. **a** Expression of EGF receptor gene in NIH/3T3 cells transfected with mutated or normal human EGF receptor cDNA. *Lanes 1–5* Single cell-derived NIH/3T3 cells transfected with mutated GL-5 EGF receptor cDNA (*lane 1* clone #5-2, *lane 3* clone #5-1). *Lane 6* NIH/3T3 cell clone overexpressing the exogenously introduced normal EGF receptor. **b** Morphology of the NIH/3T3 cells overexpressing the mutated or normal EGF receptor. Control NIH3T3 cells (*1*), #5-2 (*2*) and #5-1 (*3*) clones, and the normal EGF receptor overexpressing NIH3T3 clone in the presence of 20 ng/ml EGF (*4*)

In other regions of the receptor cDNA molecule, including the transmembrane domain and the tyrosine kinase domain, no substitution of amino acids was found, although two silent base changes were observed (Fig. 3). Since the structurally altered EGF receptor in the membrane fraction of GL-3 and GL-5 cells showed a constitutive tyrosine kinase activity without its ligand EGF, we concluded that the single deletion in the ligand-binding domain is responsible for the functional activation of an EGF receptor molecule in a human glioblastoma cell line. A similar activation mechanism of the EGF receptor gene in animals, i.e., a deletion in the extracellular domain without other point mutations in the receptor molecule, has been reported in cases of chicken erythroblastosis which were induced by integration of avian retrovirus provirus DNA within the middle portion of the EGF receptor gene [15].

Transforming Activity of Deletion-Carrying EGF Receptor cDNA Obtained from a Glioblastoma Multiforme

This cDNA molecule was introduced into the *Bam*HI site of the pZIPneo retrovirus vector and transfected to NIH/3T3 fibroblast cells in order to examine the transforming activity of the structurally altered GL-5 EGF receptor cDNA. In a regular focus-formation assay, no clearly transformed foci were detected with the GL-5 cDNA-pZIP.

To detect a weak transforming activity, NIH/3T3 cells transfected with GL-5 cDNA-pZIP were screened with a G418 resistance marker, and the resistant cells were examined in terms of the morphological alteration and the expression of the exogenously introduced GL-5 EGF receptor, mRNA. Among 20 colonies tested, 1 colony was found to express a significant amount of GL-5 mRNA. From this colony, 5 clones, each derived from a single cell, were established and the levels of the GL-5 EGF receptor mRNA in these cells were further examined. As shown in Fig. 4, clone #5-1 expressed a high level of GL-5 EGF receptor mRNA and clone #5-2 showed a moderate level. These 2 clones, especially the #5-1, showed a morphological transformation, although the degree was lower compared with that of normal EGF receptor-overexpressing NIH/3T3 cells in the presence of a high concentration of EGF (Fig. 4). As a control, normal EGF receptor-overexpressing cells without the ligand EGF did not show any morphological transformation in this culture condition. From these results, we consider that an intermediate transforming activity is associated with the mutated GL-5 EGF receptor gene carrying a large and single deletion within the ligand binding domain (Fig. 5).

Characterization of Cellular Oncogenes Involved in Human Glioblastoma other than EGF Receptor Genes

Although activation of EGF receptor genes is relatively frequent in glioblastoma multiforme, about two–thirds of these tumors do not carry amplification of the EGF receptor gene. Since double minute chromosomes, which indicate the existence of gene amplification, have been reported to be present in about 55% of near-diploid glioblastomas [16], the in-gel renaturation method appears to

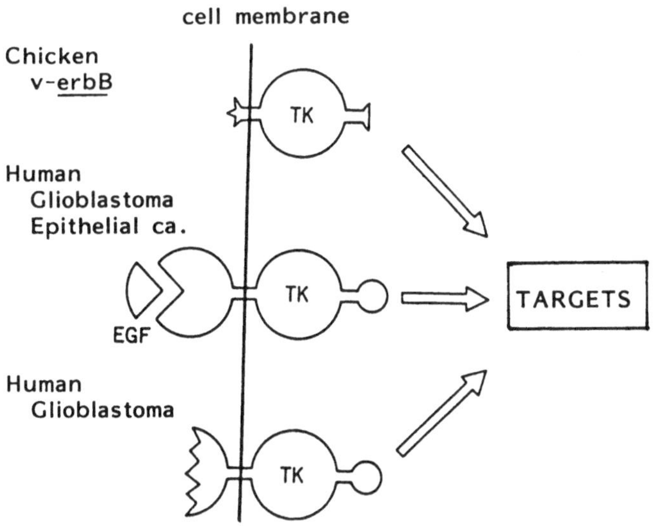

Fig. 5. A possible model for the activation of EGF receptor gene in various tumors

be one of the useful techniques for identifying amplification of other cellular genes.

Discussion

In our attempt to isolate amplified genes in glioblastoma using this method, we found one case which carried amplified genomic DNA fragments. The amplified gene was identified by Southern blot experiments to be a known cellular gene, c-*myc*. Although the amplified gene was not a novel one, we were able to clone a variety of DNA fragments which appeared to be randomly distributed in the c-*myc* amplicon in this glioblastoma. These fragments may be useful in characterizing the range of amplicon in the genomic DNA and to elucidate the molecular mechanism of c-*myc* gene amplification. These data might also be important for understanding the mechanism of EGF receptor gene amplification.

Taken together, human glioblastoma multiforme carry a variety of activated cellular oncogenes, from receptor tyrosine kinase to nuclear oncogenes (Fig. 6). In association with inactivation of suppressor oncogenes located on chromosomes 10 and 17, these activated oncogenes may play a crucial role in the progression of glioblastoma. Data on these altered genes also provide a tool for new classifications of glioblastoma, which may further contribute to the establishment of new therapeutic procedures to treat this malignancy.

Conclusion

We showed that two transplantable cell lines of human glioblastoma multiforme, GL-3 and GL-5, carried an amplification and overexpression of the

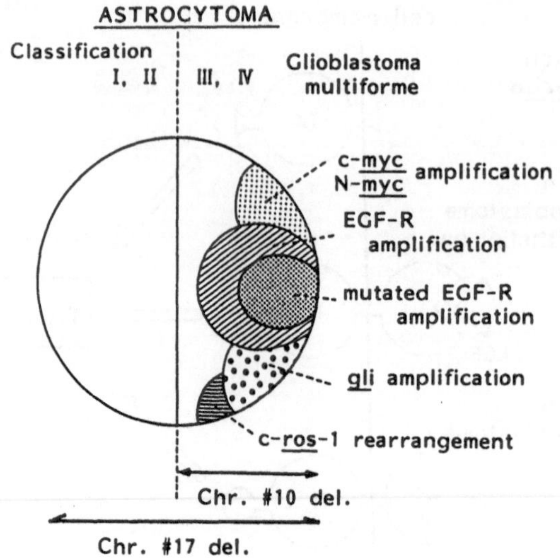

Fig. 6. Activation and inactivation of cellular genes responsible for the initiation and progression of glioblastoma (a model). *Chr. #10 del.* Chromosome 10 deletion, *Chr. #17 del* chromosome 17 deletion

structurally altered epidermal growth factor (EGF) receptor gene: the 140-kd EGF receptors in these cases exhibited a constitutively expressed tyrosine kinase activity without the ligand. The abnormal EGF receptor cDNA isolated from GL-5 cell line contained a single large intramolecular deletion mutation 801-bp long within the ligand binding domain of the EGF receptor. At the level of genomic DNA, this deletion appeared to start from the 1st intron and to terminate in the 6th intron of the EGF receptor gene. However, in the two lines of glioblastoma, GL-3 and GL-5, the positions of the start and the end of the deletion mutation in these introns were not identical, suggesting the involvement of a unique recombination mechanism in the formation of deletion mutation. A weak but ligand-independent transforming activity was observed in the deletion-carrying EGF receptor cDNA. An approach to characterize the molecular mechanism of gene amplification was also discussed.

References

1. Libermann TA, Nusbaum HR, Razon N, Kris R, Lax I, Soreq H, Whittle N, Waterfield MD, Ullrich A, Schlessinger J (1985) Amplification, enhanced expression and possible rearrangement of EGF receptor gene in primary human brain tumours of glial origin. Nature 313:144–147
2. Wong AJ, Bigner SH, Bigner DD, Kinzler KW, Hamilton SR, Vogelstein B (1987) Increased expression of the epidermal growth factor receptor gene in malignant gliomas is invariably associated with gene amplification. Proc Natl Acad Sci USA 84:6899–6903

3. Trent J, Meltzer P, Rosenblum M, Harsh G, Kinzler K, Mashal R, Fleiberg A, Vogelstein B (1986) Evidence for rearrangement, amplification, and expression of c-*myc* in a human glioblastoma. Proc Natl Acad Sci USA 83:470–473
4. Garson JA, Mcintyre PG, Kemshead JT (1985) N-myc amplification in malignant astrocytoma. Lancet 28:718–719
5. Kinzler KW, Bigner SH, Bigner DD, Trent JM, Law ML, O'Brien SJ, Wong AJ, Vogelstein B (1987) Identification of an amplified, highly expressed gene in a human glioma. Science 236:70–73
6. Birchmeier C, Sharma S, Wigler M (1987) Expression and rearrangement of the ROS1 gene in human glioblastoma cells. Proc Natl Acad Sci USA, 84:9270–9274
7. Yamazaki H, Fukui Y, Ueyama Y, Tamaoki N, Kawamoto T, Taniguchi S, Shibuya M (1988) Amplification of the structurally and functionally altered epidermal growth factor receptor gene (c-*erbB*) in human brain tumors. Mol Cell Biol 8:1816–1820
8. Yamazaki H, Ohba Y, Tamaoki N, Shibuya M (1990) A deletion mutation within the ligand binding domain is responsible for activation of epidermal growth factor receptor gene in human brain tumors. Jpn J Cancer Res 81:773–779
9. Humphrey PA, Wong AJ, Vogelstein B, Friedman HS, Werner MH, Bigner DD, Bigner SH (1988) Amplification and expression of the epidermal growth factor receptor gene in human glioma xenografts. Cancer Res 48:2231–2238
10. Humphrey PA, Wong AJ, Vogelstein B, Zalutsky MR, Fuller GN, Archer GE, Friedman HS, Kwatra MM, Bigner SH, Bigner DD (1990) Anti-synthetic peptide antibody reacting at the fusion junction of deletion-mutant epidermal growth factor receptors in human glioblastoma. Proc Natl Acad Sci USA 87:4207–4211
11. Kawai S, Nishizawa M (1984) New procedure for DNA transfection with polycation and dimethyl sulfoxide. Mol Cell Biol 4:1172–1174
12. Ullrich A, Coussens L, Hayflick JS, Dull TJ, Gray A, Tam AW, Lee J, Yarden Y, Libermann TA, Schlessinger J, Downward J, Mayes ELV, Whittle N, Waterfild MD, seeburg PH (1984) Human epidermal growth factor receptor cDNA sequence and aberrant expression of the amplified gene in A431 epidermoid carcinoma cells. Nature 309:418–425
13. Ishii S, Xu Y-H, Stratton RH, Roe BA, Merlino, GT, Pastan I (1985) Characterization and sequence of the promotor region of the human epidermal growth factor receptor gene. Proc Natl Acad Sci USA 82:4920–4924
14. Haley J, Whittle N, Bennett P, Kinchington D, Ullrich A, Waterfield M (1984) The human EGF receptor gene: Structure of the 110kb locus and identification of sequences regulating its transcription. Oncogene Res 1:375–396
15. Nilsen TW, Maroney PA, Goodwin RG, Rottman F, Crittenden LB, Raines MA, Kung, H-J (1985) c-*erbB* activation in ALV-induced erythroblastosis: Novel RNA processing and promoter insertion result in expression of an amino-truncated EGF receptor. Cell 41:719–726
16. Bigner SH, Mark J, Burger MP, Mahaley MS Jr, Bullard DE, Muhlbaier LH, Bigner DD (1988) Specific chromosomal abnormalities in malignant human giomas. Cancer Res 88:405–411

Gene Structure and Regulatory Mechanism of Gene Expression

Katsuji Hori[1]

Introduction

The genomes of higher eukaryote are much bigger than those of bacteria. It is estimated that the human haploid genome is composed of about 3×10^9 nucleotides with a total length of 1,000 mm, and that only 10% of it is utilized as coding and regulatory sequences. The largest elucidated gene in a human chromosome contains as many as 2×10^6 nucleotides pairs (dystrophin gene, the gene for Duchenne and Becker muscular dystrophy diseases), and genes of more than 100,000 nucleotides pairs in length are not unusual [1]. Assuming that a gene is $3–6 \times 10^4$ nucleotides in length, which includes the coding region and the non-coding and flanking sequences, this estimate would predict that there are about $5–10 \times 10^4$ human genes coding for different proteins (Table 1). To date, more than 1,600 human genes have been mapped to specific sites on 24 different nuclear chromosomes [2]. Thus, the number of genes mapped corresponds to approximately 3% of all human genes in a haploid genome. The extrachromosomal 54 loci have been mapped on the mitochondrial DNA. Many genes in human genomes belong to multigene families, which can be either dispersed in different chromosomes or clustered into a single or tandemly repeated array. Intensive studies have indicated that genomic organization, gene structure, gene expression, and its regulation in eukaryotic cell would be more complex than that in prokaryotes, and have shown that higher eukaryote genomes have some unexpected features: interrupted structure, pseudogenes which are an inactive but stable component of the genome derived by mutation of an ancestral active gene, and genome rearrangement which occurs during B- and T-lymphoid cell differentiation. In this article, I describe the regulatory mechanism of eukaryotic gene expression with special reference to the transcriptional regulatory sequences (cis-elements) on a gene, general and tissue-specific transcription factors, and their interaction in activating gene expression.

General Features of Eukaryotic Genes

In general, eukaryotic genes are composed of the coding and regulatory sequences (Fig. 1). Most genes in eukaryotes are also characterized as having an

[1] Department of Biochemistry, Saga Medical School, Saga, 849 Japan

Table 1. The size of some human genes. (Modified from [1])

Gene	Gene size (kb)	mRNA (kb)	Number of exons
β-Globin	1.5	0.6	3
Insulin	1.7	0.4	3
Aldolase A [40]	6.5	1.7	12
Protein kinase C	11.0	1.4	8
Albumin	25.0	2.1	15
Catalase	34.0	1.6	13
LDL receptor	45.0	5.5	18
Factor VIII	186.0	9.0	26
Thyroglobulin	300.0	8.7	37
Dystrophin	>2000	17.0	>60

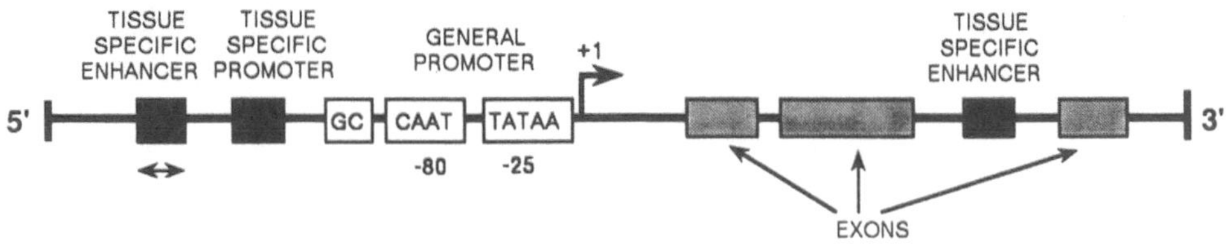

Fig. 1. Schematic representation of the location of the regulatory regions, exons, and introns of eukaryotic genes

interrupted structure [3]: the exon-intron structure which was first observed with the human adenovirus 2 genome, and the chicken ovalbumin and rabbit β-globin genes. The exons comprise the sequence represented in the mature mRNA, rRNA, and tRNA and may not necessarily have a protein-coding function. The introns comprise the interrupting sequences that are removed when primary transcripts are processed to give mRNA. A gene starts and ends with exons (corresponding to the 5′- and 3′-ends of the RNA), but there may be any number of introns within it.

In addition to the transcribable sequences, genes also have *promoters*, the sequences required for RNA polymerase binding to initiate transcription, and *regulatory sequences*, those required for transcriptional regulation (Fig. 1). Promoters for RNA polymerase I and II are located mostly upstream of the transcriptional initiation site, but the promoter for RNA polymerase III lies downstream of the initiation site. Promoters for RNA polymerase II contain a variety of short nucleotide sequences (*cis-acting elements*), each of which is recognized by a transcriptional protein factor (*trans-acting factor*) and/or RNA polymerase (Table 2). Most promoters for RNA polymerase II have a sequence called the TATA box [3], usually located about 25 bp upstream of the initiation site. It is the promoter element that has a relatively fixed location with respect to the initiation sites. It has been found in a wide variety of eukaryotic genomes of mammals, birds, amphibians, insects, and plants [1]. The TATA box is responsible for the selection of the exact initiation site. Promoters that lack TATA boxes usually lack a unique starting point. Initia-

Table 2. Transcriptional cis-elements and trans-acting factors. (Modified from [4])

Module	Consensus	Factor	Distribution
TATA Box	TATAAAA	TFIID	General
CAAT Box	GGCCAATCT	CTF/NF-1	General
GC Box	GGGCGG	SP1	General
CCAAT/Enhancer site	TGTGGAAAG	C/EBP	General
CCAAT/Enhancer site	TGTGGAAAG	C/EBP5	General
CCAAT/Enhancer site	TGTGGAAAG	C/EBP18	General
kB	GGGACTTTCC	H2-TF1	General
kB	GGGACTTTCC	NFkB	Lymphoid
Octamer	ATTTGCAT	Oct-1(OTF-1)	General
Octamer	ATTTGCAT	Oct-2(OTF-2)	Lymphoid
Pit-1 Binding site	TATNCAT	Pit-1/GHF-1	Pituitary
LF-B1 Binding site	TGGTTAATNATTAACAA	LF-B1/HNF-1	Hepatocyte
Eryf-1 Binding site	(A/T) (GAT(A/T) (A/G)	Eryf-1	Erythroid
MyoD Binding site	AGACATGTGGCT	MyoD	Muscle

tion is accomplished by a complex of RNA polymerase and several different general transcription factors that assemble at the region around the initiation sites. The role of the TATA box could be to align the RNA polymerase via the interaction with TFIID, a general transcription initiation factor, and other general factors, so that it initiates at the proper site. Some promoters have two other sequences called the CAAT box and GC box [3] (Fig. 1). The CAAT box is conserved in several known promoters and is located close to −80. It plays a role in determining the efficiencies of the promoter. The GC box contains the sequence GGGCGG and is found in genes that are expressed constitutively (housekeeping genes) and lack the TATA box. Often, multiple copies are present in the promoter. Some promoters lack a TATA box; others lack a CAAT box and have no GC boxes.

Eukaryotic promoters do not necessarily function alone. In some cases, the activity of a promoter is enormously increased by the presence of an *enhancer*, a sequence that increases the utilization of some eukaryotic promoters (Table 2). The enhancer can function in either orientation and in any location (upstream or downstream) relative to the promoter. Cellular enhancers stimulate the use of a nearby promoter in a specific tissue. For example, the immunoglobulin enhancer is downstream of the promoter that it stimulates, and appears to be active only in the B lymphocytes in which the immunoglobulin genes are expressed.

Modules that uniquely identify particular groups of genes responding to certain transcription factors are called *responsive elements* (REs). There are several responsive elements in some genes (Table 3). CRE (cAMP responsive element), HSE (heat shock responsive element), GRE (glucocorticoid responsive element), MRE (metal responsive element), TRE (thyroid responsive element), TPARE (12-0-tetradecanoyl phorbol ester 13-acetate [TPA] responsive element), and SRE (serum responsive element) are modules that uniquely identify particular groups of genes. REs are recognized by factors that coordinate the transcription of particular groups of genes. They contain a short

Table 3. Responsive elements for hormone receptors and other ligand-binding factors. (Modified from [4])

Regulatory agent	Module	Consensus	Factor
Cyclic-AMP	CRE	GTGACGT	CREB/ATF
Estrogen	ERE	GGTCAN TG(A/T)CC	Receptor
Glucocorticoid	GRE	GGTACAN TGTTCT	Receptor
Heat shock	HSE	CNNGAANNTCCNNG	HSTF
Cadmium	MRE	CGNCCCGGNCNC	Binding protein
Serum	SRE	GATGTCCATATTAGGACATC	SRF
Thyroid	TRE	CAGGGACGTGACCGCA	Receptor
Phorbol esters	TPARE	TGACTCA	AP1/Jun
Retinoic acid, TPA	AP2 Site	CCCCAGGC	AP2

consensus sequence that can be recognized in the appropriate promoters and may be located in promoters or in enhancers.

The common mode of regulation of eukaryotic transcription appears to be positive. However, regulation by specific repression of a target promoter or of distal regulatory sites (referred to as a *silencer* or *dehancer*) has also been reported with various genes [5–11], such as human interleukin-3, PEPCK (phosphoenol pyruvate carboxykinase), insulin, factor IX, gastrin, collagenase II genes, and rat growth hormone gene. A silencer is a cis-acting element which turns off or reduces transcription activity. Some silencers contain a short consensus sequence, 5′-NNGGAGANNN-3′ (Table 4).

Regulatory Mechanism of Eukaryotic Gene Expression

(1) Transcription Initiation Complex

RNA polymerase II does not initiate transcription by itself, but depends upon the general transcription factor TFIID, which is the factor that binds to the TATA box present in most promoters transcribed by RNA polymerase II. Several other transcriptional initiation factors might contact TFIID; after TFIID is bound to the promoter, TFIIA, TFIIB, RNA polymerase II, and TFIIE/F can be incorporated into the initiation complex (*basal transcription complex*) [12,13]. Transcription by RNA polymerase II is regulated by sequence-specific DNA binding proteins (Tables 2, 3). These proteins, even when bound at considerable distances from the transcriptional initiation site, cause RNA polymerase II to initiate more frequently and efficiently (*activated transcription complex*) [13]. It is predicted that the DNA between the bound activator protein and the transcription initiation site probably loops out, allowing the activator protein to contact RNA polymerase II or a general initiation factor at the promoter. Initiation is accomplished by a complex of RNA polymerase and these general transcription factors that assemble at the core region around the starting point. The role of the TATA box could be to align the RNA polymerase via interaction with TFIID and other factors so that it initiates at the proper site.

Table 4. Localization of silencer sequences in various genes

Gene	Sequence	Position, bp	Module	Reference
Human interleukin-3 (h-IL-3)	5′-GCTGCCATG-3′	−271 – −250	NIP	[5]
Phosphoenolpyruvate carboxykinase (PEPCK)	5′-TGGTGTTTTGACAAC-3′	−416 – −402	IRS (distal)	[6]
Human insulin	5′-GGAGAGACATTTG-3′	−273 – −258	GAGA Box	[7]
Human factor IX	5′-GGAGAGGAT-3′	−1.7 kb – −1.4 kb	GAGA Box	[8]
Human gastrin	5′-AGGCGAGAGGAAT-3′	−108 – −82		[9]
Collagen II	5′-GGAGGTG-3′	−700 – −620	Distal	[10]
		−460 – −360	Proximal	
Rat growth hormone	5′-AGGAGAGCA-3′	−169 – −152	PRE	[11]
Consensus	5′-NNGGAGANNN-3′			

(2) General- and Cell-Specific Transcription Factors

Initiation of the transcription of protein mRNA precursors is a complex process in which RNA polymerase II and a number of other transcription factors proteins are required. These factors can be divided into two classes depending upon their function: the general factors that are required for transcription of all RNA polymerase II-dependent genes, and the sequence-specific (promoter selective) factors that are required for optimal transcription of only a set of these genes. These factors act by recognizing cis-acting sites that are classified as comprising parts of promoters or enhancers (Tables 2, 3). The TATA-binding factor, TFIID, plays a central role in the initiation of eukaryotic mRNA synthesis. CTF/NF-1 consists of a family of CAAT box-binding proteins (CTF1, CTF2, and CTF3), which is produced by alternative splicing, and activates both transcription and adenovirus DNA replication [4]. The Sp1, a GC box-binding protein, could be involved in allowing RNA polymerase II to recognize a certain class of promoters. The factor requires TFIID and additional factors called "coactivators" to stimulate transcription at the TATA-containing promoter. At promoters lacking a TATA box, an additional activity distinct from coactivators is required for Sp1 activation of transcription [14]. C/EBP is the CAAT- and enhancer-binding protein of genes involved in lipid and carbohydrate metabolism and is composed of a family (C/EBP, C/EBP5, and C/EBP18). Ectopic expression of C/EBP can catalyze the differentiation of 3T3-L1 cells into mature adipocytes. Oct-1, a ubiquitous transcription factor, is an octamer-binding factor in non-lymphoid cells which binds to the octamer sequence (ATTTGCAT) to activate many genes including the histone H2B genes. In lymphoid cells, a different factor, Oct-2, is expressed mainly in B and T lymphocytes and binds to the octamer to activate the immunoglobulin k light gene [15]. Presumably the same factor acts at the immunoglobulin heavy-gene enhancer, making Oct-2 a tissue-specific activator of more than one gene. NFkB, immunoglobulin k gene-specific nuclear factor, Pit-1 (or GHF-1), a pituitary-specific transcription factor for prolactin and growth hormone genes [16,17], LF-B1, a liver-specific transcription factor [18], Eryf-1, erythroid specific factor [19], and MyoD1, the transcription factors required for myogenesis [20] recognize cell-type specific upstream sequences to activate transcription initiation (Table 2). Similarly, there are many RE-binding factors [4] (Table 3), such as CREB/ATF, cAMP, a responsive element binding protein, steroid hormone receptors (glucocorticoid and estrogen receptors), SRF, (serum responsive factor), Jun/AP1, and TPA, a responsive element binding protein. As will be described later, a factor may recognize another factor or it may recognize RNA polymerase.

A comparison between the sequences of many transcription factors suggests that common types of domains can be found that are responsible for binding to DNA at the upstream, to the gene-specific activating sequence (*DNA binding domain*), and that are responsible for the activation of the transcriptional machinery (*transcription activation domain*) [21]. The DNA-binding domain of the factors are of various classes, which have been termed (a) *zinc finger*,

(b) *helix-turn-helix*, (c) *helix-loop-helix*, and (d) *leucine zipper*. The zinc finger motif comprises a DNA-binding domain. There are two types of zinc finger motifs, the Cys_2/His_2 motif consisting of about 30 amino acids with two cycteine and two histidine residues that stabilize the domain by coordinating a $zinc^{2+}$ ion, and the Cys_2/Cys_2-type motif bearing two pairs of cysteine. The zinc finger motif was originally recognized in factor TFIIIA, which is required for RNA polymerase III to transcribe 5S rRNA genes. The Cys_2/His_2-type motif has since been identified in several other transcription factors [4,21] such as Sp1, the *Drosophila ADR1*, *Krueppel* (an embryonic segmentation gene product with transcriptional repressor activity), and *Hunchback*, an embryonic segmentation gene. Vertebrate glucocorticoid and estrogen receptors, Eryf-1, the yeast regulatory factor GAL4, and adenovirus E1A are the Cys_2/Cys_2-type factors. The helix-turn-helix motif, which is composed of about 60 amino acid residues and is required for the factors to bind to DNA, was originally identified as the DNA-binding domain of prokaryotic repressors. A related form of the motif may be present in the homeobox, a sequence first characterized in several regulatory proteins coded by genes concerned with developmental regulation in the *Drosophila* [4] and nematode, and was soon found in mammalian transcription factors [4,21]. Homeodomain-containing proteins can bind and directly activate transcription of target genes. A structural motif referred to as the POU (Pit-1, Oct-2, and Unc-86) domain [22] has been identified in a large family of tissue-specific transcription factors. This motif contains two regions, 67–70 and 60 amino acids in length, and is separated by a nonconserved sequence, termed the POU-specific domain and the POU homeodomain, respectively. It has now been identified in genes for several mammalian transcription factors such as Pit-1 (GHF-1), the B cell-specific Oct-2 (OTF-2), the related, widely expressed transcription factor Oct-1, and the *Caenorhabditis elegans* gene product, unc-86, a developmental regulatory protein required for accurate neuronal lineage formation. It has been shown with Pit-1 that the POU homeodomain is sufficient for low-affinity binding with relaxed specificity, whereas the POU-specific domain confers site-specific, high-affinity binding and contributes to DNA-dependent Pit-1-Pit-1 interactions [23]. The amphipathic helix-loop-helix motif has been identified in some developmental and differentiation regulators, and in genes coding for eukaryotic DNA-binding proteins [21]. Each amphipathic helix presents a face of hydrophobic residues on one side and charged residues on the other side. The factors bearing this motif are kE2, an immunoglobulin k chain enhancer-binding protein, MyoD1, Myc protein encoded by c-*myc* proto-oncogene, and *Drosophila daughterless* gene-binding proteins. The motif has two functions: it is involved in protein dimerization and in DNA-binding. The relative roles of the helices and the loop have yet to be identified. The leucine zipper, which was first described for the mammalian C/EBP [24], consists of a stretch of amino acids rich in leucine residue which could form an amphipathic α-helix or a coiled coil. A leucine zipper in one polypeptide may interact with a zipper in another polypeptide to form a dimer. Adjacent to each zipper is a stretch of positively charged residues that may be involved in binding to DNA. C/EBP, Jun and Fos, the proteins of the AP1 family that bind AP1 sites, Oct-2, Myc, CREB, and interleukin-6 protein (IL-6) are typical leucine zipper proteins [21].

Some trans-acting factors also have single or multiple transcriptional activation domains. A domain consists of 30–100 amino acid residues separated from the DNA-binding domain and is needed for the transcriptional activation of a gene through direct or indirect interaction with TFIID or transcription initiation complexes [4,21] (Table 5). A major class has an *acidic domain* enriched in glutamate and aspartate (negatively charged amphipathic α-helix-forming domain). This domain has been described with the yeast factors, GAL4 and GCN4 [25], and then the mammalian AP1-binding protein (Jun) [21]. Other factors have non-acidic domains including the glutamine-rich activation domain of Sp1 [26] and the proline-rich CTF/NF-1 [27]. The *glutamine-rich domain* is found to work in conjunction with other domains in some transacting factors such as *Drosophila Antennapedia*, *Ultrabithorax*, and *Zeste* proteins, mammalian Oct-1, Oct-2, Jun, AP-2, SRF, and human TFIID. The *proline-rich domain* is found in CTF/NF-1, AP-2, Jun, Oct-2, and SRF. In some cases, certain residues around the zinc finger of the DNA-binding domain may play a more direct role in the activation of transcription. The three different motifs that characterize the transcriptional activation domains are likely to show regions that function by contacting other proteins.

Table 5. Features of selected transcription factors. (Modified from [4, 21])

Factor	DNA Binding domain	Transcriptional activation domain
TFIID	Basic region	Glutamine-rich domain
TFIIIA	Zinc-finger (Cys2/His2)	
CTF/NF-1	Basic domain (α-helix)	Proline-rich domain
SP1	Zinc-finger (Cys2/His2)	Glutamine-rich domain
C/EBP	Leucine-zipper and basic region	
GAL4	Zinc-finger (Cys2/Cys2)	
	Leucine-zipper and basic region	Acidic domain
CREB	Leucine-zipper and basic region	
ERBP	Zinc-finger (Cys2/Cys2)	
GREBP	Zinc-finger (Cys2/Cys2)	
Eryf-1	Zinc-finger (Cyc2/Cys2)	
Myf5		Acidic domain
MyoD	Basic and HLH myc homology regions	Acidic domain
Pit-1 (GHF-1)	POU-homeo and POU-specific domains	
Oct-1	POU-homeo and POU-specific domains	
Oct-2	POU-homeo and POU-specific domains	Glutamine-rich, proline-rich
Unc-86	POU-homeo and POU-specific domains	
LF-B1 (HNF-1)	POU-homeo and POU-specific domains	
Fos	Leucine-zipper and basic region	
Jun (AP1)	Leucine-zipper and basic region	Acidic domain
Myc (C,L,N)	Leucine-zipper and basic region	Glutamine-rich, proline-rich
HSV VP16		Acidic domain
Ad2 E1A		

(3) Interaction of Cis-Acting Elements with Trans-Acting Factors

So far, transcriptional activators are categorized into two classes [25,28]: members of one work universally (*universal activators*), whereas members of the other work only in certain cells (*non-universal activators*). A universal activator bears two functions on a single polypeptide: a DNA-binding surface and an acidic-activating region that interacts with TFIID, a target protein (Fig. 2). An example of the universal activators is the yeast transcriptional activator GAL4 [25,28]. It bears two functions on a single polypeptide: a DNA-binding surface and an acidic-activating region that interacts with a target protein. The non-universal activator bears just one of the two required functions and, therefore,

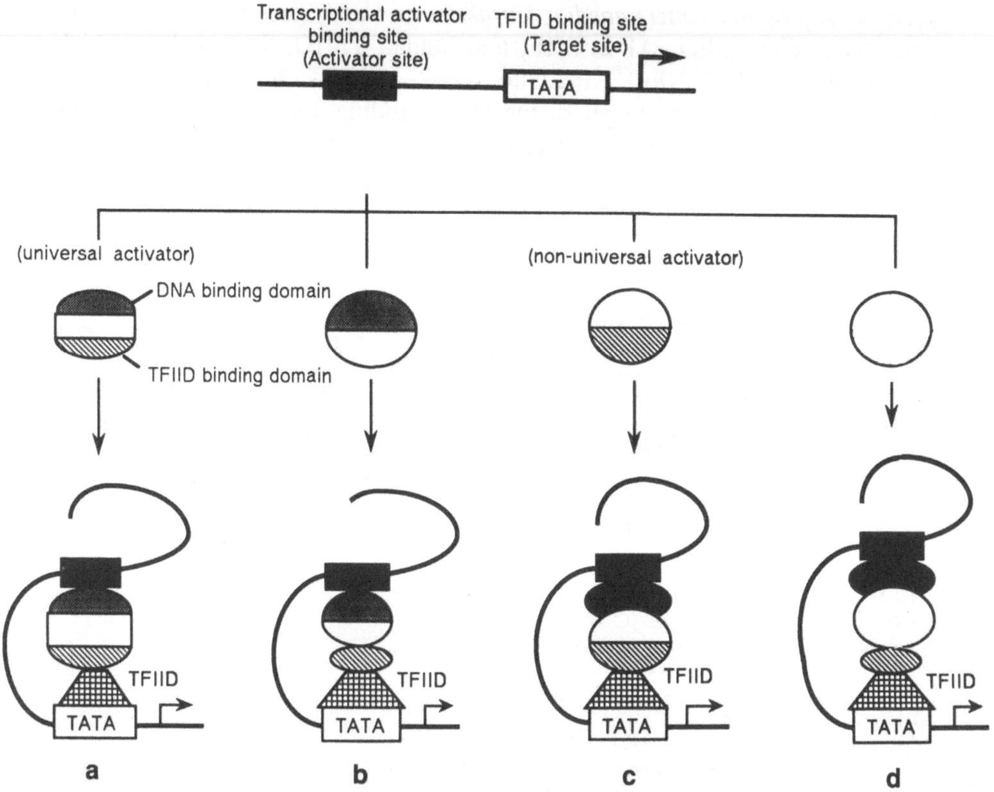

Fig. 2. Possible mechanisms for activation of transcription initiation complexes. **a** Transcription activators which bear two functions on a single polypeptide (universal activator) interact directly with both DNA-binding site (activator site) and TFIID. **b,c** Those which bear just one of the two domains (non-universal activators), DNA-binding domain, or acidic domain interact via intermediates bearing the missing domain. **d** Those which bear neither DNA-binding domain nor acidic activating domain (non-universal activators) interact with DNA-binding protein (*screen*) by one surface and attach by another surface to a third component (*hatching*) that could bear an acidic activating region

can work only in cells bearing molecules that provide the missing function (Fig. 2). The mammalian DNA-binding protein Oct-1 and the herpes virus protein VP16 are examples of this type [28]. VP16, which bears an acidic-activating domain, is unable to bind to DNA directly [29]. It can bind to a complex of DNA-bound proteins that bear a DNA binding domain. On the other hand, Oct-1, which lacks an acidic-activating domain, activates genes only in cells containing a protein which bears an acidic-activating region such as the VP16 protein [28].

Assuming that all of the transcriptional activators exert their effects by interacting with TFIID, sequence-specific DNA-binding factors which also bear acidic domain work directly, and hence universally, and others, which lack the acidic domains (Oct-1 and Sp1, for example), do so via intermediates bearing acidic-activating regions [14]. There are many protein factors which do not bear acidic domains. Many viral early gene products are specialized transcription regulators that activate or repress transcription of specific viral and cellular genes without direct binding to target promoters. The effects of viral trans-activators are mediated through protein-protein interactions with DNA-binding factors. The adenovirus E1A protein bears neither a DNA-binding domain nor an acidic-activating region. Thus, this protein is considered to attach by one surface to a DNA-binding protein such as CREB/ATF-2, and, in turn, to attach by another surface to a third component that could bear an acidic-activating region [28].

Sp1 recognizes the DNA sequence GGGCGG, found singly and in multiple in many cellular and viral promoters, and activates transcription through a domain rich in glutamine residues. This general transcription factor stimulates transcription at a TATA containing promoters in the presence of TFIID and an additional factor called "coactivators", that are dispensable for basal transcription but are required as molecular adaptors between trans-acting factors and a general transcription initiation machinery [13]. At promoters lacking a TATA box, an additional factor, termed the "tethering" factor, which is distinct from coactivators, is required for Sp1 activation of transcription [14].

(4) Autoregulation of Trans-Acting Factors

Evidence for autoregulatory mechanisms has been obtained for the distantly related class of developmental factors—the *Drosophila* homeodomain proteins such as those encoded by *Ultrabithorax*, *fushitarazu* and *deformed*, and mammalian factors—demonstrating that these proteins are capable of binding and activating their own promoters [30–33]. The myogenic determination factors MyoD1 [34], Pit-1 (GHF-1) [35,36] which is a member of a large family of genes that encode proteins which are involved in development and contain a highly homologous region referred to as the "POU domain". Jun [37] can also autoregulate their own expressions. As shown for these gene expressions, positive autoregulation may be a common way to regulate the activity of genes encoding certain regulatory proteins. Since expression precedes the appearance of the factor protein during development or differentiation activation of a trans-acting factor gene, at least one other factor should be required for initial activation. However, the molecular basis for the initial activation of the factor genes remains to be elucidated.

(5) Cellular Functions and Regulation of Gene Expression by Signal Transduction

Transcriptional initiation is a key control step in the expression of many eukaryotic genes. Diversed signals, such as heat-shock, glucocorticoid, steroid, lymphokins, growth factors, heavy metals, inflammation, and injury, regulate the expression of genes by controlling a step in which RNA polymerase II initiates and synthesizes their mRNA.

Cellular responses are initiated when extracellular signals are recognized by target cells and may directly activate the intracellular signaling apparatus to initiate the response. Hormones, growth factors, and more specific signals interact with their receptors and trigger the response. The signal from the outside to the inside of the cell, transduced through the membrane-bound receptor complex, generates second messengers. The level of the second messengers in the cell regulates the activity of relevant kinases, a cAMP-dependent protein kinase A and protein kinase C. Activation of protein kinase A by cAMP or activation of protein kinase C by phorbol ester stimulates transcription of selective genes. For example, CRE, a cAMP responsive element, was shown to mediate the cAMP response. The CRE is located within 100–120 bp upstream of the transcription initiation site and is required not only for cAMP responsiveness but also for maintaining a basal level of transcription from the promoter it controls (Table 3). CREB is a leucine zipper protein that binds to the CRE (Table 5). Phosphorylation promotes dimerization and DNA binding, and enhances the transcriptional activity of the factor [38]. Monomeric forms are no longer capable of binding to the CRE. Protein kinase C, but not protein kinase A, appears to facilitate dimerization of the factor in vitro. The ability of protein kinase A to stimulate CRE-dependent transcription without influencing dimerization suggests dual regulation of CREB-binding activity and transcriptional efficacy [38].

Phorbol esters have been shown to induce the expression of many genes, including the c-*fos* and c-*myc* genes. A TPA responsive element (TPARE) was initially found in the phorbol ester-resposive collagenase gene promoter and later with the metallothioneine IIA gene, SV40 promoter, interleukin-2, and glutathione-S-transferase gene. TPARE was also found in cellular proto-oncogenes, c-*fos*, c-*myc*, and c-*sis*. The proto-oncogene *jun* appears to occupy a central role in cellular signal transduction and regulation of cell proliferation. Jun, the AP1 DNA-binding protein (AP1/Jun) encoded by *jun*, recognizes TPARE which mediates a transcriptional response to phorbol ester tumor promoters such as TPA [37]. The binding of such factors to their cell surface receptors results in the activation of protein kinase C, which is also the cellular target for phorbol ester tumor promoters [39].

Signal transduction is a multistep process, and the steps downstream of the kinase reaction are likely to consist of a cascade of biochemical events. The research on a signal-dependent transcription system should provide critical insight into the biochemical nature of the components involved in the signal transduction pathway that connects cellular signal transduction systems to the regulation of gene expression, and will be important for our understanding of various cellular functions such as growth, development, differentiation, and oncogenesis.

References

1. Alberts B, Bray D, Lewis J, Raff M, Roberts K, Watson JD (1989) Molecular biology of the cell, 2nd edn. Garland, New York
2. Human Gene Mapping 10 (1989) 10th International Workshop on Human Gene Mapping. New Haven Conference. Cytogenet Cell Genet 51
3. Watson JD, Hopkins NH, Roberts JW, Steitz JA, Weiner AM (1987) Molecular biology of the gene, 4th edn. Benjamin/Cummings, Menlo Park, California
4. Lewin B (1990) Gene IV. Oxford University Press, Oxford
5. Mathey-Prevot B, Andrew NC, Murphy HS, Kreissman SG, Nathans DG (1990) Positive and negative elements regulate human interleukin 3 expression. Proc Natl Acad Sci USA 87:5046–5050
6. O'Brien RM, Lucas PC, Forest CD, Magnuson MA, Granner DK (1990) Identification of a sequence in the PEPCK gene that mediates negative effect of insulin on transcription. Science 249:533–537
7. Boam DSW, Clark AR, Docherty K (1990) Positive and negative regulation of the human insulin gene by multiple trans-activating factors. J Biol Chem 265:8285–8296
8. Salier J-P, Hirosawa S, Kurachi K (1990) Functional characterization of the 5′-regulatory region of human factor IX gene. J Biol Chem 265:7062–7068
9. Wang TC, Brand SJ (1990) Islet cell-specific regulatory domain in the gastrin promoter contains adjacent positive and negative DNA elements. J Biol Chem 265:8908–8914
10. Savagner P, Miyashita T, Yamada Y (1990) Two silencers regulate the tissue-specific expression of the collagen II gene. J Biol Chem 266:6669–6674
11. Pan WT, Liu Q, Bancroft C (1990) Identification of a growth hormone gene promoter repressor element and its cognate double- and single-stranded DNA binding proteins. J Biol Chem 265:7022–7028
12. Buratowski S, Hahn S, Guarente L, Sharp A (1989) Five intermediate complexes in transcription initiation by RNA polymerase II. Cell 56:549–561
13. Lewin B (1990) Commitment and activation at pol II promoters: A tail of protein-protein interactions. Cell 61:1161–1164
14. Pugh BF, Tjian R (1990) Mechanism of transcriptional activation by Spl: Evidence for coactivators. Cell 61:1187–1197
15. Scheidereit C, Cromlish JA, Gerster T, Kawakami K, Balmaceda CG, Currie RA, Roeder RG (1988) A human lymphoid-specific transcription factor that activates immunoglobulin genes is a homeobox protein. Nature 336:551–557
16. Ingrahm HA, Chen R, Mangalm HJ, Elsholtz HP, Flynn SE, Lin CR, Simmons DM, Swanson L, Rosenfeld MG (1988) A tissue-specific transcription factor containing a homeodomain specifies a pituitary phenotype. Cell 55:519–529

17. Bodner M, Castrillo J-L, Theill LE, Deerink T, Ellisman M, Karin M (1988) The pituitary-specific factor GHF-1 is a homeobox-containing protein. Cell 55:505–518
18. Frain M, Swart G, Monaci P, Nicosia A, Stampfli X, Frank R, Cortese R (1989) The liver-specific transcription factor LF-B1 contains a highly diverged homeobox DNA binding domain. Cell 59:145–157
19. Evans T, Felsenfeld G (1989) The erythroid-specific transcription factor Eryfl: A new finger protein. Cell 58:877–885
20. Lassar AB, Buskin JM, Lockshon D, Davis RL, Apone S, Hauschka SD, Weintraub H (1989) MyoD is a sequence specific DNA binding protein requiring a region of *myc* homology to bind to the muscle creatin kinase enhancer. Cell 58:823–831
21. Mitchell PJ, Tjian R (1989) Transcriptional regulation in mammalian cells by sequence-specific DNA binding proteins. Science 245:371–378
22. Herr W, Sturm RA, Clerc RG, Covcoran LM, Baltimore D, Sharp PA, Ingrahm HA, Rosenfeld MG, Finnay M, Rubkun G, Horvitz HR (1988) The POU domain: A large conserved region in the mammalian pit-1, oct-1, oct-2, and *Caenorgabditis elegans* unc-86 gene products. Genes Dev 2:1513–1516
23. Ingraham HA, Flynn SE, Voss Jm, Albert VR, Kapiloff MS, Wilson L, Rosenfeld MG (1990) The POU-specific domain of Pit-1 is essential for sequence-specific, high affinity DNA binding and DNA-dependent Pit-1–Pit1 interactions. Cell 61:1021–1033
24. Landschulz WH, Johnson PF, McKnight SL (1988) The leucine zipper: A hypothetical structure common to a new class of DNA binding proteins. Science 240:1759–1764
25. Ptashne M (1988) How eukaryotic transcriptional activators work. Nature 335:683–689
26. Courey AJ, Tjian R (1988) Analysis of Sp1 in vivo reveals multiple transcriptional domains including a novel glutamine–rich activation motif. Cell 55:887–898
27. Mermod N, O'Neil EA, Kelly TJ, Tjian R (1989) The prolin-rich transcriptional activator of CTF/NF-1 is distinct from the replication and DNA binding domain. Cell 58:741–753
28. Ptashne M, Gann AA (1990) Activators and targets. Nature 346:329–331
29. Berger SL, Cress WD, Cress A, Triezenberg SJ, Guarente L (1990) Selective inhibition of activated but not basal transcription by the acidic activation domain of VP16: Evidence for transcriptional adaptors. Cell 61:1199–1208
30. Nakano Y, Guerrero I, Hidalgo A, Taylor A, Whittle JRS, Ingham PW (1989) A protein with several possible membrane-spanning domains encoded by the *Drosophila* segment polarity *patched* gene. Nature 341:508–513
31. Hooper JE, Scott MP (1989) The *Drosophila* patched gene encodes a putative membrane protein required for segmental patterning. Cell 59:751–765
32. Dolle P, Izpisua-Belmonte J-C, Falkenstein H, Renucci A, Duboule D (1989) Coordinate expression of the murine Hox-5 complex homoeobox-containing genes during limb pattern formation. Nature 342:767–772
33. Lewis J, Martin P (1989) Limbs: A pattern emerges. Nature 342:734–735
34. Thayer MJ, Tapscott SJ, Davis RL, Wright WE, Lassar AB, Weitraub H (1989) Positive autoregulation of the myogenic determination gene MyoD1. Cell 58:241–248
35. Chen R, Ingrahm HA, Treacy MN, Albert VR, Wilson L, Rosenfeld MG (1990) Autoregulation of pit-1 gene expression mediated by two cis-active promoter elements. Nature 346:583–586

36. McCormick A, Brady H, Theill LE, Karin M (1990) Regulation of the pituitary-specific homoeobox gene GHF-1 by cell autonomous and environmental cues. Nature 345:829–832
37. Angel P, Hattori K, Smeal T, Karin M (1988) The *jun* proto-oncogene is positively autoregulated by its product, JUN/AP-1. Cell 55:875–885
38. Yamamoto KK, Gonzalez GA, Biggs III WH, Montminy MR (1988) Phosphorylation-induced binding and transcriptional efficacy of nuclear factor CREB. Nature 334:494–498
39. Nishizuka Y (1986) Studies and perspectives of protein kinase C. Science 233:305–310
40. Mukai T, Arai Y, Yatsuki H, Joh K, Hori K (1991) Eur J Biochem 195:781–787

In Situ Hybridization Using T-T Dimerized Non-Radioactive Probes

Paul K. Nakane, Hidekatsu Matsumura, and Takehiko Koji[1]

Introduction

DNA labeled with non-radioactive markers have been used for in situ hybridization of specific DNA or RNA in cells and tissues. The presence of protruding markers on the probe DNA has been attributed to be the cause for the loss of sensitivity and specificity of hybridization. In search of a non-protruding marker, we investigated the possibility of the use of a T-T dimer which can be generated easily in DNA while being a potent hapten as a marker for DNA [1]. A T-T dimer in DNA was generated by UV irradiation (254 μm). Following hybridization with complementary DNA or RNA in cells and tissues, the T-T dimerized DNA (T-T DNA) was detected immunohistochemically using rabbit anti-T-T DNA and peroxidase-labeled goat anti-rabbit IgG. It was found that the use of T-T as a marker offers several advantages over other markers: it appears not to interfere with hybridization efficiency, is simple to make, and can be detected with high sensitivity.

Using this method, various DNA and mRNA, such as human simplex virus type I DNA in the latent phase of the virus infection, the viral mRNA in the replicating phase [2], and c-*myc* mRNA in HL60 cells, were localized [3,4]. Quantitation of mRNA, such as c-*myc* mRNA in HL60, was also possible [5]. Human hepatitis virus, RNA, was found in hepatocytes as expected, but appeared unexpectedly in the infiltrating leucocytes [6]. More recently, attempts were made to localize mRNA at the electron microscopic level using the T-T dimerized probes. As with immuno-electron microscopy, the steps of in situ hybridization may be performed either on several micron-thick sections or on ultrathin sections; we selected to work with the thick sections. A major reason for this choice is as follows: an average length of mRNA is about 2,000 bases and, when it is stretched, the length of mRNA will exceed over 680 nm, but when mRNA is in a complex of circinate polyribosome, the diameter of the whirl will be about 200 nm. When the whirls are dispersed on a cytoplasmic surface of rough endoplasmic reticulum, as is the case when exportable pro-

[1] Department of Anatomy III, Nagasaki University School of Medicine, Nagasaki, 852 Japan

teins are synthesized, the distance between the centers of the whirls is about 200 nm. Hence, unlike that of antigens in the lumen of endoplasmic reticulum, the local concentration of any given specific mRNA is extremely low. Under this condition, the frequency that a stretch of a specific sequence of 20–25 nucleotides in mRNA to be present in a 100 nm thickness ultrathin section is extremely rare. Furthermore, the incidence in which the stretch will be on or near the surface of an ultrathin section is even less, which may result in not recognizing the presence of specific mRNA in a cell when the ultrathin sections are used. To circumvent this problem, we opted to use relatively thick sections, i.e., more than a 2 µm thickness, mounted on a light microscopic glass slide. Two different approaches were employed in our laboratory. One involved embedding fixed tissues in JB4, and sections with a 2 µm thickness were obtained from the blocks. The sections were adhered onto glass slides, exposed to a mixture of chrologform and isoarmyl alcohol to partially dissolve the JB4, and further treated with diluted HC1 and digested with proteinase K to remove proteins. On such a treated section, *in situ* hybridization was carried out using the T-T dimerized oligo-nucleotide probes. The sites of T-T dimers were then localized immunohistochemically using peroxidase-labeled antibodies. The reaction products of peroxidase was finally visualized by a back scattered electron detection mode of the scanning electron microscope [7]. This was found to be a convenient way to localize specific mRNA, since the tissue sections could be observed directly both at the light and electron microscopic levels. The second approach was similar to "pre-embedding immunoelectron microscopy" [8]. Some details of this method will be described below.

Materials and Methods

The DNA Probes Used

Anti-sense oligo-nucleotides DNA (ON-DNA) and sense ON-DNA probes corresponding to the nucleotides from #382 to #420 of alpha-subunit of mouse nicotinic acetylcholine receptors [9] (Fig. 1) were synthesized by Model 391 PCR-MATE DNA SYNTHESIZER, Applied Biosystems. At the time of synthesis, a sequence of A-T-T was added three times at the 3′ ends of the probes since these ON-DNA sequences did not contain the sites for T-T dimerization (indicated by *asterisks*, Fig. 1). ON-DNA were dissolved in 10 mM Tris/HC1 buffer, pH 7.4, containing 1 mM EDTA (TE) and were kept frozen at −20°C until used.

Method of UV Irradiation

From 20 to 40 µl ON-DNA (50 µg/ml in TE) were placed on a flat siliconized quartz dish, type AB 10 (cat. #CA 06102, Gasukuro Kogyo Inc., Tokyo) with a light path of 0.1 mm. The quartz dish with sample was irradiated with a 253.7 nm wave length ultraviolet (UV) light. The source of the ultraviolet was two UV 15 W Toshiba GL-15 lamps (Toshiba Ltd., Tokyo) placed 36.1 cm

```
Sense probe (382-420):
                                                ********
5'-TGTGAGATCATTGTCACTCACTTTCCCTTCGATGAGCAGATTATTATT-3'

Anti-sense probe (420-382):
  *********
3' TTATTATTAACACTCTAGTAACAGTGAGTGAAAGGGAAGCTACTCGTC 5'
```

Fig. 1. Synthetic oligo-nucleotides used for the localization of mRNA of alpha-subunit of mouse nicotinic acetylcholine receptor. A segment from 382 to 420 was utilized since the segment did not contain T-T and had a high homogeneity with the receptors mRNA of other species. TTATTATT was added on to the 3′ end of the sense probe and 5′ end of the anti-sense probe to provide dimerizable sites. (After [9])

from the surface of the quartz dish. The dose of UV irradiation was monitored using a Topcon U.V. radiometer UVR-254 (Tokyo Kougaku Kikai, Ltd., Tokyo). The monitor was placed at the same distance from the light source as the quartz dish. With the above irradiation set-up, the rate of irradiation was 5 joules/m^2 per s. An optimal dose of ultraviolet was found to be about 7,000 joules/m^2.

Antibody Used

Antiserum against T-T dimer was obtained from rabbits immunized with T-T dimerized salmon sperm DNA with methyl-bovine serum albumin [10]. IgG was purified from the antiserum first by precipitating immunoglobulin with ammonium sulfate, then by 2-diethylaminoethanol (DEAE) affinity chromatography. The isolated IgG was used as the first antibody. Fragment antigen binding (FAB) of goat anti-rabbit IgG antibody conjugated with horseradish peroxidase (HRP) (Sigma, type VI) was prepared according to the method of Wilson and Nakane [11] and was used as the second antibody. The immunoreactivity and specificity of the rabbit anti-T-T dimer DNA antibody (R anti-T-T) and the goat anti-rabbit IgG conjugated with HRP (HRP-G anti-R IgG) were determined utilizing T-T dimerized salmon sperm DNA dotted on nitro cellulose disks [1]. The optimal concentrations of the first and second antibodies determined in the experiment were used throughout these experiments [1].

Dot Hybridization

Various quantities (8 pg–8 ng of DNA in 2 μl of TE per dot) of non-irradiated single-stranded sense or anti-sense ON-DNA were dotted on strips of nitrocellulose filters as above. The filter was dried and heated at 80°C for 2 h and pre-hybridized at 24°C for 2 h with the following mixture: 10 mM Tris/HCl (pH 7.3), 1 mM EDTA, 0.6 M NaC1, 1 × Denhardt's solution (0.02% (BSA), 0.02%

Ficoll-400, 0.02% poly-vinylpyrrolidone), 20% deionized formamide, 500 μg/ml yeast tRNA, and 250 μg/ml salmon sperm DNA which was boiled for 10 min and quickly chilled in an ice bath. Hybridization was done at 42°C for 15 h with 250 μl of the following mixture: 10 mM Tris/HCl (pH 7.3), 1 mM ethylenediaminetetraacetate (EDTA), 0.6 M NaCl, 1 × Denhardt's solution, 20% deionized formamide, 10% dextran sulfate, 250 μg/ml yeast tRNA, 125 μg/ml salmon sperm DNA, and 0.8 μg/ml T-T dimerized ON-DNA, all of which was boiled for 10 min and quickly chilled. Then, the filters were washed successively with 2 × SSC for 1 h, twice with 1 × SSC for 30 min, 0.1 SSC for 30 min and phosphate buffered saline (pH 7.2) (PBS) for 30 min. To block the nonspecific binding of antibody to the filter, the filter was treated with PBS containing 5% BSA, 500 μg/ml normal goat IgG, 100 μg/ml salmon sperm DNA, 100 μg/ml yeast tRNA and 0.05% NaN_3 for 1 h at 25°C. The filter was then reacted with rabbit anti-T-T IgG (40 μg/ml) dissolved in PBS containing 5% BSA, 100 μg/ml salmon sperm DNA, 100 μg/ml yeast tRNA, and 0.05% NaN_3 for 3 h. After washing for 15 h with PBS, the filter was reacted for 3 h with HRP-G anti-R IgG dissolved in PBS containing 5% BSA, 100 μg/ml salmon sperm DNA, and 100 μg/ml yeast tRNA. Following further washing with PBS for 3 h, horseradish peroxide (HRP) was visualized with 3,3′diaminobenzidine [12] in the presence of nickel and cobalt ions [13].

In Situ Hybridization

A mouse anesthetized by intraperitoneal injection of nembutal (50 μg/mouse) was perfused through the heart first by 10 ml (50 units/ml) heparin sodium in PBS and then by about 15 ml of 4% para-formaldehyde in PBS. Pieces of skeletal muscle were removed and further fixed in the fixative for an additional 2 h and then were washed by PBS. The tissues were impregnated with 0.02% ditheyl pyrocarbonate in 30% sucrose solution for 2 h at 4°C and frozen in O.C.T. compound (Miles Inc. Elkhart, IN, USA) by a mixture of isopentane and liquid nitrogen. The frozen tissues were then sectioned in a cryostat at 6 μm thickness. The sections were thawed and air dried for 1 h at room temperature, and the dried sections were further dried at 45°C overnight and were used for in situ hybridization [14]. During *in situ* hybridization, the sections were rehydrated with PBS and treated with 0.2 N HCl for 20 min to remove some basic proteins. The sections were digested for 30 min at 37°C by 0.02 units/ml proteinase K in order to expose mRNA, and washed three times by PBS for 5 min each. The sections were again fixed in 4% para-formaldehyde in PBS for 5 min and washed with PBS. The remaining aldehyde was quenched by immersion in 2 mg/ml glycine in PBS for 30 min. Twenty μl of the hybridization mixture such as that used in the dot hybridization was applied to each slide, mixed, and incubated for 15 h at 45°C. The slides were washed five times in 20% formamide in 2 × SSC at 37°C for 1 hr each, and twice with 2 × SSC at room temperature for 15 min each. The slides were then processed for immunohistochemical localization of T-T dimers as was done for the filter. The stained sections were then osmicated as was done for the localization of antigens at the ultrastructural level and ultrathin sections were obtained from the Epon block and examined by an electron microscope.

Enzyme-Histochemical Localization of Acetylcholine Esterase

Some frozen sections prepared for in situ hybridization were also used to localize acetylcholine esterase. The sections were thawed and air dried for 1 h at room temperature. The dried sections were then processed according to the method of Karnovsky [15].

Results

At least 10 pg of non-irradiated sense ON-DNA blotted on a strip of nitrocellulose filter could be recognized by the T-T dimerized anti-sense probe (Fig. 2).

The acetylcholine esterase was localized in patches near the edge of muscle bundles much like that of the motor endplate (Fig. 3 *top*). At the light microscopic level, the reaction products of peroxidase were deposited at the areas near the edge of muscle bundles in a fashion similar to the localization of acetyl-choline esterase when T-T dimerized antisense ON-DNA was used as the probe (Fig. 3 *middle*). The T-T dimerized sense ON-DNA did not hybridize with the sections of muscles (Fig. 3 *bottom*).

At the ultrastructural level, when an unstained ultrathin section which was hybridized with T-T dimerized anti-sense ON-DNA was examined, the reaction products of peroxidase were found as electron dense speckles in the sole plasma of the motor endplate and in areas between muscle fibers situated near the motor endplates (Fig 4 *top*). When the ultrathin section was counterstained with lead and uranium and examined, the sites of the reaction products coin-

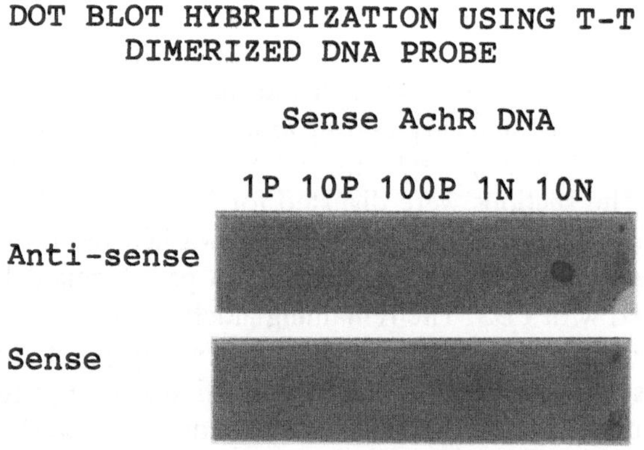

Fig. 2. Dot blot hybridization of T-T dimerized anti-sense ON-DNA probe with non-irradiated sense ON-DNA and anti-sense ON-DNA. Spots blotted with more than 10 pg of sense ON-DNA were stained. No staining was observed with the spots blotted with anti-sense ON-DNA

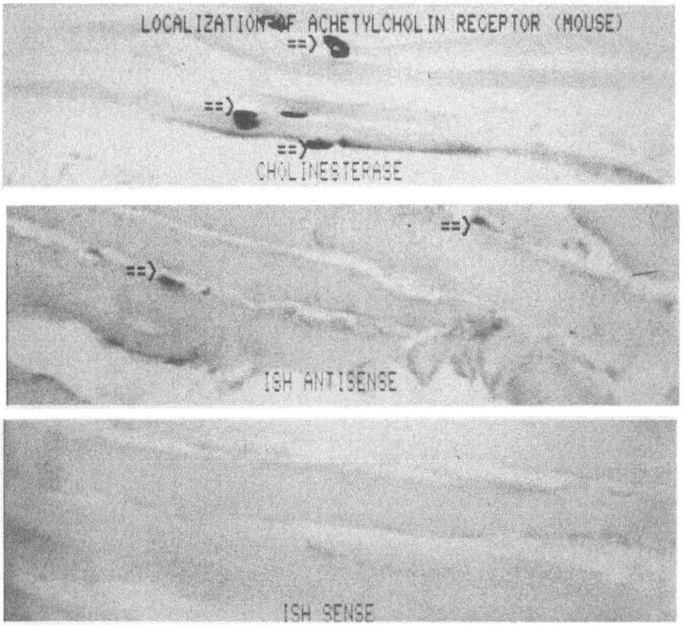

Fig. 3. Skeletal muscle of a mouse. Acetylcholine esterase was localized enzyme histochemically [15] at the motor endplate (*top*). Acetylcholine receptor mRNA was localized near the motor endplate when the T-T dimerized anti-sense probe was used (*middle*), but not with T-T dimerized sense probe (*bottom*). ==> indicates motor endplates

cided with that of polyribosome in the sole plasma and sarcoplasmic reticulum (Fig. 4 *bottom*).

Discussion

This study demonstrated the usefulness of a T-T dimer as a haptenic marker for a non-radioactive probe to be used in *in situ* hybridization both at the light and electron microscopic levels. This method had several advantages over other ligands used for non-radioactive probes. When 5-allylaminobiotin-labeled uridine triphosphate (bio-UTP) or 5-allylaminobiotin-labeled deoxyuridine triphosphate (bio-dUTP) was used as a ligand, the introduction of the ligands into probe RNA or DNA by the nick translation steps, as well as steps to separate the unincorporated ligand from the probes [16] were required. With acetylaminofluorene as the ligand, the nick translation steps were not required, although the separation steps were still needed [17]. Furthermore, with this ligand, strict environmental controls are required since acetylaminofluorene is a potential carcinogen. Photobiotin, a ligand introduced more recently [18], still requires the separation steps, and the labeling procedures must be carried

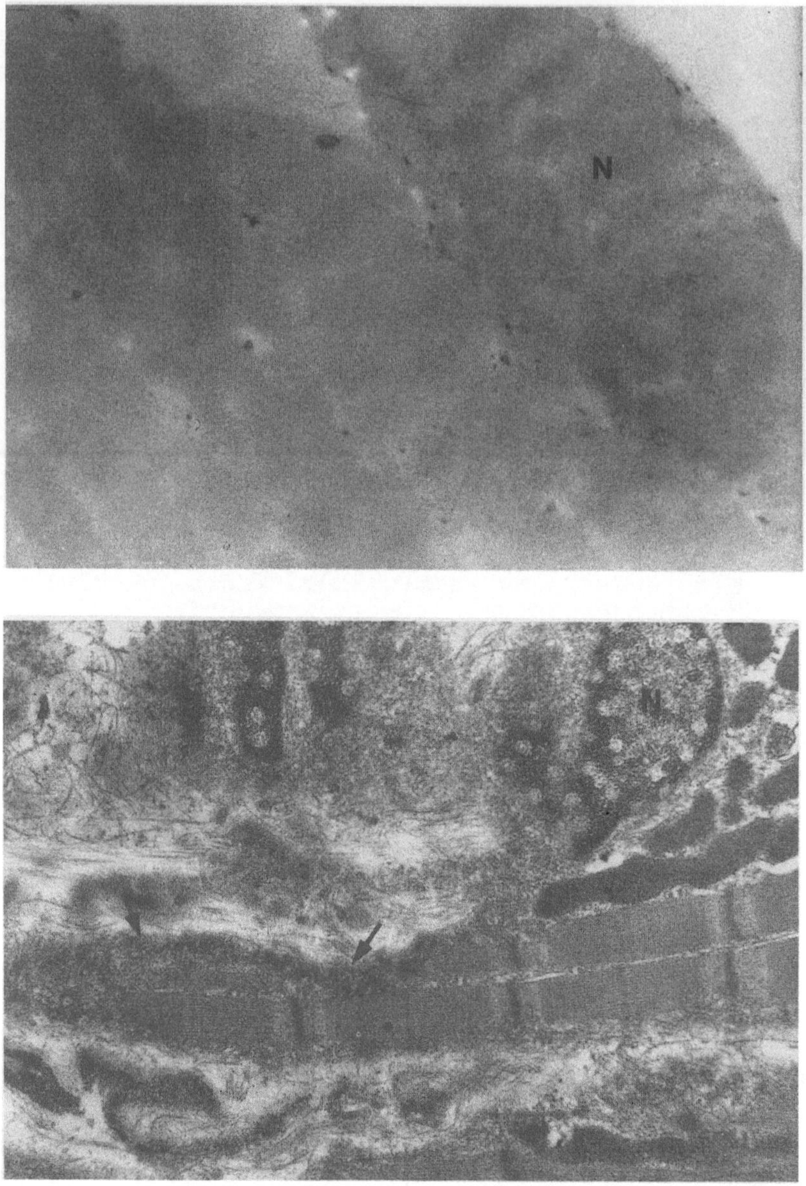

a

b

Fig. 4. Skeletal muscle of the mouse hybridized with T-T dimerized antisense ON-DNA. **a** The reaction products of peroxidase were found as electron dense speckles in the sole plasma of motor endplate and in areas between muscle fibers situated near the motor endplates. **b** A section counter stained with lead and uranium. The sites of the reaction products (*arrows*) coincided with that of polyribosome in sole plasma and sarcoplasmic reticulum, ×14,000. *N*, nucleus of a Schwann cell out in the dark, whereas there is only one required step for the preparation of the probe with T-T dimer, i.e., to UV irradiate the probe DNA, which can be done in a conventional environment. The T-T can be dimerized either in single-stranded DNA or in double-stranded DNA, as long as there are some thymines adjacent to each other in the DNAs. This is an added advantage of the use of T-T dimerization. In recent years, more synthetic oligo-nucleotides have begun to be utilized, and if modified nucleotides are to be introduced into the sequence, it requires separate special reagents and a DNA synthesizer must be set to handle the special reaction. On the other hand, the T-T dimerizable probes may be synthesized by the routine manner.

Some negative effects of the artificially introduced residues on the efficiency of hybridization have been anticipated. Langer et al. [16] observed that the melting temperature of DNA duplexes decreased as the Bio-dUMP content of the polymer increased, but there was little or no effect on the melting temperature or on the efficiency of hybridization when about 20 bases/kilobase was substituted with Bio-dUMP. With the acetylaminofluorene modified DNA, there was a slight decrease in the melting temperature when about 10 bases/kilobase was modified [17], but with this degree of modification they found no effect on the efficiency of hybridization. Up to about 10 base/kilobase of DNA labeled with photobiotin also did not show the expected negative effect on the efficiency of hybridization [18]. Although Landegent et al. [19] found that the use of DNA or cRNA probes labeled with about 50 acetylaminofluorene per kilo-base gave the best results, it is generally agreed upon that at least up to 2% of chemical modification of the bases will not have a significant effect on the efficiency of hybridization and a higher degree of modifications should be avoided. In order to achieve the optimal labeling index (a lower index will reduce the sensitivity and a higher index will reduce the specificity), several preliminary experiments are required for each probe, since with all three ligands mentioned above the labeling indexes are expected to fluctuate depending upon the guanine-cytosine (G-C) content of each probe. With the UV T-T dimerization, the number of T-T dimerizable sites also varies from one probe to another, but the number can be estimated from the nucleotide sequence of each probe. Even when all dimerizable sites (about 20% of sites where one thymine is found adjacent to another thymine [20]) are dimerized it does not exceed 2%. Thus, no preliminary experiment is required with the T-T dimerization method.

In our recent study, we demonstrated that the T-T dimerized ON-DNA may be used to quantitate mRNA in a given cell [5]. Since, at least in theory, an amount of mRNA present in a given cell is proportional to the rate of synthesis of protein of which the amino acid sequence is derived from the mRNA nucleotide sequence, quantitative information on mRNA is required to understand the physiology of the cells. In our experience, the mRNA quantitation appears to be more amenable than that of antigens. During the past decades, many investigators have attempted to quantify antigens in cellular and histological preparations, but they faced practical as well as theoretical difficulties. It has been our experience, as well as that of others, that the retention of antigenicity of a given antigen varied considerably, depended upon the type of fixatives used, and that the retention of antigenicity of one antigen differed from that of another in a given fixative. Furthermore, it has been a common finding that sensitivity to a given fixative varies, depending upon the location of antigens in cells. These variabilities have hindered the quantitation of antigens. On the other hand, mRNAs, although differing from one another in the nucleic acid sequences, are chemically similar, if not identical, the effect of fixatives upon them are expected to be same, since most of the mRNAs are situated in cytosol. Because of the similarities, one should be able to better control the hybridization in situ between the complementary nucleic acid probes and cytoplasmic mRNAs when the condition of fixation, conditions for the removal of mRNA-associated proteins, an optimal size of the probes, and conditions for an equal accessibility of the probe to cytoplasmic mRNA are established. We attempted to determine the numbers of copies of c-*myc* mRNA present in HL60 cells in vitro [5] as a model system, since the HL60 are known to contain about 20 times the normal copies of c-*myc* DNA and express about 10 times the normal copies of c-*myc* mRNA [8]. In our HL60 cell line, an average of 439 copies of c-*myc* mRNA per cell was found [5] and most of the HL60 cells contained between 0 and 50 copies of c-*myc* mRNA with some having between 100 and 300 copies. Occasional cells contained more than 1,000 copies of the RNA. The activation of the c-*myc* gene is known to take place at the boundary between the G0 and G1 phase [21] and those cells containing about 200 copies may be considered to be with in the boundary, since a population of ATL cells which expresses normal copies of c-*myc* mRNA maximally expressed about 200 copies. Whether those HL60 cells which contained an unusually high number of c-*myc* mRNA copies differ from those HL60 cells with a normal number of copies remains to be established.

In order to visualize the sites of mRNA at the ultrastructural level, most investigators have utilized the so-called "pre-embedding method". Hatchison et al. [22] demonstrated the localization of mouse satellite DNA in whole mount chromosomes using colloidal gold as the electron dense ligand. A group of investigators in R. H. Singer's laboratory [23] used whole mounts of fibroblasts to demonstrate the sites of actin and vementin mRNA at the ultrastructural level. Silva et al. [24] first hybridized fixed myoblast with a biotinylated cDNA probe and followed it by rabbit anti-biotin and colloidal gold conjugated anti-rabbit IgG. The hybridized cells were then embedded in Epon by the reversed capsule method and ultrathins section were obtained from the Epon blocks. By this method they were successful in localizing myosin heavy chain mRNA at the ultrastructural level. Since cDNAs and the colloidal gold were too large to penetrate freely into fixed cells and tissues, these investigators utilized detergents such as Triton X, and the procedure usually resulted in poor ultrastructural preservation. Using a special embedding medium such as Lowicryl, the so-called "post-embedding method" was used by some investigators. Binder et al. [25] localized mitochondrial rDNA and Webster et al. [26] localized Po glycoprotein on ultrathin sections. By using ON-DNA and peroxidase-labeled antibodies (which are smaller than cDNA) and colloidal gold-labeled antibodies, we were able to utilize the "pre-embedding method" much in the same way as that used for immunoelectron microscopy. Since the reaction products of peroxidase are also visible by a light microscope, and the method utilizes sections of tissues as well as monolayers of cells, this technique has the advantage of examining the hybridized sections by light microscope and then being able to trim desired areas for the electron microscopic examination. Although an extensive investigation on the opitimalization of conditions remains to be carried out, our results on the localization of mRNA at the ultrastructural level are quite encouraging.

References

1. Nakane PK, Moriuchi T, Koji T, Tanno M, Abe K (1987) *In situ* localization on mRNA using thymine-thymine dimerized cDNA. Acta Histochem Cytochem 20: 229–243
2. Takahashi S, Nakane K (1988) Detection of viral genes in the tissues by in situ hybridization. Clin Immunol 20:172–178
3. Izumi S, Moriuchi T, Koji T, Tanno M, Terashima K, Iguchi K, Mochizuki T, Yanaihara C, Yanaihara T, Abe K, Nakane PK (1988) Localization of c-*myc* in HL-60 cells, neoplastic and normal tissues: An immunohistochemistry and in situ hybridization study. Acta Histochem Cytochem 20:327–342
4. Koji T, Sugawara I, Kimura M, Nakane PK (1989) *In situ* localization of c-*myc* in HL60 cells using non-radioactive synthetic oligonucleotide probes. Acta Histochem Cytochem 22:295–307
5. Nakane PK (to be published) Modern histochemical methods in mucosal immunology. In: Proc VIth International Congress of Mucosal Immunology, Elsevier, Amsterdam
6. Yamada G, Takahashi M, Endo H, Takaguchi K, Nishimoto H, Tsuji T (to be published) Pathogenesis and interferon treatment in chronic hepatitis C. In: Proc VIth International Congress of Mucosal Immunology, Elsevier, Amsterdam
7. Izumi S, Koji T, Nakane PK (1990) *In situ* localization of mRNA visualized by backscattered electron imaging. J Histochem Cytochem 38:1052
8. Mazurkiewicz JE, Nakane PK (1972) Light and electron microscopic localization of antigens in tissues embedded in polyethene glycol with a peroxidase-labeled antibody method. J Histochem Cytochem 20:967–974
9. Isenberg KE, Mudd J, Shah V, Merlie JP (1986) Nucleotide sequence of the mouse muscle nicotinic acetylcholine receptor alpha subunit. Nucleic Acids Res 14:5111
10. Levine L, Seaman E, Hammerschlag E, Van Vunakis H (1966) Antibodies to photoproducts of deoxyribonucleic acids irradiated with ultraviolet light. Science 153:1666–1667
11. Wilson, MB, Nakane PK (1978) Recent developments in the periodate method of conjugating horseradish peroxidase (HRPO) to antibodies. In: Knapp W, Holubar K, Wick G (eds) Immunofluorescence and related staining techniques. Elsevier/ North-Holland Biomedical, 215–224
12. Graham RC, Karnovsky MJ (1966) The early stages of injected horseradish peroxidase in the proximal tubules of mouse kidney: Ultrastructural cytochemistry by a new technique. J Histochem Cytochem 14:291–302

13. Adams JC (1981) Heavy metal intensification of DAB-based HRP reaction product. J Histochem Cytochem 29:775
14. Brigati DJ, Myerson D, Leary JJ, Spalholz B, Travis SZ, Fong CKY, Hsiung GD, Ward DC (1983) Detection of viral genomes in cultured cells and paraffin-embedded tissue sections using biotin-labeled hybridization probes: General method for *in situ* hybridization. Virology 126:32–50
15. Karnovsky MJ (1964) The localization of cholinesterase activity in rat cardiac muscles by electron microscopy. J Cell Biol 23:217–232
16. Langer PR, Waldrop AA, Ward DC (1981) Enzymatic synthesis of biotin-labeled polynucleotides: Novel nucleic acid affinity probes. Proc Natl Acad Sci USA 78:6633–6637
17. Tchen P, Fuchs RPP, Sage E, Leng M (1984) Chemically modified nucleic acids as immunodetectable probes in hybridization experiments. Proc Natl Acad Sci USA 81:3466–3470
18. Forster AC, McInnes JL, Skingle DC, Symons RH (1985) Nonradioactive hybridization probes prepared by the chemical labelling of DNA and RNA with a novel reagent, photobiotin. Nucleic Acids Res 13:745–759
19. Landegent JE, Jansen in de Wal N, Baan RA, Hoeijmakers JHJ, Van der Ploeg M (1984) 2-acetylaminofluorene-modified probes for the indirect hybridocytochemical detection of specific nucleic acid sequences. Exp Cell Res 153:61–72
20. Franklin WA, Ming Lo K, Haseltine WA (1982) Alkaline lability of fluorescent photoproducts produced in ultraviolet lightirradiated DNA. J Biol Chem 257:13535–13543
21. Campisi J, Gray HE, Pardee AB, Dean M, Sonenshein GE (1984) Cell-cycle control of c-*myc* but c-*ras* expression is lost following chemical transformation. Cell 36:241–247
22. Hutchison NJ, Langer-Safer PR, Ward DC, Hamkalo BA (1982) *In situ* hybridization at the electron microscope level: Hybrid detection by autoradiography and colloidal gold. J Cell Biol 95:609–618
23. Singer RH, Lawrence JB, Silva F, Langevin GL, Pomeroy M, Billings-Gargliardi S (1989) Strategies for ultrastructural visualization of biotinated probes hybridized to messenger RNA *in situ*. In: Current topics in microbiology and immunology, vol. 143. Springer, Berlin Heidelberg, pp 55–69
24. Silva FG, Lawrence JB, Singer RH (1989) Progress toward ultrastructural idenfication of individual mRNAs in thin section: Myosin heavy-chain mRNA in developing myotubes. In: Techniques in immunohistochemistry, vol 4. Academic, New York, pp 147–165
25. Binder M, Tourmente S, Roth J, Renaud M, Gehring W (1986) In situ hybridization at the electron microscopic level: Localization of transcripts on ultrathin sections of Lowcryl K4M-embedded tissue using biotinated probes and protein A-gold complexes. J Cell Biol 102:1646–1653
26. Webster H de F, Lamperth L, Favilla J T, Lemke G, Tesin D, Manuelidis L (1987) Use of a biotinylated probe and in situ hybridization for light and electron microscopic localization of Po mRNA in myelin-forming Schwann cells. Histochemistry 86:441–444

A Molecular Basis for Multidrug-Resistance and Reversal of the Resistance

Shin-ichi Akiyama, Akihiko Yoshimura, Misako Ichikawa, Tomoyuki Sumizawa, and Tatsuhiko Furukawa[1]

Introduction

The development of multidrug-resistance (MDR) is a serious problem during treatment of various malignant tumors. Multidrug-resistant cells were isolated from human carcinoma cell lines and studied to elucidate the molecular basis for their multidrug resistance properties [1–4].

Overexpression of a 170- kilodalton transmembrane glycoprotein called P-glycoprotein (P-gp), or P170, has been observed in various multidrug-resistant cells [5–8]. The genetic analysis of the P-gp encoded by the MDR1 gene [9–11] and evidence that P-gp binds anticancer and multidrug-resistance-reversing agents [12–17] and adenosine triphosphate (ATP) [18] indicate that P-gp acts as an energy-dependent drug-efflux pump [19].

Since recent studies have shown that P-gp-associated MDR occurs clinically, agents that inhibit P-gp activity at concentrations with little or no cytotoxic effect may be useful in reversing MDR in clinical chemotherapy when they are administered in combination with anti-cancer drugs. Extensive studies are underway throughout the world to find new agents that reverse MDR with fewer and less extreme side effects.

P-gp Expression in Tumors and Clinical Drug Resistance

Expression of the P-gp was measured to evaluate the implications of P-gp in clinical drug resistance. We first examined the expression of P-gp in fresh leukemia cells from patients with chronic myelogenous leukemia (CML) in blast crisis. By using immunoblotting with a monoclonal antibody against P-gp, C219, we showed that leukemia cells from three patients with CML in blast crisis were P-gp negative at the stage when they were in complete remission, and that the cells showed high levels of P-gp expression at times when the same patients had relapsed and had not responded to chemotherapy. Six out of 11

[1] Department of Cancer Chemotherapy, Institute of Cancer Research, Faculty of Medicine, Kagoshima University, Kagoshima, 890 Japan

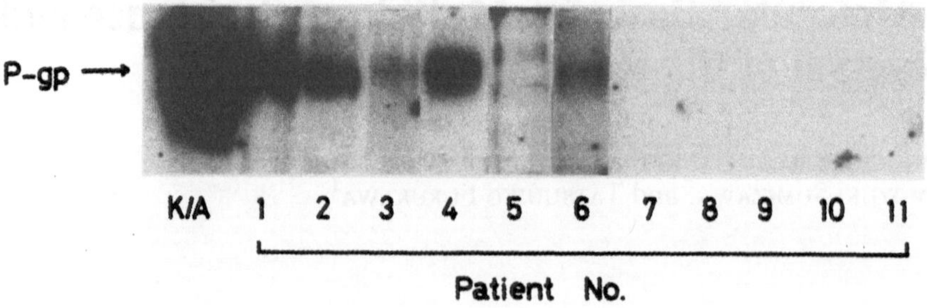

Fig. 1. Immunoblotting of leukemia cells from 11 patients with CML and K562/ADM cells. Membrane fractions (100 µg protein/lane) from leukemia cells were prepared and subjected to 7.5% SDS-PAGE and immunoblotting

patients (nine in the refractory state) were P-gp positive (Fig. 1) and rarely responded to chemotherapy. These data suggest that the expression of P-gp is closely associated with drug-resistance in CML [20].

We then examined the expression of P-gp in leukemia cells from patients with acute myelogenous leukemia (AML) and acute lymphoblastic leukemia

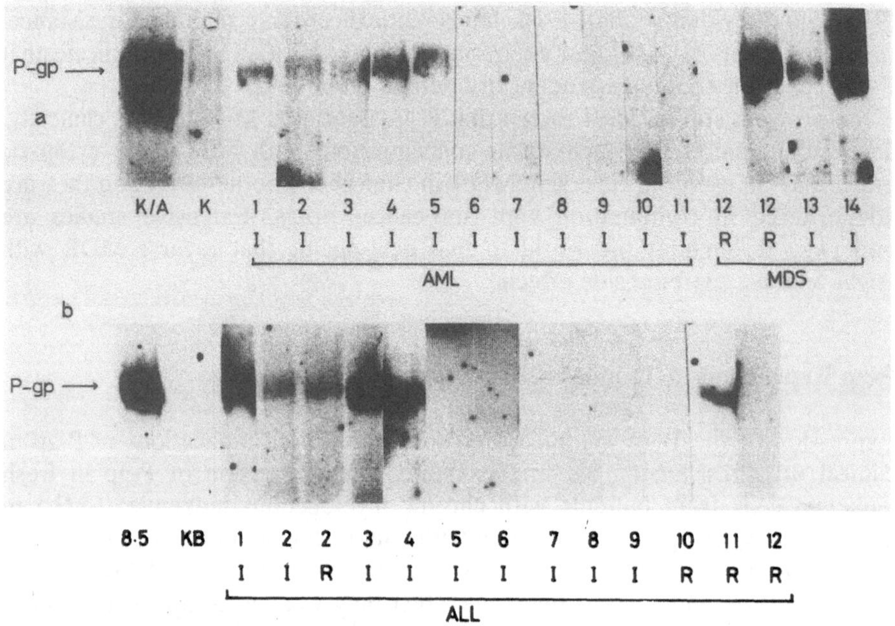

Fig. 2. Immunoblotting of leukemia cells from patients with acute leukemia. Membrane fractions (100–200 µg protein/lane) from leukemia cells were prepared and subjected to 7.5% SDS-PAGE and immunoblotting. **a** AML and MDS, **b** ALL. The patient number and collected stage of leukemia cells (*I*, initial presentation; *R*, relapsed state) are shown. The *arrow* indicates the position of *P-gp*. *PB*, peripheral blood; *BM*, bone marrow; 8.5: KB-8-5; K: K562; K/A: K562/ADM

(ALL) at initial presentation and relapse. Nine out of 17 patients with AML and four out of 11 patients with ALL were P-gp positive at the initial presentation (Fig. 2), and most P-gp positive patients did not respond to chemotherapy (Table 1). Three out of five patients at the relapsed stage and all three patients with a preceding myelodysplastic syndrome were P-gp positive. The expression of P-gp and the clinical resistance to treatment by chemotherapy were highly correlated. These data indicate that the expression of P-gp is closely related to clinical durg resistance in acute leukemia. [21]

Adult T-cell leukemia (ATL), a particular type of T-cell malignancy, is quite common in parts of Japan and in the Caribbean. Several lines of evidence strongly implicate the human T-cell leukemia virus type I (HTLV-I) as the cause of ATL. The prognosis of patients with advanced ATL is poor. In order to develop a more effective treatmen program, it is important to analyze

Table 1. Correlation between the expression of P-glycoprotein and response to chemotherapy

	CR + PR (%)	NR (%)	Total (%)
P-gp (+)	4(23.5)	13(76.5)	17(100)
P-gp (−)	14(73.7)	5(26.3)	19(100)
Total (%)	18(50.0)	18(50.0)	36(100)

CR, complete remission; *PR*, partial remission; *NR*, no response

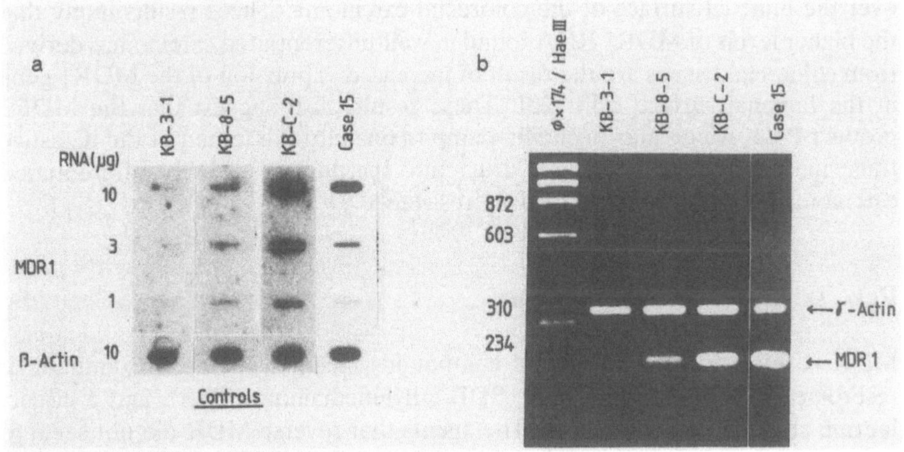

Fig. 3a,b. Analysis of MDR1 mRNA by PCR. The reaction products were analyzed by 2% agarose gel electrophoresis and ethidium bromide staining. DNA fragments generated from single-stranded cDNA synthesized from RNA by reverse transcriptase were amplified by 30 cycles of PCR with each primer pair. Fragments of 200 bp were generated from cDNA of multidrug-resistant cell lines, KB-8-5 and KB-C2, and leukemia cells, by using MDR1 set1 primers. Equal amounts of fragments of 300 bp were generated from cDNA of KB, KB-8-5, KB-C2 and leukemia cells from case 15 by using γ-actin set1 primers.

factors contributing to the poor prognosis as well as the refractory nature of ATL to chemotherapy.

The expression of P-gp in adult T-cell leukemia samples from 25 patients was examined. Eight out of 20 patients with ATL were P-gp positive at the initial presentation. All eight patients at the relapsed stage were P-gp positive, and refractory to chemotherapy. The expression of MDR1 mRNA in P-gp-positive ATL cells was increased in one patient at the relapsed stage (Fig. 3). The P-gp of this patient was photolabeled with [^{3}H] azidopine, and the labeling was inhibited with nimodipine, vinblastine, and progesterone. These results suggest that P-gp expressed in ATL cells from patients at the relapsed stage has the same binding site(s) for the drugs as that in multidrug-resistant cells, and is correlated with the refractory nature of the cells to chemotherapy. [22]

We also measured the expression of the MDR1 gene in the human gastrointestinal tract. MDR1 RNA levels were elevated in 13 out of 15 colorectal carcinoma specimens, and in 6 out of 13 gastric carcinoma specimens. Well-differentiated colorectal carcinomas contained significantly higher levels of MDR1 RNA than moderately differentiated colorectal carcinomas. Similarly, moderately differentiated gastric carcinomas contained higher levels of MDR1 RNA than poorly differentiated gastric carcinomas. MDR1 gene expression in normal colorectal and gastric tissues adjacent to carcinomas was similar to that in the carcinomas. The MDR1 gene expression in xenografts of colorectal and gastric carcinomas in nude mice was also investigated. Elevated expression of the MDR1 gene was seen in only 4 out of 18 xenografts of colorectal carcinoma, and was not seen in any xenografts of gastric carcinoma. P-gp was distributed over the lumenal surface of the colorectal carcinoma. These results imply that the higher levels of MDR1 RNA found in well-differentiated carcinomas derived from colorectal tissues are the result of increased expression of the MDR1 gene in the lumenal surface cells [23]. These results also suggest that the MDR1 product P-gp, which may normally pump toxins into the lumen of the digestive tract, may also pump anticancer drugs into the duct of a highly differentiated carcinoma and thus increase its drug resistance.

Reversal of Multidrug Resistance

MDR is reversed by a variety of compounds including verapamil, quinidine, reserpine, a synthetic isoprenoid, SDB-ethylenediamine (SDB), and a biscoclaurine alkaloid, cepharanthine. The agents that reverse MDR did not seem to have any common features. However, it appears that hydrophobicity at physiological pH, cationic charge, and molar refractivity are important physical properties for modulators of MDR. They are supposed to inhibit the pump activity of P-gp. When the activity of the pump is inhibited, anticancer agents accumulate in MDR cells and this may be why MDR is reversed.

Ten synthetic dihydropyridine analogs were investigated for their ability to reverse drug resistance in a multidrug-resistant human carcinoma cell line, KB-C1. Four dihydropyridine analogs completely reversed the resistance, three lowered the resistance, and three had little effect.

The radioactive photoactive dihydropyridine calcium channel-blocker, [^{3}H]azidopine, photolabels P-gp in membrane vesicles from KB-C1 cells. This photolabeling was almost completely inhibited by excess dihydropyridine analogs that reversed or lowered drug resistance. In contrast, the labeling was not significantly inhibited by analogs that do not reverse resistance. Among other reversing agents, cepharanthine and reserpine inhibited the [^{3}H]azidopine photolabeling, but thioridazine did not. SDB slightly inhibited the labeling at 100 μM. An anticancer agent, vinblastine, also inhibited the labeling.

The correlation between the reversing of the drug resistance and the inhibition of the [^{3}H]azidopine photolabeling of P-gp by dihydropyridine analogs suggests a role for P-gp in multidrug resistance as well as the reversing of the resistance by dihydropyridine analogs [24].

Pyridine analogs are known to have lower calcium channel-blocking activity and higher lipid solubility than their dihydropyridine analog counterparts. Thus, we synthesized four pyridine analogs and their dihydropyridine analog counterparts, and investigated their MDR-reversing activity. Two pyridine analogs were more capable of reversing drug resistance than their dihydropyridine counterparts. The other two pyridine analogs had an effect on drug resistance similar to their dihydropyridine counterparts. The calcium channel-blocking activity of all of the pyridine analogs was considerably lower than that of the dihydropyridine analogs.

Of the pyridine analogs, 2-[4-(diphenylmethyl)-1-piperazinyl]ethyl 5-(trans-4,6-dimethyl-1,3,2-dioxaphosphorinan-2-yl)-2,6-dimethyl-4-(3-nitrophenyl)-3-pyridinecarboxylate P-oxide (PAK-104P) was the most effective in reversing multidrug resistance. PAK-104P (1 and 5 μM) completely reversed the drug resistance in KB-8-5 and KB-C2 cells, respectively. The reversing effect of PAK-104P was greater than that of other multidrug resistance-reversing agents, cepharanthine, verapamil, nimodipine, and nicardipine. PAK-104P at 1 μM increased by about 10-fold the accumulation of vinblastine in KB-C2 cells, whereas verapamil at the same concentration increased the accumulation by about twofold.

The inhibition of [^{3}H]azidopine photolabeling of P-gp by the pyridine and dihydropyridine analogs except 2-[methyl(phenyl-methyl)amino]ethyl 4-(2-chlorophenyl)-5-(4-methyl-1,3,2-dioxaphosphorinan-2-yl)-1,4-dihydro-2,6-dimethyl-3-pyridinecarboxylate P-oxide correlated with the reversing of drug resistance by the analogs. Some newly synthesized pyridine analogs seemed to have lower calcium channel-blocking activity and more potent resistance-reversing ability than verapamil and other calcium channel blockers [25].

The Molecular Basis for the Reversal of Multidrug-Resistance

It has been demonstrated that a photoaffinity analog of vinblastine, ^{125}I-NASV, specifically labels P-gp [26]. Most drugs that reverse multidrug resistance, such as the calcium channel-blocker verapamil and the synthetic isoprenoid SDB, block drug efflux from cells and also inhibit the photoaffinity labeling of P-gp by the vinblastine analog [14].

Agents that reverse multidrug resistance appear to compete with hydrophobic anticancer agents for a binding site on P-gp. SDB is known to reverse drug resistance in human multidrug-resistant KB cells. SDB inhibits the photolabeling of P-gp with the photoaffinity analog of vinblastine. We synthesized photoactive radioactive SDB and used it to photolabel membrane vesicles from human KB cells and their multidrug-resistant subline KB-C2 cells. A 150–170 kDa protein in membrane vesicles from KB-C2 cells was specifically labeled by the photoanalog of SDB. The labeled band was not detectable in parenteral drug-sensitive cells. The photolabeled 150–170 kd protein was immunoprecipitated with a monoclonal antibody (C219) specific to P-gp. Our data show that P-gp is an acceptor of a synthetic isoprenoid that has no calcium channel-blocking activity. P-gp labeling was inhibited by anticancer agents, vinblastine, vincristine, actinomycin D, and daunomycin, with half-maximal inhibition at 2.0, 2.3, 18, and 23 μM, respectively. Only 33% and 18%

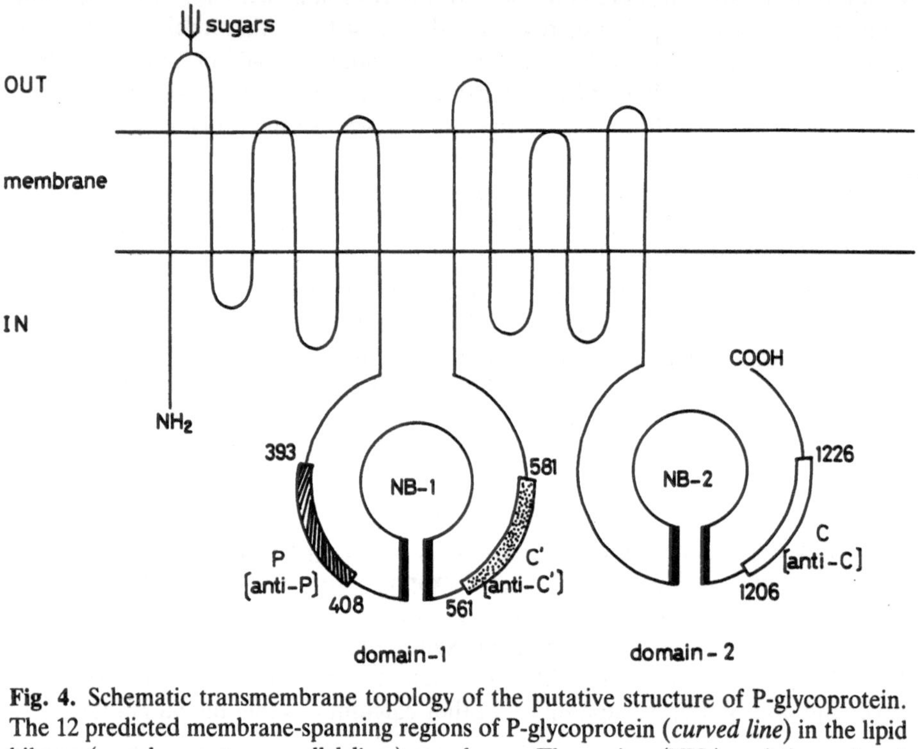

Fig. 4. Schematic transmembrane topology of the putative structure of P-glycoprotein. The 12 predicted membrane-spanning regions of P-glycoprotein (*curved line*) in the lipid bilayer (*membrane, two parallel lines*) are shown. The amino (NH_2) and the carboxyl (COOH) terminus and extracellular (*OUT*) and intracellular (*IN*) space are shown. *Domains 1* and *2* represent the first and second halves of duplicate segments, respectively. The predicted glycosylation sites are marked by a branch (*Sugars*). NB-1 and NB-2 (*bold lines*) are the predicted consensus ATP-binding sites. *Numbers* indicate the positions of amino acid residues, 393–408 (*P*) and 1206–1226 (*C*) are the sites for synthetic peptides, and 561–581 (*C′*) was the corresponding sequence of the first half to anti-C recognition site (1206–1226) of the second half

of the labeling was inhibited by 100 μM Adriamycin and colchicine, respectively. The labeling was also inhibited by agents that reverse multidrug resistance, such as verapamil, reserpine, cepharanthine, and SDB. The existence of other molecules that specifically bind to ^{125}I-SDB-photoanalog was suggested in both KB and KB-C2 membrane vesicles. The fact that we could identify the synthetic isoprenoid acceptor in membrane vesicles from multidrug-resistant cells confirms that P-gp plays a role in the multidrug resistance phenotype and provides an explanation for the fact that SDB reverses multidrug resistance [17].

Recently, the photoactive dihydropyridine calcium channel-blocker, azidopine, has been shown to photolabel P-gp [27]. Vinblastine and nimodipine inhibited this labeling. P-gp seems to be an acceptor for some calcium channel-blockers, such as verapamil, diltiazem, and dihydropyridine analogs, that are reported to reverse multidrug resistance.

In order to identify azidopine binding sites, we synthesized peptides corresponding to amino acid residues, Glu^{393}-Lys^{408} (P-site) and Leu^{1206}-Thr^{1226} (C-site) in P-gp from human mdr1 cDNA and used these peptides to produce polyclonal antibodies (Fig. 4). From the primary structure of P-gp, anti-C antibody is expected to recognize another position, Leu^{561}-Thr^{581}, in the duplicate structure of P-gp, but anti-P recognizes only one site. These antibodies bind to multidrug-resistant cells (KB-C2) with permeabilized plasma membrane, but do not bind to nonpermeabilized KB-C2 cells or parental KB cells,

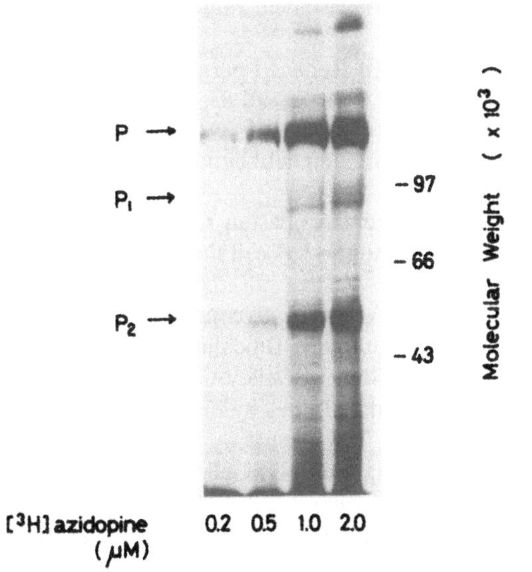

Fig. 5. Dose dependence of photoaffinity labeling of P-glycoprotein and its tryptic fragments with [^{3}H]azidopine. Membrane vesicles which were treated with 10 μg/ml trypsin for 1 h were photolabeled with [^{3}H]azidopine at indicated concentrations. The samples were subjected to SDS-PAGE and fluorography. *P* 140-kDa native P-glycoprotein, *P*$_1$ and *P*$_2$ 95- and 55-kd tryptic fragments, respectively

supporting the predicted cytoplasmic orientation of these sequences. With immunoblotting of the membrane fractions from KB-C2 cells, a major 140-kDa polypeptide of the P-gp was detected with both anti-P and anti-C. Two minor polypeptides with molecular masses of 95 and 55 kd were also detected. When membrane vesicles were digested mildly with trypsin, the amount of these two polypeptides increased. Anti-P detected only the 95-kd polypeptide, while anti-C detected both of the 95- and 55-kd polypeptides. *Achromobacter lyticus* protease I (lysyl endopeptidase) and *Staphylococcus aureus* V8 protease also produced two polypeptides with similar molecular weights. Absorption into lectin-agarose beads and labeling with [^{3}H]glucosamine indicated that the 95 kd polypeptide was glycosylated but that the 55-kd polypeptide was not. These two polypeptides as well as P-gp were photoaffinity-labeled with a calcium channel-blocker, [^{3}H]azidopine, but most of the label was found in the 55-kd polypeptide (Fig. 5). The yield of labeled fragments from membrane vesicles photolabeled after digestion with trypsin was similar to that from membrane vesicles digested with trypsin after photolabeling. These data indicate that (1) the 95-kd polypeptide is the fragment corresponding to the amino-terminal half of P-gp containing sugar chains, and (2) the 55-kd polypeptide is the carboxyl-terminal half which was mainly labeled with [^{3}H]azidopine [28].

References

1. Biedler JL, Riehm H (1970) Cellular resistance to actinomycin D in Chinese hamster cells in vitro: Cross-resistance, radioautographic, and cytogenetic studies. Cancer Res 30:1174–1184
2. Ling V, Thompson LH (1973) Reduced permeability in CHO cells as a mechanism of resistance to colchicine. J Cell Physiol 83:103–116
3. Beck WT, Mueller TJ, Tanzer LR (1979) Altered surface membrane glycoproteins in Vinca alkaloid-resistant human leukemic lymphoblasts. Cancer Res 39:2070–2076
4. Akiyama S, Fojo A, Hanover JA, Pastan I, Gottesman MM (1985) Isolation and genetic characterization of human KB cell lines resistant to multiple drugs. Somatic Cell Mol Genet 11:117–126
5. Juliano RL, Ling V (1976) A surface glycoprotein modulating drug permeability in Chinese hamster ovary cell mutants. Biochim Biophys Acta 455:152–162
6. Kartner, N, Evernden-Porelle D, Bradley G, Ling V (1985) Detection of P-glycoprotein in multidrug-resistant cell lines by monoclonal antibodies. Nature 316:820–823
7. Kartner N, Riordan JR, Ling V (1983) Cell surface P-glycoprotein associated with multidrug resistance in mammalian cell lines. Science 221:1285–1288
8. Shen DW, Cardarelli C, Hwang J, Cornwell MM, Richert N, Ishii S, Pastan I, Gottesman MM (1986) Multiple drug resistant human KB carcinoma cells independently selected for high-level resistance to colchicine, Adriamycin, or vinblastine show changes in expression of specific proteins. J Biol Chem 261:7762–7770
9. Chen CJ, Chin JE, Ueda K, Clark DP, Pastan I, Gottesman MM, Roninson IB (1986) Internal duplication and homology with bacterial transport proteins in the mdrl (P-glycoprotein) gene from multidrug-resistant human cells. Cell 47:381–389

10. Gros P, Croop J, Housman D (1986) Mammalian multidrug resistance gene: Complete cDNA sequence indicates strong homology to bacterial transport protein. Cell 47:371–380
11. Gerlach JH, Endicot A, Juranka R, Henderson G, Sarangi F, Deuchars KL, Ling V (1986) Homology between P-glycoprotein and a bacterial haemolysin transport protein suggests a model for multidrug resistance. Nature 324:485–489
12. Cornwell MM, Safa AR, Felsted RL, Gottesman MM, Pastan I (1986) Membrane vesicles from multidrug-resistant human cancer cells contain a specific 150 to 170 kDa protein detected by photoaffinity labeling. Proc Natl Acad Sci USA 83: 3847–3850
13. Safa AR, Glover CJ, Meyers MB, Biedler JL, Felsted RL (1986) Vinblastine photoaffinity labeling of a high molecular weight surface membrane glycoprotein specific for multidrug-resistant cells. J Biol Chem 26:6137–6140
14. Akiyama S, Cornwell MM, Kuwano M, Pastan I, Gottesman MM (1988) Most drugs that reverse multidrug resistance also inhibit photoaffinity labeling of P-glycoprotein by a vinblastine analog. Mol Pharmacol 33:144–147
15. Safa AR, Glover CJ, Sewell JL, Meyers MB, Biedler JL, Felsted RL (1987) Identification of the multidrug resistance-related membrane glycoprotein as an acceptor for calcium channel blockers. J Biol Chem 262:7884–7888
16. Safa AR (1988) Photoaffinity labeling of the multidrug-resistance related P-glycoprotein with photoactive analogs of verapamil. Proc Natl Acad Sci USA 85:7187–7191
17. Akiyama S, Yoshimura A, Kikuchi H, Sumizawa, T, Kuwano M, Tahara Y (1989) Synthetic isoprenoid photoaffinity labeling of P-glycoprotein specific to multidrug-resistant cells. Mol Pharmacol 36:730–735
18. Cornwell MM, Tsuruo T, Gottesman MM, Pastan I (1987) ATP-binding properties of P-glycoprotein from multidrug-resistant KB cells. FASEB J 1:51–54
19. Gottesman MM, Pastan I (1988) The multidrug transporter, a double-edged sword. J Biol Chem 263:12163–12166
20. Kuwazuru Y, Yoshimura A, Hanada S, Ichikawa M, Saito T, Uozumi K, Utsunomiya A, Arima T, Akiyama S (1990) Expression of the multidrug transporter, P-glycoprotein, in chronic myelogenous leukemia cells in blast crisis. Brit J Haematol 74:24–29
21. Kuwazuru Y, Yoshimura A, Hanada S, Makino T, Terada A, Utsunomiya A, Arima T, Akiyama S (1990) Expression of the multidrug transporter, P-glycoprotein, in acute leukemia cells and correlation to clinical drug resistance. Cancer 66:868–873
22. Kuwazuru Y, Hanada S, Furukawa T, Yoshimura A, Sumizawa T, Utsunomiya A, Ishibashi K, Saito T, Arima T, Akiyama S (1990) Expression of P-glycoprotein in adult T cell leukemia cells. Blood 76:2065–2071
23. Mizoguchi T, Yamada K, Furukawa T, Hidaka K, Hisatsugu T, Shimazu H, Tsuruo T, Sumizawa T, Akiyama S (1990) Expression of the MDR1 gene in human gastric and colorectal carcinomas. J Natl Cancer Inst 82:1679–1683
24. Kamiwatari M, Nagata Y, Kikuchi H, Yoshimura A, Sumizawa T, Shudo N, Sakoda R, Seto K, Akiyama S (1989) Correlation between reversing of multidrug resistance and inhibiting to [^{3}H]azidopine photolabeling of P-glycoprotein by newly synthesized dihydropyridine analogues in a human cell line. Cancer Res 49:3190–3195
25. Shudo N, Mizoguchi T, Kiyosue T, Arita M, Yoshimura A, Seto K, Sakoda R, Akiyama S (1990) Two pyridine analogues with more effective ability to reverse

multidrug resistance and with lower calcium channel blocking activity than their dihydropyridine counterparts. Cancer Res 50:3055–3061
26. Cornwell MM, Safa AR, Felsted RL, Gottesman MM, Pastan I (1986) Membrane vesicles from multidrug resistant human cancer cells contain a specific 150 to 170 kDa protein detected by photoaffinity labeling. Proc Natl Acad Sci USA 83:3847–3850
27. Safa AR, Glover CJ, Sewell JL, Meyers MB, Biedler JL, Felsted RL (1987) Identification of the multidrug resistance-related membrane glycoprotein as an acceptor for calcium channel blockers. J Biol Chem 262:7884–7888
28. Yoshimura A, Kuwazuru Y, Sumizawa T, Ichikawa M, Ikeda S, Uda T, Akiyama S (1989) Cytoplasmic orientation and two-domain structure of the multidrug transporter, P-glycoprotein, demonstrated with sequence-specific antibodies. J Biol Chem 264:16282–16291

The Extracellular Matrix: Cues from the Microcellular Environment Which Can Inhibit or Facilitate Glioma Cell Growth

JAMES T. RUTKA[1]

Introduction

The extracellular matrix (ECM) is the naturally occurring substrate upon which cells migrate, proliferate, and differentiate *in vivo* [1,2]. The ECM functions as a biological adhesive that maintains the normal cytoarchitecture of different tissues and defines the key spatial relationships among dissimilar cell types. A loss of coordination and an alteration in the interactions between mesenchymal cells and epithelial cells separated by an ECM are thought to fundamental steps in the development and progression by an ECM are thought to fundamental steps in the development and progression of cancer. The interested reader can now refer to a number of key review articles in this field [2–4].

The ECM can be defined biochemically as the sum of its component parts (Table 1). These parts include the collagen types, the noncollagenous glycoproteins such as laminin and fibronectin, the glycosaminoglycans (GAGs) such as hyaluronic acid and heparin sulfate, and the proteoglycans. In most organ systems, the ECM forms a series of extracellular proteins that have fairly specific spatial relationships with each other and with the cells to which they bind.

There are at least 11 different collagen molecules whose amino acid sequences have been well described. Types I–III collagen are the intersitial collagens found in skin, bone, blood vessels, and connective tissue septae. Type IV collagen is found exclusively in basement membranes (BMs), and usually forms a scaffolding to which linking proteins such as laminin and fibronectin bind cells [2,5–7]. The distribution of types V–XI collagen in tissues has not been completely determined.

The noncollagenous glycoproteins are relatively large compounds that either bind directly to cells to mediate their effects, or link cells to other ECM macromolecules. Examples of these proteins include laminin, fibronectin, entactin, and vitronectin.

The GAGs were formerly known as the "mucopolysaccharides", and are linear carboyhydrate polymers of high molecular weight. Except for hyaluronic

[1]Hospital for Sick Children, University of Toronto, Toronto, Ontario, M5G 1X8 Canada

Table 1. Primary components of the ECM

Collagens
Noncollagenous glycoproteins (laminin, fibronectin)
Glycosaminoglycans (GAGs)
Proteoglycans

acid, all GAGs in their native state are covalently bound to proteins forming larger complexes known as proteoglycans. Examples of GAGs include dermatan, chondroitin, keratan, and heparan.

Proteoglycans in different tissues have similar structures, but differ with respect to protein content, molecular size, and the number of types of GAG side chains per molecule. Proteoglycans are closely associated with fundamental cellular processes such as cell growth, adhesiveness, receptor binding, and transformation [8–11].

What is the Distribution of ECM Proteins in Human Brain and Brain Tumors?

Despite recent interest in the field of ECM research by investigators in the neurosciences, the extracellular space of the central nervous system (CNS) has yet to be completely characterized. Whereas the parenchyma of the CNS appears to be filled with a relatively amorphous matrix that is largely free of collagens and other fibrous proteins, a well-defined ECM exists in the form of a true basement membrane around all cerebral blood vessels and at the glial limitans externa. As a delimiting basement membrane, the glial glimitans externa invests the entire cortical surface of the brain and separates astrocytic foot processes from pia-arachnoid cells. Thus, it forms an interface between cellular CNS elements derived embryologically from neuroepithelium and leptomeningeal elements presumably derived from the neural crest. Immunohistochemical studies of normal and pathological human CNS specimens have shown that ECM proteins are predominantly deposited at the junction between glial and mesenchymal elements [5,12–16].

We and others have shown that the glial limitans externa immunostains positively for laminin, fibronectin, type IV collagen, and type III collagen [14,15] Interestingly, the glial limitans externa usually remains as an intact barrier which is not destroyed by malignant glioma cells even when the glioma originates near the cortical surface of the brain. For poorly understood reasons, malignant gliomas rarely metastasize extracranially. In only 10%–12% of cases does the glioblastoma multiforme spread into cerebrospinal fluid (CSF) pathways. The success of malignant tumor cells in penetrating the glial limitans externa and other basal laminae probably depends in part on the ability of these cells to produce specific proteases capable of degrading extracellular matrix proteins [17,18]. We have previously shown that malignant glioma cells secrete both metalloproteinases and inhibitors of metalloproteinases (infra vide).

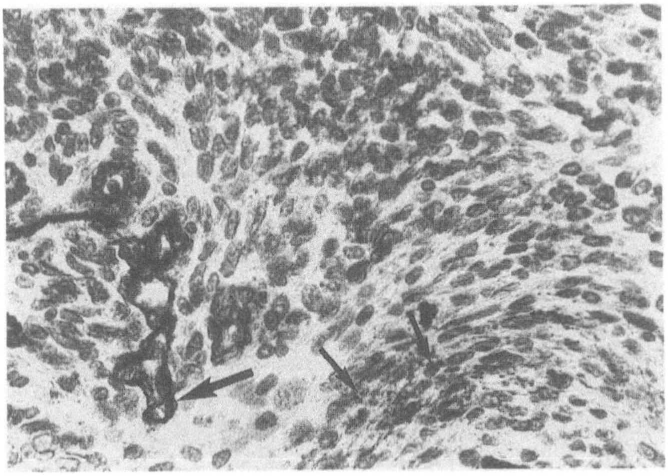

Fig. 1. Meningotheliomatous meningioma immunstained for laminin. The subendothelial basement membrane of the blood vessels (*large arrow*) and the cytoplasm of the meningioma cells are positively indentified in a whorl formation (*straight arrows*). Light microscopy, × 200

Laminin has been immunolocalized to hyperplastic blood vessels and glomerular vascular formations in gliomas [5,13,15], in the sarcomatous elements of some gliosarcomas [16], the vasculature and fibrillary extracellular spaces of some meningiomas, and intracytoplasmically in some meningioma cells (Fig. 1) [15,19].

Fibronectin has been found to stain all layers of both normal and tumor-associated blood vessels, the leptomeninges, meningiomas cells in whorl formations, the border between gliomatous and sarcomatous elements in gliosarcomas, and corpora amylacea in the normal brain [13,20–22].

Type IV collagen has been immunolocalized to the subendothelial basement membrane of blood vessels in gliomas and meningiomas. Neuroepithelial derivatives (glia, neurons, and glimoa cells) rarely if ever stain positively for type IV collagen. The interstitial collagens, types I and III, have been immunolocalized to the leptomeninges, the fibromuscular coats of large cerebral blood vessels, and the glia limitans externa [12].

GAGs have been found in the normal CNS, but their nature and role have yet to be determined. Studies of the ECM with ruthenium red have shown that GAGs are present in the extracellular space of the normal human brain [23]. Hyaluronic acid, dermatan sulfate, and chondroitin sulfate have all been found in the human brain [9,10,24]. It has been suggested that GAGs may be important in the myelination process. There is increased concentration of GAGs at the nodes of Ranvier [25,26].

Based on published data, we have arrived at a tentative model of the spatial arrangement of ECM macromolecules in the CNS (Fig. 2).

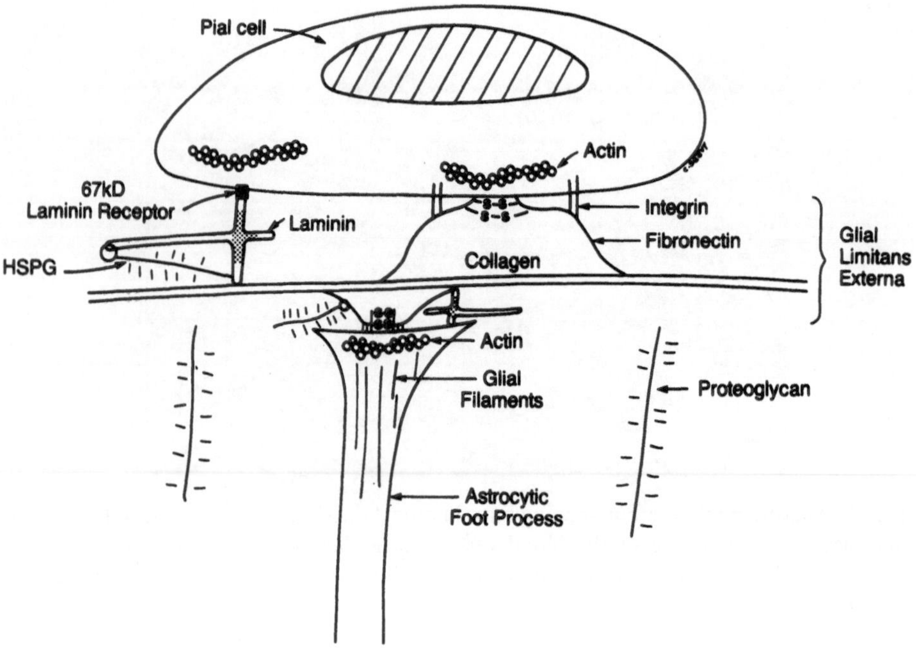

Fig. 2. The glial limitans externa as shown here in molecular detail contains *laminin, fibronectin, heparan sulfate proteoglycan*, and *collagen*. *Pial cells* attach to the glial limitans through specific ECM receptors, such as the *67-kd laminin receptor* and the *integrin receptor*. Through mechanisms not yet established, the interactions of an extracellular matrix molecule with its specific receptor triggers conformational changes in the cell cytoskeleton, one component of which is *actin*. *Astrocytic foot processes* are shown to adhere to the *glial limitans externa* in a similar fashion. Interestingly, *astrocytic foot processes* abutting this basal lamina are highly enriched in glial fibrillary acidic protein

What is the Interaction Between ECM Proteins and Glioma Cells?

In a variety of tissues, proteins of the ECM are known to influence cell kinetics and modulate the expression of normal and tumor phenotypes [1,27–29]. After we had characterized the ECM of normal leptomeningeal cell in vivo and in vitro [15,19], we were interested in studying the effects of leptomeningeal ECM proteins on glioma cell growth and differentiation [30].

In our model system, we found that U 343 MG-A glioma cells seeded onto a well-characterized leptomeningeal ECM were profoundly growth inhibited, had morphological features, such as stellate cell induction, that were suggestive of normal astrocytes, and had increased expression of glial fibrillary acidic protein (GFAP), an astrocytic marker of differentiation (Fig. 3) [30].

We were convinced that a protein complex from the ECM was responsible for the growth inhibition and differentiating effects of the glioma cell line because pre-treatment of the leptomeningeal ECM with trypsin or collagenase

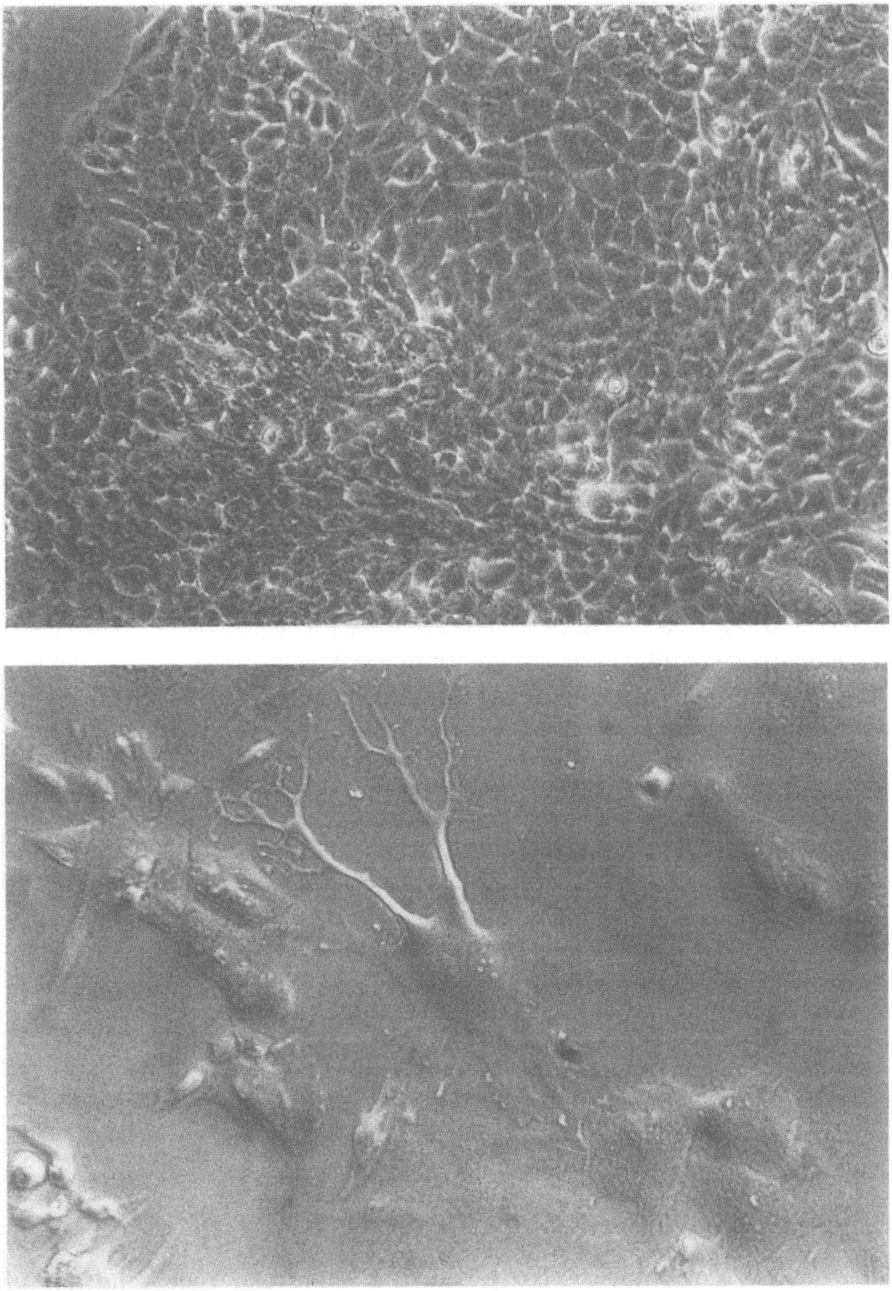

a

b

Fig. 3. **a** U-343 MG-A tumor cells grown on plastic alone are cuboidal and show signs of crowding and piling. Phase microscopy, × 250. **b** U 343 MG-A tumor cells grown on an extracellular matrix from normal pia-arachnoid cells. There is no colony formation and the cells have an increased cytoplasmic: nuclear ratio. Many of the cells have multiple, thin cytoplasmic processes and resemble normal astrocytes in culture. Phase microscopy, × 500 allowed the glioma cells to grow at their normal rate. We then did a series of experiments of test whether a single component of the leptomeningeal ECM was responsible for the inhibition of glioma cell growth in our system. We studied the effects of purified fibronectin, laminin, type IV collagen, and type I collagen as individual substrata onto which U 343 MG-A cells were seeded in a number of different proliferation assays. Of these glycoproteins, only type I and type IV collagen inhibited glioma cell proliferation and induced formation of stellate cells. Laminin and fibronectin had no effect on glioma cell growth.

We used an enzyme-linked immunosorbent assay (ELISA) to quantitate the amount of GFAP produced by glioma cells, and found that GFAP increased 20-fold in glioma cells grown on an ECM when compared to glioma cells growing on plastic alone. In addition, indirect immunofluroescence microscopy demonstrated more intensely staining networks of filaments within glioma cells grown on ECM-coated flasks than in controls.

The mechanism by which normal leptomeningeal ECM proteins exert their effects on the growth and differentiation of malignant glioma cells has not yet been elucidated. One possibility is that the active moeity of the leptomeningeal ECM binds to a specific ECM receptor within the plasma membrane of U 343 MG-A cells. In support of this concept is the recent identification and characterization of the 67,000 Dalton laminin receptor [31] which has been localized immunohistochemically to a variety of normal and carcinomatous human tissues. There is increasing evidence that specific cell receptors also exist for fibronectin and the collagen types [32]. A family of transmembrane glycoproteins, known as the "integrin receptors", interact with a wide variety of ligands, including ECM glycoproteins. These integrin receptors recognize ligands bearing the tripeptide sequence Arg-Asp-Gly [33,34]. Ruoslahti and Pierschbacher demonstrated that the binding capacity of fibronectin to cells is determined by the presence of this tripeptide sequence on the cell-binding domain of fibronectin [35,36]. How cellular proliferation and differentiation are mediated through the interaction between ECM macromolecules and their specific receptors is speculative. In another report, addition of fibronectin to transformed cells increased cell: substratum adhesion and cell size and resulted in a more orderly arrangement of filaments in the cytoskeleton [37].

How Do Glioma Cells Migrate Through the ECM?

Clues from Neuroembryogenesis

The primitive neural tube is comprised of a ventricular zone consisting of relatively undifferentiated, pseudostratified, and columnar epithelial cells. With increasing gestational age and migration away from the ventricular zone, the primitive epithelial precursor cells differentiate and acquire phenotypes that permit accurate characterization.

The embryology of the CNS is exceedingly complex, but important steps include the migration of cells and the extension of cellular processes to their

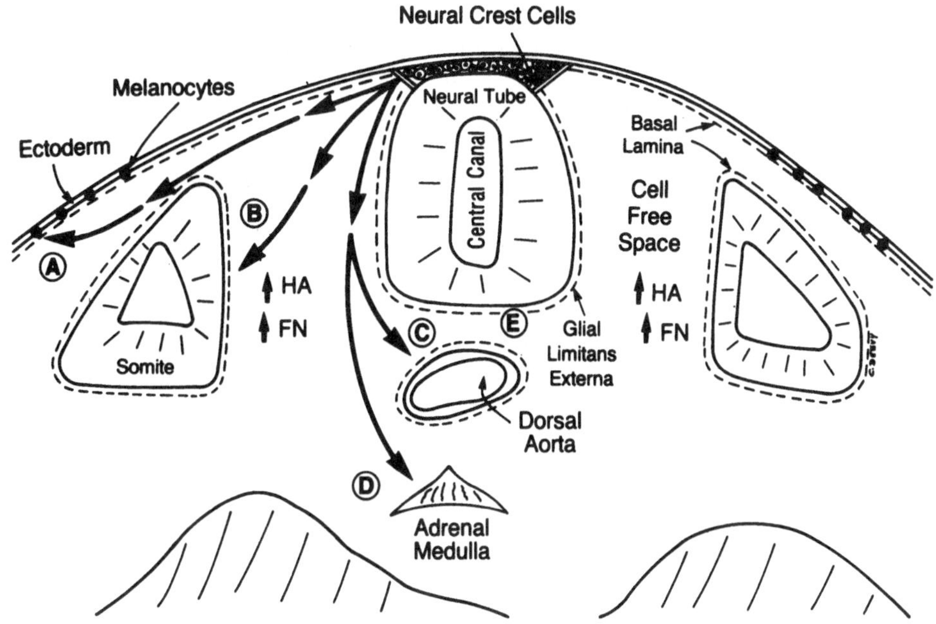

Fig. 4. Neuroembryology of the neural crest. Primitive neural crest cells leave the dorsolateral margins of the neural tube and migrate ventrally or laterally to become leptomeningeal cells (*E*), Schwann cells, melanocytes (*A*), dorsal root ganglia, or adrenal medulla cells (*D*). Neural crest cells may also play important roles in the genesis of the somite (*B*), and dorsal aorta (*C*) basal lamina. Cues for the final migration and differentiation of these different cell types are thought to be derived from the extracellular matrix (*arrows*). Areas enriched in fibronectin (*FN*) and hyaluronic acid (*HA*) are shown. In many ways, malignant cells emulate the migratory potential and invasiveness of neural crest cells

appropriate locations, the acquisition of distinctive phenotypes by neurons and glia, and the formation of synapses between neurons and their targets. These steps probably require fundamental communication between developing cells and their extracellular environment. It has been proposed that ECM macromolecules are involved in directing the migration of neuroblasts away from the primitive germinal matrix [38] (Fig. 4).

The neural crest is a transitory aggregate of cells that forms on the dorsal rim of the neural tube as the tube separates from the overlying ectoderm. Neural crest cells migrate along defined pathways to target sites throughout the embryo and give rise to a variety of cell types, including autonomic and sensory neurons, leptomeningeal cells, Schwann cells, and melanocytes [39]. It is thought that through the specific distribution of ECM components, neural crest cells become associated with a particular tissue and differentiate.

Increasing evidence, mostly from transplant studies, has shown that the migration of neural crest cells to their final destination is guided by components of the ECM with which they come in contact. The tissue through which the neural crest cells migrate is relatively acellular, but is abundant in ECM macromolecules [39]. Just before migration, the cell-free space becomes rich in hyaluronic acid, a highly hydrated molecule that occupies a large domain relative to its mass and provides an attractive migratory environment. Hyaluronic acid exerts a swelling pressure that alters the size of intercellular spaces and separates cell and connective tissue layers, thereby opening avenues for cell migration. In the neural crest, high concentrations of hyaluronic acid, high levels of hydration, and increased matrix volume are closely correlated with cell migration.

Fibronectin also plays a key role in the migration of neural crest cells [40]. Fibronectin levels in the cell-free space increase before migration and decrease as migration ends [41]. The fibronectin observed in the cell-free space is though to be derived from primitive mesenchymal cells, as neural crest cells appear not to produce fibronectin [39].

Expression of Proteinases and Proteinase Inhibitors by Fetal Astrocytes and Glioma Cells

Proteinases are important in the remodeling of the ECM during development, growth, and tissue repair [42,43]. Uncontrolled degradation of the ECM has been implicated in the pathogenesis of many diseases and in tumor invasion and metastasis [44,45]. The dissolution of basement membranes facilitates the migration, penetration, and hematogenous dissemination of tumor cells. In many connective tissue cells, proteinase activity can be modulated by a variety of stimuli, including hormones, monokines, endocytosis, phorbol esters, and agents that affect cell shape.

Proteinases can be characterized in part by their active moieties, the conditions needed for their activation, and by the types of inhibitors that prevent their action. Several known proteases are listed in Table 2.

Since gliomas are locally invasive neoplasms that would require proteinases to breach connective tissue barriers in the brain, and since these enzymes may also be important in increasing our understanding of how fetal astrocytes are able to migrate in the developing central nervous system, we tested a variety of different glioma cells lines and fetal human astrocytes for their ability to secrete metalloproteinases [47].

In one of our earlier reports, we identified a major proteolytic species with a molecular weight of 65,000 in the conditioned medium (CM) of U 343 MG-A,

Table 2. Classification of proteinases. (Modified from [46])

Type of proteinase	Active moiety	Examples	Inhibitors
Serine	Hydroxyl	Trypsin	DFP, MNSF
Metallo	Metal group	Collagenase	EDTA
Cysteine	Thiol	Papain	NEM
Aspartic	Aspartatyl	Pepsin	Pepstatin

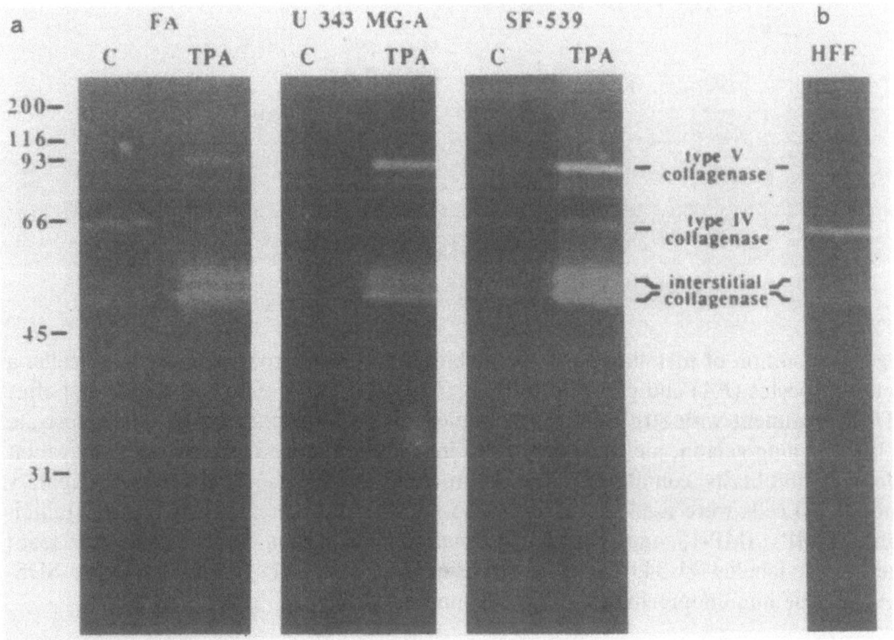

Fig. 5. Detection of proteinase activity in fetal astrocytes and glioma cell lines by SDS-substrate gel analysis. **a** Fetal astrocytes (*FA*), *U 343 MG-A* and *SF-539* cells grown in serum-free DME, either in the absence (*C*) or presence (*TPA*) of 80 nM TPA. The CM was subjected to electrophoresis on a 9% SDS-polyacrylamide gel containing gelatin. Zones of clearing represent proteinase activity. **b** *TPA*-treated human foreskin fibroblasts analyzed by substrate gel electrophoresis and used as a standard to indicate three well-characterized proteinases present in these cells

a human glioma cell line [30]. It is a metalloproteinase, active at pH 8.0, that is capable of degrading gelating but not casein on substrate gels. Interestingly, U 343 MG-A CM was unable to degrade azocoll, a nonspecific gelatin substrate covalently coupled to an azo dye. Because azocoll is a general substrate for several proteinases, including metalloproteinases, and similar to the gelatin used in the substrate gel analysis, we hypothesized that U 343 MG-A cells may be secreting *endogenous inhibitors* that mask azocollytic activity in its CM.

Several inhibitors of metalloproteinases have been described. Alpha-2 macroglobulin is a general proteinase inhibitor found in serum which will inhibit metalloproteinases. Serum also contains a tissue inhibitor of metalloproteinase (TIMP, Mr 28,000) which has inhibitory activity against many metalloproteinases, including the interstitial collagenases. TIMP-2, an inhibitor that shares amino acid homology with TIMP, has recently been purified from human melanoma conditioned medium [48].

From our most recent report [47], we demonstrated that malignant glioma cell and fetal astrocytes secrete a number of metalloproteinases (Fig. 5) and metalloproteinase inhibitors. We have identified several major proteolytic species (Mr 92,000, 65,000, 57,000, and 52,000) which are secreted by human

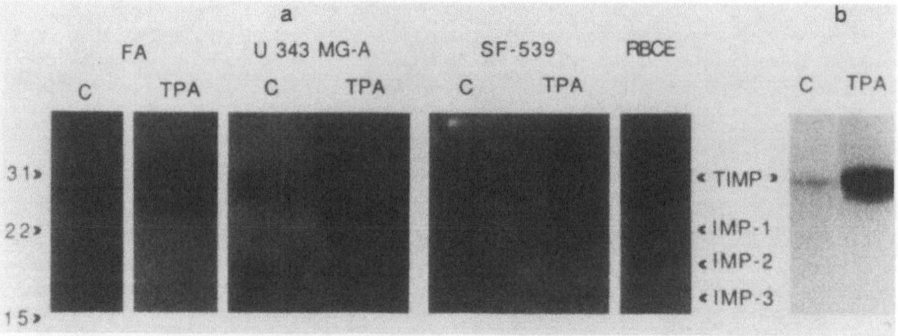

Fig. 6. Secretion of metalloproteinase inhibitors by fetal astrocytes and glioma cells. **a** Fetal astrocytes (*FA*) and glioma cell lines (*U 343 MG-A, SF-539*) before (*C*) and after (*TPA*) treatment with 80 nM TPA was subjected to electrophoresis on 10% substrate gels containing gelatin, and then incubated in conditioned medium derived from rabbit synovial fibroblasts containing activated metalloproteinases. Rabbit brain capillary endothelial cells were used as a standard to indicate three previously described inhibitors, TIMP, IMP-1, and IMP-2. **b** Immunoprecipitation of TIMP from [35S] methionine-labeled U 343 MG-A cells using an anti-TIMP IgG antibody on SDS-PAGE. The immunoprecipitated TIMP is marked at the *left*

gliomas. These proteinases have proved to be gelatinases and collagenases. Some of these enzymes are capable of degrading type IV collagen. A type IV collagenase might be important in the invasion of basement membranes by tumor cells, and there is a correlation between secretion of this type of enzyme and metastatic potential [18]. We found that we could induce human glioma cells to produce interstitial collagens (Mr 57,000 and 52,000) only after phorbol ester treatment with TPA.

All of the fetal human astrocyte cultures we examined contained proteinases that were similar to those found in glioma cells. Proteinase secretion by fetal astrocytes may facilitate their migration through the developing nervous system in a manner similar to the enhanced migration described for malignant cells that secrete tumor-associated proteinases [17]. We would have liked to test whether adult human astrocytes, which under normal conditions do not migrate, produce any proteinases. However, at present there is no reliable model for studying adult human astrocytes in a monolayer culture.

Both glioma cell lines and fetal human astrocyte cultures produced TIMP constitutively (fig. 6). The glioma cell lines also secreted a number of smaller metalloproteinase inhibitors, IMP-1 (Mr 22,000), IMP-2 (Mr 19,000), and IMP-3 (Mr 16,500). Interestingly, glioma and fetal astrocytes appear to produce enough inhibitors to prevent the detection of their proteinases by a general assay of proteolytic activity, degradation of azocoll.

The expression of metalloproteinase inhibitors may help to explain certain histopathological features of the malignant gliomas. Malignant gliomas are locally invasive, infiltrative neoplasms that rarely metastasize extracranially [49]. The local invasion could be mediated by the proteolysis of the ECM of the parenchyma of the brain. This would occur only if the balance of proteinases and inhibitors were shifted in favor of proteolysis. Although local invasion of brain tissue could be purely mechanical, in about 12% of the cases, the glioma does spread into CSF pathways; in such cases, spread often occurs as a result of leptomeningeal involvement following the disruption of the glial limitans externa by glioma cells.

Other investigators have shown that metalloproteinase inhibitors can regulate the invasive potential of a cell [50]. Experimentally, the down regulation of TIMP RNA levels by expression of antisense TIMP RNA in Swiss 3T3 cells, a normally noninvasive cell line, results in cells that are invasive in an amnion invasion assay and both tumorigenic and metastatic when injected into nude mice [51].

How the balance of proteinases and inhibitors in cells like gliomas and astrocytes is swayed in favor of proteolysis is not known. It could be regulated by exogenous stimuli from inflammatory cells such as macrophages or lymphocytes, from cues such as expression of a growth factor during development, growth or tumorigenesis, or by the temporal or spatial partitioning of secretion of proteinases and inhibitors. Although much is known about stimuli that increase proteinase production, little is known about how levels of proteinase inhibitors are modulated. It is clear that the programmed degradation of ECM by cells requires the careful balancing of proteinases and inhibitors.

Conclusions

We have reviewed the current knowledge about the structure and function of the ECM in the CNS. It is clear that we can no longer explain cell function without reference to the important role played by the cellular microenvironment in normal, reparative, and neoplastic states. Once the factors that contribute to the synthesis and deposition of the ECM between different cell types are better understood, efforts to manipulate the microcellular environment may prove useful in altering the course of important complex biological processes, such as axonal regeneration and cerebral neoplasia.

References

1. Gospodarowicz D, Greenburg G, Birdwell CR (1978) Determination of cellular shape by the extracellular matrix and its correlation with the control of cellular growth. Cancer Res 38:4155–4171
2. Reid LM, Jefferson DM (1984) Cell culture studies using extracts of ECM to study growth and differentiation in mammalian cells. In: Mather JP (ed) Mammalian cell culture. Plenum, New York, pp 239–280
3. Carbonetto S (1984) The extracellular matrix of the nervous ststem. Trends Neurosci 7:382–387
4. Rutka JT, Apodaca G, Stern R, Rosenblum M (1988) The extracellular matrix of the central and peripheral nervous system. JNS 69:155–170

5. Giordana MT, Giaccone G, Mauro A, et al. (1985) The distribution of laminin in human brain tumors: An immunohistochemical study. Acta Neuropathol (Berl) 67:51–57
6. Timpl R (1982) Antibodies to collagens and procollagens. Methods Enzymol 82: 472–498
7. Laurie GW, Bing JT, Kleinman HK, et al. (1986) Localization of binding sites for laminin, heparan sulfate proteoglycan and fibronectin on basement membrane (type IV) collagen. J Mol Biol 189:205–216
8. Iozzo RV (1984) Proteoglycans and neoplastic-mesenchymal cell interactions. Hum Pathol 15:2–10
9. Margolis RK, Thomas MD, Crockett CP, et al. (1979) Presence of chondroitin sulfate in the neuronal cytoplasm. Proc Natl Acad Sci USA 76:1711–1715
10. Margolis RU, Margolis RK (1977) Metabolism and function of glycoproteins and glycosaminoglycans in nervous tissue. Int J Biochem 8:85–91
11. Turley EA (1984) Proteoglycans and cell adhesion: Their putative role during tumorigenesis. Cancer Metastasis Rev 3:325-339
12. Bellon G, Caulet T, Cam Y, et al. (1985) Immunohistochemical localization of macromolecules of the basement membrane and extracellular matrix of human gliomas and meningiomas. Acta Neuropathol (Berl) 66:245–252
13. Mauro A, Bertolotto A, Germano I, et al. (1984) Collagenase in the immunohistochemical demonstration of laminin, fibronectin, and factor VIII/RAg in nervous tissue after fixation. Histochemistry 80:157–163
14. McComb RD, Bigner DD (1985) Immunolocalization of laminin in neoplasms of the central and peripheral nervous system. J Neuropathol Exp Neurol 44:242–253
15. Rutka JT, Myatt CA, Giblin JR, et al. (1987) Distribution of extracellular matrix proteins in primary human brain tumors: An immunohistochemical analysis. Can J Neurol Sci 14:20–30
16. Schiffer D, Giordana MT, Migheli A (1984) GFAP, FVIII/RAg, laminin and fibronectin in gliosarcomas: An immunohistochemical study. Acta Neuropathol 63: 108–116
17. Kramer RH, Vogel KG, Nicholson GL (1982) Solubilization and degradation of subendothelial matrix glycoproteins and proteoglycans by metastatic tumor cells. J Biol Chem 257:2678–2686
18. Liotta LA, TryggvasonK, Garbisa S, et al. (1980) Metastatic potential correlates with enzymatic degradation of basement membrane collagen. Nature 284: 67–68
19. Rutka JT, Giblin J, Dougherty DV, et al. (1985) An ultrastructural and immunocytochemical analysis of leptomeningeal and meningioma cultures. J Neuropath Exp Neurol 44:242–253
20. Kochi N, Tani E, Morimura T, et al. (1983) Immunohistochemical study of fibronectin in human glioma and meningioma. Acta Neuropathol (Berl) 59:119–126
21. Paetau A, Mellstrom K, Vaheri A, et al. (1980) Distribution of a major connective tissue protein, fibronectin, in normal and neoplastic human nervous tissue. Acta Neuropathol (Berl) 51:47–51
22. Schachner M, Schoomaker G, Hyner RO (1978) Cellular and subcellular localization of LETS protein in the nervous system. Brain Res 158:149–155
23. Tani E, Ametani T (1971) Extracellular distribution of ruthenium red-positive substance in the cerebral cortex. J Ultrastruct Mol Struct Res 34:1–14
24. Singh M, Bachawat BK (1968) Isolation and characterization of glycosaminoglycans in human brain of different age groups. J Neurochem 15:249–258

25. Aquino DA, Margolis RU, Margolis RK (1984) Immunocytochemical localization of a chondroitin sulfate proteoglycan in nervous tissue I. Adult brain, retina, and peripheral nerve. J Cell Biol 99:1117–1129
26. Aquino DA, Margolis RU, Margolis RK (1984) Immunocytochemical localization of a chondroitin sulfate proteoglycan in nervous tissue II. Studies of the developing brain. J Cell Biol 99:1130–1139
27. Vlodavsky I, Levi A, Lax I, et al. (1982) Induction of cell attachment and morphological differentiations in a pheochromocytoma cell line and embryonal sensory cells by the extracellular matrix. Dev Biol 93:285–300
28. Vlodavsky I, Lui GM, Gospodarowicz D (1980) Morphological appearance, growth behavior, and migratory activity of human tumor cells maintained on extracellular matrix versus plastic. Cell 19:607–616
29. Wicha MS, Lowrie G, Kohn E, et al. (1982) Extracellular matrix promotes mammary epithelial growth and differentiation in vitro. Proc Natl Acad Sci USA 79: 3213–317
30. Rutka JT, Giblin JR, Apodaca G, et al. (1987) Inhibition of growth and induction of differentiation in a malignant human glioma cell line by normal leptomeningeal extracellular matrix proteins. Cancer 47:3515–3522
31. Terranova VP, Rao CN Kalebic T, et al. (1983) Laminin receptor on human breast carcinoma cells. Proc Natl Acad Sci USA 80:444–448
32. Yamada KM, Akiyama SK, Hasegawa T (1985) Recent advances in research on fibronectin and other cell attachment proteins. J Cell Biochem 28:79–97
33. Hynes RO (1987) Integrins: A family of cell surface receptors. Cell 48:549–554
34. Yamada KM (1983) Cell surface interactions with extracellular materials. Annu Rev Biochem 52:761–799
35. Pierschbacher MD, Ruoslahti E (1984) Variants of the cell recognition site of fibronectin that retain attachment promoting activity. Proc Natl Acad Sci USA 81: 5985–5988
36. Ruoslahti E, Pierschbacher MD (1986) Arg-Gly-Asp: A versatile cell recognition signal. Cell 44:517–518
37. Ali IU, Mautner V, Lanza R, et al. (1977) Restoration of normal morphology, adhesion and cytoskeleton in transformed cells by addition of transformation-sensitive surface protein. Cell 11:115–126
38. Lander AD, Fujii DK, Gospodarowicz D, et al. (1982) Characterization of a factor that promotes neurite outgrowth: Evidence linking activity to a heparan sulfate proteoglycan. J Cell Biol 94:574–585
39. Sanes JR (1983) Roles of extracellular matrix in neural development. Annu Rev Physiol 45:581–600
40. Greenberg JH, Seppa S, Seppa H, et al. (1981) Role of collagen and fibronectin in neural crest cell adhesion and migration. Dev Biol 87:259–266
41. Feigin I (1980) The mucopolysaccarhides of the ground substance of the human brain. J Neuropathol Exp Neurol 39:1–12
42. Murphy G, Reynolds JJ (1985) Progess towards understanding the resorption of connective tissues. Bioessays 2:55–60
43. Peterson PH (1985) On the role of proteases, their inhibitors and the extracellular matrix in promoting neurite outgrowth. J Physiol (Lond) 80:207–211
44. Goldfarb RH, Liotta LA (1986) Proteolytic enzymes in cancer invasion and metastasis. Semin Thromb Hemost 12:294–307
45. Thorgeirsson UP, Turpeenniemi-Hujanen T, Liotta LA (1985) Cancer cells, components of basement membranes, and proteolytic enzymes. Int Rev Exp Pathol 27: 203–234

46. Barrett AJ (1980) The classification of proteinases. In: Evered D, Whelan I (eds) Protein degradation in health and disease. Ciba Foundation Symposium 75. Excerpta Medica, Amsterdam, pp 1–13
47. Apodaca G, Rutka JT, Bouhana K, et al. (1990) Expression of metalloproteinases and metalloproteinase inhibitors by fetal astrocytes and glioma cells. Cancer Res 50:2322–2329
48. Stetler-Stevenson WG, Krutzch HC, Liotta LA (1989) Tissue inhibitor of metalloproteinase (TIMP-2): A new member of the metalloproteinase inhibitor family. J Biol Chem 264:17374–17378
49. Cerame MA, Guthikonda M, Kohli CM (1985) Extraneural metastases in gliosarcoma: A case report and review of the literature. Neurosurgery 17:413–418
50. Mignatti P, Robbins E, Rifkin DB (1986) Tumor invasion through the human amniotic membrane: Requirement for a proteinase cascade. Cell 47:487–498
51. Khokha R, Waterhouse P, Yagel S, et al. (1989) Antisense RNA-induced reduction in murine TIMP levels confers oncogenicity on Swiss 3T3 cells. Science 243:947–950

Part II. Selected Papers

Section 1. Growth Activity of Brain Tumor

Cell Kinetics of Brain Tumors and Its Clinical Relevance

Takao Hoshino[1]

Introduction

Brain tumors are unique in their cell kinetics. They grow within the cranium, a limited space in which the proliferative capacity is minimal. Most patients with brain tumors die from cerebellar or cerebral herniation caused by increased intracranial pressure when the weight of the tumor reaches from 250 to 300 g. Thus, any patient whose brain contains a tumor of that size may die, whether it is histopathologically benign or malignant. Thus, the prognosis for patients with brain tumors depends largely upon the size of the lesion and rate of tumor growth.

The rate of tumor growth is usually estimated by the frequency of mitosis in tumor tissue; however, mitoses are very infrequent and uneven, even in highly malignant gliomas, including glioblastomas. Thus, quantitation of growth rate by mitotic index is very difficult. In addition, the number of mitoses observed in gliomas does not necessarily correlate with the rapidity of growth. For example, a glioblastoma multiforme may fail to show mitoses, whereas an oligodendroglioma, a slow-growing tumor, may show frequent mitoses. Thus, more quantitative measurements of the proliferative activity are needed to predict survival.

The development of a monoclonal antibody that can identify 5-bromo-2′-deoxyuridine, or BUdR, is a breakthrough for quantitating the proliferative potential of individual tumors [1]. BUdR is an analogue of thymidine and, like 3H-thymidine, it is incorporated into nuclear DNA of cells during DNA synthesis [2]. An anti-BUdR antibody identifies these cells and can be readily detected by the immunocytochemical method [3–5].

After a series of experiments, we set up the following protocol in order to study the 5-bromodeoxyuridine (BrdU) labeling index (LI) in human brain tumors in situ. The patients were given a 30 m intravenous infusion of BUdR, 200 mg/sqm, at the time of surgery, but before biopsy of the tumor. The biopsied specimen was stained for BUdR by means of immunoperoxidase [4,5].

[1] Department of Neurosurgery, Kyorin University School of Medicine, Mitaka, Tokyo, 181 Japan

Table 1. BUdR Labeling indices of 463 neuroectodermal tumors

Tumor type	No. of cases	Labeling index (%) Median	Range	No. of cases of LI (%) <1	1–5	>5
Medulloblastoma	24	9.5	3.9–38.2	0	2	22
Glioblastoma multiforme	157	6.7	<1.0–30.5	3	55	98
Malignant astrocytoma	82	2.1	<1.0–38.1	24	40	18
Astrocytoma	77	<1.0	<1.0–9.3	53	21	3
Ependymoma	32	<1.0	<1.0–18.9	19	11	2
Juvenile pilocytic astrocytoma	35	<1.0	<1.0–4.3	22	13	0
Mixed glioma	45	1.3	<1.0–15.1	22	18	5
Ganglioglioma	11	<1.0	<1.0–2.8	7	4	0
Total	463	—	—	151	164	148

(UCSF 9/90)

Labeling Index Study

To date we have studied over 1,000 patients with various brain tumors. Table 1 summarizes the results of 463 neuroectodermal tumors studied at the Brain Tumor Research Center, University of California, San Francisco. The median-labeling indices for medulloblastomas and glioblastomas were 9.5% and 6.7%, respectively, while low-grade astrocytomas demonstrated a median labeling index of less than 1%. Malignant astrocytomas showed a median labeling index of 2.1%. Thus, generally speaking, malignant gliomas have higher labeling indices reflecting faster growth. Over 60% of glioblastomas had labeling indices of over 5%. On the other hand, 60% of astrocytomas showed a labeling index of less than 1%; however, one-third of these tumors showed higher labeling indices, similar to either malignant astrocytomas or glioblastomas. This is an important observation, since it demonstrates that one-third of histologically similar-appearing low-grade astrocytomas, for example, may behave differently from other tumors even though such discrepancies may be explained on the basis of sampling errors in the biopsied materials.

Prognosis and Labeling Index

It is necessary to elucidate whether or not the BUdR-labeling index correlates with the survival of individual patients (a denominator of proliferative potential), and if the BUdR-labeling index gives more information than pathology can provide. In order to address these questions, patients were grouped into quartiles based upon the increasing percent of labeling index, and the survival rates of each quartile of patients were analysed.

The Kaplan-Meier survival analysis [6] of each quartile of 172 patients with intracranial astrocytomas or glioblastomas [7]) showed that the lowest quartile (43 patients), those whose tumors had a labeling index of less than 1%, showed the best 3-year survival rate of 80% and the second lowest quartile (44 patients), whose tumors showed a labeling index of less than 1%–3.7%, showed the survival rate of 50%, while the third (44 patients with LIs of 3.7%–7.6%) and the highest (46 patients with LIs > 7.6%) quartiles demonstrated similar poor survival rates of 15%. This result confirms that the BUdR-labeling index is strongly correlated with the survival rate of patients and reflects the proliferative potential of individual tumors.

To determine whether the BUdR-labeling index gives more information than that provided by pathology, a similar survival analysis, by quartile, was performed for each tumor type. In the low-grade astrocytoma and malignant astrocytoma groups, patients with BUdR LIs in the upper quartile had significantly poorer survival than those with LIs in the lower quartiles. Among patients with glioblastomas however, those in the lowest quartile (BUdR LIs < 5.9%) had a 2-year survival probability of 40%, compared with only 15% in each of the other three quartiles. Because most patients with glioblastomas had LIs > 5% and very few had LIs < 1%, even the lowest quartile included many patients with LIs close to 5%. The analysis could not, therefore, show the influence of LI on survival in these cases.

Analysis with the univariate Cox proportional hazards step-wise model [8] revealed (1) the BUdR labeling index did not improve the predication of survival for patients with glioblastomas once the age was entered in the model, but, (2) for patients with malignant and low grade astrocytomas, the BUdR-labeling index was the best single predictor of survival. Multivariate analysis, however, demonstrated that: (1) distinguishing between glioblastomas and malignant astrocytomas did not significantly improve the prediction once age and the BUdR-labeling index were entered, (2) the survival rate is a function of age and the BUdR-labeling index among patients with glioblastomas or malignant astrocytomas, and (3) the survival rate is a function of the BUdR-labeling index alone in patients with low-grade astrocytomas.

With the implementation of the proportional hazards model, a probability of survival can be estimated. An interaction term of BUdR LI for low-grade astrocytomas was significantly different from either malignant astrocytomas or glioblastomas and showed that a different coefficient was needed to generate survival curves for low-grade astrocytomas according to their BUdR LIs. Therefore, two equations for estimating the probability of survival in these patients were devised:

1. Malignant astrocytomas and glioblastomas

$$S(t) = So(t)^{\exp(0.024 \times \text{Age} + 0.034 \times \text{BUdR LI})}$$

2. Low-grade astrocytomas

$$S(t) = So(t)^{\exp(0.284 \times \text{BUdR LI})}$$

In both equations, $S(t)$ is the probability of survival at time "t" and So (t) is the probability of survival when all covariates = 0, thus the curves can be calculated from the survival of all malignant astrocytomas and glioblastomas or of low-grade astrocytomas.

These equations indicate that low-grade astrocytomas grow differently from either glioblastomas or malignant astrocytomas. The slope of the curve for low-grade astrocytomas is more influenced by increasing the labeling index.

The equations proposed also indicate a substantial difference between the two groups: the same labeling index for low-grade tumor versus glioblastoma or malignant astrocytoma results in different probabilities of survival. Therefore, it is very important to differentiate low-grade astrocytomas from either glioblastomas or malignant astrocytomas because their growth patterns are different. Of course, this does not negate the importance of differentiating glioblastomas from malignant astrocytomas. They may be phenotypically different, but their growth patterns appear to follow the same principle. Without any highly effective treatment toward any specific tumor phenotype, at present, the survival of patients with intracranial gliomas appears to be strongly dependent upon the proliferative potential of individual tumors.

Nevertheless, it is not always appropriate to correlate the proliferative potential with survival in individual cases. In most cases, the natural growth of gliomas is disrupted by postoperative treatment. For example, medulloblastomas, like glioblastomas, have high LIs and grow very fast [9]. Unlike glioblastomas, they respond very well to radiation therapy. The higher rates of survival of patients with medulloblastomas [10–15] is primarily due to improved radiation therapy and to the greater sensitivity of medulloblastomas to radiation. Therefore, histopathologic analysis is important in characterizing the phenotype of each tumor, and the usefulness of labeling studies should be judged only within certain categories of tumors. The clinical significance of the BUdR LI in other gliomas, such as ependymomas, juvenile pilocytic astrocytomas, and mixed gliomas cannot be assessed until more patients have been studied.

Thus, the BUdR-labeling index study helps estimate the proliferative potential of individual tumors; however, it represents only a fraction of cells in DNA synthesis and does not indicate their actual growth rate.

Recently, a new monoclonal antibody, Br-3, which recognizes only BUdR was created [16]. This is in contrast to the currently available anti-BUdR antibodies which recognize both BUdR and another thymidine analogue, IUdR or iododeoxyuridine. Differential staining with these two antibodies makes possible double-labeling studies with BUdR and IUdR as probes, and we can measure the duration of DNA synthesis and potential doubling time from a single specimen of biopsy material [16,17]. The actual application of this technique is presented in the following chapter.

With further elaboration of this technique, we will be better able to understand cell kinetic characteristics of individual brain tumors from a single biopsy.

BUdR labeling is not the only method for predicting the proliferative potential of tumors. Monoclonal antibodies to proliferating cell nuclear antigen or cyclin [18], thymidylate synthase [19], deoxyribonucleic acid polymerase α [20], Ki-67 [21,22], and nucleolar organizing region [23] are also potentially useful for cell kinetic studies. So far, BUdR-labeling studies have provided more reliable results than studies with other monoclonal antibodies currently available. The development of any method to quantitate the proliferative potential depending either on BUdR or other methods will be of great theoretical and practical importance in order to understand the biological and clinical malignancy of individual gliomas.

Summary

The development of monoclonal antibodies against bromodeoxyuridine (BUdR) has made it possible to study cell kinetics of individual brain tumors more extensively and rapidly. The results of in situ labeling of brain tumors with BUdR done at the Brain Tumor Research Center, University of California San Francisco were reviewed. The study demonstrated that: (1) BUdR-labeling indexes (LI or percentage of cells in DNA synthesis) were generally higher in malignant gliomas, (2) histologically similar tumors may have different proliferative potentials, demonstrated by differences in LIs, and (3) a higher LI indicates a higher proliferative potential and demonstrates a shorter interval of recurrence and survival. Thus, the need for improved methods of predicting the proliferative potential of individual gliomas is clear, since such studies could elucidate the complex cell kinetics of various types of gliomas and benefit individual patients as well.

Acknowledgement. This work was supported in part by grants CA 13525, CA 50210 from the National Cancer Institute and by Grants-in Aid for Scientific Research (A) #02404058 from the Ministry of Education, Science and Culture of Japan.

References

1. Gratzner HG (1982) Monoclonal antibody to 5-bromo- and 5-iododeoxyuridine: A new reagent for detection of DNA replication. Science 218:474–476
2. Goz B (1978) The effects of incorporation of 5-halogenated deoxyuridines into the DNA of eukaryotic cells. Pharmacol Rev 29:249–272
3. Dolbeare F, Gratzner H, Pallavicini MG, Gray JW (1983) Flow cytometric measurement of total DNA content and incorporated bromodeoxyuridine. Proc Natl Acad Sci USA 80:5573–5577
4. Hoshino, T, Nagashima T, Murovic J, Levin EM, Levin VA, Rupp SM (1985) Cell kinetic studies of *in situ* human brain tumors with bromodeoxyuridine. Cytometry 6:627–732
5. Nagashima T, DeArmond SJ, Murovic J, Hoshino T (1985) Immunocytochemical demonstration of S-phase cells by anti-bromodeoxyuridine monoclonal antibody in human brain tumor tissues. Acta Neuropathol (Berl) 67:155–159
6. Kaplan EL, Meier P (1958) Nonparametric estimation from incomplete observations. J Am Stat Assoc 53:457–481
7. Hoshino T (1991) Proliferative potential of astrocytomas and glioblastomas. In: Paoletti P, Takakura K, Walker MD, Butti G, Pezzotta S (eds)., Neuro-oncology, Kluwer Academic, Dordrecht. p 33–39
8. Cox DR (1972) Regression models and life tables. J R Statist Soc 34[B]:187–220
9. Hoshino T, Kobayashi S, Townsend JJ, Wilson CB (1985) A cell kinetic study on medulloblastomas. Cancer 55:1711–1713
10. Bloom HJG, Wallace ENK, Henk JM (1969) The treatment and prognosis of medulloblastoma in children. AJR 105:43–62

11. Bongartz EB, Bamberg M, Nau HE, Schmitt G, Bagindin E (1979) Optimal therapy in medulloblastoma. Acta Neurochir (Wien) 50:117–125
12. Chin HW, Maruyama Y (1983) Early response and long-term results in the radiotherapy of childhood medulloblastoma. J Neurooncol 1:53–59
13. Cumberlin R, Luk KH, Wara WM, Sheline GE, Wilson CB (1979) Medulloblastoma. Treatment results and effect on normal tissues. Cancer 43:1014–1020
14. Hirsh JF, Renier O, Czerniehow P, Benveniste L, Pierr-Kahn A (1979) Medulloblastoma in childhood. Survival and functional results. Acta Neurochir (Wien) 48:1–15
15. Park TS, Hoffman HJ, Hendrick EB, Humphreys RP, Becker LE (1983) Medulloblastoma: Clinical presentation and management. J Neurosurg 58:543–552
16. Shibui S, Hoshino T, Vanderlaan M, Gray JW (1989) Double labeling with iodo- and bromodeoxyuridine for cell kinetic studies. J Histochem Cytochem 37:1007–1011
17. Asai A, Shibui S, Barker M, Vanderlaan M, Gray JW, Hoshino T (1990) Cell kinetics of the 9L rat brain tumor determined by double labeling with iodo- and bromodeoxyuridine. J Neurosurg 73:254–258
18. Tabuchi K, Honda C, Nakane P (1987) Demonstration of proliferating cell nuclear antigen (PCNA/Cyclin) in glioma cells. Neurol Med Chir (Tokyo) 27:1–5
19. Shibui S, Hoshino T, Iwasaki K, Nomura K, Jastreboff MM (1989) Cell cycle phase dependent emergence of thymidylate synthase studied by monoclonal antibody (M-TS-4). cell Tissue Kinet 22:259–268
20. Mushika M, Miwa T, Suzuoki Y, Hayashi K, Masaki S, Kaneda T (1988) Detection of proliferative cells in dysplasia, carcinoma *in situ*, and invasive carcinoma of the uterine cervix by monoclonal antibody against DNA polymerase α. Cancer 61: 1182–1186
21. Gerdes J, Schwab U, Lemke H, Stein H (1983) Production of a mouse monoclonal antibody reactive with a human nuclear antigen associated with cell proliferation. Int J Cancer 31:13–20
21. Nishizaki T, Orita T, Furutani Y, Ikeyama Y, Aoki H, Sasaki K (1989) Flow-cytometric DNA analysis and immunohistochemical measurement of Ki-67 and BUdR labeling indices in human brain tumors. J Neurosurg 70:379–384
22. Kajiwara K, Nishizaki T, Orita T, Nakayama H, Aoki H, Ito H (1990) Silver colloid staining technique for analysis of glioma malignancy. J Neurosurg 73:113–117

Double-Labeling Method with BUdR and IUdR for Cell Kinetic Studies of Brain Tumors

SOICHIRO SHIBUI[1], RYO NISHIKAWA[1], KAZUHIRO NOMURA[1], KEIKO IWASAKI[2], TATSUHIRO MAEDA[3], and TAKAO HOSHINO[3]

Introduction

Bromodeoxyuridine (BUdR) and iododeoxyuridine (IUdR) are known to be incorporated into cellular DNA during DNA synthesis, and can be recognized by immunohistochemical or immunofluorescent techniques utilizing anti-BUdR or anti-IUdR monoclonal antibodies [1–4]. Recently, two new monoclonal antibodies were developed by Vanderlaan *et al.*: Br-3[5], which recognizes only BUdR, and IU-4[6], which recognizes both BUdR and IUdR. By administering IUdR and BUdR at different time sequences, it is possible to determine not only the S-phase fraction but also to measure the rate of cell cycle progression and thus calculate the duration of S-phase, the cell cycle time or growth fraction of an individual tumor from a single tumor biopsy. This report describes double-labeling and staining techniques for estimating the duration of S-phase and the doubling time of biopsied materials.

Materials and Methods

In Vitro Labeling

Patients with malignant brain tumors (one metastatic lung carcinoma and one medulloblastoma) were each given an intravenous injection of 200 mg/m^2 BUdR preoperatively [4]. The biopsied tumors were immediately minced into 2–3 mm pieces and incubated in a complete medium containing 100 μM IUdR under 3 atmospheric pressure of carbogen (95% O_2, 5% CO_2) for 1 h [7]. Then, the specimens were rinsed, fixed with 70% ethanol, and embedded in paraffin.

[1] Department of Neurosurgery and [2] FCM Analysis Room, National Cancer Center, Chuo-Ku, Tokyo, 104 Japan
[3] Department of Neurosurgery, Kyorin University School of Medicine, Mitaka, Tokyo, 181 Japan

In Situ Labeling

Two patients with glioblastomas each received an intravenous injection of IUdR (200 mg/m^2) 2 h before another injection of BUdR (200 mg/m^2) prior to surgery. Biopsied materials were fixed with 70% ethanol and embedded in paraffin.

Immunohistochemistry

The 5 µm-thick sections prepared from the paraffin blocks were deparaffinized with xylene and rehydrated in 100% ethanol and phosphate buffered saline (PBS). After blocking endogenous peroxidase with 0.3% H_2O_2, they were incubated in 4N HCI for 10 min to denature DNA. They were then reacted with a 1:2000 dilution of anti-BUdR monoclonal antibody (Br-3, Caltag Lab., Inc., San Francisco), and stained with avidin-biotin complex method (ABC) (Vectorstain ABC kit, Vector Laboratories, Burlingame, Calif.). The slides stained by the ABC method were incubated with 5% acetic acid overnight to remove the excessive Br-3. They were rinsed with Tris HCI buffer solution (TBS), reacted with a 1:5000 dilution of anti-IUdR monoclonal antibody (IU-4, Caltag Lab., Inc.), and stained with the alkaline phosphatase-anti-alkaline phosphatase (APAAP) method (Universal DAKO APAAP kit, DAKO Corporation, Santa Barbara, Calif.) using a fast blue BB base. Thus, the cells labeled only with IUdR were stained blue and those labeled with BUdR or with BUdR and IUdR were stained either brown or brown against a blue background [8,9]. Several kinds of double-staining methods were also tried: APAAP using cobalt for BUdR, APAAP using fast red or fast blue for IUdR, and immunogold silver staining (AuroProbe LM GAM IgG kit, Janssen Life Science Products, Piscataway, NJ) for BUdR and APAAP using fast red dye for IUdR.

Estimation of the Duration of S-phase, Turnover Time, and Potential Doubling Time

The doubly stained slides were analyzed to determine the ratio of BUdR-positive (stained brown) or only IUdR-positive (stained blue) cells. When stained by immunogold silver/APAAP with the fast red technique or APAAP with cobalt/APAAP with the fast red technique, IUdR-labeled nuclei were stained red while BUdR-labeled nuclei showed black reaction products on the nuclei. The duration of S-phase (Ts) was estimated from the following equation [9]: $Ts = t/\partial S$, where t is the interval between administration of IUdR and BUdR, and ∂S is the fraction of S-phase cells that entered or left the S-phase during time t (Fig. 1). For example, ∂S can be calculated as the number of cells stained blue/the number of cells stained brown in the double-staining method of ABC for BUdR and APAAP for IUdR. Turnover time (Tover) is the theoretical time for a given number of cells to replace their original population, and can be calculated as $100 \times Ts/BUdR\ LI$, where *LI* is percent labeling

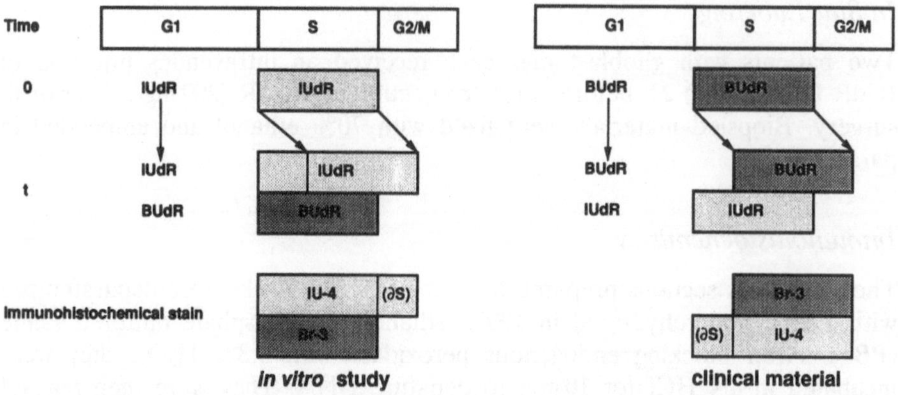

Fig. 1. Cell cycle progression during the time interval (*t*) between administration of BUdR and IUdR. *Left* Cultured cells labeled first with IUdR and then BUdR. Delta S (∂S) represents the fraction of S-phase cells that left S-phase during time *t*. *Right* Clinical materials labeled first with BUdR in situ and then with IUdR in vitro. Delta S (∂S) represents the fraction of S-phase cells that entered S-phase during time *t*

index. Potential doubling time (Tp) is the time required for a tumor to double its size in the absence of cell loss and is calculated as k × Tover, where *k* is approximately 0.7 for a tumor with an expected doubling time of over 50 h and 0.8 for expected doubling time of 30 h [11].

Results

The paraffin-embedded clinical materials labeled with IUdR and BUdR could be stained satisfactorily with ABC for BUdR and APAAP for IUdR, as well as by the immunogold silver method for BUdR and APAAP for IUdR (Fig. 2). The cells which incorporated only IUdR were clearly discriminated from the cells which incorporated BUdR. BUdR LI was 18.1% and ∂S was 0.11 in the metastatic lung cancer sample. Ts calculated from the ∂S and the interval between administration of BUdR and IUdR (1.5 h) was 17.9 h, and Tover and Tp were 4.1 days and 2.9 days, respectively. In the case of the medulloblastoma, BUdR LI was 3.33% and ∂S was 0.114. Ts calculated from the interval (1.5 h) and ∂S was 13.2 h, and Tp was 11.6 days. The BUdR LIs were 19.8% and 9.4% in the two glioblastomas, and their ∂Ss were 0.193 and 0.228. Ts and Tp were 10.5 h and 37.6 h in the former case and were 8.8 h and 65.5 h (2.7 days), respectively, in the latter case.

Discussion

Thymidine analogues such as BUdR or IUdR are incorporated into cellular DNA during DNA synthesis and can be detected rapidly by immnohistoche-

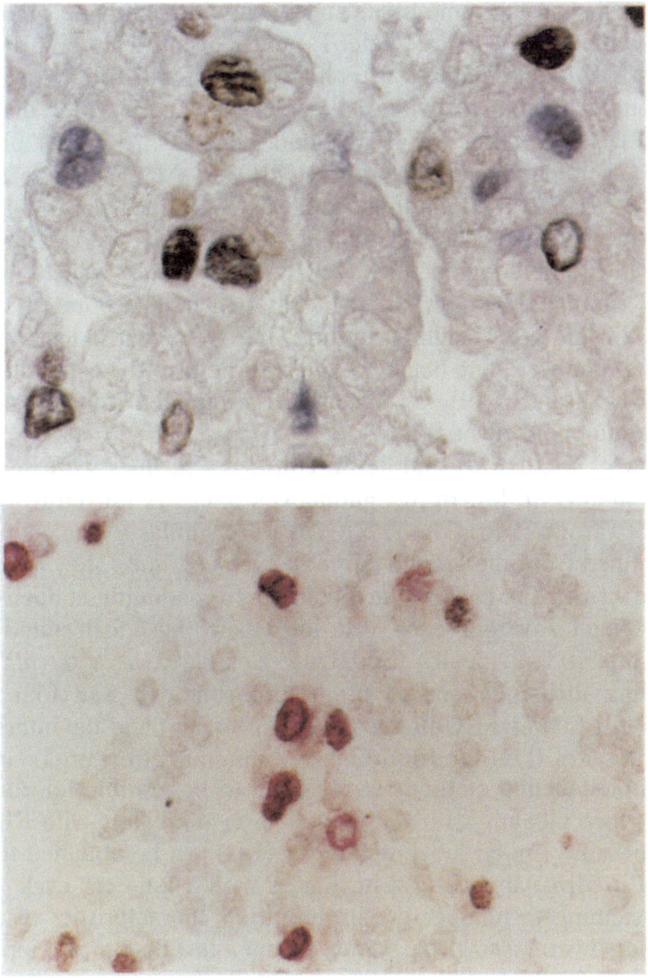

a

b

Fig. 2. **a** Photomicrograph of metastatic brain tumor from lung carcinoma stained with ABC for BUdR and with APAAP for IUdR. Nuclei stained blue indicate the cells labeled only with IUdR. Nuclei stained brown indicate the cells labeled with BUdR, × 400. **b** Photomicrograph of glioblastoma stained with immunogold silver for BUdR and APAAP using fast red for IUdR, × 400

mical staining. Measuring the percent of labeling nuclei after a pulse of these agents, the proliferative potential of individual tumors can be estimated. However, in order to characterize the growth of a tumor, other parameters such as the duration of S-phase and potential doubling time are very important for study. Double labeling with tritium and ^{14}C-thymidine has been used to analyze cell cycle progression [10]. Although the cells which incorporated tritium or ^{14}C-thymidine were clearly discriminated by their energy differences, this technique poses a radiation hazard, is laborious to perform, and is time-consuming for obtaining the results.

Double labeling of the same tissue specimen with BUdR and IUdR is quick and an efficient method to calculate Ts and Tover or Tp. We tried several combinations of double staining to enhance the visual distinction, and found that two double-staining techniques demonstrated good color discrimination for such studies: (1) ABC for BUdR and APAAP using fast blue dye for IUdR, and (2) immunogold silver for BUdR and APAAP using fast red for IUdR. In the ABC/APAAP method, the cells which incorporated BUdR were stained brown while the cells which incorporated IUdR were stained blue. In the methods of immunogold silver/APAAP, the cells which incorporated BUdR were stained black, while the cells which incorporated IUdR were stained red. In the latter staining method, the reaction products by immunogold silver staining were fine black granules, therefore, the cells which incorporated both BUdR and IUdR were clearly discriminated from the cells stained only with immunogold silver (Fig. 2).

Calculation of Ts, Tover, and Tp in cultured cell lines were reported previously by Shibui *et al.* [8]. In five glioma cell lines, Ts ranged from 8 to 13 h, and Tp ranged from 26 to 33 h. These Tps were similar to the actual doubling times determined from the growth curve of each cell line. They concluded that the standard errors for each value obtained from doubly stained specimens were much smaller within each cell line than those calculated from the specimens stained individually for BUdR or IUdR. Asai *et al.* applied a double-labeling technique on rat brain tumor model, and found that the sequence (IUdR first and BUdR second or vice versa) and the interval (2–3 h) of administration of IUdR and BUdR had a minimal effect on Ts and Tp [9].

These double-labeling methods were found to be feasible for clinical investigations. In vitro labeling with IUdR after in vivo labeling with BUdR is also applicable, because similar labeling indexes (LIs) can be obtained from in vivo labeling and in vitro labeling [12] in tumors with a long cell-cycle time. With our double-staining technique, the proliferation characteristics of the tumors can be estimated from a single specimen within a few days after biopsy, and the information obtained can be used to predict the prognosis and to select the treatment for individual patients.

Acknowledgments. This work was supported in part by a grant-in-aid for cancer research from the Ministry of Health and Welfare (2–14) and Scientific Research (A) 0240458 from the Ministry of Education, Science, and Culture of Japan.

References

1. Dolbeare F, Gratzner HG, Pallavicini MG, Gray JW (1983) Flow cytometric measurement of total DNA and incorporated bromodeoxyuridine. Proc Natl Acad Sci USA 80:5573-5577

2. Gratzner HG (1982) Monoclonal antibody to 5-bromo- and 5-iododeoxyuridine: A new reagent for detection of DNA replication. Science 218:474–475
3. Gray JW, Mayall BH (1986) Monoclonal antibodies against bromodeoxyuridine. Alan R. Liss, New York
4. Hoshino, T, Nagashima T, Cho KG, Murovic JA, Hodes JE, Wilson CB, Edwards MSB, Pitts LH (1986) S-phase fraction of human brain tumors *in situ* measured by uptake of bromodeoxyuridine. Int J Cancer 38:369–374
5. Dolbeare F, Kuo WL, Vanderlaan M, Gray JW (1988) Cell cycle analysis by flow cytometric analysis of the incorporation of iododeoxyuridine (IdUrd) and bromodeoxyuridine (BrdUrd). Proc Am Assoc Cancer Res 29:1896
6. Vanderlaan M, Watkins B, Thomas C, Dolbeare F, Stanker L (1986) Improved high-affinity monoclonal antibody to iododeoxyuridine. Cytometry 4:499–507
7. Sasaki K (1977) Measurement of tritiated thymidine labeling index by incubation *in vitro* of surgically removed cervical cancer. Jpn J Cancer Research 68:307–313
8. Shibui S, Hoshino T, Vanderlaan M, Gray JW (1989) Double labeling with iodo- and bromodeoxyuridine for cell kinetic studies. J Histochem Cytochem 37: 1007–1011
9. Asai A, Shibui S, Barker M, Vanderlaan M, Gray JW, Hoshino T (1990) Cell kinetics of 9L brain tumors determined by double labeling with iodo- and bromodeoxyuridine. J Neurosurg 73: 254–258
10. Hoshino T, Barker M, Wilson CB, Boldrey EB, Fewer, D (1968) Cell kinetics of human gliomas. J Neurosurg 37:15–26
11. Steel GG (1968) Cell loss from experimental tumors. Cell Tissue Kinet 1:193–207
12. Riccardi A, Danova M, Wilson G, Ucci G, Dormer P, Mazzini G, Brugnatelli S, Girino M, McNally NJ, Ascari E (1988) Cell kinetics in human malignancies studied with *in vitro* administration of bromodeoxyuridine and flow cytometry. Cancer Res 48:6238–6245

Heterogeneous Cell Growth in Human Brain Tumors; an Analysis of the BrdU-Labeling Index and the NOR Histogram

Toshiki Yoshimine, Koji Tokiyoshi, Motohiko Maruno, Akira Murasawa, Hiroyuki Nakata, and Toru Hayakawa[1]

Introduction

Nucleolar organizer regions (NORs) are segments of DNA which encode ribosomal RNA (rRNA) and form loops within the nucleoli of cells [1]. Recently, many pathologists have begun to pay much attention to this region since the acidic proteins bound here can be visualized with the silver colloidal technique on histologic sections [2,3], and their increase in number seems to be related to the malignancy of tumors [1,4]. In order to study the significance of the number of silver-stained regions (AgNORs) in the evaluation of tumor malignancy, the AgNOR count per cell and the bromodeoxyuridine labeling index (BrdU LI) have been compared in human brain tumors [5,6]. These studies demonstrated a linear relationship between these two parameters in meningiomas [5] and in glial tumors [6]. On a cytological basis, however, evidence that indicates a direct connection between the increased AgNOR count and the cellular proliferative activity are not yet clear. Therefore, in the present study, we tried to re-evaluate the implications of AgNOR count in brain tumors, especially in relation to the growth activity of the cells. Special attention was paid to whether or not the AgNOR histogram may change in accordance to the regional heterogeneity of the BrdU LI, which is noted in human as well as in experimental brain tumors [7].

Materials and Methods

Twenty surgical specimens of brain tumors and of infarcted brain tissues were fixed in either formalin or ethanol and embedded in paraffin. When malignant glial tumors were suspected before surgery, 10 mg/kg of BrdU (Takeda Chemical Industry, Ltd., Osaka) were administered intravenously 1–3 h before tumor removal. Three serial sections of 6 μm thickness were stained for hematoxylin-eosin, for avidin biotin peroxidase-complex (ABC) method with antibody to

[1]Department of Neurosurgery, Osaka University Medical School, Fukushima, Osaka, 553 Japan

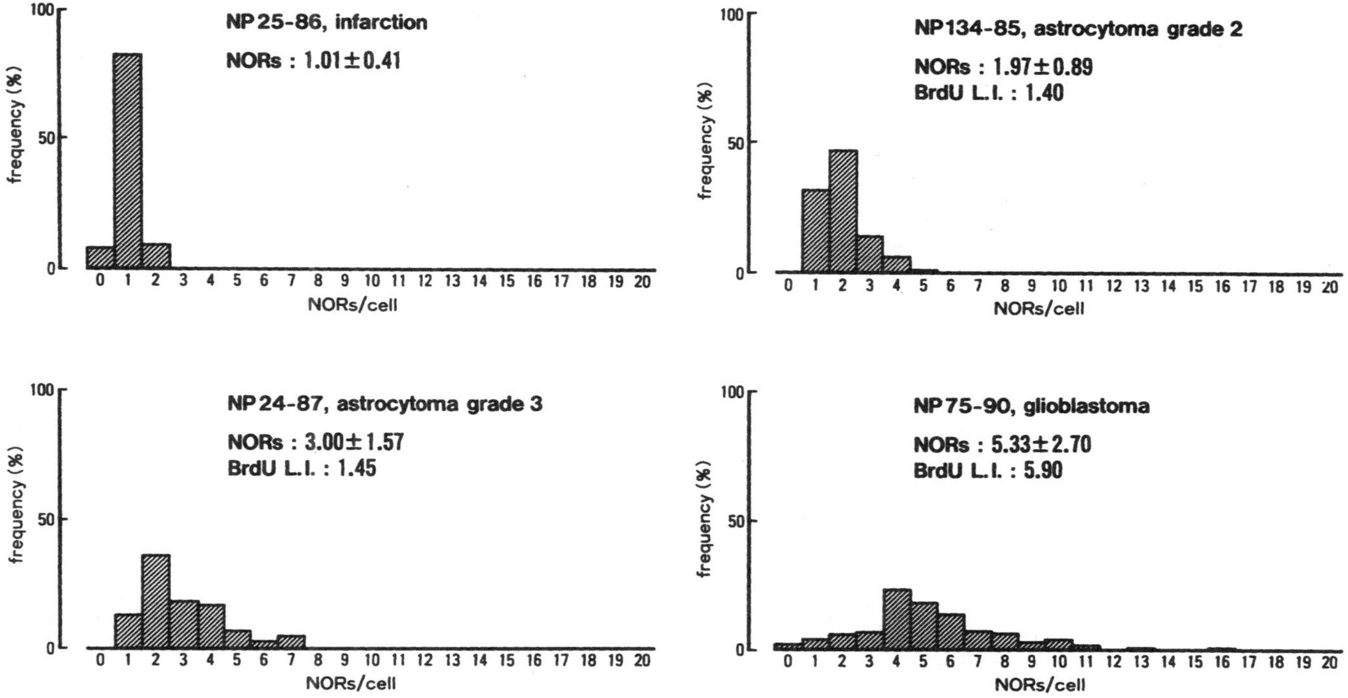

Fig. 1. AgNOR histograms of infarcted brain and astrocytic tumors with various degrees of malignancy. In tumors, the number of AgNORs increased as the histologic grade and the BrdU LI were increased

BrdU [7], and for the silver-colloidal technique [2]. The number of cellular AgNORs was counted in various areas, each of which contained 200 cells, and the frequency of AgNORs per cell was analyzed with a histogram. The number of BrdU-positive cells per 100 background cells was expressed as BrdU LI (%).

In order to evaluate the relationship between cell proliferation and the AgNOR count in vitro, the growth of T98G human glioma cells were suppressed by x-irradiation with a single dose of 20 Gy, and the BrdU LI and AgNOR count were examined 24 h later.

Results

Most of the normally looking neurons or non-neoplastic astrocytes had only one or two large AgNORs, while astrocytoma cells contained AgNORs which were smaller in size and greater in number. Grossly, the number of AgNORs increased as the malignancy of tumors increased (Fig. 1). In a few cases of glioblastomas with focal necrosis, the frequency of BrdU-positive cells differed significantly from region to region. Therefore, we examined several different areas of the specimen in one case of glioblastoma (NP75–90). The BrdU LI of tissue closer (0–1 mm) to the surface of the tumor was very high (10.4%), but that of deeper (1–2 mm) tissue was very low (1.3%). When the AgNOR counts were obtained from the corresponding areas on the adjacent section, the difference was less significant, giving mean AgNOR counts of 6.37 ± 2.89 and 4.14 ± 2.10 per cell, respectively (Fig. 2). Similarly, the BrdU LI of areas adjacent to (0–200 μm) and remote from (200–400 μm) a small intratumoral vessel were significantly different (11.0% and 4.5%, respectively), while the AgNOR histograms were grossly similar, giving mean AgNOR counts of 8.07 ± 3.08 and 7.64 ± 2.70 per cell, respectively (Fig. 2). In T98G cells, the BrdU LI of irradiated cells was very low (0.3%) compared to non-irradiated cells (13.9%), but the AgNOR counts were not significantly different (Fig. 3).

Discussion

Since NORs are located on each of the short arms of chromosomes 13, 14, 15, 21, and 22 in mammalian cells, normal cells theoretically contain 10 regions during the G_0 to G_1 phase and 20 regions after DNA duplication (S phase). Practically, however, only one or two AgNORs can be demonstrated in most normal cells. A tight aggregation of AgNORs may hinder fine discrimination of each AgNOR on histologic sections [4]. In the tumor cells, the number of AgNORs tended to increase. This increase in AgNOR count could be explained by the following possibilities: (1) nucleoli are dispersed throughout the cell nucleus in the actively proliferating tumors, which leads to easier discrimination of each AgNOR, (2) a defect in nucleolar association results in AgNOR dispersion, (3) increased cell ploidy leads to a real increase in AgNOR-bearing chromosomes, or (4) increased transcriptional activity may result in prominence of otherwise inconspicuous AgNORs [4]. Thus, the in-

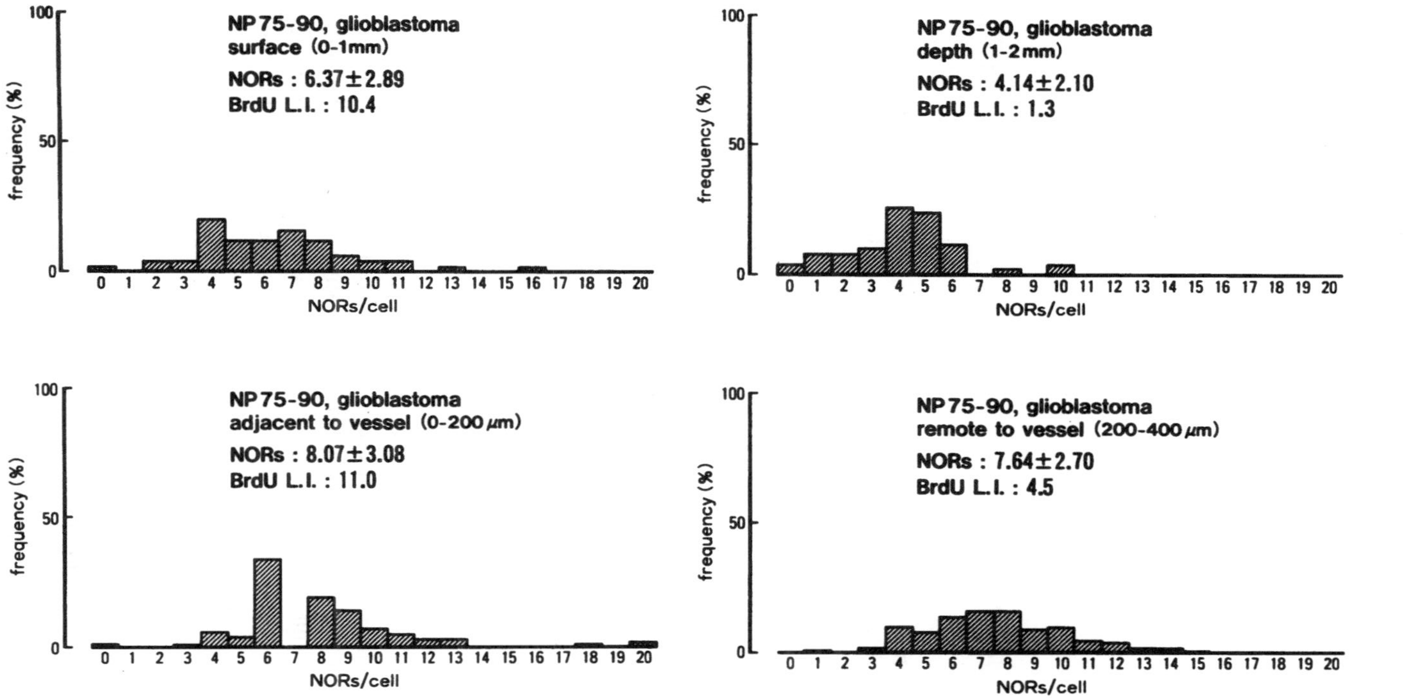

Fig. 2. AgNOR histograms of different areas of a specimen of a glioblastoma. The regional BrdU LI is significantly decreased in areas remote from the surface of the tumor or remote from the intratumoral small vessel, while the AgNOR histogram was not significantly changed

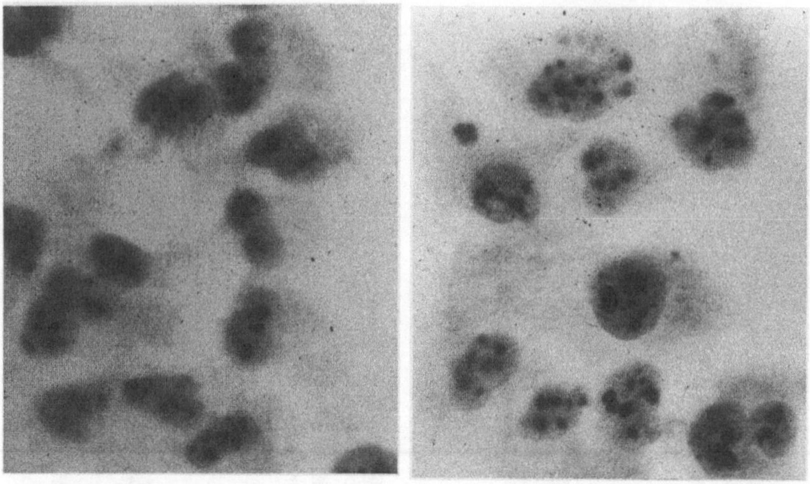

Fig. 3. Although x-irradiaiton nearly completely suppressed the proliferation of T98G cells, the AgNOR counts of irradiated cells (*right*) and non-irradiated cells (*left*) were similar

creased AgNOR count may be related in part to the increased proliferative activity of tumors. Our present study, however, demonstrated an evolution of discrepancy between those two parameters in tumors with regional heterogeneity of proliferative activity. These results contrasted with those in the previous papers that demonstrated a linear relationship between the AgNOR count and the BrdU LI [5,6]. Commonly, the BrdU LI of given tumors is obtained from areas with most typical, i.e., most malignant-looking, histology. In the present study, however, we paid special attention to areas with an unusually low BrdU LI within the tumor; a marked decrease in the BrdU LI was observed in areas with possible hypoxia or hyponutrition, but the AgNOR count was not significantly decreased. In vitro study with T98G glioma cells demonstrated that the AgNOR count was not affected in spite of nearly complete cessation of cell proliferation after irradiation. Thus, the number of AgNORs does not always reflect the proliferative activity of the tumor cells. We speculated that the increased number of AgNORs is more likely an expression of inherent malignancy of tumor cells, rather than the indicator of the proliferative activity itself.

Conclusion

The AgNOR count tended to increase as the malignancy of gliomas increased. Regional heterogeneity in the proliferative activity of tumor cells was, however, demonstrated by the BrdU LI in a case of glioblastoma, in which the AgNOR histogram was not changed significantly. Those results suggested that the increased AgNOR count seems to be an expression of the inherent malignancy of tumor cells rather than an absolute indicator of activated cell proliferation.

References

1. Crocker J, Nar Paramjit (1987) Nucleolar organizer regions in lymphomas. J Pathol 151:111–118
2. Howell WH, Black DA (1980) Controlled silver-staining of nucleous organizer regions with a protective colloidal developer: A 1-step method. Experimentia 36:1014–1016
3. Ploton D, Menager M, Jeannesson P, Himber G, Pigeon F, Adnet JJ (1986) Improvement in the staining and in the visualization of the argyrophilic proteins of the nucleolar organizer region at the optimal level. Histochem J 18:5–14
4. Underwood JCE, Giri DD (1988) Nucleolar organizer regions as diagnostic discriminants for malignancy (editorial). J Pathol 155:95–96.
5. Orita T, Kajiwara K, Nishizaki T, Ikeda N, Kamiryo T, Aoki H (1990) Nucleolar organizer regions in meningioma. Neurosurg 26:43–46
6. Kajiwara K, Nishizaki T, Orita T, Nakayama H, Aoki H, Ito H (1990) Silver colloid staining technique for analysis of glioma malignancy. J Neurosurg 73:113–117
7. Yoshimine T, Ushio Y, Hayakawa T, Takemoto O, Maruno M, Mogami H (1986) Growth activity of tumors at different intracranial structures, immunohistochemical study with bromodeoxyuridine. Acta Neuropathol (Berl) 71:15–18

Nucleolar Organizer Regions in Cultured Brain Tumor Cells

Tetsuya Shiraishi[1], Kazuo Tabuchi[1], Toshihiro Mineta[1], Nobuaki Momozaki[1], Masashi Takagi[1], and Keith L. Black[2]

Introduction

Nucleolar organizer regions (NORs), segments of ribosomal DNA (rDNA) which transcribe to ribosomal RNA (rRNA), contribute to the regulation of cellular protein synthesis [1]. Since NORs-associated proteins are argyrophilic, recent modification of a silver staining technique makes it possible for NORs to be visualized (AgNORs) in chromosomal preparations and conventional paraffin sections [2]. We have proposed that the number and size of AgNORs correlate with cellular activity in general and may be indicators of the degree of proliferative potential or malignancy of human brain tumors [3,4].

It has been reported that cellular differentiation related to NOR activity in leukemic cells [5] as well as the number and location of NORs were changed during a cell cycle in lymphocytes [6]. The present study was performed to determine the location of AgNORs during the cell cycle and to investigate the activity of the AgNORs following treatment with differentiating agents. NORs are located on the five acrocentric chromosome pairs [7]. However, NORs in abnormal locations (ectopic NORs) have been reported in human testicular tumors [8]. We also examined the expression of NORs in the chromosomes of human brain tumor cultured cells.

Materials and Methods

Cell Culture

C6 rat glioma cells were maintained in a monolayer culture in an F-12 medium (Gibco Laboratories, Grand Island, N.Y.) supplemented with 10% heat-inactivated calf serum (Gibco), penicillin, and streptomycin (Gibco) in humidified 5% CO_2/95% air at 37°C. The culture medium was replaced with fresh

[1] Department of Neurosurgery, Saga Medical School, Saga, 849 Japan
[2] Division of Neurosurgery, University of California at Los Angeles, School of Medicine, Los Angeles, CA 90024-1761, USA

material every 3 days. Experiments were started from the exponential phase stocks.

Treatment of Cells

Differentiation. Exponentially growing cells were treated in the medium with 1.0 mM of dibutyryl cyclic AMP (dBcAMP, Sigma) for 48 h.

Cell Cycle Study. Cells in the G_1 phase were estimated by their transition into the G_1 phase after mitotic selection (shaking method). After the medium was centrifuged, the cell pellets were incubated for 2 h (early G_1 phase) or 6 h (late G_1 phase). Exponentially growing cells were treated in the medium with 0.5 mg/ml aphidicholin (Sigma) for 24 h (S phase). After incubation with a chemical-free medium for 2, 4, and 6 h (G_2 phase), AgNORs staining was performed. Mitotic cells were distinguished from the cells in the interphase on the basis of the difference in chromatic structure observed under a microscope.

AgNORs Staining

The cells were detached from the surface of culture flasks with phosphate buffered saline (PBS) containing 0.25% trypsin and 0.2% EDTA and plated on Lab Tek chamber slides (Nunc, Inc., Naperville, Ill., USA) at a concentration of 2×10^5 cells/well. After several treatments, chamber slides were fixed with 10% neutral buffered formalin. The AgNORs staining was carried out by the one-step method of Howell and Black [2]. Briefly, a colloidal developer solution (freshly made each time) consisting of one volume of 2% gelatin in 1% aqueous formic acid and two volumes of 50% aqueous silver nitrate solution were reacted on the surface of the sections for 60 min under safelight conditions at room temperature. The sections were washed with deionized water and dehydrated in ascending ethanol concentrations. The sections were immersed in xylene and mounted in a synthetic medium. No counterstain was applied.

About 200 nuclei were examined using a ×100 oil immersion objective lens. Multiple regions from each section were examined. The silver-stained dots were counted and the mean number of AgNORs per nucleus was determined for each case. Careful focusing was used for visualization all of the AgNORs in a nucleus.

Chromosomal Analysis

In order to obtain cells in metaphase from established glioma cell lines and primary cultured tumor cells, the cells were incubated in Eagle's minimum essential medium (MEM) containing 0.5 µg/ml of Colcemid (Sigma) for 6 h. After hypotonic treatment (0.56% KCl) and triple fixation (3:1 methanol-acetic acid), slides were made and flame-dried. AgNORs staining was performed on the slides which were then rinsed several times in distilled water and counterstained with Giemsa solution for 2–3 min.

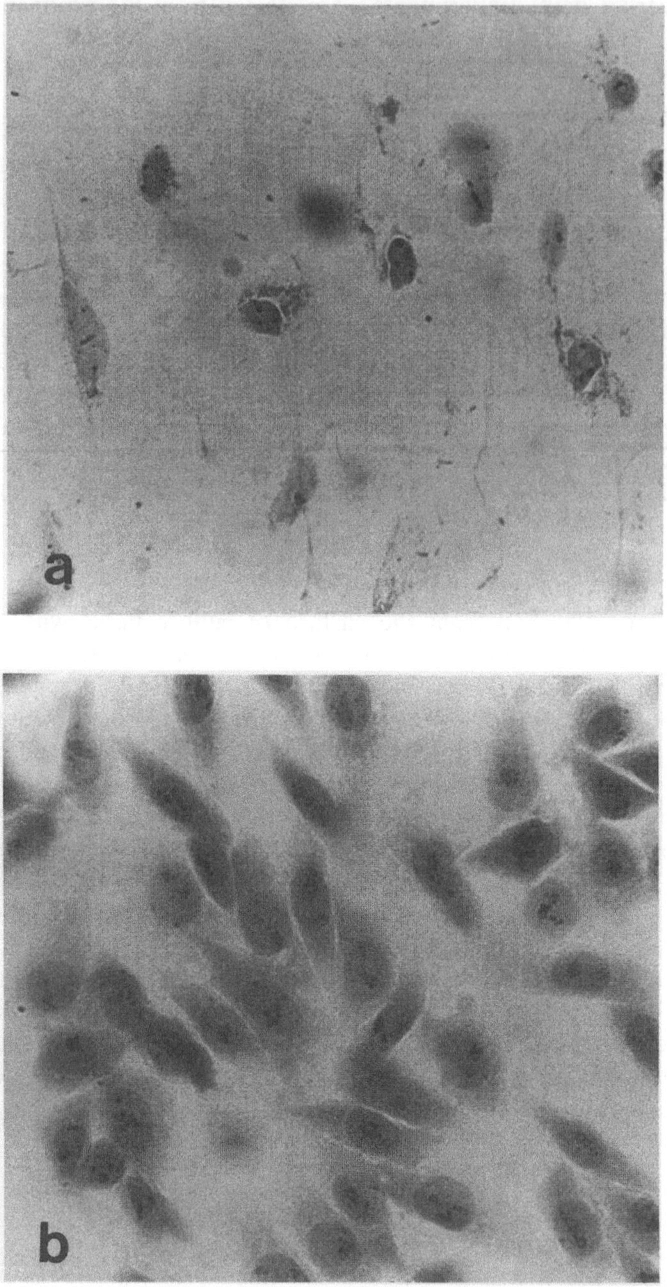

Fig. 1. AgNORs staining of C6 cell (× 400). **a** Exponentially growing C6 cells demonstrated a mean AgNORs number of 5.3. AgNORs were located on the center of nucleus and small granules aggregated to one large nucleolus. **b** Bipolar cells with long processes were increased in number in the dBcAMP treated cells. The mean AgNORs number is 3.1 and the size of each granules were small. They were located on the peripheral side of nucleus

Results

Effect of Differentiating Agents on AgNORs Activity

Exponentially growing C6 cells demonstrated a mean AgNORs number of 5.3. AgNORs were located on the center of the nucleus and small granules aggregated to one large nucleolus (Fig. 1a). Bipolar cells with long processes were increased in number in the dBcAMP-treated cells (Fig. 1b). The mean AgNORs number was 3.1 and the size of each of the granules was small. They were located on the peripheral side of the nucleus.

Cell Cycle Study

Schematic illustration of the AgNORs during various cell cycle phases observed in cultured C6 cells are shown in Fig. 2. Postmitotic daughter nuclei displayed compact large AgNORs. Two, four, and six h after M-phase synchronization (G_1 phase), the cells demonstrated a mean AgNORs number of 5.8, 5.2, and 4.3 per nucleus, respectively, in a clustered distribution. Following 0, 2, and 6 h S-phase synchronization by incubation with aphidicholin, the cells demonstrated a mean AgNORs number of 4.2, 5.4, and 5.5 per nucleus, respectively. They were located on the center of the nucleus. In the M phase, each AgNOR was generally small in size and scattered throughout the chromosome.

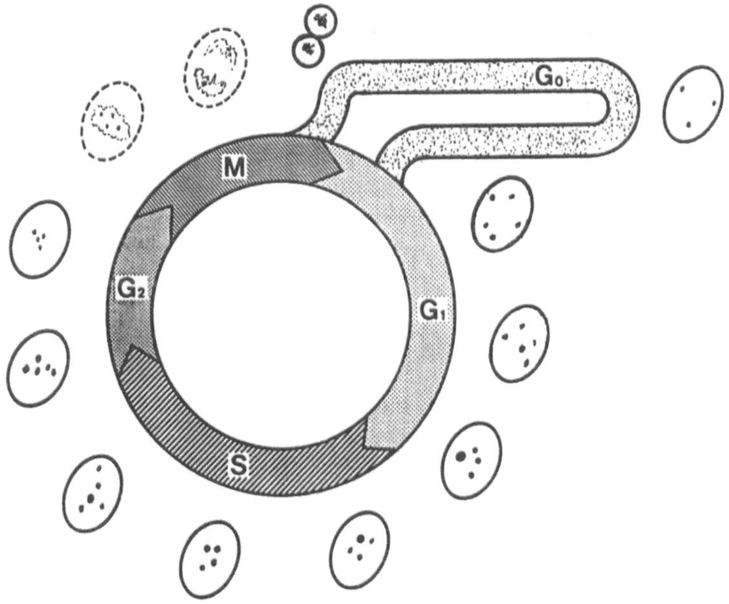

Fig. 2. Schematic illustration of the AgNORs during various cell cycle phases observed in cultured C6 cells

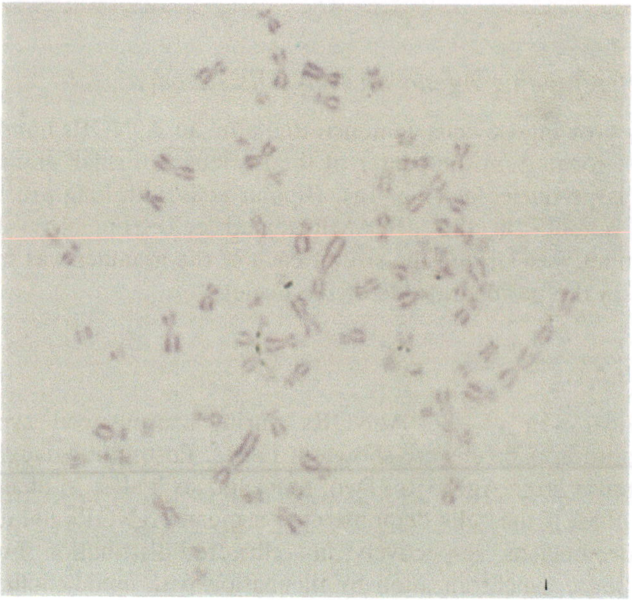

Fig. 3. Silver-stained human metaphase chromosomes from T-98G glioma cell line (× 1,000). AgNORs appear as *black dots* above the satellite stalks of the short arms of the acrocentric chromosomes

Chromosome Analysis

In chromosomal preparations, all cultured cells except for T-98G expressed 5–8 AgNORs on the acrocentric chromosomes. T-98G glioma cells expressed 12 AgNORs and 3 constant ectopic AgNORs (Fig. 3). These ectopic sites were located near the centromere of A-, B-, and C-group-sized chromosomes (Fig. 4). Abstracts of karyotypes and AgNORs of the cultured cells are shown in Table 1.

Discussion

Nucleolar Organizer Regions and NOR-Associated Proteins

The nucleolus is a subcellular organelle producing ribosomal RNA (rRNA) and is composed of three components, the fibrillar center, the dense fibrillar component, and the granular component. [1] Of these components, the fibrillar centers are the so-called "nucleolar organizer regions" (NORs) which consists of loops of DNA transcribing to 18S and 28S rRNA subunits by RNA polymerase I [1,9].

Several proteins, such as RNA polymerase I [10], C_{23} protein (nucleolin) [11], B_{23} protein [12], 100 K protein [13], and 80 K protein [14] are thought to be NORs-associated proteins. They act as regulators of ribosomal DNA

Table 1. Abstracts of karyotypes and AgNORs of the cultured cells

Cell line	Origin	No. of cells counted	Modal no. of chromosomes	Modal no. of D + G group	Modal no. of AgNORs	Ectopic AgNORs
A172	Glioblastoma	20	81	15	8	Often (B**,E)
T98G	Glioblastoma	30	130	22	12	Constant (A,B,C)
GM-1	Glioblastoma, P*	25	44	9	6	Often (A)
ME-1	Meningioma, P	20	43	8	7	None
ME-2	Meningioma, P	24	46	9	6	None
ME-3	Meningioma, P	20	44	9	7	Often (B)

**P*, primary culture; ***B*, B-group sized chromosomes

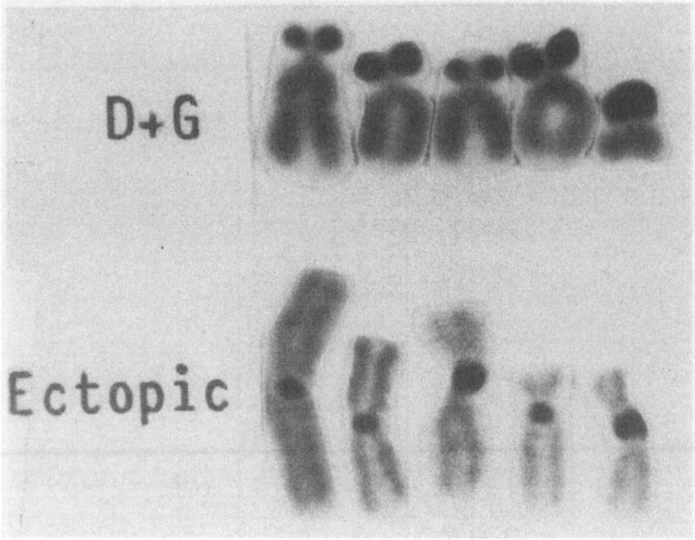

Fig. 4. Ectopic AgNORs were located near the centromere of A-, B-, and C-group-sized chromosomes. AgNORs and Giemsa stain × 1,000

(rDNA) [15] and maintain the extended configuration of rDNA [16]. They have carboxyl- and sulphur-containing groups that are of essential importance in the reactions of the AgNORs [17]. These proteins are present on only transcribed units but not on non-transcribed spacer regions [18].

AgNORs and Cellular Activity

The exact significance of changes in the number and distribution of AgNORs is not fully understood. However, since NORs are transcribed to ribosomal RNA and thus ultimately to ribosomes and finally to protein, it has been speculated that an increased number of AgNORs might reflect an increased rDNA transcriptional activity or potential [19] and is thought to indicate increased nucleolar and cellular activities [6,20].

Some hormones such as the thyroid hormone [21], the growth hormone and steroids [22] trigger NOR activity and increase AgNORs numbers. Phytohemagglutinin-stimulated lymphocytes [6] and rapidly growing fibroblasts contain more AgNORs than nonstimulated cells [23].

Cellular differentiation has been related to NOR activity in the HL 60 human promyelocytic leukemic cell line [5] and in erythroid cells [24]. The gradual decrease in the number of NORs is apparently related to the decrease of nucleolar RNA synthesis in differentiating and maturing blood cells. We also observed a decreased number of AgNORs in differentiated C6 cells treated in dBcAMP. The number of NORs may be related to malignant cell differentiation.

AgNOR numbers are affected by aging. Das *et al.* [20] showed that the numbers of AgNORs in PHA-stimulated human peripheral blood lymphocytes were diminished in elderly individuals compared to newborns and neonates. It has been suggested that the decrease in Ag staining was due to an age-dependent irreversible repression of rDNA [25].

AgNORs and Cell Cycle

It mitosis, the nucleolus diminishes in size and is invisible in the prophase. Then, in the telophase, the fibrillar component becomes apparent [26]. In the interphase, the fibrillar centers are equivalent to NORs. The numbers of fibrillar centers in a cell nucleus might be expected to be related to the numbers of chromosomes possessing NORs. Field *et al.* [6] have reported that the cell phase was related to the size and position of the NORs, as was the number of divisional generations. Resting (G_0) lymphocytes had a single argyrophilic nucleolar area. This became enlarged in the G_1 phase, sometimes accompanied by smaller associated granules. In the first generation in culture, this pattern persisted in the S and G_2 phases. However, in the second and third generation divisions, multiple smaller granules appeared.

Our findings showed that in the M phase small AgNORs were scattered throughout the chromosome. In the interphase, approximately 4–6 AgNORs tended to be located on the central (S and G_2 phase) and on the peripheral (G_1 phase) side of the nucleus. However, it is difficult to distinguish cell cycles by the number and distribution of the AgNORs.

AgNORs on Chromosomes

NORs are located on the satellite stalks of short arms (secondary constriction regions) of the five acrocentric chromosome pairs (Nos. 13, 14, 15, 21, and 22) in human diploid cells [7,27,28]. The five acrocentric chromosomes together contain approximately 200 rRNA gene copies [29].

The amount of rDNA is highly variable from chromosome to chromosome and from individual to individual [30,31]. These variations probably result from the unequal crossing-over or duplication. Unusually large-sized short arms with dupliate and triplicate NORs and/or satellites have been reported [32]. It has been reported that each individual has a characteristic pattern and model number of AgNORs which are inherited from generation to generation [33].

NOR activity will be influenced by somatic chromosomal changes. Increased rDNA has been detected biochemically in the trisomy 21 [29]. A specific chromosome, 14p+, has been noted in a human family, which has 6–8 times more rDNA than the normal 14 chromosome [30].

The nucleolar abnormalities in malignant cells probably reflect modifications in rRNA activity which influences the metabolic rate and growth of malignant cells. There have been several reports and descriptions of abnormal NORs in malignant cells. Crossen and Godwin [34] described rearrangement and amplification of rRNA genes in the chronic myeloid leukemia cell line, K562.

Cytogenic studies showed ectopic AgNORs or unusual AgNORs patterns in certain malignancies [8,35]. DeLozier-Blanchet *et al.* [8] have identified qualitative abnormalities in chromosomal preparations from malignant testicular tumors, with AgNORs residing on chromosomes that normally do not contain AgNORs. Such heterotopic AgNORs may result from translocations or derepression of previously existing but inactive NOR sites on nonacrocentric chromosomes.

Our findings showed that cultured brain tumor cells, except for T-98G, expressed 5–8 AgNORs on acrocentric chromosomes. T-98G glioma cells possessed increased numbers of AgNORs on chromosomes. Except for T-98G cells, the number of AgNORs was similar to that reported in normal cells in spite of their increased modal chromosome number and increased number of acrocentric chromosomes. Five out of eight cell lines demonstrated inconstant ectopic AgNORs. T-98G glioma cells have 3 constant ectopic AgNORs on chromosome and their increased AgNORs may be ascribed to these ectopic AgNORs. Such active ectopic NORs may be due to the participation of short arm acrocentric chromosomes in translations or derepression of previously existing, but inactive, NORs sites on nonacrocentric chromosomes [8]. It would be worthwhile to investigate the biological role of ectopic NORs in brain tumors.

Conclusion

A silver colloid staining technique for the demonstration of NORs-associated proteins (AgNORs) was applied to cultured brain tumor cells and to chromosomal preparations. Differentiated C6 cells treated in dBcAMP showed a decreased number of AgNORs which were located on the center of the nucleolus. In the M phase, small AgNORs were scattered throughout the chromosome. In the interphase, approximately 4–6 AgNORs tended to be located on the center (S and G_2 phase) and on the peripheral (G_1 phase) side of the nucleus. In chromosomal preparations, the cultured cells displayed 5–12 AgNORs on acrocentric chromosomes. Five out of the eight cell lines examined demonstrated ectopic AgNORs. The AgNORs method can be used as a convenient procedure for the simple evaluation of the cellular activity of cultured brain tumor cells and chromosomal changes.

Acknowledgement. We wish to thank Miss Yumiko Saho for her skillful technical assistance.

References

1. Alberts B, Bray D, Lewis J, Raff M, Roberts K, Watson JD (1989) The cell nucleus. In: Alberts B, Bray D, Lewis J, Raff M, Roberts K, Watson JD (eds) Molecular biology of the cell, 2nd edn. Garland New York, pp 541–544

2. Howell WM, Black DA (1980) Controlled silver-staining of nucleolus organizer regions with a protective colloidal developer: A 1-step method. Experientia 36:1014–1015
3. Shiraishi T, Tabuchi K, Mineta T, Momozaki N, Takagi M (1989) Analysis of proliferating potential of brain tumors by silver staining technique of the nucleolar organizer regions on paraffin sections. Igaku no Ayumi 148:125–126
4. Shiraishi T, Tabuchi K, Mineta T, Momozaki N, Takagi M. (to be published) Nucleolar organizer regions in various human brain tumors. J Neurosurg
5. Reeves BR, Casey G, Honeycombe JR, Smith S (1984) Correlation of differentiation state and silver staining of nucleolar organizers in the promyelocytic leukaemia cell line HL-60. Cancer Genet Cytogenet 13:159–166
6. Field DH, Fitzgerald PH, Sin FYT (1984) Nucleolar silver-staining patterns related to cell cycle phase and cell generation of PHA-stimulated human lymphocytes. Cytobios 41:23–33
7. Cheuug SW, Sun L, Featherstone T (1989) Visualization of NORs in relation to the precise chromosomal localization of ribosomal RNA genes. Cytogenet Cell Genet 50:93–97
8. DeLozier-Blanchet CD, Walt H, Engel E (1986) Ectopic nucleolus organizer regions (NORs) in human testicular tumors. Cytogenet Cell Genet 41:107–113
9. Fakan S, Hernandez-Verdun D (1986) The nucleolus and the nucleolar organizer regions. Biol Cell 56:189–206
10. Scheer U, Rose KM (1984) Localization of RNA polymerase I in interphase cells and mitotic chromosomes by light and electron microscopic immunocytochemistry. Proc Natl Acad Sci USA 81:1431–1435
11. Ochs RL, Busch H (1984) Further evidence that phosphoprotein C_{23} (110kD/pI5.1) is the nucleolar silver staining protein. Exp Cell Res 152:260–265
12. Lischwe MA, Smetana K, Olson MOJ, Busch H (1979) Proteins C_{23} and B_{23} are the major nucleolar silver staining proteins. Life Sci 25:701–708
13. Hernandez-Verdun D (1983) The nucleolar organizer regions. Biol Cell 49:191–202
14. Courvalin JC, Maunoury R, Hernandez-Verdun D, Maro B, Bornens M (1983) Une proteine de 80 kD est associée à l'organisateur nucléolaire (NOR) des cellules humaines. Biol Cell 49:10a
15. Olson MOJ, Thompson BA (1983) Distribution of proteins among chromatin components of nucleoli. Biochemistry 22:3187–3193
16. Hernandez-Verdun D, Derenzini M, Bouteille M (1984) Relationship between AgNOR proteins and ribosomal chromatin *in situ* during induced RNA synthesis inhibition. J Ultrastruct Mol Struct Res 88:55–65
17. Smith PJ, Skilbeck NQ, Harrison A, Crocker J (1988) The effect of a series of fixatives in the AgNOR technique. J Pathol 155:109–112
18. Angelier N, Hernandez-Verdun D, Bouteille M (1982) Visualisation of Ag-NOR proteins on nucleolar transcriptional units in molecular spreads. Chromosoma 86:661–672
19. Derenzini M, Farabegoli F, Pession A, Novello F (1987) Spatial redistribution of ribosomal chromatin in the fibrillar centers of human lymphocytes after stimulation of transcription. Exp Cell Res 170:31–41
20. Das BC, Rani R, Mitra AB, Luthra UK (1986) The number of silver-staining NORs (rDNA) in lymphocytes of newborns and its relationship to human development. Mech Ageing Dev 36:117–123
21. Zankl, H, Mayer C, Zang KD (1980) Association frequency and silver staining of nucleolus organizing regions in hyperthyroid patients. Hum Genet 54:111–114

22. de Capoa A, Baldini A, Marlekaj P, Natoli C, Rocchi M, Archidiacono N, Cianfarani S, Spasoni GL, Boscherini B (1985) Hormone-modulated rRNA gene activity is visualized by selective staining of the NOs. Cell Biol Int Rep 9:791–796
23. Schwarzacher HG, Wachtler F (1983) Nucleolus organizer regions and nucleoli. Hum Genet 63:89–99
24. Smetana K, Likovsky Z (1984) Nucleolar silver-stained granules in maturing erythroid and granulocytic cells. Cell Tissue Res 237:367–370
25. Denton TE, Liem SL, Cheng KM, Barrett JV (1981) The relationship between ageing and ribosomal gene activity in humans as evidenced by silver staining. Mech Ageing Dev 15:1–7
26. Goessens G, Thiry M, Lepoint A (1987) Relations between nucleoli and nucleolus-organizing regions during the cell cycle. In: Stahl A, Lucini JM, Vagner-Capodano AM (eds) Chromosomes today, vol 9. Allen and Unwin, London, pp 261–271
27. Henderson AA, Warburton D, Atwood KC (1972) Location of ribosomal DNA in the human chromosome complement. Proc Natl Acad Sci USA 69:3394–3398
28. Hsu TC, Spirito SE, Pardue ML (1975) Distribution of 18 + 28 S ribosomal genes in mammalian genomes. Chromosoma 53:25–36
29. Crocker J (1990) Nucleolar organizer regions. In: Underwood JCE (ed) Current topics in pathology 82. Springer, Heidelberg, pp 91–149
30. Miller DA, Breg WR, Warburton D, Dev VG, Miller OJ (1978) Regulation of rRNA gene expression in a human familial 14p+ marker chromosome. Hum Genet 43:289–297
31. Babu KA, Verma RS (1985) Structural and functional aspects of nucleolar organizer regions (NORs) of human chromosomes. Int Rev Cytol 94:151–176
32. Sofuni T, Tanabe K, Awa AA (1980) Chromosome heteromorphisms in the Japanese. II. Nucleolus organizer regions of variant chromosomes in D and G groups. Hum Genet 55:265–270
33. Taylor EF, Delcon PAM (1981) Familial silver staining patterns of human nucleolus organizer regions (NORs) Am J Hum Genet 33:67–76
34. Crossen PE, Godwin JM (1985) Rearrangement and possible amplification of the ribosomal RBA gene sites in the human chronic myelogenous leukemia cell line K562. Cancer Genet Cytogenet 18:27–30
35. Hubbel HR, Hsu TC (1977) Identification of nucleolus organizer regions (NORs) in normal and neoplastic cells by the silver-staining technique. Cytogenet Cell Genet 19:185–196

Rapid Assessment of Malignancy in Human Brain Tumors on Squash Preparations Using Nucleolar Organizer Region Staining

Akira Hara[1], Noboru Sakai[1], Shuji Nijkawa[1], Hiroshi Hirayama[1], Yasuaki Nishimura[1], Takashi Ando[1], Hiromu Yamada[1], Takuji Tanaka[2], and Hideki Mori[2]

Introduction

The intraoperative histologic diagnosis on conventional rapid frozen sections is very helpful in deciding the area to be resected during the operation of a brain tumor. However, the inadequately conserved construction of frozen tissues sometimes makes the histological diagnosis difficult. Therefore, the development of new convenient methods that can assist the rapid diagnosis of brain tumors and the estimation of their proliferative potential, even during surgery, is needed.

Nucleolar organizer regions (NORs) have been shown to reflect the cellular proliferation or malignancy [1,2]. NORs are loops of ribosomal DNA which are present in the nucleoli. The NOR DNA possesses ribosomal RNA genes which are transcribed by RNA polymerase I [3]. NORs are demonstrated by means of the argyrophilia of their associated proteins (AgNORs) such as RNA polymerase I, C23 protein [4], and B23 protein [5]. These proteins are thought to play some roles in the transcription of ribosomal RNA. Newly developed one-step silver colloid staining for NORs is simple and needs neither pretreatments nor troublesome techniques [6,7]. Recently, a number of studies analyzing the proliferative potentials using the AgNOR score in various brain tumors have been reported [6–8]. A linear correlationship between the mean number of AgNORs and the Ki-67 labeling index [6,7] or the bromodeoxyuridine (BrdU) labeling index [8] was demonstrated.

The AgNOR-staining method is usually applied to conventional formalin-fixed and paraffin-embedded sections. In the present study, we applied this method to squash preparations for brain tumors and attempted to achieve a rapid detection of the proliferative potential in neoplastic cells. The required staining time was less than 1 h.

Materials and Methods

A total of 38 specimens of tumor tissues was used for this study. These tumors included 7 meningiomas, 2 recurrent meningiomas, 1 meningeal sarcoma, 4

Departments of [1]Neurosurgery and [2]Pathology, Gifu University School of Medicine, Gifu, 500 Japan neurinomas, 7 pituitary adenomas, 1 recurrent craniopharyngioma, 2 ependymomas, 1 benign astrocytoma, 3 anaplastic astrocytomas, 5 glioblastoma multiforme, 1 adenoma of the lachrymal gland, and 4 metastatic brain tumors. These diagnoses were made on H and E-stained cryostat sections and confirmed on H and E-stained paraffin-embedded sections.

Each small (about 1 mm^3) solid specimen of fresh brain tumor was placed between two slide glasses and moderately pressed. Then, two squash preparations were provided by drawing two slides. Immediately following this, the preparations were fixed in 95% ethanol for 5 min. After being rinsed in distilled water, the specimens were stained by the one-step silver colloid method for AgNORs. The silver colloid solution for AgNOR staining was prepared by dissolving gelatin in 1% aqueous formic acid at a concentration of 2%, and this solution was mixed, 1:2 volumes, with 50% aqueous silver nitrate [1,2,6–8]. This solution was dropped over the slides which were left for about 30 min under safelight conditions at room temperature, and quickly rinsed in distilled water. No counterstaining was performed. The specimens were immersed in xylene for dehydration and mounted in a synthetic medium. The positive AgNORs were clearly present as black dots in the cell nuclei. The mean number of AgNORs in a total of 200 neoplastic cell nuclei was calculated in each case.

It was possible for the process of squashing a small piece of brain tumor between two slide glasses to be done in the operation room. The specimens were then fixed in 95% ethanol on the way from the operating room to the laboratory, where the AgNOR staining was done. The above procedure can shorten the processing time in order to provide more rapid information about AgNORs in each case.

The Student's *t*-test was used for the statistical evaluation of the data.

Results

On the squash preparations, AgNORs were clearer than those seen on the usual formalin-fixed and paraffin-embedded sections. This made it easy to count them rapidly (Fig. 1).

The mean number of AgNORs per cells in each case is shown in Table 1. The mean scores of AgNORs in various histological types of brain tumors were as follows: meningioma, 1.67; recurrent meningioma, 2.18; meningeal sarcoma, 5.66; neurinoma, 1.74; pituitary adenoma, 1.86; recurrent craniopharyngioma, 3.55; ependymoma, 2.74; benign astrocytoma, 1.84; anaplastic astrocytoma, 3.40; glioblastoma multiforme, 3.33; adenoma of the lachrymal gland, 1.71; metastatic brain tumors, 5.14. The mean AgNOR score of malignant brain tumors was 4.08 ± 1.28 (mean ±SD). The mean AgNOR score of recurrent brain tumors was 2.64 ± 0.65, and that of both malignant and recurrent brain tumors was 3.81 ± 1.31. The AgNOR score of benign brain tumors, including meningiomas, neurinomas, pituitary adenomas, benign astrocytoma, ependymomas, and adenoma of lachrymal gland, was 1.86 ±

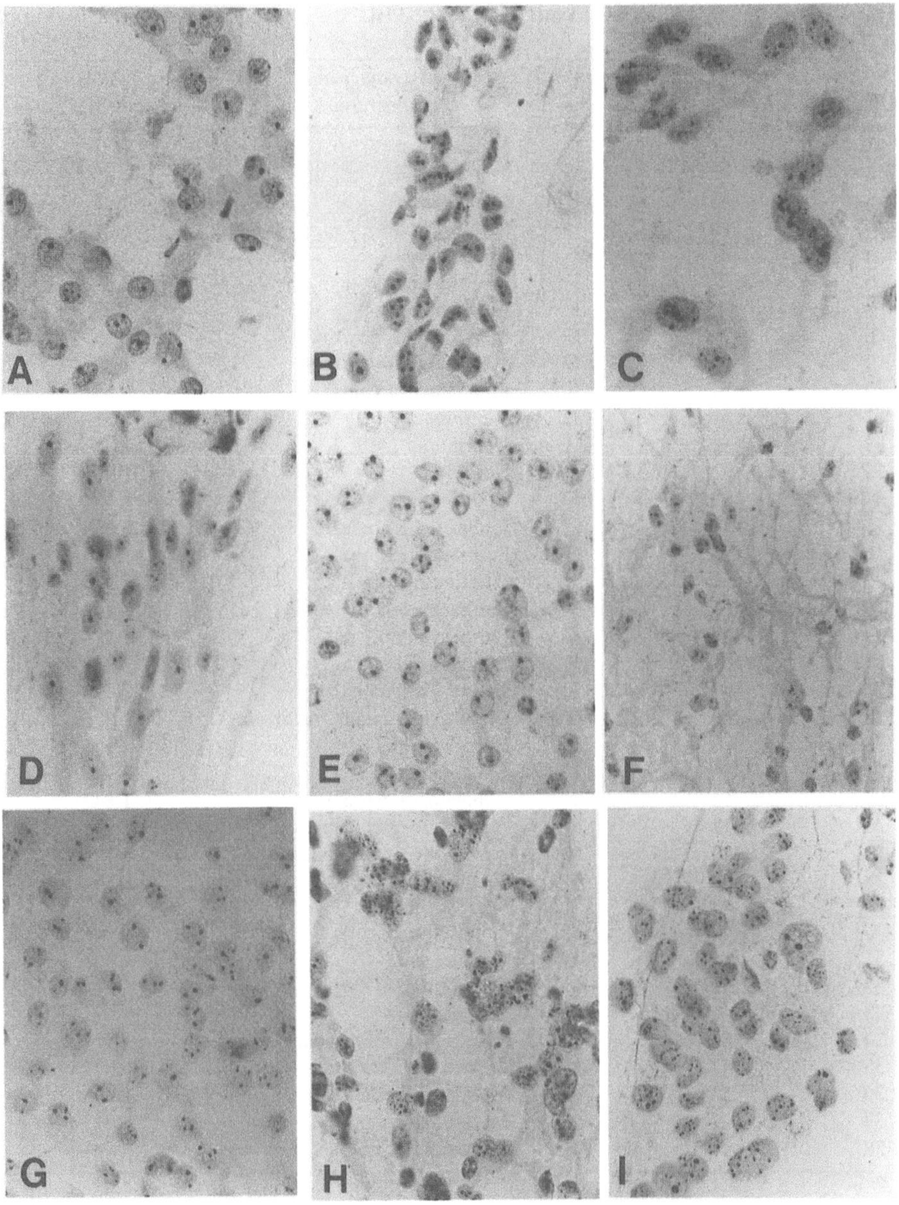

Fig. 1A-I. Photomicrographs of squash preparations of brain tumors. Silver colloid staining for AgNOR, × 500. **A** Meningioma (case 3) containing one or two AgNORs in cell nuclei. **B** Recurrent meningioma (case 9) having more AgNORs than case 3. **C** Meningeal sarcoma (case 10) containing many more AgNORs, compared with meningioma. **D** Acoustic neurinoma (case 11) containing one or two AgNORS. **E** Pituitary adenoma (case 15) containing one or two AgNORs. **F** Benign astrocytoma (case 25) containing about two AgNORs. **G** Anaplastic astrocytoma (case 26) have more AgNORs than benign astrocytoma. **H** Glioblastoma (case 31) have numerous AgNORs in cell nuclei. **I** Metastatic brain tumor (case 35) containing numerous AgNORs

Table 1. Summary of mean numbers of AgNORs on squash preparations by rapid AgNOR staining

Case	Age (years)	Sex	Histological diagnosis	Mean number of AgNORs
1	56	M	Meningioma	1.73
2	50	M	Meningioma	1.58
3	44	F	Meningioma	1.48
4	51	F	Meningioma	1.55
5	70	F	Meningioma	1.51
6	49	F	Meningioma	2.39
7	69	F	Meningioma	1.43
8	76	F	Meningioma-recurrent	2.16
9	41	F	Meningioma-recurrent	2.20
10	28	F	Meningeal sarcoma	5.66
11	34	M	Neurinoma	1.51
12	52	M	Neurinoma	1.84
13	62	F	Neurinoma	1.96
14	63	F	Neurinoma	1.63
15	58	M	Pituitary adenoma	1.66
16	75	M	Pituitary adenoma	1.74
17	64	M	Pituitary adenoma	1.49
18	66	M	Pituitary adenoma	2.14
19	57	F	Pituitary adenoma	1.92
20	61	F	Pituitary adenoma	2.22
21	50	F	Pituitary adenoma	2.02
22	25	M	Craniopharyngioma-recurrent	3.55
23	6	M	Ependymoma	2.54
24	56	F	Ependymoma	2.93
25	54	F	Benign astrocytoma	1.84
26	17	M	Anaplastic astrocytoma	3.52
27	48	M	Anaplastic astrocytoma	4.15
28	44	M	Anaplastic astrocytoma	2.53
29	73	M	Glioblastoma	2.34
30	73	M	Glioblastoma	4.01
31	54	M	Glioblastoma	4.60
32	48	M	Glioblastoma	3.01
33	62	M	Glioblastoma	2.69
34	57	M	Adenoma of lachrymal gland	1.71
35	47	M	Metastatic brain tumor	6.85
36	58	M	Metastatic brain tumor	5.43
37	47	F	Metastatic brain tumor	4.27
38	47	F	Metastatic brain tumor	3.99

0.38. The mean AgNOR scores of malignant brain tumors and that of recurrent brain tumors were significantly higher than that of benign brain tumors ($P < 0.001$ and $P < 0.02$, respectively) (Fig. 2). The mean value of both malignant and recurrent brain tumors was also significantly greater than that of benign brain tumors ($P < 0.001$).

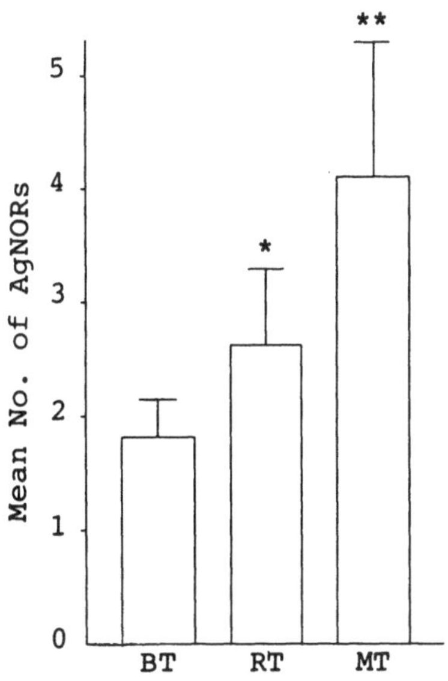

Fig. 2. Mean AgNOR scores in benign brain tumors (meningioma, neurinoma, pituitary adenoma, ependymoma, benign astrocytoma, and adenoma of lachrymal gland), recurrent brain tumors (recurrent meningioma and recurrent craniopharyngioma) and malignant brain tumors (meningeal sarcoma, anaplastic astrocytoma, glioblastoma, and metastatic brain tumor). A statistically significant difference between malignant brain tumors or recurrent brain tumors and benign brain tumors was found with $P < 0.02$(*) or $P < 0.001$(**). *BT*, benign brain tumor, *RT*, recurrent brain tumor, *MT*, malignant brain tumor

Discussion

Rapid information about the proliferative potential in brain tumors during surgery is considered to be important for deciding the area for resection. Neurosurgeons usually judge the degree of malignancy of brain tumors preoperatively by means of the data provided by the patient's past history, the findings of neurological abnormalities, image analyses such as CT-scan, MRI, angiography, and various other evaluations. Before the operation, the area to be resected is determined and the operating procedure is planned. However, according to the degree of malignancy of the brain tumors confirmed by histology on rapid frozen sections, unexpected changes in the operation procedure may occur abruptly, and precise and rapid information of whether or not the tumor is malignant or benign is required. Usually, routine stainings on cryostat sections are used for rapid diagnosis. The construction of tissues on frozen sections, however, is not always conserved satisfactorily, so that the histological diagnosis is sometimes difficult.

In the present study, rapid detection of the proliferative potential of brain tumors on silver colloid-stained squash specimens was developed and revealed to provide useful information for the assessment of malignancy in brain tumors during surgery. Our previous study demonstrated that the mean number of AgNORs in human gliomas and of the Ki-67 labeling index, which indicates the percentage of proliferating cells in all cell cycles except in the G_0 phase, were well correlated, and that both indexes reflected the histological grade [6,7]. A linear correlationship between the number of AgNORs and the bromodeoxyuridine (BrdU) labeling index, which indicates the percentage of

S-phase cells, was also demonstrated [8]. The results of the above studies and of the present study clearly indicate that the enumeration of AgNORs is useful for estimating the proliferative activity of brain tumor cells.

The major advantage of the AgNOR score for assessment of cell proliferation is that this method requires neither pretreatments nor troublesome techniques. Furthermore, this method could be applied to squash preparations with the easy and simple procedure shown in the present study. Recently, the squash preparations have been adopted for Ki-67 immunocytochemistry to assess proliferative potential [9,10]. However, the Ki-67 immunocytochemistry on squash specimens requires at least 3 h [9]. On the other hand, AgNOR staining on squash materials needs only 1 h. Thus, the present method for the estimation of the proliferative nature of neoplasms enables the surgeon to get rapid information about the malignancy of a brain tumor during the operation.

In conclusion, this convenient method can be easily performed, and provides rapid and clear information about brain tumor malignancy.

References

1. Crocker J, Nar P (1987) Nucleolar organizer regions in lymphomas. J Pathol 151:111–118
2. Hall PA, Levison DA (1990) Review: Assessment of cell proliferation in histological material. J Clin Pathol 43:184–193
3. Williams MA, Kleinschmidt JA, Krohne G, et al. (1982) Argyrophilic nuclear and nucleolar proteins of *Xenopus laevis* oocytes identified by gel electrophoresis. Exp Cell Res 137:341–351
4. Ochs RL, Busch H (1984) Further evidence that phosphoprotein C23 (110 kD/pH5.1) is in nucleolar silver staining protein. Exp Cell Res 152:260–265
5. Lische MA, Smetana K, Olson MOJ, et al. (1984) Protein C23 and B23 are the major nucleolar silver staining proteins. Life Sci 25:701–708
6. Hara A, Hirayama H, Sakai N, et al. (1990) Correlation between nucleolar organizer region staining and Ki-67 immunostaining in human gliomas. Surg Neurol 33:320–324
7. Hara A, Hirayama H, Sakai N, et al. (1991) Nucleolar organizer region scores and Ki-67 labeling index in high-grade gliomas and metastatic brain tumors. Acta Neurochir (Wien) 109:37–41
8. Kajiwara K, Nishizaki T, Orita T, et al. (1990) Silver colloid technique for analysis of glioma malignancy. J Neurosurg 73:113–117
9. Burger PC, Shibata T, Kleihues P (1986) The use of the monoclonal antibody Ki-67 in the identification of proliferating cells. Am J Surg Pathol 10:611–617
10. Ostertag CB, Volk B, Shibata T, et al. (1987) The monoclonal antibody Ki-67 as a marker for proliferating cells in stereotactic biopsies of brain tumors. Acta Neurochir (Wien) 89:117–121

A Preliminary Report on the Use of Nucleolar Organizer Regions (NORs) Counting for Improved Surgical Resection of Glioblastomas

Hideichi Takayama, Yuichi Hirose, Masahiro Toda, Yukiteru Nakano, Takeshi Kawase, Mitsuhiro Otani, Yoshihiro Ogawa, and Shigeo Toya

Introduction

Since 1982 we have tried gross total removal of gliomas when the tumor appeared as a circumscribed lesion on preoperative CT or MRI scans, using intraoperative histopathological examinations of the marginal to determine the extent of the excision. However, it is sometimes difficult to detect tumor cells among normal brain parenchyma by means of routine histological procedures. Recently, nucleolar organizer regions (NORs), chromosomal segments which transcribe to ribosomal RNA, could be visualized by a simple silver-staining method, and the number and/or intranuclear distribution of NORs have been found to be related to malignancy in gliomas [1,2]. Assessment of the number of NORs may reflect cellular activity and, possibly, proliferation, and make it possible to distinguish isolated glioma cells for normal or reactive glial elements.

The purpose of this preliminary study was to investigate the usefulness of NORs counting for the improved intraoperative identification and delineation of gliomas from adjacent normal brain tissues, in order to facilitate more complete tumor removal.

Material and Methods

Six cases of supratentorial circumscribed glioblastoma in which we attempted total tumor removal were investigated. There were three males and three females with an average age of 41.8 years (range 17–59 years). In each case the surgical specimens were obtained from the tumor itself as well as frorm several marginal locations.

Paraffin-embedded samples of tissue fixed in 10% formaldehyde in phosphate-buffered saline were cut into a 4μm thickness. The argyrophilic method

[1]Department of Neurosurgery, School of Medicine, Keio University, Shinjuku-ku, Tokyo, 160 Japan
[2]Department of Pathology, Minami-Tama Hospital, Saitama Children's Medical Center, Iwatsuki, 339 Japan

for the demonstration of nucleolar organizer regions (AgNORs) was applied according to Orita et al. [3]. Briefly, sections were deparaffinated in successive baths of xylene and ethanol. After being washed in distilled water, they were postfixed in a 3:1 ethanol-acetic acid mixture for 10 min and then rehydrated. Sections were then incubated with a solution containing one volume of 2% gelatin in 1% aqueous formic acid mixed with two volumes of 50% aqueous silver nitrate for 30 min in a dark room at room temperature. The slides were carefully rinsed with distilled water and mounted in PermaFluor. No counter-staining was used.

All sections were examined by one observer. The numbers of AgNORs were counted on three photomicrographs of each specimen, taken at a 400-fold

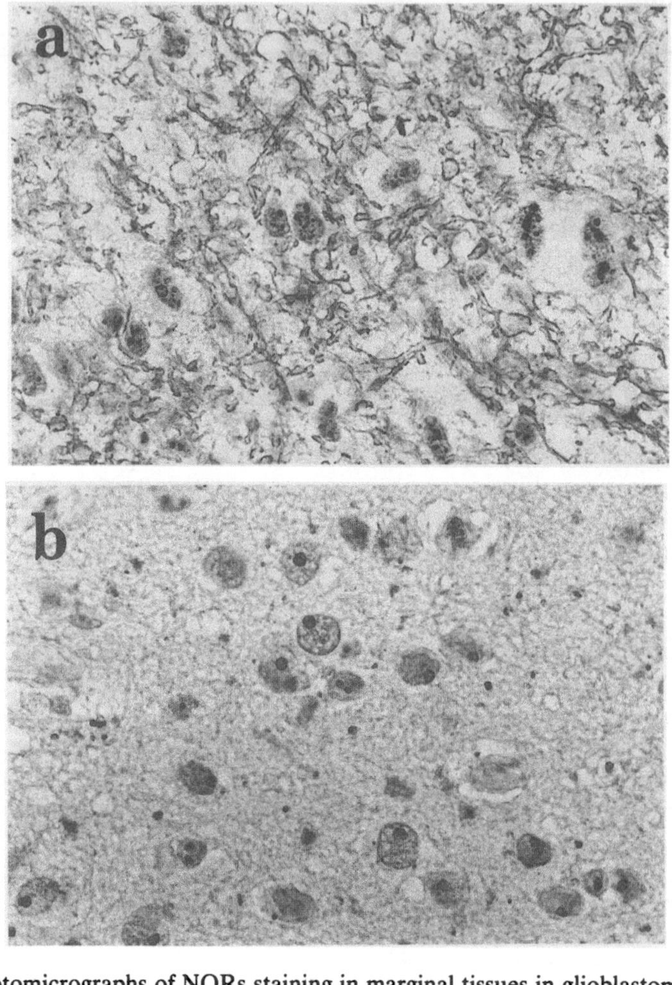

Fig. 1. Photomicrographs of NORs staining in marginal tissues in glioblastomas, × 200. **a** In this case with tumor cells invasion the mean number of AgNORs is 2.30 per nucleus. **b** In this case without tumor cells invasion the mean number of AgNORs is 1.39 per nucleus

magnification. The mean number of AgNORs per cell was determined. Data were analyzed using Wilcoxon's test.

Results

AgNORs are visible as black dots not only in tumor cells but also in neuronal cells, astrocytes, and oligodendrocytes of normal cerebral tissue. The mean AgNORs number was 1.22 for normal gray matter and 1.16 for white matter. The number was 1.22 for normal gray matter and 1.16 for white matter. The number of AgNORs ranged from 1.40 to 3.30 (mean 2.32 ± 0.27 standard error of the mean value) for glioblastoma (n = 6), and from 1.28 to 2.30 (1.63 ± 0.11) for marginal tissues (n = 10). In the latter the mean number for the part of reactive gliosis was 1.66. The number of for glioblastoma showed a tendency to be higher than that for marginal tissues (Wilcoxon T = 72.00, $P <$ 0.05).

The number of AgNORs ranged from 1.49 to 2.30 (1.86 ± 0.20) in marginal tissues with tumor cells invasion (n = 4) (Fig. la), and from 1.28 to 1.94 (1.48 ± 0.11) in those without it (n = 6) (Fig. 1b). There were significant differences between the mean numbers of AgNORs per cell in marginal tissues with tumor cell invasion and in that without (Wilcoxon T = 31.00, $P < 0.05$) (Fig. 2). These results show that the number of AgNORs may be useful in determining whether or not marginal tissues contain tumor cells.

In the marginal tissues of cases with subsequent tumor recurrence (n = 4), the number of AgNORs ranged from 1.28 t 2.30 (1.82 ± 0.32), whereas in

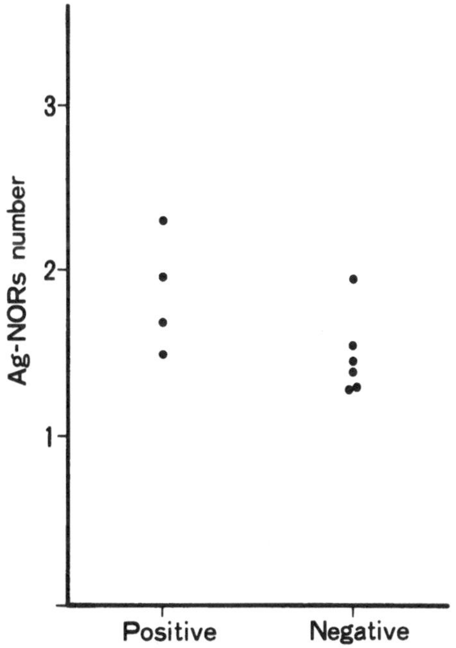

Fig. 2. Mean number of AgNORs in each marginal tissue grouped according to the presence (*positive*) or absence (*negative*) of tumor cells, as determined histologically. There were significant differences between the two groups (Wilcoxon T = 31.00, $P < 0.05$)

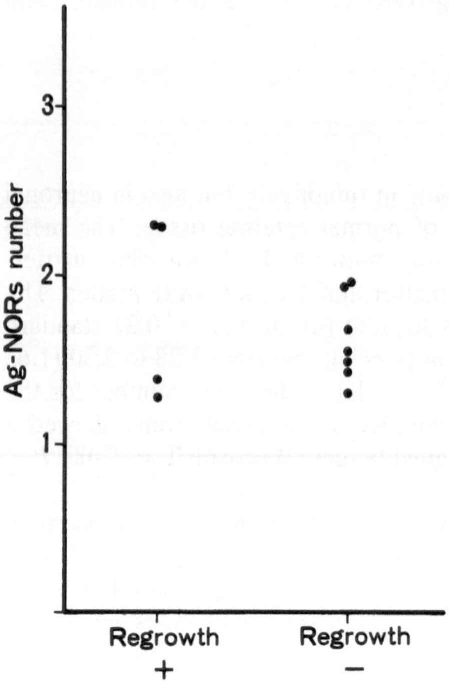

Fig. 3. Mean number of AgNORs in each marginal tissue, grouped by the occurrence of tumor regrowth. The mean numbers of AgNORs in marginal tissues are not correlated with tumor regrowth

those of cases where no recurrence has been observed ($n = 7$), it varied between 1.29 and 1.96 (1.62 ± 0.10) (Fig. 3.). However, this difference was not significant.

Discussion

In considering what should be the extent of cytoreductive surgery in the treatment of malignant gliomas, grossly total resection is recommended because it is associated with longer and better survival, compared to subtotal resection [4,5]. Definition of tumor margins is essential for achieving good surgical results and for estimating the amount of residual tumor, which in turn, facilitates adjunctive treatment plans. During surgery, surgeons usually determine the transition between normal brain and tumor material according to tissue color and constancy, but these may be unreliable guides. Even with currently available intraoperative techniques, such as CT and/or MRI-guided stereotactic localization of tumors [6], intraoperative ultrasonography [7], or intraoperative use of fluorescein [8], tumor margins often remain difficult to delineate precisely. Tumor cells are not limited to areas of contrast enhancement. They frequently extend beyond an area of hypodensity on CT scans and beyond a region of abnormal signals on MRI scans. Histological examination during an operation may reveal isolated tumor cells located at the boundaries of gliomas, according to traditional criteria; they may show nuclear pleomorphism and hyperchromasia as cytologic features of malignant lesions, and lack regular cell arrangement and symmetric stellate processes of reactive cells [9]. However, this technique requires an expert for interpretation, thus a more simple, rapid, reproducible, and quantitative method has been investigated intensively.

Recently, the evaluation of nucleolar organizer regions (NORs) by simple silver staining has been recognized to be a method of great value because NORs show a significantly higher frequency in the nuclei of malignant cells [1,2,10]. NORs are loops of DNA which possess ribosomal ribonucleic acid genes, and are thus involved in protein synthesis, cell growth, cell differentiation, and perhaps malignant transformation.

The present study on cases of glioblastoma showed that the mean number of AgNORs per cell in marginal tissues with tumor cells invasion is significantly higher than those without. It is suggested in cases of glioblastoma that residual tumor cells seem to be present in marginal tissues with a mean number of 1.9 AgNORs or more, and in contrast, those with less than a mean number of 1.5 AgNORs seem to be free from tumor cells.

The AgNORs technique can be easily performed on small amounts of tissue samples, and is applicable not only to routine paraffin sections but to frozen sections as well [2]. Moreover, AgNORs are better distinguishable in smear preparations of cytological specimens [10]. The procedure is composed simply of a one-step silver colloid solution staining that takes less than 1 h. These data show that the AgNORs technique may be valuable for detecting tumor cells at the boundaries of gliomas and delineating gliomas from normal brain tissue during an operation.

In attempting to establish the estimation of probability of tumor recurrence from the peripheries of gliomas, we were unable to observe any correlation between the mean number of AgNORs in marginal tissue specimens and tumor recurrence. This may be due to the variable sensitivity of tumors to postoperative radiotherapy and/or chemotherapeutic agents.

Because most gliomas are heterogeneous with regard to cell populations, and are highly infiltrative in terms of invasion, the AgNORs technique bears the problem of tissue sampling unevenness and inappropriateness. Further studies of the AgNORs in a large series of gliomas are necessary in order to resolve this problem.

Conclusion

NORs counting in marginal tissues of glioblastomas during surgery is an efficient method for identification of infiltrative tumor cells and for determining the boundaries of gliomas, facilitating more complete tumor removal.

References

1. Kajiwara K, Nishizaki T, Orita T, Nakayama H, Aoki H, Ito H (1990) Silver colloid staining technique for analysis of glioma malignancy. J Neurosurg 73:113–117
2. Hara A, Hirayama H, Sasaki N, Yamada H, Tanaka T, Mori H (1990) Correlation between nucleolar organizer region staining and Ki-67 immunostaining in human gliomas. Surg Neurol 33:320–324
3. Orita T, Kajikawa K, Nishizaki T, Ikeda N, Kamiryo T, Aoki N (1990) Nucleolar organizing regions in meningioma. Neurosurgery 26:43–46
4. Ammirati M, Vick N, Liao Y, Ciric I, Mikhael M (1987) Effect of the extent of surgical resection on survival and quality of life in patients with supratentorial glioblastomas and anaplastic astrocytomas. Neurosurgery 21:201–206
5. Winger MJ, Macdonald DR, Cairncross JG (1989) Supratentorial anaplastic gliomas in adults. The prognostic importance of extent of resection and prior low-grade glioma. J Neurosurg 71:487–493
6. Kelly PJ, Kall BA, Goerss S, Earnest F (1986) Computer-assisted stereotaxic laser resection of intra-axial brain neoplasms. J Neurosurg 64:427–439
7. Leroux PD, Berger MS, Ojemann GA, Wang K, Mack LA (1989) Correlation of intraoperative ultrasound tumor volumes and margins with preoperative computerized tomography scans. An intraoperative method to enhance tumor resection. J Neurosurg 71:691–698
8. Murray KJ (1982) Improved surgical resection of human brain tumors: Part 1. A preliminary study. Surg Neurol 17:316–319
9. Daumas-Duport C, Scheithauer BW, Kelly PJ (1987) A histologic and cytologic method for the spatial definition of gliomas. Mayo Clin Proc 62:435–449
10. Plate KH, Ruschoff J, Behnke J, Mennel HD (1990) Proliferative potential of human brain tumours as assessed by nucleolar organizer regions (AgNORs) and Ki67-immunoreactivity. Acta Neurochir (Wien) 104:103–109

Evaluation of the Proliferation on Brain Tumor Cells and the Endothelial Cells of Tumor Vessels Using Immunohistochemical Study with Anti-BrdU Monoclonal Antibody and Factor VIII-Related Antigen

MITSUSUKE MIYAGAMI, EISHI KASAHARA, and TAKASHI TSUBOKAWA[1]

Introduction

Malignant brain tumors, especially those of the astrocytic series, are characterized by neovascularity and endothelial proliferation. To understand the biology of these tumors, it is important to study the properties of the abnormal intratumoral endothelial cells. Cytokinetic studies of human brain tumors, using bromodeoxyuridine (BrdU), provide a far more reliable method to determine the proliferative rate of cells than the measurement of angiogenesis and counts of mitotic figures by light microscopy [1]. Tissue culture studies have confirmed the synthesis of factor VIII-related antigen (FVIIIR:Ag) in endothelial cells [2,3]. The immunohistochemical demonstration of FVIIIR:Ag has recently been used as a marker for endothelial cells in neoplastic diseases [4–6].

In this paper vascular proliferation and malignancy have been studied by the measurement of the BrdU labeling index (LI) and the distribution of Factor VIIIR:Ag in the vascular components of human brain tumors.

Materials and Methods

Of the 62 cases of histologically diagnosed human brain tumors, there were 27 cases of glial tumors, 27 cases of non-glial tumors, and 8 cases of metastatic brain tumors. The immunohistochemical staining method was used in order to detect BrdU-labeled cells with the same procedure as previously reported [7]. Briefly, after denaturation with 2N HCl and 0.1M $Na_2B_4O_7$, sections were immersed for 45 min in a 1:30 dilution of purified anti-BrdU monoclonal antibodies (Becton Dickinson, Oxnard, Calif.) in phosphate-buffered saline (PBS). Then, they were covered for 30 min with PBS solution containing a 1:200 dilution of peroxidase-conjugated anti-mouse IgG antibodies. Most of the sections were counterstained with periodic acid-schiff (PAS) to enhance the

[1] Department of Neurological Surgery, School of Medicine, Nihon University, Chiyoda-ku, 101 Japan

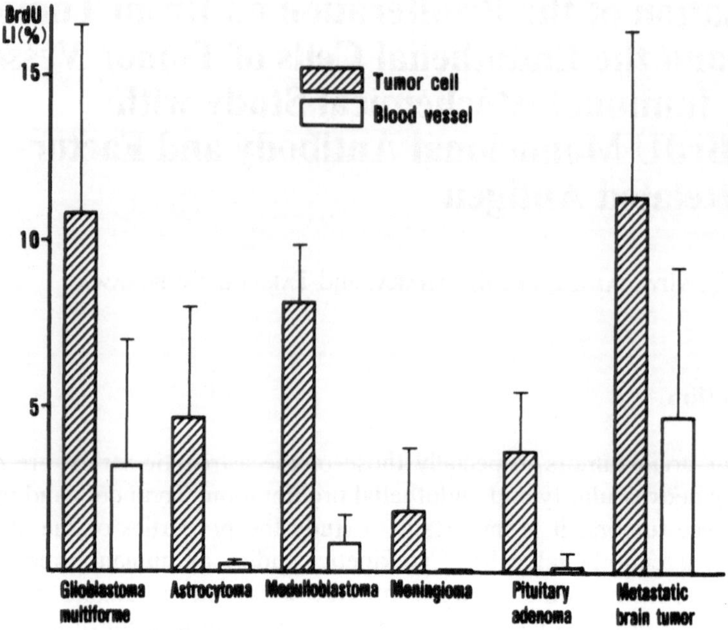

Fig. 1. Graph demonstrating mean and standard deviation of BrdU LI(%) in the tumor cells and vascular components

basement membrane of the vessel walls. Finally, all of the nuclei were stained with hematoxylin. The BrdU LI of the vascular components, which were surrounded by the PAS-positive basement membrane, was calculated as the ratio of labeled cells to the total number of vascular cells and expressed as a percentage. The BrdU LI for tumor cells was also measured as the ratio of labeled cells to the total number of tumor cells.

For immunohistochemical localization of Factor VIIIR:Ag in 6 μ sections of formalin-fixed and paraffin-embedded tissue, the peroxidase-antiperoxidase complex (PAP) method was used with a kit. The sections were incubated with rabbit anti-human factor VIII R:Ag (DAKO, Copenhagen, Denmark).

Results

The BrdU LI(%) of the tumor cells and vascular components in each brain tumor are indicated in Table 1. The BrdU LI in 12 cases of glioblastoma multiforme ranged from 3.1 to 24.0 (mean ±SD; 10.73 ± 5.79) in the tumor cells and from 0 to 15.0 (3.1 ± 3.92) in their blood vessel walls. Six cases of astrocytoma demonstrated BrdU LIs ranging from 2.8 to 7.1 (4.17 ± 1.38) in the tumor cells and from 0 to 0.6 (0.1 ± 0.22) in their blood vessel walls. The BrdU LIs (min. – max. mean ±SD) in the tumor cells and blood vessels of other brain tumors were as follows: medulloblastomas, 6.3 – 10.5 (8.17 ± 1.75) in the tumor cells and 0.0 ~ 1.7 (0.83 ± 0.69) in the blood vessel walls;

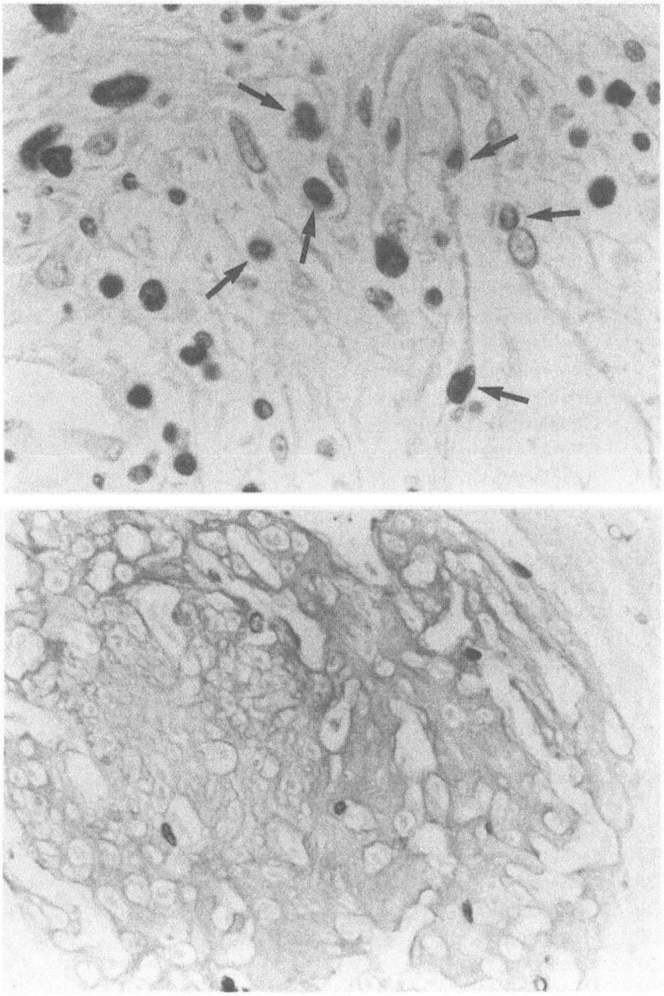

a

b

Fig. 2. **a** Note immunostaining by labeling of BrdU in the cell nuclei of tumor cells nuclei of endothelial cells (*arrows*) and tumor cells around the microvessels in the glioblastoma multiforme, 10 × 40. **b** Note labeling of BrdU in the cell nuclei of endothelial cells in the accumulated microvessels of the glioblastoma multiforme with connective tissues counterstained by PAS, 10 × 40

metastatic brain tumors, 2.8 – 18.0 (11.45 ± 4.91) in the tumor cells and 0.3 – 14.3 (4.73 ± 4.57) in the blood vessel walls; pituitary adenoma, 0.8 – 7.2 (3.58 ± 1.86) in the tumor cells and 0.0 – 1.2 (0.17 ± 0.42) in the blood vessel walls. The labeling index of the vascular components was calculated as the percentage of all labeled vascular cells in relation to the total number of vascular cells in the selected areas. The BrdU LI in the blood vessel walls was high in the vascular components of glioblastoma multiforme, medulloblastoma, and metastatic brain tumors which revealed BrdU LIs of more than 5% in their

Table 1. BrdU LI(%) in the tumor cells and blood vessel walls of human brain tumors

Case	Tumor type	BrdU LI(%)	
		Tumor cell	Blood vessel wall
1.	Glioblastoma multiforme	24.0	15.0
2.	Glioblastoma multiforme	15.0	3.2
3.	Glioblastoma multiforme	15.7	5.0
4.	Glioblastoma multiforme	15.0	4.8
5.	Glioblastoma multiforme	10.6	2.0
6.	Glioblastoma multiforme	7.1	1.2
7.	Glioblastoma multiforme	7.0	1.8
8.	Glioblastoma multiforme	6.3	0.7
9.	Glioblastoma multiforme	4.2	0
10.	Glioblastoma multiforme	13.3	1.0
11.	Glioblastoma multiforme	3.1	0
12.	Glioblastoma multiforme	7.5	2.5
13.	Anaplastic astrocytoma	1.4	0
14.	Anaplastic astrocytoma	1.9	0
15.	Anaplastic astrocytoma	6.9	0
16.	Astrocytoma	3.7	0
17.	Astrocytoma	3.6	0
18.	Astrocytoma	3.5	0
19.	Astrocytoma	2.8	0
20.	Astrocytoma	7.1	0
21.	Astrocytoma	4.3	0.6
22.	Oligodendroglioma	2.8	0
23.	Oligodendroglioma	3.7	1.0
24.	Undifferentiated glioma	1.8	0
25.	Medulloblastoma	7.7	0
26.	Medulloblastoma	10.5	1.7
27.	Medulloblastoma	6.3	0.8
28.	Germ cell tumor	2.4	1.2
29.	Germ cell tumor	5.4	0
30.	Meningioma	2.1	0
31.	Meningioma	1.3	0
32.	Meningioma	1.1	0
33.	Meningioma	3.0	0
34.	Meningioma	3.1	0
35.	Meningioma	1.1	0
36.	Meningioma	1.2	0
37.	Meningioma	7.2	0
38.	Meningioma	0.5	0
39.	Meningioma	0.7	0
40.	Meningioma	1.8	0
41.	Meningioma	2.2	0
42.	Meningioma	0.5	0
43.	Neurinoma	1.2	0
44.	Neurinoma	0.0	0
45.	Craniopharyngioma	0.8	0
46.	Malignant lymphoma	8.1	0
47.	Malignant lymphoma	4.7	0
48.	Pituitary adenoma	3.9	0
49.	Pituitary adenoma	3.5	0
50.	Pituitary adenoma	2.0	0

Table 1. *Cont.*

Case	Tumor type	BrdU LI(%)	
		Tumor cell	Blood vessel wall
51.	Pituitary adenoma	3.2	0
52.	Pituitary adenoma	4.4	0
53.	Pituitary adenoma	0.83	0
54.	Pituitary adenoma	7.2	1.2
55.	Metastatic brain tumor	18.0	14.3
56.	Metastatic brain tumor	10.7	9.0
57.	Metastatic brain tumor	7.0	5.5
58.	Metastatic brain tumor	8.0	0.7
59.	Metastatic brain tumor	2.8	0.3
60.	Metastatic brain tumor	14.0	1.8
61.	Metastatic brain tumor	14.3	1.2
62.	Metastatic brain tumor	16.8	5.0

tumor cells. However, the BrdU-labeling indexes in tumor vessels were variable and different within the area of the tumor. BrdU-labeled cells were observed mostly in the microvessels with endothelial proliferation and/or hyperplasia. BrdU-labeled endothelial cells did not always appear even in areas in which microvessels were increased, such as in menin gioma. Human brain tumors with tumor cells showing an LI of less than 5% provided scarcely any BrdU in the cell nuclei of their tumor vessels.

The immunohistochemical staining pattern for factor VIII R:Ag were not dependent upon tumor type. A diffuse, linear, or sometimes slightly granular staining reaction pattern indicated the presence of FVIIIR:Ag in the endothelial cell layer of the blood vessel walls. The capillaries with endothelial proliferation or hyperplasia in malignant brain tumors were characterized by the

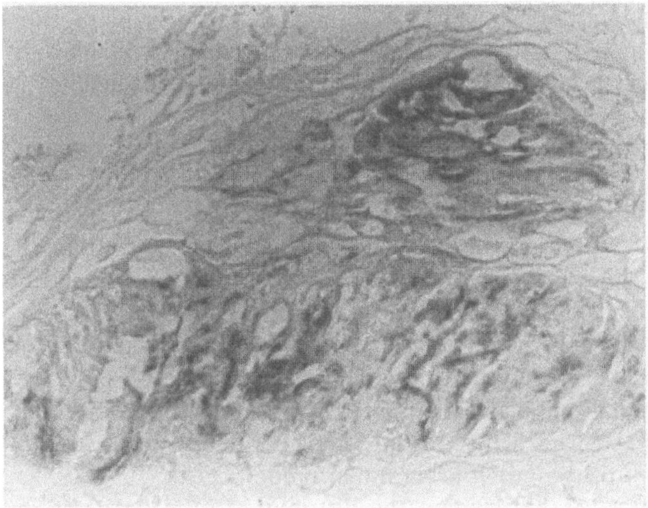

Fig. 3. Note immunostaining for Factor VIII-related antigen (FVIIIR:Ag) in the endothelial cell layers of the microvessels in the glioblatoma multiforme, 10 × 40

intensity and thickness of the immunostaining for FVIIIR:Ag in the vascular walls. In glioblastoma multiforme and metastatic brain tumors, there was an increase in the total number of blood vessels, with prominent capillary proliferation in the tumor tissues. These tumor vessels, demonstrating BrdU LIs of more than 5% in their tumor cells, revealed strong immunostaining for FVIIIR:Ag in most of the endothelial cell layer. In general, capillaries showed stronger positive staining than larger blood vessels in the tumor tissues. Even if there were an increase of microvessels with thin walls in the tumor tissues, as in meningioma, FVIIIR:Ag was neither remarkable nor linear in the blood vessel walls.

Discussion

Previous studies of cell kinetics of human brain tumors in situ have revealed evidence that the BrdU LI reflects proliferative activity or biological malignancy, that histologically similar tumors may have different proliferative potentials, and that this can be demonstrated by differences in the BrdU LIs [1]. Quantitation of vascular cytokinetics using BrdU LIs had been studied in glioblastoma multiforme [8] and in experimentally induced rabbit brain tumor [9]. Tannock [10] reported that the ^{3}H-TdR LI of capillary endothelial cells (11.4%) in transplanted C3H mouse mammary tumors was much lower than that of tumor cells (35%). In a large number of experimental non-glial tumors studied by Denekamp and Hobson [11] and in the human glioblastomas reported by Nagashima et al. [8], the BrdU LI of vascular components in the tumors was considerably lower than that of the tumor cells themselves. In our series of human brain tumors, the BrdU LIs of blood vessels provided about 10% to 30% of those of tumor cells in glioblastomas, metastatic brain tumors, and medulloblastomas, which were higher than those of the other brain tumors. In human brain tumors with BrdU LIs of lower than 5% of their tumor cells had scarce immunostaining for BrdU in the cell nuclei of their vascular components.

The heterogeneity of BrdU-labeling could be due to variable blood flows [12], thymidine transport [13], or insufficient intravenous delivery of the drug BrdU. In order to minimize the effect of restricted delivery of BrdU, we selected viable areas in which labeled cells were evenly distributed or appeared abundantly. The mean BrdU LIs of vascular components and tumor cells in twelve glioblastomas were 3.1 ± 3.9% (mean ±SD) and 10.7 ± 5.8% in our study, similar to the results of Nagashima et al. [8]. The LI of the endothelial cell component in the tumor periphery was high in both experimental gliomas [14] and human glioblastomas [15]. Brien et al. [9] indicated that the LI of endothelial cells was 25.8% at the tumor periphery, compared to 1.7% in the tumor center of the rabbit brain tumor model.

Miyagami et al. [4] studied the distribution of FVIIIR:Ag in 12 cases of human brain tumors with immunoelectron microscopic techniques and found that one characteristic of malignant tumors was a strongly positive dilated endoplasmic reticulum. This may reflect an increased FVIIIR:Ag in the endothelial cells which was broader and denser in the malignant brain tumors with proliferative potential of high BrdU LI in their endothelial cells. These findings suggested that the endothelial cells with high proliferative potential for BrdU might contain an increased synthesis of FVIIIR:Ag of malignant brain tumors.

Conclusion

The proliferative potential on the tumor cells and vascular components in 62 cases of human brain tumors were evaluated using BrdU LI, and the distribution of FVIIIR:Ag as an endothelial cell marker were studied with an immunohistochemical technique. The BrdU LI of vascular components has been shown to be lower than that of tumor cells, and is about 10%–30% of that in the tumor cells of glioblastomas, metastatic brain tumors and medulloblastomas. Therefore, human brain tumors with BrdU LIs of their cells lower than 5% have evidenced little BrdU in the cell nuclei of their vascular components. The endothelial cells with a high proliferative potential for BrdU might contain an increased synthesis of FVIIIR:Ag of malignant brain tumors.

References

1. Hoshino T, Nagashima T, Murovi JA, Wilson CB, Edwards MSB, Gutin PH, Davis RL, DeArmond SJ (1986) In situ cell kinetics studies on human neuroectodermal tumors with bromodeoxyuridine labeling. J Neurosurg 64:453–459
2. Jaffe EA, Hoyer LW, Nachman RL (1973) Synthesis of antihemophilic factor antigen by cultured human endothelial cells. J Clin Invest 52:2757–2764
3. Shearn SAM, Peake IR, Giddings JC, Humphreys J, Bloom AL (1977) The characterization and synthesis of antigens related to Factor VIII in vascular endothelium. Thromb Res 11:43–56
4. Miyagami M, Smith BH, Mckeever PE, Chronwall BM, Greenwood MA, Kornblith PL (1987) Immunocytochemical localization of factor VIII-related antigen in tumors of the human central nervous system. J Neurooncol 4:269–285
5. Mukai K, Rosai J, Burgdorf WHC (1980) Localization of Factor VIII-related antigen in vascular endothelial cells using a immunoperoxidase method. Am J Surg Pathol 4:273–275
6. Sehested M, Hou-Hensen K (1981) Factor VIII-related antigen as an endothelial cell marker in benign and malignant diseases. Virchows Arch [A] 391:217–225
7. Hoshino T, Wilson CB (1978) Cell kinetic analyses of human malignant brain tumors (gliomas). Cancer 44:956–962
8. Nagashima T, Hoshino T, Cho KG (1987) Proliferative potential of vascular components in human glioblastoma multiforme. Acta Neuropathol (Berl) 73:301–305
9. Brien SE, Zagzag D, Brem S (1989) Rapid in situ cellular kinetics of intracerebral tumor angiogenesis using a monoclonal antibody to bromodeoxyuridine. Neurosurgery 25:715–719

10. Tannock IF (1970) Population kinetics of carcinoma cells, capillary endothelial cells and fibroblasts in a transplanted mouse mammary tumor. Cancer Res 30:2470–2476
11. Denekamp J, Hobson B (1982) Endothelial cell proliferation in experimental tumors. Br J Cancer 46:711–720
12. Yamada K, Hayakawa T, Ushio Y, Arita N, Kato A, Mogami H (1981) Regional blood flow and capillary permeability in the ethylnitrosourea-induced rat glioma. J Neurosurg 55:922–928
13. Molnar P, Groothuis D, Blasberg R, Zaharko D, Owens E, Fenstermacher J (1984) Regional thymidine transport and incorporation in experimental brain and subcutaneous tumors. J Neurochem 43:421–432
14. Groothuis DR, Fischer JM Vick NA, Bigner DD (1980) Experimental gliomas: An autoradiographic study of the endothelial component. Neurology 3:297–301
15. Yoshii Y. Sugiyama K (1988) Intercapillary distance in the proliferating area of human glioma. Cancer Res 48:2938–2941

Weibel-Palade Bodies as a Marker for Endothelial Proliferative Potential of Human Glioma Capillaries

SHINGO TAKANO, YOSHIHIKO YOSHII, and TADAO NOSE[1]

Introduction

We studied whether quantitative assessment of Weibel-Palade bodies may represent the proliferative potential of the endothelial cells in human gliomas using the following parameters: histopathological malignancy, blood vessel proliferation, and growth fraction of the endothelial cells.

Materials and Methods

Source of Tissue Samples

Tissues from 31 patients who were operated upon for various gliomas were studied. The lesions were comprised of 11 low-grade astrocytomas, 7 anaplastic astrocytomas, and 13 glioblastomas. Twelve patients of the 31 received iv. infusion of $200\,mg/m^2$ body surface of BrdU for 30 min every 8 h for 3 days before craniotomy (a total of 9 infusions). Samples were obtained from the marginal area of the tumors which had no necrosis. Each sample was classified into 3 specimens: the first for formalin fixation, the second for alcohol fixation, and the third for glutaraldehyde fixation.

Light Microscopic Study

The first specimen was fixed in 10% formalin and was embedded in paraffin. Sections were stained with hematoxyline and eosin for pathological study, or treated with reticulin stain for vessel density. In order to determine the vessel density of the tumors in each patient, we manually counted the vessels in 10 microscopic fields using × 400 magnification on reticulin-stained sections. Vessel density was expressed as an average number of vessels in one microscopic field. The second specimen was fixed in chilled 70% ethanol and was embedded in paraffin. Sections were treated with immunoperoxidase stain for BrdU.

[1]Department of Neurological Surgery, Institute of Clinical Medicine, University of Tsukuba, Tsukuba, 305 Japan

In order to estimate the growth fraction (GF) of endothelial cells, we manually counted the BrdU-labeled endothelial cells in 10 microscopic fields containing a total population of 22–228 endothelial cells in each case. GF was expressed as a ratio of the BrdU-labeled cells to the total cell count.

Electron Microscopic Study

The third specimen was processed for electron microscopic studies. We chose blocks that were composed entirely of tumor cells and vessels without necrosis. Thin sections were examined using a JEM-100CX electron microscope. The vessels, which were cut transversely (luminal diameter ≦10μm), were photographed at low magnification (× 10,000) in order to check their general features, and Weibel-Palade bodies (WPB) were counted at high magnification (× 33,000). A total of 113 vessel profiles (31 from low-grade astrocytomas, 36 from anaplastic astrocytomas, and 46 from glioblastomas) was analyzed. The ratio of the endothelial cells (ECs) with WPB to whole ECs and the number of WPB per one EC were measured in each vessel. Also, in the 12 patients infused with BrdU, more than 5 vessels in each patient were analyzed, and an incidence of WPB was similarly measured in each patient.

Results

Figure 1 shows a typical case of glioblastoma. At low manification the capillary shows lumen narrowed by hypertrophied ECs (Fig. 1a), and at high magnification, the capillary shows many WPB in the cytoplasm (Fig. 1b). Vessel density is high (Fig. 1c) and many ECs and tumor cells are labeled for BrdU by immunoperoxidase stain (Fig. 1d).

The average incidence of WPB in 31 vessels from low-grade astrocytoma (Astro), 36 from anaplastic astrocytoma (AA) and 46 from glioblastoma (GM) are shown in Table 1. The average ratio of the ECs with WPB was significantly higher in AA and GM than in Astro (47.2% and 53.5% vs 12.8%, $P < 0.01$). The average number of WPB per one EC was 0.35 in Astro, 1.14 in AA, and 1.89 in GM. The difference among them is significant (0.35 vs 1.14, $P < 0.01$; 1.14 vs 1.89, $P < 0.05$).

Vessel density, GF in ECs, and incidence of WPB in 12 patients are shown in Table 2. The ratio of ECs with WPB to whole ECs showed a significant

Table 1. Incidence of Weibel-Palade bodies

Diagnosis[1]	Endothelial cells with WPB/ whole endothelial cells (%)	Number of WPB/ one endothelial cell (no.)
Astro ($n = 31$)	12.8 ± 21.3	0.35 ± 0.60
AA ($n = 36$)	47.2 ± 35.5**	1.14 ± 1.22*
GM ($n = 46$)	53.5 ± 31.3	1.89 ± 1.99**

[1] *astro*, low grade astrocytoma; *AA*, anaplastic astrocytoma; *GM*, glioblastoma; *, $P < 0.01$; **, $P < 0.05$. Means are given ± standard deviation

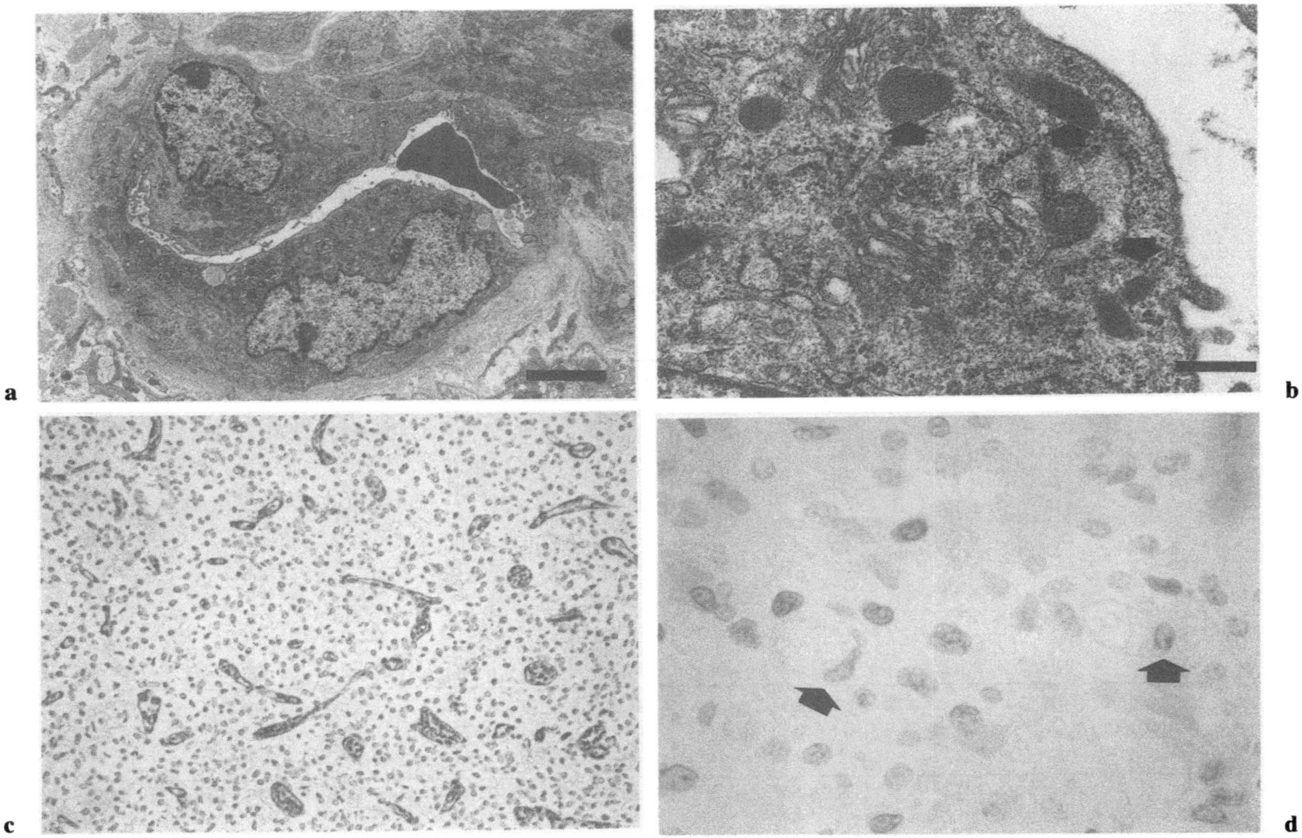

Fig. 1a–d. Glioblastoma multiforme. **a** Low magnification view of capillary showing narrowed lumen by hypertrophied endothelial cells. Bar = 5 μm. **b** High magnification view of capillary showing many Weibel-Palade bodies (*arrow*). Bar = 0.5 μm. **c** Vessel density is high. Reticulin stain × 100. **d** Tissue section stained with immunoperoxidase stain for bromodeoxyuridine. Proliferating phase cells of endothelial cells are labeled (*arrow*). Many of the tumor cells are also labeled. × 400

Table 2. Summary of light and electron microscopic studies in 12 gliomas

	Light microscopic				Electron microscopic					
Diagnosis[1]	Vessel density	end[2] (*n*)	BrdU (+)[3] (*n*)	GF[4] (%)	Vessel (*n*)	End (*n*)	WPB (+)[5] (*n*)	WPB-1[6] (%)	WPB[7] (*n*)	WPB-2[8] (*n*/end)
Astro	6.8	109	8	7.3	7	38	8	21.1	14	0.37
Astro	6.8	53	4	7.5	5	13	1	7.7	3	0.23
Astro	6.1	145	10	6.9	5	29	1	3.4	2	0.07
AA	24.8	52	17	32.7	7	26	21	80.8	59	2.27
AA	24.8	51	21	41.2	5	29	17	58.6	57	1.97
AA	12.8	120	20	16.7	9	22	10	45.5	23	1.05
AA	11.5	22	4	18.2	6	20	6	30.0	11	0.55
GM	23.5	49	16	32.7	6	36	24	66.7	97	2.69
GM	30.9	216	49	22.7	5	27	4	14.8	7	0.26
GM	23.5	139	23	16.5	10	26	13	50.0	34	1.31
GM	25.2	228	50	21.9	5	38	24	63.2	53	1.39
GM	30.8	59	21	35.6	7	19	16	84.2	65	3.42

[1] *Astro*, low grade astrocytoma; *AA*, anaplastic astrocytoma; *GM*, glioblastoma
[2] *end*, number of observed endothelial cells
[3] *BrdU* (+), number of immunohistochemically labeled endothelial cells
[4] *GF*, growth fraction = BrdU (+)/end × 100
[5] *WPB* (+), number of endothelial cells with WPB
[6] *WPB-1*, number of endothelial cells with WPB/whole endothelial cells = WPB (+)/end × 100
[7] *WPB* number of total WPB of each case
[8] *WPB-2*, number of WPB per one endothelial cell = WPB/end

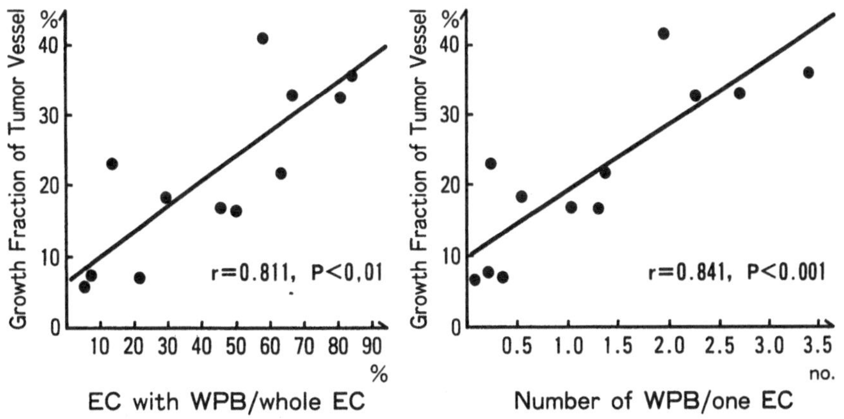

a b

Fig. 2a,b. Scatter plot of the growth fraction of the endothelial cells versus incidence of Weibel-Palade bodies (**a** ratio of the endothelial cells with WPB to whole endothelial cells, **b** number of WPB per one endothelial cell) for each of the 12 gliomas. A linear relationship is demonstrated between these factors

correlation with vessel density ($r = 0.690$, $P < 0.02$). The number of WPB per one EC also showed a significant correlation with vessel density ($r = 0.674$, $P < 0.02$).

The GF of ECs ranged from 6.9% to 41.2% in each case, and was higher than the GF of tumor cells in 10 out 12 patients. The ratio of ECs with WPB to whole ECs showed a significant correlation with the GF of ECs (Fig. 2a, $r = 0.811$, $P < 0.01$). The number of WPB per one EC showed a more significant correlation with the GF of ECs (Fig. 2b, $r = 0.841$, $P < 0.001$).

Discussion

WPB [1] is characteristic of endothelial cells, and is widely distributed in the endothelial cells of inflammatory or tumorous abnormal tissue as well as in the normal tissue of humans. However, it is rarely observed in normal brain blood vessels [2,3]. Although WPB is frequently found in brain tumors, such as medulloblastoma, ependymoblastoma, and pituitary adenoma [4,5], it has not been sufficiently examined on human glioma. Furthermore, the incidence of WPB has not been studied in relation to other parameters representing the proliferative potential of the endothelial cells.

The incidence of WPB was the highest in glioblastoma and the lowest in low-grade astrocytoma, and increased according to the degree of histopathological malignancy: this result was similar to that obtained by Miyagami et al. [3].

Angiogenesis is necessary to the growth of the glioma tissue and is considered to be the vascular response of the angiogenesis factor [6]. Although vessel density increases on the occasion of angiogenesis [7], the morphological changes in the nucleus and the cytoplasm of the endothelial cells are not well known. Our studies showed that the incidence of WPB increased with vessel density. Therefore, we can agree with some reports which state that a large number of WPB may be a marker for proliferating endothelial cells [3,5].

Recently, the proliferative potential of endothelial cells has been studied by measurement of the labeling index and growth fraction using BrdU or 3H-thymidine. It was reported that the proliferative potential of the endothelial cells in brain tumors was far higher than that of the endothelial cells in normal blood vessels [8,9], and higher than that of the tumor cells themselves [10,11]. When the relation between the incidence of WPB and the growth fraction of the endothelial cells was examined, a significant correlation was found to exist between them. This result confirms that the incidence of WPB may represent the degree of proliferative potential of the endothelial cells [3,5]. However, we do not know exactly why WPB in the cytoplasm closely correlates with the GF that expresses the proliferation in the nucleus. Further study of this question is needed.

Conclusion

1. Incidence of WPB was the highest in glioblastoma and was the lowest in low grade astrocytoma.
2. There was significant correlation between the incidence of WPB and the vessel density.
3. There was significant correlation between the incidence of WPB, especially the number of WPB per one endothelial cell, and the growth fraction of the endothelial cells.
4. It is suggested that the value of WPB can represent the degree of proliferative potential of the endothelial cells in the human glioma.

References

1. Weibel ER, Palade GE (1964) New cytoplasmic components in arterial endothelia. J Cell Biol 23:101–112
2. Herrlinger H, Anzil AP, Blinzinger K, Kronski D (1974) Endothelial microtubular bodies in human brain capillaries and venules. J Anat 118:205–209
3. Miyagami M, Tsubokawa T, Smith BH, Kornblith PL (1985) Tubular bodies (Weibel-Palade) in the endothelial cell of glioblastoma. No To Shinkei (Brain and Nerve) 37:277–285
4. Hirano A, Matsui T (1975) Vascular structures in brain tumors. Hum Pathol 6:611–621
5. Kumar P, Kumar S, Marsden HB, Lynch PG, Earnshaw E (1980) Weibel-Palade bodies in endothelial cells as a marker for angiogenesis in brain tumors. Cancer Res 40:2010–2019
6. Folkman J, Cotran R (1976) Relation of vascular proliferation to tumor growth. Int Rev Exp Path 16:207–248
7. Schiffer D, Chio A, Giordana T, Mauro A, Migheli A, Vigliani C (1989) The vascular response to tumor infiltration in malignant gliomas. Acta Neuropathol 77:369–378

8. Nagashima T, Hoshino T, Cho KG (1987) Proliferative potential of vascular components in human glioblastoma multiforme. Acta Neuropathol (Berl) 73:301–305
9. Brien SE, Zagzag D, Brem S (1989) Rapid in situ cellular kinetics of intracerebral tumor angiogenesis using a monoclonal antibody to bromodeoxyuridine. Neurosurgery 25:715–719
10. Groothuis DR, Fischer JM, Vick NA, Bigner DD (1980) Experimental gliomas: An autoradiographic study of the endothelial component. Neurology 30:297–301
11. Yoshii Y, Sugiyama K (1988) Intercapillary distance in the proliferating area of human glioma. Cancer Res 48:2938–2941

The Proliferative Potential After Hyperthermia and Irradiation on a Human Glioma Cell Line

Hideaki Shigematsu, Kazuyuki Tsuno, Takashi Matsuhisa, Tomohide Maeshiro, Nobuya Mishima, Kengo Matsumoto, Tomohisa Furuta, Minoru Arimori, and Akira Nishimoto[1]

Introduction

The lethal effects of hyperthermia and irradiation on glioma cells have been demonstrated both in vitro and in vivo. In general, cells in the S-phase are the most resistant to X-rays, whereas they are the most sensitive to hyperthermia. In this report, the effect of hyperthermia or irradiation on cultured glioma cells was examined by colony formation assay. The effect of these treatments on the proliferative potential of the glioma cells was investigated with an immunohistochemical technique using monoclonalantibody (MoAb) against bromodeoxyuridine (BrdU) and MoAb Ki-67.

Materials and Methods

Cell Line

Cultured human glioma cells (KC cells) were used in this study. The 5×10^5 cells were cultured on $25\,cm^2$ plastic flasks (Falcon 3013 tissue culture flask) in modified Eagle's medium (MEM) supplemented with 10% fetal calf serum in a humidified incubator with a mixture of 95% air and 5% CO_2. The exponentially growing cells were submitted either to the hyperthermia or irradiation experiment on the 3rd day after being newly inoculated.

Hyperthermia

The monolayer cells in plastic flasks were heated in a water bath at 43°C or 44°C for up to 120 min. The pH of the media was maintained at 7.4 during the experiments.

Irradiation

The cells were irradiated with single doses of 2, 4, 6, or 8 Gy at 37°C in a 165 kVp X-ray unit (Toshiba KXC-18-3, Toshiba Corp., Tokyo). The X-ray parameters were 165 kVp, 20 mA, and 35.28 R/min.

---

[1]Department of Neurological Surgery, Okayama University Medical School, Okayama, 700 Japan

Colony Formation Assays

About 1 h after undergoing hyperthermia or irradiation, the cells were harvested by trypsinization and 200 cells were plated in 6 cm-diameter tissue culture dishes (Falcon 3002 tissue culture dish) for 10 days at 37°C in MEM supplemented with 10% fetal calf serum. The macroscopic colonies, which were composed of more than 50 cells, were counted after appropriate fixation and staining. The planting efficiencies averaged 58%.

Immunohistochemical Studies

1×10^5 cells were cultured on tissue chamber slides (Lab-Tek tissue chamber slide, Nunc Inc. Naperville, USA) and treated in the same way as described above. After the hyperthermia or irradiation, the cells were fixed with chilled methanol and stained with MoAb against BrdU or MoAb Ki-67 using the peroxidase-anti-peroxidase method. For BrdU staining, the cells were pretreated with 1.25 μM BrdU for 1 h. Labeling indexes (LIs) were determined as the percentage of labeled cells by counting 1000 cells.

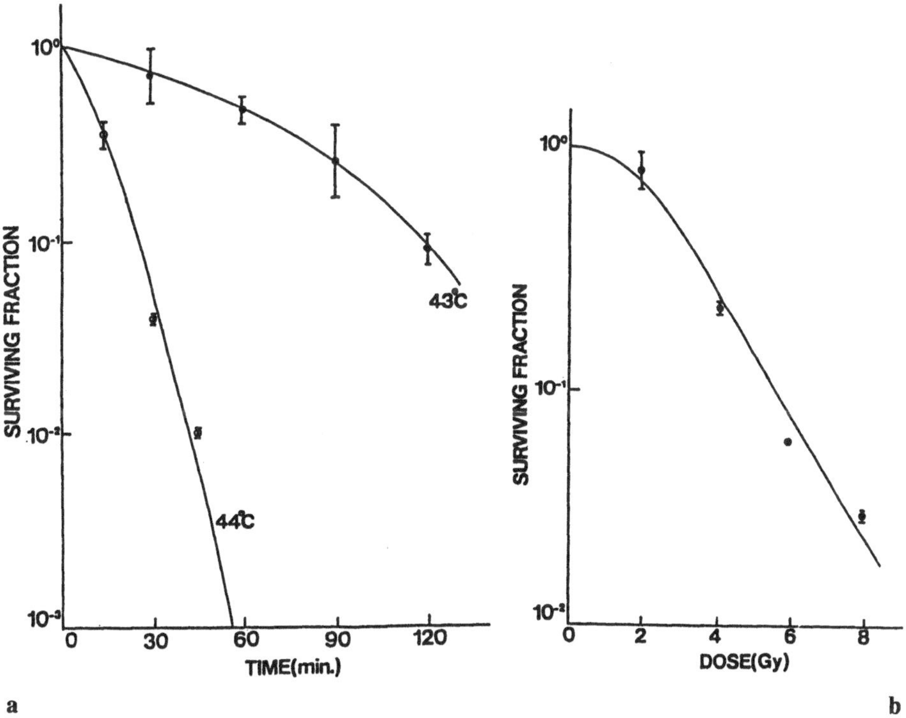

Fig. 1a,b. Graphs showing the survival of exponentially growing KC cells. **a** Cell survival after hyperthermia at 43°C and 44°C. **b** Cell survival after irradiation of up to 8 Gy

Table 1. BrdU and Ki-67 labeling indexes in KC cell after hyperthermia

LI	Control	30 min	60 min	90 min	120 min
Ki-67 (%) 43°C	81.4	80.3	67.2	67.5	55.6
44°C	81.4	60.0	49.9	41.6	44.4
BrdU (%) 43°C	35.6	30.7	27.6	19.1	12.7
44°C	35.6	22.8	14.2	7.6	2.2

Results

Colony Formation Assay

The survival curve after hyperthermia at 43°C decreased exponentially with shoulders, but at 44°C the curve was almost linear. The survival fraction of KC cells treated by hyperthermia decreased in proportion to the time length of the treatment and the degree of temperature (Fig. 1a). The ratio of D_0 was 77 min at 43°C and 14 min at 44°C. Irradiation also suppressed the survival rate correlating to the radiation doses (Fig. 1b). The ratio of D_0 was 3.7 Gy.

Immunohistochemical Studies

The changes of the LIs of BrdU and Ki-67 after hyperthermia are shown in Table 1. Both LIs decreased in proportion to the time of hyperthermia and heating temperature, but the decrease of the BrdU LI was significantly greater than that of the Ki-67 LI. The photomicrograph of the cells which stained Ki-67 after irradiation are shown in Fig 2. The Ki-67 LI decreased in proportion to irradiation doses, but the BrdU LI was not affected by irradiation of up to 8 Gy (Table 2).

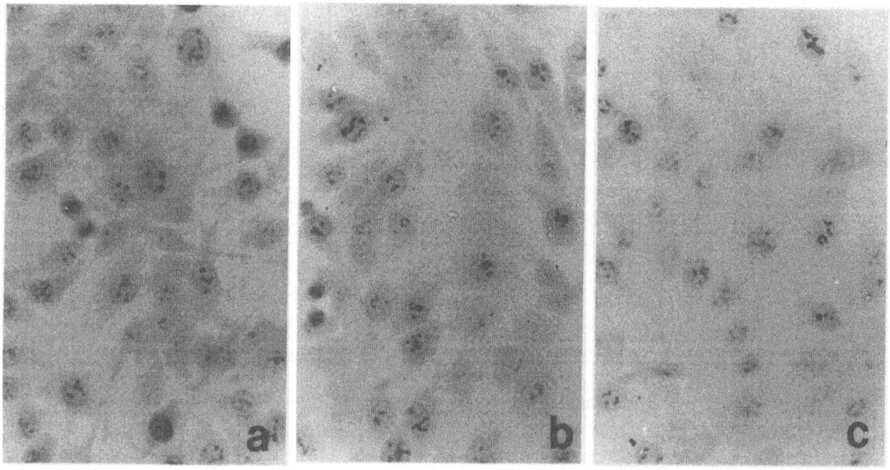

Fig. 2a–c. Photomicrograph of KC cells stained by Ki-67 after irradiation. **a** Control, **b** 4 Gy, **c** 8 Gy (× 400)

Table 2. BrdU and Ki-67 labeling indexes in KC cell after irradiation

LI	Control	2 Gy	4 Gy	6 Gy	8 Gy
Ki-67 (%)	74.6	62.7	61.9	59.3	57.5
BrdU (%)	30.5	31.0	29.2	30.4	30.9

These results suggested that both treatments suppressed cell survival, that the cells in the S-phase were more vulnerable to hyperthermia than those in the other phases, and that irradiation affected all of the cells except for those in the S-phase.

Discussion

In this study, both hyperthermia and irradiation inhibited the survival of cultured human glioma cells, and the effects of these treatments were dependent upon the time of hyperthermia and heating temperature, or upon the irradiation doses, respectively. These results fundamentally coincide with previous reports on this subject [1,2]. In terms of cell cycles, the cells of the S-phase are reported to be more sensitive to hyperthermia than those of the other phases [3,4], and irradiation is believed to be effective upon the cells of the G_2-M phases. We applied an immunohistochemical technique for the evaluation of the effect of hyperthermia and irradiation on human glioma cells. This is a very simple and useful method for this purpose. BrdU is an analogue of thymidine and is incorporated into the proliferating cells only in the S-phase [5]. The antigen recognized by MoAb of Ki-67 is still unclear, but is immunohistochemically stained in all of the phases of the cell except in the G_0 phase, and relates with the processing of preribosome and cell proliferation [6].

The fact that the decrease of the BrdU LI was significantly greater than that of Ki-67 suggests that hyperthermia mainly affects the cells in the S-phase. Contrarily, irradiation seems to affect the cells in all of the phases other than those in the S-phases, because the Ki-67 LI decreased as irradiation doses increased. Immunohistochemically, these results suggested that the combination of hyperthermia and irradiation can have a synergistic effect in the treatment of malignant gliomas.

Conclusions

1. Hyperthermia and irradiation inhibit cell growth and proliferation.
2. The lethal effect of hyperthermia or irradiation is dependent upon time and temperature of hyperthermia and irradiation doses.
3. The cells in the S-phase are more sensitive to hyperthermia than the cells in other phases while all of the cells except for those in the S-phase are more affected by irradiation.

4. The immunohistochemical technique which we used in the present study is simple and useful for investigating thermosensitivity and radiosensitivity of cultured cells.

References

1. Dewey WC, Hopwood LE, Sapareto SA, Gerwech LE (1977) Cellular responses to combination of hyperthermia and radiation. Rad Biol 123:463–474
2. Nielsen OS (1983) Influence of thermotolerance on the interaction between hyperthermia and radiation in L1A2 cells in vitro. Int J Radiat Biol 43:665–673
3. Machey MA, Dewey WC (1989) Cell cycle progression during chronic hyperthermia in S-phase CHO cells. Int J Hyperthermia 3:405–415
4. Westra A, Dewey WC (1971) Variation in sensitivity to heat shock during the cell-cycle of Chinese hamster cells in vitro. Int J Radiat Biol 5:467–477
5. Ramsay J, Suit HD, Preffer FI, Sedlacek R (1988) Changes in bromodeoxyuridine labeling index during radiation treatment of an experimental tumor. Radiat Res 116:453–461
6. Shiraishi T, Tabuchi K, Kunishio K, Furuta T, Nishimoto A (1989) The antigen recognized by the monoclonal antibody Ki-67. Brain Tumor Pathol 6:149–156

Section 2. Metabolism of Brain Tumor

PET Measurement of Tumor Metabolism in Patients with Gliomas

Katsuyoshi Mineura[1], Toshio Sasajima[1], Masayoshi Kowada[1], Fumio Shishido[2], and Kazuo Uemura[2]

Introduction

Brain tumors are considered to have well-integrated metabolic systems, because each tumor survives and maintains an adenosine triphosphate (ATP) level and energy charge. Diversity of metabolic patterns was noted in specimens of human brain tumors [1]. Biochemical assay may not always reflect in vivo enzyme activities and the metabolites of resected tumor tissues: it is not pure and is usually contaminated with heterogenous materials such as necroses and stromal tissues.

Recent advances in positron emission tomography (PET) enable us to visualize *in vivo* metabolic images of brain tumors. We have applied 0–15-oxygen, F-18-fluorodeoxyglucose (FDG), C-11-L-methionine (Met), and F-18-fluorophenylalanine tracers for quantitative measurement of the hemodynamics and metabolism in tumors, mainly gliomas [2–6]. In our preliminary reports, hemodynamics differed widely among gliomas, and oxygen metabolism fell considerably compared with the normal brain. The metabolic rate of glucose (rCMRGl) increased with malignancy [2]. We have scanned additional patients using PET and in the present paper, we summarize the results of metabolic images in gliomas compared to other brain tumors and non-tumorous CNS lesions, and test the prognostic significance of metabolic values and ratios.

Subjects and Methods

Fifty-three patients with glioma were examined with the PET apparatus, Headtome III or IV. Twenty-seven patients (with 8 low-grade and 19 high-grade tumors) were entered into the FDG study, 25 patients (11 low-grade, 14 high-grade) into the Met study, and one patient into both studies. Forty-eight patients had been diagnosed histologically as having mostly astrocytoma and glioblastoma. Three patients, whose tumors were unchanged or grew slowly

[1] Neurosurgical Service, Akita University Hospital, Akita, 010 Japan
[2] Department of Radiology and Nuclear Medicine, Research Institute for Brain and Blood Vessels-Akita, Akita, 010 Japan

over several years, had low-grade glioma. The remaining two patients were clinically diagnosed as having high-grade glioma, on the basis of neuroradiological findings and rapid growth of the tumors.

rCMRGl was measured after an intravenous injection of 185 MBq FDG according to the methods of Phelps [2]. Met was intravenously administrated at a dose of 22.2 MBq/kg. The uptake of the tracer was calculated on PET images scanned at 45 min after the injection. The tracer accumulation in tumors was quantitatively or visually compared to the contralateral gray matter on PET images. Regions of interest were placed over the tumors including peak values, the contralateral gray matter, and the white matter.

To determine whether or not rCMRGl values and ratios were significant for biological activity of the tumors, we analyzed their relationship with survival in 18 evaluable patients with histologically proven malignant astrocytoma or glioblastoma. Survival from the time of the PET study was compared according to the rCMRGl values and ratios of tumor/gray matter, regardless of the types of therapy. The follow-up time after the PET study ranged from 20 to 80 months with a mean of 62 months.

Results

Results of the FDG and the Met studies in comparison with other brain tumors and central nervous system (CNS) pathology are summarized in Tables 1 and 2, respectively.

Of the 19 high-grade gliomas examined with FDG, 17 (89%) had a higher peak activity than that of the contralateral white matter, and 10 (53%) had a higher value than that of the gray matter. All cases with a peak high activity showed inhomogeneous patterns of FDG uptake within the tumors. Two cases with low FDG uptake had either a tiny tumor or a cystic tumor. Of the 9 low-grade gliomas, 8 cases revealed a homogeneously lower uptake in the

Table 1. Results of the FDG PET study

		Level				Level	
Diagnosis	No.	+	−	Diagnosis	No.	+	−
Glioma	28	11	17	Radiation necrosis	3	0	3
Low grade	(9	1	8)	Infection	1	1	0
High grade	(19	10	9)	Sarcoidosis	1	1	0
Pituitary tumor	1	0	1	Heterotopic gray matter	1	1	0
Meningioma	3	1	2	Pineal cyst	1	0	1
Metastasis	2	1	1	Behçet's disease	1	0	1
Germ cell tumor	2	0	2				
Chordoma	1	0	1				
Angioma	2	0	2				
Tumorous	39	13 (33%)	26	Non-tumorous	8	3 (38%)	5

The FDG uptake of tumors was quantitatively compared to the contralateral gray matter: +, higher; −, lower; *PML*, progressive multifocal leucoencephalopathy tumor than that in the contralateral white matter. Only one case, which was oligodendrocytic and mainly infiltrative, indicated a higher uptake than that of the contralateral white matter.

The uptake of FDG was compared between the low-grade and high-grade gliomas. The mean value of rCMRGl in the high-grade gliomas was 5.76 ± 1.27 (SD) mg/100 ml/min, marginally but significantly higher than the 3.65 ± 2.05 mg/100 ml per min in the low-grade gliomas.

In the 18 patients with malignant astrocytoma or glioblastoma, the ones with rCMRGl values higher than the median (5.3 mg/100 ml per min) had a median survival time of 7.5 months; in contrast, patients with lower values (below the median) had a relatively long median survival time of 12.9 months. When comparing the tumor/gray matter ratio, the median survival time between the two groups of patients with higher and lower ratios than the median (1.0) differed more apparently and significantly ($P = 0.004$ by the generalized Wilcoxon test). The patients with higher ratios had a median survival time of only 6.0 months, whereas the patients with lower ratios had a survival time of 13.4 months. On the basis of histological diagnosis, patients with malignant astrocytoma (10.6 months) and glioblastoma (9.5 months) showed only a small difference in median survival time after PET was studied (Fig. 1).

In other CNS diseases, FDG increased in the lesions of brain abscess and cerebral sarcoidosis as well as in non-glial tumors, such as meningioma and metastasis.

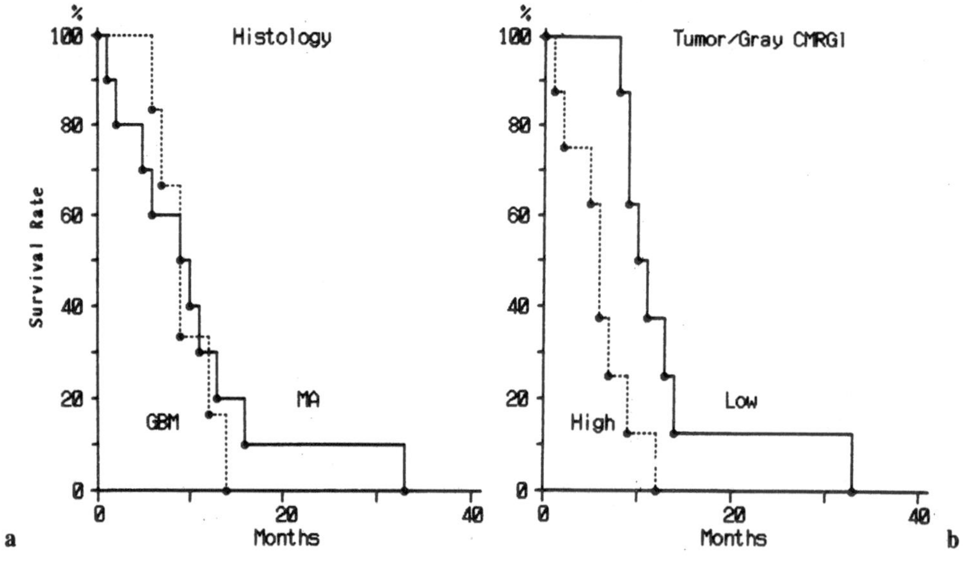

Fig. 1. **a** Survival curves according to the histological diagnosis and **b** the tumor/gray matter ratios of rCMRG1. The difference in survival rates is apparent and significant between groups with higher ratios and lower ratios of rCMRG1 ($P = 0.004$ by the generalized Wilcoxon test)

Table 2. Results of the Met PET study

Diagnosis	No.	Level +	Level −	Diagnosis	No.	Level +	Level −
Glioma	26	23	3	Radiation necrosis	2	0	2
Low grade	(12	9	3)	Infection	2	1	1
High grade	(14	14	0)	Arachnoid cyst	1	0	1
Pituitary tumor	4	4	0	PML	1	0	1
Meningioma	1	1	0				
Lymphoma	1	1	0				
Plasma cell granuloma	1	1	0				
Tumorous	33	30 (91%)	3	Non-tumorous	6	1 (17%)	5

Tumor images were visually compared to the contralateral gray matter on PET images: + higher accumulation, − lower accumulation.

In all 14 high-grade gliomas, the Met tracer accumulated in the tumor more intensely than in the contralateral gray matter. In 12 low-grade gliomas, 9 cases (75%) showed tracer accumulation. Three cases with no tracer accumulation had either a cystic or a small lesion.

Non-glial tumors (pituitary tumor, meningioma, lymphoma, and plasma cell granuloma) studied with Met had high-uptake lesions. All non-tumorous lesions (radiation necrosis, infection, arachnoid cyst, and progressive multiple leukodystrophy) showed no accumulation of the tracer, except for one case of cerebritis which had a moderate increase in tracer uptake.

Discussion

The present FDG study in gliomas supports the preliminary results and reports of other groups [7–9]. The FDG uptake in the high-grade gliomas was variedly nonhomogeneous, reflecting mixture of heterogeneous tissue components, e.g., viable portions of tumor cells, necroses, and perifocal edema. Contrarily, the FDG-uptake patterns in the low-grade gliomas appeared uniformly low.

Areas with high FDG uptake represented metabolically active portions or tumor cell aggregations within tumors determined on the basis of CT and autopsy findings of brains in many cases of the present study. Preoperative recognition of viable and proliferative zones enables us to choose an appropriate route to retrieve tumor tissues adequate for histological examination and for prediction of prognosis, because highly malignant cells determine prognosis and therapeutic effectiveness.

A single FDG study was not always convincing to make a differential diagnosis between high-grade gliomas and other high FDG-uptake lesions such as brain abscess and cerebral sarcoidosis. The FDG PET was examined together with hemocirculation and oxygen metabolism in most cases of the present study. Regional oxygen extraction fraction (rOEF) and metabolic rate of oxygen ($rCMRO_2$) decreased considerably in each grade of glioma [2].

Unlike glioma, brain abscess or cerebral sarcoidosis showed high $rCMRO_2$ values in the lesions. A combined PET study with oxygen metabolism was very effective in differentiating these diseases.

Met images clearly depicted the existence and localization of the tumors. In the previous report on quantitative analysis, the Met uptake index for both the low-grade and high-grade gliomas increased markedly and significantly compared with that of the contralateral gray matter ($P < 0.01$) [5]. The accumulation of Met in cases of gliomatosis cerebri was a good example of the utility of metabolic imaging in the detection of diffuse tumor involvement where the anatomic methods of CT and MRI failed to show significant abnormalities [4,6].

Met tracers accumulated in the non-glial tumors as well as in gliomas, whereas most non-tumorous CNS lesions showed inappreciable uptake. Further clinical application and basic research studies are warranted to clarify the mechanism of high Met uptake and to understand metabolic differences among CNS diseases.

Despite aggressive application of combined therapy, gliomas have remained lethal. PET quantifies the in vivo metabolism of gliomas, and offers information on metabolic differences among gliomas. The elucidation of metabolic features in gliomas may lead us to more accurate diagnosis and more appropriate therapy on the basis of metabolic characteristics of an individual tumor.

Conclusion

We have employed positron emission tomography (PET) with F-18-fluorodeoxyglucose (FDG) and C-11-L-methionine (Met) for in vivo measurement of metabolism in gliomas. In 17 out of 19 (89%) high-grade gliomas, tumors had a higher peak activity than the contralateral white matter, while the pattern of FDG uptake within the tumor was heterogenous. Among histologically verified malignant astrocytoma or glioblastoma, patients showing higher metabolic rates of glucose (rCMRGl) (the median ratio of tumor/gray matter and more) had a median survival time of 6 months after the time of PET, in contrast to 13.4 months for those showing a lower rCMRGl ratio (generalized Wilcoxon test, $P = 0.004$). FDG PET study combined with oxygen metabolism was valuable in differentiating gliomas from other high-FDG-uptake diseases such as brain abscess and cerebral sarcoidosis. Met PET images clearly disclosed the existence and the localization of the tumors in all 14 high-grade gliomas and in 9 out of 12 low-grade gliomas.

References

1. Lowry OH, Berger SJ, Carter JG, Chi MMY, Manchester JK, Knor J, Pusateri ME (1983) Diversity of metabolic patterns in human brain tumors: Enzymes of energy metabolism and related metabolites and cofactors. J Neurochem 41:994–1010

2. Mineura K, Yasuda T, Kowada T, Shishido T, Ogawa T, Uemura K (1986) Positron emission tomographic evaluation of histological malignancy in gliomas using oxygen-15 and fluorine-18-fluorodeoxyglucose. Neurol Res 8:164–168
3. Mineura K, Kowada M, Shishido F (1989) Brain tumor imaging with synthesized 18F-fluorophenylalanine and positron emission tomography. Surg Neurol 31: 468–469
4. Mineura K, Sasajima T, Suda Y, Kowada M, Shishido F, Uemura K (1989) Early and accurate detection of primary cerebral glioma with interfibrillary growth using ^{11}C-L-methionine positron emission tomography. J Med Imag 3:192–196
5. Mineura K, Sasajima T, Suda Y, Kowada M, Shishido F, Uemura K (1990) Amino acids study of cerebral gliomas using positron emission tomography: Analysis of (^{11}C-methyl)-L-methionine uptake index. Neurol Med Chir (Tokyo) 30:997–1002
6. Mineura K, Sasajima T, Kowada M, Uesaka Y, Shishido F (1991) Innovative approach in the diagnosis of gliomatosis cerebri using ^{11}C-L-methionine positron emission tomography. J Nucl Med 32:726–728
7. DiChiro G, DeLaPaz RL, Brooks RA, Sokoloff L, Kornblith PL, Smith BH, Patronas NJ, Kufta CV, Kessler RM, Johnston GS, Manning RG, Wolf AP (1982) Glucose utilization of cerebral gliomas measured by [^{18}F]fluorodeoxyglucose and positron emission tomography. Neurology 32:1323–1329
8. Alavi JB, Alavi A, Chawluk J, Kushner M, Powe J, Hickey W, Reivich M (1988) Positron emission tomography in patients with glioma. A predictor of prognosis. Cancer 62:1074–1078
9. Patronas NJ, DiChiro G, Kufta C, Bairamian D, Kornblith PL, Simon R, Larson SM (1985) Prediction of survival in glioma patients by means of positron emission tomography. J Neurosurg 62: 816–822

Malignancy of Glioma Estimated by PET-^{18}F-FDG, PET-^{11}C-Methionine, and SPECT-^{201}Thallium

Masaru Tamura[1], Takashi Shibasaki[1], Satoru Horikoshi[1], and Noboru Oriuchi[2]

Introduction

The detection of malignancy in glioma by histological studies and by the bromodeoxyuridine labeling index (BUdR-LI) have been well documented [1]. Increased glucose and amino acid uptake in glioma measured by positron emission tomography (PET) with fluorine-18-fluorodeoxyglucose (FDG) [2] and with carbon-11-methionine (Met) [3] have been reported capable of identifying the malignant grade of lesions. Single photon emission CT (SPECT) with 201-thalium chlòride (Tl) is also valuable for determining the grade of malignancy [4]. A method of predicting malignancy preoperatively could alert the operating surgeon to the extent of tumor removal that will be required.

We retrospectively analyzed 28 cases of glioma with variable malignancy using these modalities and correlated the results.

Clinical Material and Methods

Between June, 1988 and May, 1990, 28 patients with supratentorial glioma (9 glioblastoma, 9 malignant glioma, and 11 low-grade glioma) underwent surgical procedures. Before the operations, PET-FDG, PET-Met, and SPECT-Tl neuroimaging was performed. PET scans were obtained on a scanner (Hitachi PCT-H1) 60 min after intravenous injection of 5–8 mCi ^{18}F-FDG. Hypo- and hypermetabolism in FDG uptake of the tumor region was evaluated by comparing contralateral corresponding and/or surrounding brain tissue. PET-Met images were also made in 4 cases 25 min after intravenous injection of ^{11}C-Met. The uptake of Met at the tumor region was evaluated. SPECT-Tl images were obtained on a scanner (Shimazu SET-031) after intravenous injection of ^{201}Tl. An early image was made 15 min after injection of the tracer, and a delayed image 3 h later. The uptake of ^{201}Tl at the tumor region was evaluated as low, moderate, or high. For the study of proliferative potential, patients were given

[1]Department of Neurosurgery and [2]Nuclear Medicine, Gunma University School of Medicine, Maebashi, 371 Japan

300 mg bromodeoxyuridine intraoperatively, and the tumor tissues obtained were fixed 70% ethanol. Immunohistochemical staining with anti-BUdR monoclonal antibody was made on histological preparations. BUdR-LI was calculated from each slide as the percentage of BUdR-labeled nuclei among the total number of tumor cell nuclei.

Results

The correlation of results from histological diagnosis, BUdR-LI, PET-FDG, and SPECT-Tl is summerized in Table 1. Most cases of glioblastoma showed more than 5% in BUdR-LI, hypermetabolism in PET-FDG, and a high uptake in SPECT-Tl. Alternatively, most cases of low-grade glioma showed less than 1% in BUdR-LI, hypometabolism in PET-FDG, and a low uptake in SPECT-Tl. Malignant glioma showed variable parameters, but the cases of higher BUdR-LIs correlated with hypermetabolism in PET-FDG and high uptakes in SPECT-Tl. PET-Met was examined in cases 18 and 19 at the time of recurrency, and on primary lesions in cases 28 and 29. PET-Met images showed positive accumulation at all of these tumor regions.

Representative Cases

Case 3. A 67-year-old female admitted with complaints of headache and vomiting. The CT scan (Fig. 1a) revealed an enhanced mass lesion in the right temporal lobe. PET-FDG (Fig. 1b) showed hypermetabolism and SPECT-Tl (Fig. 1c) revealed a high uptake at the tumor region. Tumor removal was performed and the histological diagnosis was glioblastoma, and the BUdR-LI was 9%.

Case 19. A 54-year-old female admitted with convulsive seizures. The CT scan revealed a non-enhanced low-density mass lesion at the left parietal region. PET-FDG (Fig. 2a) showed hypometabolism, and SPECT-Tl had a low uptake at the tumor. Tumor removal was performed, and the histological diagnosis was an astrocytoma grade 2, however, the BUdR-LI was 3%. The patient received 50 Gy linac X-ray irradiation at the tumor site. Twenty-two months later she had a right hemiparesis. It was difficult to differentiate by CT scan and MRI between tumor recurrence and radiation necrosis. PET-Met (Fig. 2b) showed high accumulation at the right parietal region, and SPECT-Tl (Fig. 2c) also showed an abnormal uptake. Tumor recurrence was highly suspected. An operation was performed, and the histologically diagnosed lesion was astrocytoma grade 3.

Case 28. A 50-year-old male admitted with the complaint of uncinate epileptic seizures. The CT scan (Fig. 3a) showed a small low-density mass lesion at the medial temporal lobe. PET-Met (Fig. 3b) showed abnormal uptake, but there was a SPECT-Tl (Fig. 3c) low uptake at the lesion. An operation was performed, and the histological diagnosis was astrocytoma grade 2 with a BUdR-LI of less than 1%.

Table 1. Summary of cases

Histological diagnosis	Case No.	BUdR-LI ≦1%	BUdR-LI <5%	BUdR-LI ≦5%	PET-FDG Hypo-metabolic	PET-FDG Hyper-metabolic	SPECT-TI Uptake Low	SPECT-TI Uptake Moderate	SPECT-TI Uptake High
Glioblastoma (9 cases)	1			●		●			●
	2			●		●			●
	3			●		●			●
	4			●		●			●
	5			●					●
	6			●					●
	7			●		●		◍	
	8		◍						●
	9		◍			●			
Malignant glioma (9 cases)	10			●		●			●
	11			●		●			
	12		◍			●			●
	13		◍			●			●
	14					●			●
	15		◍		○		○		
	16		◍		○		○		
	17	○			○		○		
	18	○					○		
Low-grade glioma (11 cases)	19		◍		○		○		
	20	○							●
	21	○			○			◍	
	22	○			○		○		
	23	○			○		○		
	24	○					○		
	25	○			○		○		
	26	○			○				
	27	○					○		
	28	○					○		
	29	○					○		

●, highly malignant glioma; ○, moderately malignant glioma; ○, benign glioma

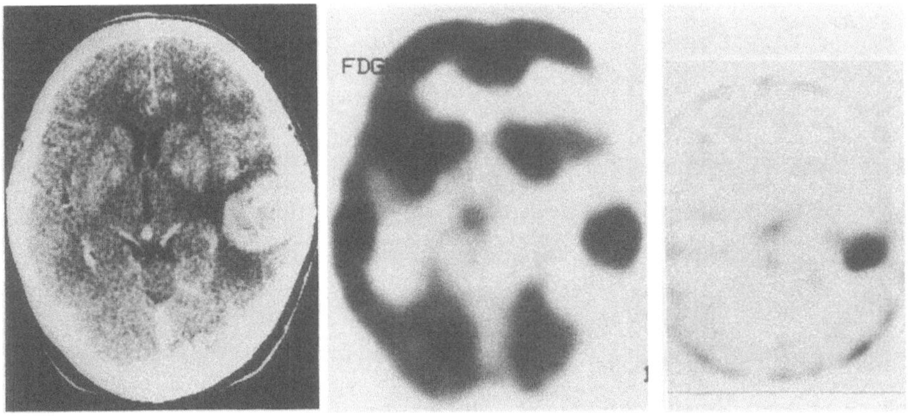

a b c

Fig. 1. Case 3. **a** CT scan with contrast medium shows enhanced mass lesion (glioblastoma) in the right temporal lobe. **b** Hypermetabolism in PET-FDG. **c** High uptake in SPECT-TI

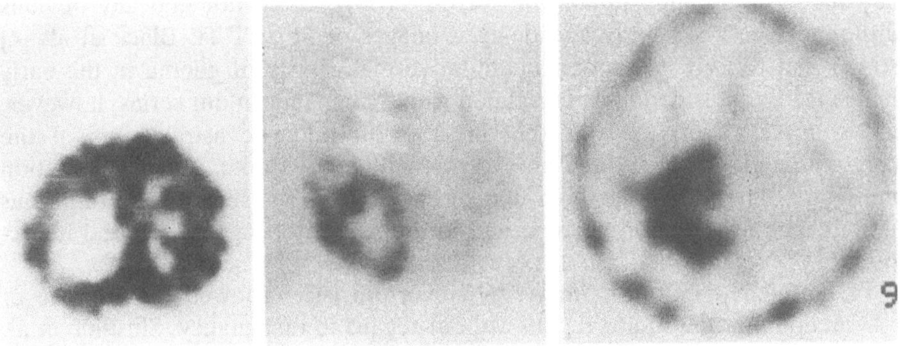

a b c

Fig. 2. Case 19. **a** PET-FDG shows hypometabolism at the left parietal tumor (astrocytoma grade 2). **b** PET-Met shows high accumulation at recurrence (astrocytoma grade 3). **c** SPECT-TI also shows high uptake

Discussion

PET-FDG has shown high activity in glucose consumption in high-grade (III and IV) astrocytoma [2]. In our series, all the glioblastoma and more than half the malignant glioma showed high BUdR-LI and hypermetabolism in PET-FDG, as well as high uptake in SPECT-Tl. Contrarily most cases of low-grade glioma and some cases of malignant glioma showed a BUdR-LI of less than 1% and hypometabolism in PET-FDG. While they showed low uptake, they rarely

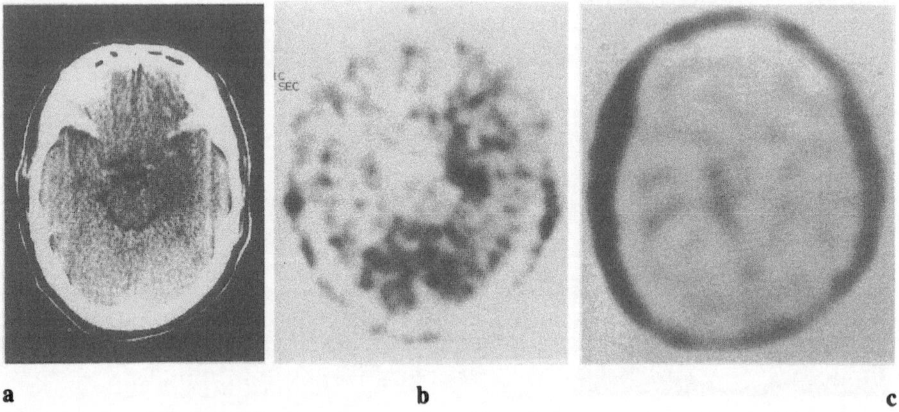

Fig. 3. Case 28. **a** Plain CT scan shows small low-density mass lesion (astrocytoma grade 2) at the right medial temporal lobe. **b** PET-Met shows abnormal uptake. **c** SPECT-Tl shows no accumulation at the lesion

had moderate or high uptake in SPECT-Tl. We could not find any obvious differences between early and delayed images of SPECT-Tl. Black et al. [4] stated that SPECT-Tl showed quantitative malignancy of glioma in the early image. Most cases definitely correlated with malignancy in our series, however, a low-grade glioma such as that in case 20 (pilocytic astrocytoma of the cerebral hemisphere) showed an exceptionally high uptake. Moreover caution must be observed, since a high uptake of SPECT-Tl is seen in non-tumorous lesions such as radiation necrosis and in the subacute stage of cerebral infarction [5].

PET-Met in our four primary and recurrent cases showed high uptake of ^{11}C-methinin at the tumor region without regard to malignancy. Shishido et al. [6] stated that high uptake in PET-Met was recognized in all of their 10 cases of low-grade glioma. From these data, PET-Met is thought to be a useful tool for tumor detection. However, decreased uptake in PET-Met in low-grade glioma has also been reported [3]. A combination of PET-Met and PET-FDG is most reliable for diagnosis of the presence and malignancy of tumors. SPECT-Tl is also useful, if PET is not available. Differential diagnosis of tumor recurrence or radiation necrosis in the course of treatment will be possible using PET-Met, PET-FDG, and SPECT-TlCl in addition to CT scan and MRI.

Conclusion

The combination of PET-Met, PET-FDG, and SPECT-Tl is promising in the diagnosis and determination of malignancy of glioma, as well as in differential diagnosis of recurrence and radiation necrosis.

References

1. Hoshino T, Nagashima T, Murovic JA, Wilson CB, Edwards MSB, Gutin PH, Davis RL, DeArmond SJ (1986) In situ cell kinetics studies on human neuroectodermal tumors with bromodeoxyuridine labeling. J Neurosurg 64:453–459
2. Di Chiro G, DeLaPaz RL, Brooks RA, Sokoloff L, Kornblith PL, Smith BH, Patronas NJ, Kufta CV, Kessler RM, Johnston GS, Manning RG, Wolf AP (1982) Glucose utilization of cerebral gliomas measured by [^{18}F] fluorodeoxyglucose and positron emission tomography. Neurology 32:1323–1329
3. Ericson K, Lilja A, Bergström M, Collins VP, Eriksson L, Ehrin E, von Holst H, Lundqvist H, Långström B, Mosskin M (1985) Positron emission tomography with ([^{11}C]methyl)-L-methionine, [^{11}C] D-glucose, and [^{68}Ga] EDTA in supratentorial tumors. J Comput Assist Tomogr 9:683–689
4. Black KL, Hawkins RA, Kim KT, Becker DP, Lerner C, Marciano D (1989) Use of thalium-201 SPECT to quantitate malignancy grade of gliomas. J Neurosurg 71:342–346
5. Araki Y, Imano Y, Hirata T, Andoh T, Sakai N, Yamada H (1989) Thalium-201 imaging of brain tumors using single photon emission CT (in Japanese). Kaku Igaku (Jpn J Nucl Med) 26:1363–1369
6. Shishido F, Uemura K, Inugami A, Tomura N, Higano S, Fujita H, Murakami M, Kanno I, Yasui N, Mineura K (1990) Value of ^{11}C-methionine and PET in the diagnosis of low-grade gliomas (in Japanese). Kaku Igaku (Jpn J Nucl Med) 27:239–302.

Metabolic Changes in a Glioma Model Following Chemotherapy

KIYOTAKA SATO[1], MOTONOBU KAMEYAMA[1], RYUICHI KATAKURA[1], TAKAMASA KAYAMA[1], TAKASHI YOSHIMOTO[1], and KIICHI ISHIWATA[2]

Introduction

Positron emission tomography (PET) has been widely used in the diagnosis of brain tumors and in the evaluation of therapy. ^{18}F-fluorodeoxyglucose (^{18}FDG) and ^{11}C-methionine have been used to diagnose the malignancy of tumors and to evaluate therapeutic effectiveness [1–3]. Moreover, tracers indicating the metabolism of nucleic acid have been investigated and ^{18}F-fluoro-2′-deoxyuridine (^{18}FdUrd) was developed for this use [4–8]. To shed light on the metabolic changes in gliomas following therapy, we have used a glioma model to study correlational changes among ^{18}FdUrd, ^{14}C-thymidine, ^{14}C-methionine, and ^{3}H-deoxyglucose uptake after chemotherapy as a means for interpreting clinical PET results, together with the changes in the bromodeoxyuridine labeling index (BUdR LI).

Materials and Methods

KEG-1 rat glioma cells were transplanted subdermally in the groin region of Wistar-King rats. The tumors attained a diameter of 8–10 mm 10 days after transplantation, at which time therapy was carried out. The chemotherapy consisted of an intraperitoneal injection of 30 mg/kg 1-(4-amino-2-methyl-5-pyrimidinyl)methyl-3-(2-chloroethyl)-3-nitrosourea hydrochloride (ACNU).

The tracers were administrated in each of the 5 animals either at 2 or 6 h or 1, 7, or 14 days after chemotherapy, and at the same time in 5 untreated control rats. The tracers were as follows: 100 μCi ^{18}FdUrd, 10 μCi L-[methyl-^{14}C]methionine (^{14}C-Met), 20 μCi 2-[1,2-^{3}H]deoxyglucose (^{3}H-DG), 10 μCi [2-^{14}C]thymidine (^{14}C-dThd), and 30 mg/kg 5-bromo-2′-deoxyuridine (BUdR). The ^{18}FdUrd was synthesized using an automatic synthesizing system and had a purity of more than 99% [9]. The tracers, with the combination of ^{18}FdUrd, ^{3}H-DG, and ^{14}C-Met or ^{14}C-dThd, were injected into the tail vein simul-

[1] Division of Neurosurgery, Institute of Brain Diseases, Tohoku University School of Medicine, Sendai, 980 Japan
[2] Division of Radiopharmaceutical Chemistry, Tohoku University, Sendai, 980 Japan

taneously, or the BUdR was administered alone intraperitoneally. The animals were sacrificed 60 min after the administration of tracers and tumor samples were obtained. Radioactivity was measured or the anti-BUdR stain was performed [10–12]. The results are expressed as differential absorption ratios (DARs) [13] for radioactive isotopes or labeling index for BUdR. The statistical analysis was done by the two-sample *t*-test.

Results (Figs. 1–5)

A significant decrease in the DAR for ^{18}FdUrd was observed at 2 and 6 h and at 1 and 7 days after treatment ($P < 0.005$, 0.001, 0.001, and 0.001, respective-

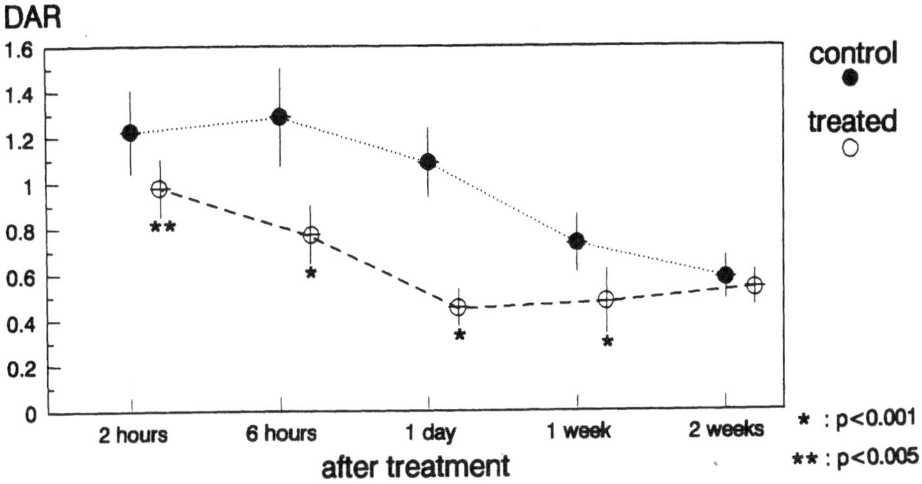

Fig. 1. Change in uptake of F18-fluorodeoxyuridine

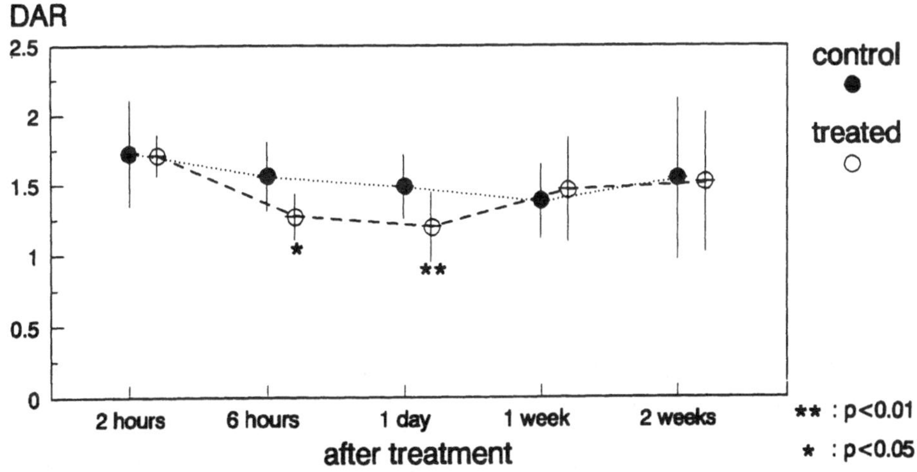

Fig. 2. Change in uptake of C14-methionine

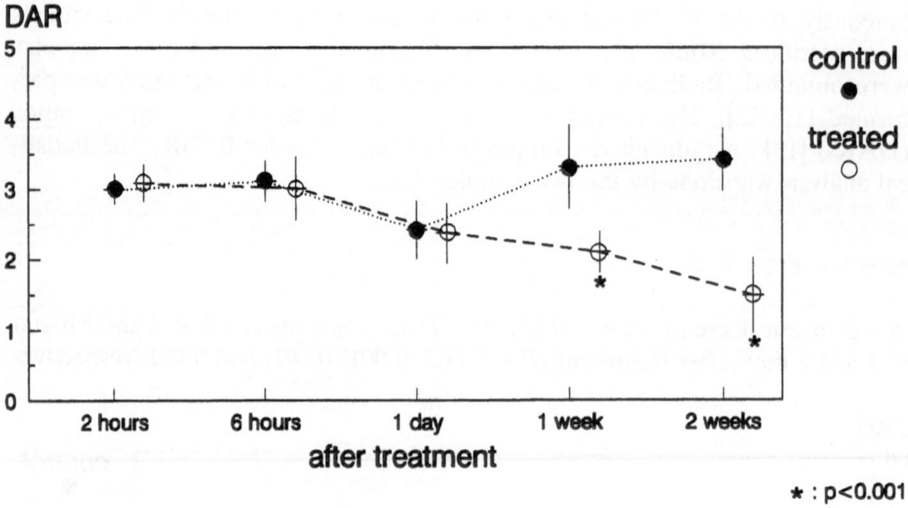

Fig. 3. Change in uptake of H3-deoxyglucose

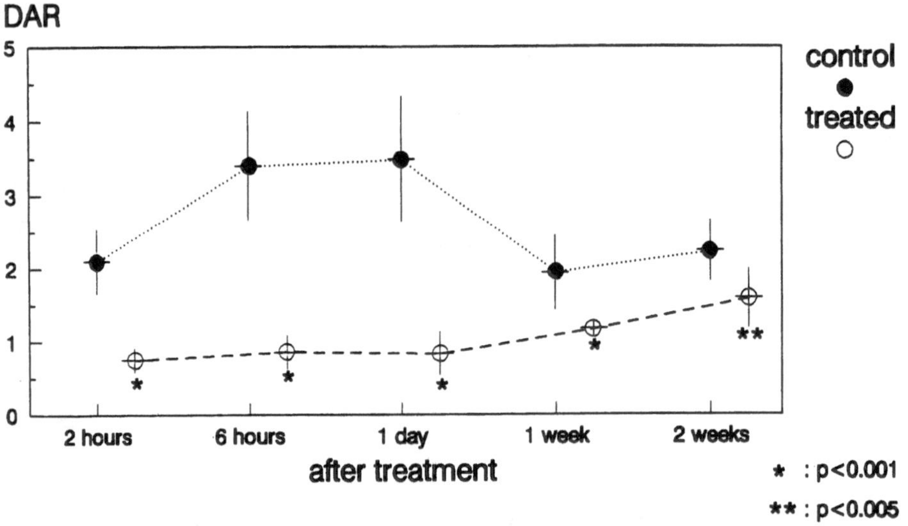

Fig. 4. Change in uptake of C14-thymidine

ly) and the DARs for ^{14}C-Met appeared after 6 h and after 1 day from therapy ($P < 0.05$ and 0.01). With regard to ^{3}H-DG, significant decreases between control and treated groups were found after 1 or 2 weeks ($P < 0.001$). Significant decreases in ^{14}C-dThd uptake were found at all time intervals ($P < 0.001$ for all points excepts for that at 2 weeks, where $P < 0.005$). The changes of the BUdR LIs paralleled the changes in the DARs for dThd and FdUrd.

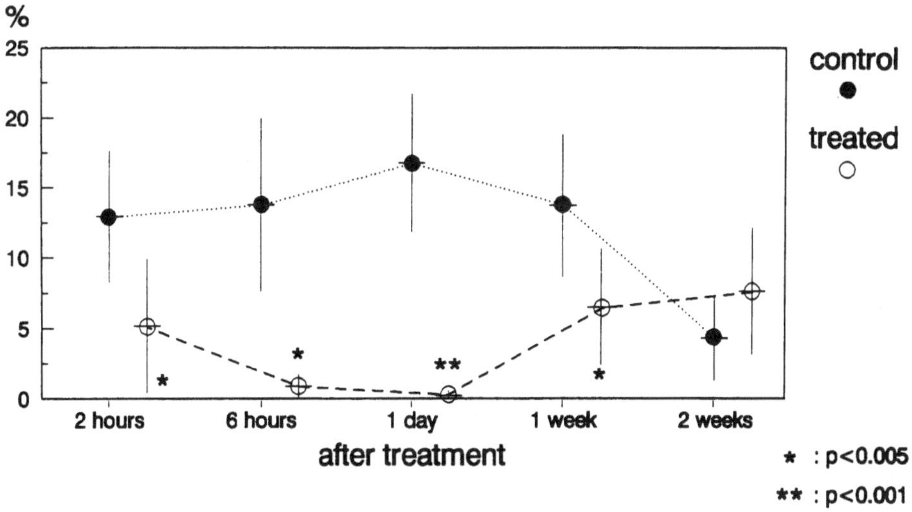

Fig. 5. Change of bromodeoxyuridine labeling index

Discussion

Using a variety of tumor models in the mouse and rat, Shani and Wolf [14], Shani et al. [15] and Visser et al. [16] studied the accumulation of ^{18}F-fluorouracil (^{18}FU) and found that the washout in FU-sensitive tumors is slow, suggesting that the effectiveness of 5-FU therapy can be predicted by ^{18}FU PET scanning. Abram et al. [17] studied the accumulation of 6-^{3}H-5-FdUrd and 6-^{3}H-5-FU in tumor tissues and showed that more of the former than the latter is accumulated. Additionally, Abe et al. [4] made a comparative study of the uptake by tumor tissue of ^{18}F-labeled fluorinated pyrimidines. They found that the uptake of ^{18}FdUrd by tumor tissue of other organs is 1.3- to 4-fold greater than ^{18}FUrd or ^{18}FU uptake, thus indicating that ^{18}FdUrd is suitable for the imaging of tumors. From an analysis of ^{18}FdUrd accumulation in tumors, Ishiwata et al. [5,6] showed that at 2 h from administration, 3%–11%, 6%–14%, 17%–34%, and 19%–24% of ^{18}F are found in the microsomal, nuclear, acid soluble, and nucleotide fractions, respectively, indicating that it had entered the nucleic acid synthesis pathway. Tsurumi et al. [8] did autoradiographic and isotope uptake (^{18}FdUrd, ^{14}C-dThd, and ^{14}C-isobutyric acid) studies using a transplanted glioma model, and found that the radioactivity of ^{18}F from tumor tissue remained constant between 30 and 120 min. In contrast, there was a steady increase in the nucleotide and acid insoluble fractions over time. On the basis of these results, they concluded that ^{18}FdUrd is suitable as a tracer of nucleic acid metabolism.

Using BUdR and its antibody, only S-phase cells are stained, and it is thought that the BUdR LI has the same significance as that using dThd [18]. In the present study, we found that changes of the BUdR LI due to therapy were similar to those for dThd and FdUrd uptakes. These findings were interpreted as indicating a decrease in the percentage of S-phase cells immediately following chemotherapy and a gradual recovery thereafter. Since the percentage of S-phase cells is taken as an indication of the proliferation of tissue, it was possible to evaluate the proliferation of tumor tissues and to interpret PET results using ^{18}FdUrd in the present tracer uptake experiment.

A comparison of the results obtained with the various tracers indicates that changes in Met and DG uptakes were not sensitive in the early period following chemotherapy. It is thought that for the PET evaluation of therapeutic effects following the administration of ACNU in clinical cases, either dThd or FdUrd labeled by a positron emitter are appropriate. The application of ^{11}C-labeled dThd to brain tumors, however, has not yet appeared in the literature, probably due to the complicated synthesizing process and a poor yielding rate. Therefore ^{18}FdUrd would be a suitable tracer in clinical PET studies. On the other hand, the rapid response does not necessarily indicate a cure of the disease, so that further studies on dThd and FdUrd, as well as on DG and Met, are still needed in order to determine whether satisfactory clinical results have been attained.

Conclusion

The metabolic changes after chemotherapy in the glioma model were investigated using ^{18}FdUrd, ^{14}C-dThd, ^{14}C-Met, and ^{3}H-DG simultaneously. It was found that the metabolism of nucleic acid, amino acid, and glucose responded differently in time course and degree. These results clearly indicate that PET scans used in conjunction with a variety of tracers should be used for clinical diagnosis and evaluation of therapy in glioma cases. Also, the fact that the pattern of ^{18}FdUrd metabolic changes was parallel to those of dThd and the BUdR LI, indicate that ^{18}FdUrd is a promising tracer of nucleic acid metabolism for evaluating the proliferative potential of brain neoplasm.

References

1. Derlon JM, Bourdet C, Bustany P, Chatel M, Theron J, Darcel F, Syrota A (1989) [^{11}C]L-methionine uptake in gliomas. Neurosurg 25:720–728
2. Kameyama M, Shirane R, Itoh J, Sato K, Katakura R, Yoshimoto T, Hatazawa J, Itoh M, Ido T (1990) The accumulation of ^{11}C-methionine and histological grade in cerebral glioma patients studied with PET. Acta Neurochir (Wien) 104:8–12
3. Patronas NJ, Brooks RA, DeLaPaz RL, Smith BH, Kornblith PL and DiChiro G (1983) Glycolytic rate (PET) and contrast enhancement (CT) in human cerebral gliomas. AJNR 4:533–535
4. Abe Y, Fukuda H, Ishiwata K, Yoshioka S, Yamada K, Endo S, Kubota K, Sato T, Matsuzawa T, Takahashi T, Ido T (1983) Studies on ^{18}F-labeled pyrimidines. Tumor uptakes of ^{18}F-5-fluorouracil, ^{18}F-5-fluorouridine, ^{18}F-5-fluorodeoxy-uridine in animals. Eur J Nucl Med 8:258–261

5. Ishiwata K, Ido T, Kawashima K, Murakami M, Takahashi T(1984) Studies on ^{18}F-labeled pyrimidines: II. Metabolic investigation of ^{18}F-5-fluorouracil, ^{18}F-5-fluoro-2′-deoxy- uridine and ^{18}F-5-fluorouridine in rats. Eur J Nucl Med 9:185–189
6. Ishiwata K, Ido T, Abe Y, Matsuzawa T and Murakami M (1985) Studies on ^{18}F-labeled pyrimidines: III. Biochemical investigation of ^{18}F-labeled pyrimidines and comparison with ^{3}H-deoxythymidine in tumor-bearing rats and mice. Eur J Nucl Med 10:39–44
7. Kameyama M, Tsurumi Y, Itoh J, Sato K, Katakura R, Yoshimoto T, Hatazawa J, Itoh M, Ido T (to be published) Clinical application of ^{18}Fluorodeoxyuridine in glioma patients–PET study of nucleic acid metabolism. J Neurol Neurosurg Psychiatry
8. Tsurumi Y, Kameyama M, Ishiwata K, Katakura R, Monma M, Ido T, Suzuki J (1990) ^{18}F-fluoro-2′-deoxyuridine as a tracer of nucleic acid metabolism in brain tumors. J Neurosurg 72:110–113
9. Ishiwata K, Monma M, Iwata R, Ido T (1987) Automated synthesis of 5-[^{18}F]fluoro-2′-deoxyuridine. Int J Radiat Isot 38:467–473
10. Hoshino T, Nagashima T, Murovic J, Levin EM, Levin VA, Rupp SM (1985) Cell kinetic studies of in situ human brain tumors with bromodeoxyuridine. Cytometry 6:627–632
11. Ikeda H, Yoshimoto T (to be published) Developmental changes in proliferative activity of cells of the murine Rathke's pouch. Cell Tissue Res
12. Nagashima T, De Rrmond SJ, Murovic J, Hoshino T (1985) Immunocytochemical demonstration of S-phase cells by anti-bromodeoxyuridine monoclonal antibody in human brain tumor tissues. Acta Neuropathol (Berl) 67:155–159
13. Moore FD, Tobin LH, Aub JC (1943) Studies with radioactive di-azo dyes: III. The distribution of radioactive dyes in tumor-bearing mice. J Clin Invest 22:161–168
14. Shani J, Wolf W (1977) A model for prediction of chemotherapy response to 5-fluorouracil based on the differential distribution of 5-[^{18}F]fluoro- uracil in sensitive versus resistant lymphocytic leukemia in mice. Cancer Res 37:2306–2308
15. Shani J, Wolf W, Schlesinger T (1978) Distribution of ^{18}F-5-fluorouracil in tumor-bearing mice and rats. Int J Nucl Med Biol 6:19–28
16. Visser GWM, Gorree GCM, Braakhuis BJM, Herscheid JDM (1989) An optimized synthesis of ^{18}F-labeled 5-fluorouracil and a re-evaluation of its use as a prognostic agent. Eur J Nucl Med 15:225–229
17. Abrams ND, Knaus EE, Lentle BC and Wiebe LL (1979) Tumor uptake of radiolabeled pyrimidine bases and pyrimidine nucleotides in animal model: II. 6-[^{3}H]-5-fluoro-2′-deoxyuridine. Int J Nucl Med Biol 6:103–107
18. Hoshino T (1973) Cell kinetics of brain tumors. Neurol Med Chir (Tokyo) 6:453–459

Quantitative Autoradiographical Evaluation of Protein Synthesis in a Brain Tumor Model Using ^{14}C-labeled Valine

SHIGERU MITSUKA[1], HIDEAKI NUKUI[1], MIRKO DIKSIC[2], Y. LUCAS YAMAMOTO[2], and WILLIAM FEINDEL[2]

Introduction

Since tumor tissue grows rapidly, it can be assumed that a large amount of protein has to be synthesized in the tissue. Previous studies have already shown evidence that a very high exogenous uptake of amino acid is present in human brain tumor [1,2]. The studies were done by positron emission tomography (PET) using ^{11}C-DL-valine, ^{11}C-DL-tryptophan [1], and L-^{11}C-methionine [2]. An autoradiographical method for the measurement of the rate of protein synthesis has also been introduced [3,4]. A variation of this method has been applied to some experimental brain tumors as well [5]. The kinetic model for L-1-^{14}C- leucine incorporation into proteins, described by Smith et al. [3], was applied to L-1-^{14}C-valine, and the rate constants were measured in several normal brain structures [6]. In this paper, we describe the measurement of the rate constants and the rate of valine incorporation into proteins in AA ascites tumors implanted into rat brains. The reliability and the applicability of the kinetic model to the tumor model is also discussed.

Materials and methods

Animal Preparation and Quantitative Autoradiography

Small pieces of a spontaneous ascites tumor (AA ascites tumor, Mason Research Institute) [7], minced by scissors from a solid tumor grown subcutaneously, were implanted into the right hemisphere of adult female Wistar rats (200–240 g) under pentobarbital anesthesia. Seven days later, polyethylene catheters (PE50) were placed into the femoral artery and vein for blood sampling and tracer injection under halothane anesthesia. The rats were immobilized with a loose-fitting plaster cast on lower halves of their bodies, they

[1] Department of Neurosurgery, Yamanashi Medical College, Nakakoma, Yamanashi, 409–38 Japan
[2] Montreal Neurological Institute, Montreal, Quebec, H3A 2B4, Canada

were taped onto a lead block, and were allowed to awake. Twenty-six animals were divided into nine groups, depending upon the killing time after tracer injection. The animals were injected intravenously with 10 μCi of L-1-^{14}C valine (specific activity = 55–56 mCi/mmol) and killed by decapitation at 1, 5, 10, 15, 20, 25, 30, 45, and 60 min after the start of injection. Timed arterial blood samplings were done during the experiment. Plasma samples were deproteinized by the addition of 10% trichloroacetic acid (TCA). The plasma concentration of ^{14}C-valine was measured by a liquid scintillation counter. The brains were removed immediately after decapitation, frozen, and cut into 20 μm sections in a cryostat at –21°C. The brain slices were then exposed to SB5 films together with ^{14}C standards for 1 week. Tissue radio-activities were determined by an image-processing system in selected regions of interest which were related to regions on hematoxyline and eosin (HE)-stained sections. Since the tumor had an inhomogenous tracer distribution, two different regions of interest were selected on the image in order to estimate the mean and maximum concentrations of the tracer in the tumor. Both sets of tumor tracer concentrations were used in the rate constants calculation. The rate constants in the contralateral parietal cortex were also estimated.

Determination of Rate Constants

The mathematical analysis in the kinetic model is essentially identical to that of the 2-deoxy-D-^{14}C-glucose method originally described by Sokoloff et al. [8]. The three-compartment model used in this study is described in Fig. 1. The total concentration of ^{14}C can be calculated by the following equation:

$$C_i^*(T) = (K_1^*/K)[k_4^* + (k_2^* + k_3^*)e^{-K \cdot t}] \otimes C_p^*(t) \qquad (1)$$

where C_p^* is the plasma concentration of ^{14}C-valine, $K = (k_2^* + k_3^* + k_4^*)$, and $\otimes$ denotes an operation of convolution. The total tissue radioactivity is a function of the time and rate constants with the plasma ^{14}C-valine concentration as an input function (Eq. 1). The contribution of blood volume was estimated by the method described by Kato et al. [9]. The rate constants were determined by fitting with the non-linear least squares routine.

The rate of valine incorporation into proteins was calculated using Eq. 2:

$$V_i = \frac{CP[C_i^*(T) - K_1^* e^{-K \cdot t} \otimes C_p^*(t)]}{[1 - e^{-K \cdot t}] \otimes C_p^*(t)} \qquad (2)$$

where V_i is the rate of valine incorporation (nmol/g per min) and C_p is the plasma concentration of valine measured by means of high performance liquid chromatography (HPLC).

Determination of the Acid Soluble Fraction

To verify the reliability of the rate constants calculated by this method, six tumor-bearing rats were prepared by the same manner as described above. Animals were decapitated at 45 min after tracer injection, and the tumor and

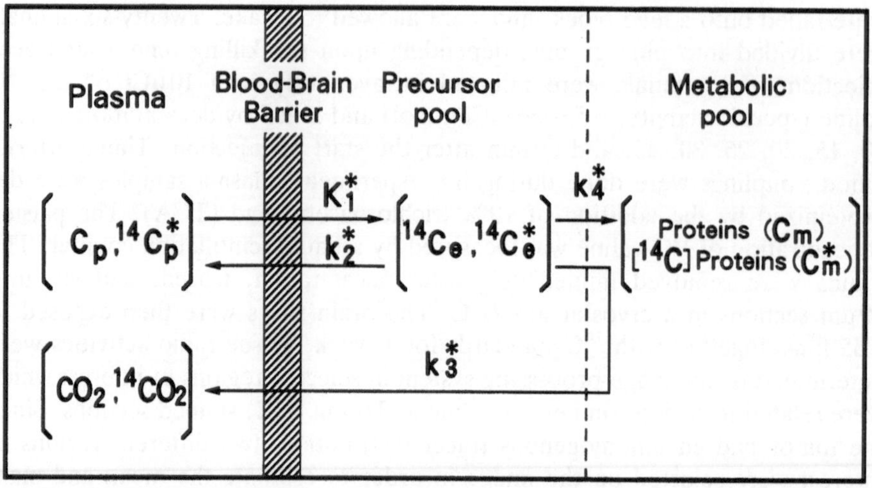

Fig. 1. Schematic representation of the model of L-1-^{14}C valine used in this work. C_p and C_p^* represent the concentration of valine and radioactively labeled valine tracer in the arterial plasma. C_e and C_e^* represent their concentration in the precursor pool. The transfer coefficients (rate constants) representing movement of labeled valine and its metabolite between diffetent compartments are K_1^* (from blood to tissue), k_2^* (from tissue to blood), k_3^* (decarboxylation of valine), and k_4^* (incorporation of valine into proteins)

contralateral cortex were sampled and homogenized with chilled 10% TCA. The supernatant (acid soluble fraction) was transferred into scintillation vials and the precipitate was digested by protosol. The radioactivity of both fractions was measured by liquid scintillation. The ratio of radioactivity of the acid soluble fraction and the total radioactivity (sum of both fractions) was compared to the ratio of $C_e^*(T)/C_i^*(T)$ calculated by using measured rate constants in whole tumor.

Results

The Rate Constants in the Tumor

The rate constants estimated by this method, half-life of precursor pool ($\ln 2/(k_2^* + k_3^* + k_4^*)$), distribution volume ($K_1^*/(k_2^* + k_3^* + k_4^*)$), and net steady-state rate of valine uptake ($Vs = K_1^* k_4^*/(k_2^* + k_3^* + k_4^*)$), are given in Table 1. For comparison, the values for normal gray matter reported by Kirikae et al. [6] are also given in Table 1. Since the mean blood volume estimated was 3.3% in whole tumor and 2.8% in peak accumulated region, the tumor rate constants show in Table 1 were calculated by setting the blood volume of 3% as the constant.

Table 1. Rate constants for L-1-^{14}C-valine

	Rat (n = 14) Normal gray (Kirikae et al. [6])	Tumor (n = 26) Whole (Present study)	Tumor (n = 26) Peak (Present study)
K_1^* (ml/g per min)	0.038 ± 0.005	0.325 ± 0.046	0.572 ± 0.083
$k_2^* + k_3^*$ (/min)	0.116 ± 0.020	0.149 ± 0.054	0.179 ± 0.074
k_4^* (/min)	0.033 ± 0.005	0.063 ± 0.019	0.091 ± 0.028
Half-life of precursor pool (min)	4.7 ± 0.59	3.27 ± 0.88	2.57 ± 0.75
Distribution volume (ml/g)	0.255 ± 0.038	1.53 ± 0.47	2.12 ± 0.69
Vs (ml/g per min)	0.0084 ± 0.0013	0.097 ± 0.009	0.193 ± 0.015

Values are mean ±SD. The half-life of the precursor pool was calculated as $\ln 2/(k_2^* + k_3^* + k_4^*)$, the distribution volume as $K_1^*/(k_2^* + k_3^* + k_4^*)$, and the steady-state rate of valine uptake (*Vs*) as $K_1^* k_4^*/(k_2^* + k_3^* + k_4^*)$. The tumor rate constants listed here were estimated using fixed blood volume (3%)

The rate constants in the tumor were greater than those in the normal gray matter. The most prominent change was noted in K_1^* which was from 8.6 times (whole tumor) to 15 times (peak region) greater. The k_4^* was from 1.9 times to 2.8 times greater, and the $(k_2^* + k_3^*)$ was from 1.3 to 1.5 times greater than that of the normal gray matter. The half-life of the precursor pool was shorter, the distribution volume was from 6 to 8 times larger and the steady-state rate of valine incorporation into proteins was 12 times greater in whole tumor and 23 times greater in the peak region of the tumor than that of the normal gray matter.

Rate of Valine Incorporation into Proteins

The plasma concentration of free valine and the rate of valine incorporation into proteins in tumor and the contralateral parietal cortex estimated in seven rats are given in Table 2. Valine incorporation rates in these structures were calculated by Eq. 2 using the regional rate constants listed in Table 1 for tumor and the rate constants for the contralateral parietal cortex (K_1^* = 0.024 ± 0.004, $k_2^* + k_3^*$ = 0.063 ± 0.027, and k_4^* = 0.029 ± 0.015) which were regionally estiamted in this study. The average concentration of plasma-free valine was 283 nmol/ml. The average rate of valine incorporation was 2.6 nmol/g per min in the contralateral parietal cortex, 24.1 nmol/g per min in whole tumor, and 47.6 nmol/g per min in the region of peak accumulation of radioactivity in the tumor.

Fraction of Tissue-free Valine

There was good agreement of percentages of the tracer present in the acid soluble fraction (precursor pool) to the total tissue radioactivity estimated by two different methods (see Materials and Methods). The acid soluble fraction in the tumor was around 10% in both direct measurement (12.5 ± 3.1%) as

Table 2. Concentration of plasma-free valine and the valine incorporation rate into proteins in tumor and contralateral parietal cortex

Rat	Plasma-free valine (nmol/min)	Valine incorporation rate (nmol/g per min)		
		Contralateral parietal cortex	Tumor Whole	Tumor Peak
A	267	3.0	16.7	39.0
B	319	2.3	17.2	38.4
C	319	2.5	33.6	58.2
D	336	3.1	29.7	60.2
E	362	3.0	26.9	55.9
F	187	1.9	20.2	42.3
G	189	2.4	24.1	39.1
Mean ±SD	283 ± 71	2.6 ± 0.4	23.6 ± 6.9	47.6 ± 10.0

The valine incorporation rates in tumor were calculated using Eq. 2 with the regional rate constants given in Table 1. For the contralateral parietal cortex, the rate constants ($K_1^* = 0.024 \pm 0.004$, $k_2^* + k_3^* = 0.063 \pm 0.027$, and $k_4^* = 0.029 \pm 0.015$) were used

well as from the calculation using rate constants for whole tumor (11.7 ± 3.0%). The acid soluble fraction in the contralateral cortex was about 20%, with a good agreement between the direct measurement (22.9 ± 3.5%) and calculation (21.1 ± 5.6%).

Discussion

Some methods for the estimation of protein synthesis rate using tracer kinetic model of labeled amino acid has been reported [1,2,3,4,5,6]. Among these, L-^{11}C-methionine has been used as a tracer for the estimation of protein synthesis in the tumor in PET study [2]. However, S-methyl labeled methionine produces other labeled amino acids like serine and cysteine by transmethylation process and these amino acids can also be incorporated into proteins. This makes the use of tracer kinetics more complex. Contrary to this, the tracer kinetics of branched chain amino acids selectively labeled at carboxyl group (in this case L-1-^{14}C-valine) is simple because the labeled carbon is removed as labeled CO_2 at the step of decarboxylation. This eliminates the effect of the labeled metabolites formed in this pathway on the estimation of the model parameters. The kinetic model used in this study has three compartments and four rate constants (Fig. 1), and is identical to the model for L-1-^{14}C-leucine described earlier [3]. The model is fairly simple and convenient to apply to the autoradiographic or PET measurement of protein synthesis. However, the validity of the assumption upon which the model is derived has to apply not only to normal tissue but also to certain pathological tissue such as tumor.

The rate constants estimated in AA ascites tumor in this study differed greatly from the values for normal gray matter [6] (Table 1). The reliability of the set of the rate constants estimated in this study, however, was confirmed by the measurement of the acid soluble fraction in homogenized tissue. The agreement between the two estimates, i.e., direct measurement and calculation using rate constants (see Results), supports the adequacy of the rate constants determined by this method, and the results also indicate that the kinetic model used in this study is applicable to tumor tissue as well as to normal tissue.

We observed a 10–20 times higher rate of valine incorporation into AA ascites tumor than into that of normal tissue (Table 2). These high rates may correlate with the characteristic of this tumor as being a fast growing one [10].

Recently, the influence of recycling of the amino acids derived from protein degradation on the tracer kinetic method has been evaluated [11]. It was reported that significant recycling of unlabeled amino acids derived from steady-state protein degradation is present both in brain and liver, and that the precursor pool for protein synthesis is diluted by these amino acids. In this case, the valine incorporation rate estimated in this study predicts the lowest level of the total rate of valine incorporation into proteins. However, our result indicate that the three-compartment model used in this study predicts at least the rate of exogenous uptake of valine correctly.

Conclusion

The three-compartment model for the estimation of valine incorporation rate into proteins is applicable not only to normal brain tissue but also to AA ascites tumor. The value of rate constants in the tumor was greater than those in normal brain tissue especially in K_1^*. This method can predict at least the rate of exogenous uptake of valine correctly.

References

1. Hübner KF, Purvis JT, Mahaley SM Jr, Robertson JT, Rogers S, Gibbs WD, King P, Partain CL (1982) Brain tumor imaging by positron emission computed tomography using ^{11}C-labeled amino acids. J Comput Assist Tomogr 6:544–550
2. Bustany P, Chatel M, Derlon JM, Darcel F, Sgouropoulos P, Soussaline F, Syrota A (1986) Brain tumor protein synthesis and histological grades: A study by positron emission tomography (PET) with C11-L-Methionine. J Neurooncol 3:397–404
3. Smith CB, Davidsen L, Deibler G, Patlak C, Pettigrew K, Sokoloff L (1980) A method for the determination of local rates of protein synthesis in brain. Trans Am Soc Neurochem 11:94
4. Dwyer BE, Donatoni P, Wasterlin CG (1982) A quantitative autoradiographic method for the measurement of local rates of brain protein synthesis. Neurochem Res 7:563–576
5. Blasberg RG, Groothius D, Molnar P (1981) Application of quantitative autoradiographic measurements in experimental brain tumor models. Semin Neurol 1:203–221
6. Kirikae M, Diksic M, Yamamoto YL (1988) The transfer coeffients for L-valine and the rate of incorporation of L-1-^{14}C-valine into protein in normal adult rat brain. J Cereb Blood Flow Metab 8:598–605

7. Aptekman PM, Bodgen AE (1955) A spontaneous ascites tumor originating and transplantable in the Wistar rat. Cancer Res 15:89–92
8. Sokoloff L, Reivich M, Kennedy C, Des Rosiers MH, Patlak CS, Pettigrew KD, Sakurada O, Shinohara M (1977) The ^{14}C deoxyglucose method for the measurement of local cerebral glucose utilization: Theory, procedure, and normal values in the conscious and anesthesized albino rat. J Neurochem 28:897–916
9. Kato A, Diksic M, Yamamoto YL, Strother SC, Feindel W (1984) An improved approach for measurement of regional cerebral rate constants in the deoxyglucose method with positron emission tomography. J Cereb Blood Flow Metab 4:555–563
10. Arita N, Yamamoto YL, Feindel W (1983) Effect of dexamethasone on rat brain with implanted tumor – changes of regional cerebral blood flow and glucose utilization (in Japanese). No To Shinkei 35:1073–1081
11. Smith CB, Deibler GE, Schmidt EK, Sokoloff L (1988) Measurement of local cerebral protein synthesis in vivo: Influence of recycling of amino acids derived from protein degradation. Proc Natl Acad Sci USA 85:9341–9345

Irradiation Effects on Tumor Blood Flow and Tumor Vascular Permeability in a Rat Transplanted Glioma Model: A Quantitative Autoradiographic Study

Shinji Sugimoto, Toshimitsu Aida, Koichi Tokuda, and Hiroshi Abe[1]

Introduction

Both radiotherapy and chemotherapy have been mainstays in the treatment of brain tumors. Because the delivery of chemotherapeutic drugs to a brain tumor is currently considered to be dependent upon tumor blood flow and/or tumor vascular permeability, it is important to have a clear understanding of irradiation effects on these transport processes. We report the preliminary results of local blood flow (F) and blood-to-tissue transfer constant (K) measurements with quantitative autoradiography (QAR) in a rat-transplanted glioma model.

Materials and Methods

Male Fischer-344 rats were inoculated with 9L gliosarcoma cells (4×10^5). The animals received 20 Gy of whole-brain irradiation when they became symptomatic or when they began losing body weight, usually 9–12 days after tumor inoculation. Control rats were sham irradiated. Two days after irradiation or sham irradiation, the animals were prepared for QAR. Briefly, the femoral artery and vein were catheterized with PE-50 polyethylene tubing under light halothane anesthesia. The animal was placed in a plaster cast and had recovered from anesthesia for at least 2 h before the following experiment. Body temperature was maintained between 35°–37°C using a heat lamp during the experiment. Hematocrit, arterial blood pressure, and arterial pO_2, pCO_2 and pH were monitored; the experiment was accomplished only when these physiological parameters were within normal ranges. F and K were measured using ^{14}C-iodoantipyrine (IAP) and ^{14}C-alpha-aminoisobutyric acid (AIB), respectively. Twenty μCi of the tracer in 1 ml saline was injected for over 1 min at a constant rate into a femoral vein. Timed arterial blood samples were obtained for over 1 min (for measuring F) or 30 min (for measuring K), at which time the animal was decapitated and the brain was rapidly removed.

[1]Department of Neurosurgery, School of Medicine, Hokkaido University, Kita, Sapporo, 060 Japan

Twenty-μm-thick brain sections were made at −20°C in a cryostat and dried on a hot plate at 60°C. Approximately 30–50 dried brain sections were selected, and exposed together with plastic ^{14}C standards (American Radiolabeled Chemicals, Inc.) to Kodak SB-5 film for 2 weeks in order to make autoradiographic images. The rest of the sections were formalin fixed, H & E stained, and preserved as adjacent histological sections. Arterial blood or plasma concentrations of the tracer were measured with a liquid scintillation counter. A microcomputer-based imaging devise (Imaging Research, Inc.) was used to digitize and analyze the autoradiographic images. Selected tissue areas in a digitized autoradiographic image were defined on the basis of a digitized image of the adjacent histological section registered in another channel of the imaging device. F and K were obtained from the autoradiographic images of the brain section with the maximum cross-sectional area of the tumor, and determined pixel-by-pixel within the regions of interest (ROIs).

The calculation of F was dependent upon the following equation [1,2]:

$$Ci(T) = F\int_0^T Ca(t)e^{-F/\lambda(T-t)}dt$$

where $Ci(T)$ is the tissue concentration of ^{14}C-IAP as determined by QAR at time T, λ is the tissue:blood partition coefficient, Ca is the arterial blood concentration of ^{14}C-IAP, and t is the variable time. In the present study, λ was taken to be 0.8, as suggested by Sakurada et al. [1] for normal rat cortex.

The calculation of K was dependent upon the following equation [3]:

$$K = Ci(T) \Big/ \int_0^T Cp(t)dt$$

where Ci is the tissue concentration of ^{14}C-AIB as determined by QAR at time T, Cp is the arterial plasma concentration of ^{14}C-AIB, and t is the variable time.

Table 1. Blood flow in brain tumor and brain adjacent to tumor (BAT)

Animal No.	Blood flow: Tumor: Whole tumor	Tumor: Area of high value	Tumor: Area of low value	BAT
Non-irradiated				
1.	17.82 ± 14.69	41.96 ± 11.55	3.60 ± 2.57	88.98 ± 30.28
2.	86.60 ± 65.62	129.71 ± 46.32	46.82 ± 5.60	123.23 ± 40.32
(Average)	52.21 ± 48.63	85.84 ± 62.04	25.21 ± 30.56	46.47 ± 42.69
Irradiated				
1.	25.18 ± 17.30	40.76 ± 10.13	7.50 ± 4.87	63.01 ± 21.73
2.	31.37 ± 24.81	81.54 ± 44.45	11.07 ± 3.44	69.24 ± 30.84
(Average)	28.82 ± 4.38	61.15 ± 28.84	9.29 ± 2.52	66.13 ± 4.41

Values are means and ±S.D. (ml/hg per min)

Table 2. Blood-to-tissue transfer constant of AIB in brain tumor and brain adjacent to tumor (BAT)

Animal No.	Blood-to-tissue transfer constant: Tumor: Whole tumor	Tumor: Area of high value	Tumor: Area of low value	BAT
Non-irradiated				
1.	54.74 ± 18.59	77.75 ± 4.05	20.30 ± 5.69	26.68 ± 11.83
2.	68.66 ± 12.75	18.41 ± 5.84	42.96 ± 4.06	12.66 ± 5.02
3.	27.53 ± 12.49	45.06 ± 7.12	9.36 ± 6.99	7.71 ± 3.47
4.	42.27 ± 15.05	46.85 ± 8.78	34.20 ± 8.85	2.11 ± 1.94
5.	26.31 ± 24.20	84.03 ± 18.03	8.84 ± 3.75	6.10 ± 4.65
(Average)	43.90 ± 18.10	67.02 ± 19.37	23.13 ± 15.15	11.05 ± 9.52
Irradiated				
1.	7.78 ± 4.92	9.29 ± 2.58	3.80 ± 1.28	4.88 ± 2.03
2.	22.78 ± 11.96	37.08 ± 11.19	9.47 ± 2.82	8.20 ± 5.02
3.	25.61 ± 10.07	41.34 ± 9.80	19.55 ± 3.56	4.03 ± 1.98
4.	20.40 ± 11,06	32.06 ± 7.65	11.17 ± 4.07	2.49 ± 1.34
(Average)	19.14 ± 7.87*	29.94 ± 14.28*	11.00 ± 6.51	4.90 ± 2.41

Values are means and ±S.D. (ml/hg per min)
*$P < 0.05$ vs non-irradiated animals

Results

Microscopically, the tumors showed several small foci of necrosis. Capillaries were sparse and thin walled. The tumor was well demarcated from the surrounding brain, except where the tumor infiltrated into the brain adjacent to the tumor (BAT). Tumors examined 2 days after 20 Gy irradiation were unchanged from the above histological features.

The mean F or K was determined in whole tumor, in the areas of high and low values within a tumor, and in the BAT. Tables 1 and 2 list the mean Fs and Ks (±S.D.), respectively, within these ROIs in the both non-irradiated and irradiated animals. Considerable local variation in F or K within a tumor was present (Figs. 1a, 2a) in both groups of animals, as indicated by a relatively large S.D. in whole tumor or by a large difference in mean F or K between the areas of high and low values (Tables 1, 2). Necrotic foci within a tumor uniformly had low Fs or low Ks, but otherwise the local variation did not necessarily correlate with histological features (Figs. 1a, 1b, 2a, 2b).

All of the tumors in which F was measured had apparently lower Fs than that in the cerebral cortices (Fig. 1a). The mean F was usually higher in the BAT than in whole tumor. Averaged mean Fs in the tumor and BAT of the irradiated animals did not differ from those of the non-irradiated animals (Table 1).

All of the tumors in which K was measured had higher Ks than did the cerebral cortices (Fig. 2a). The mean K was usually lower in the BAT than in

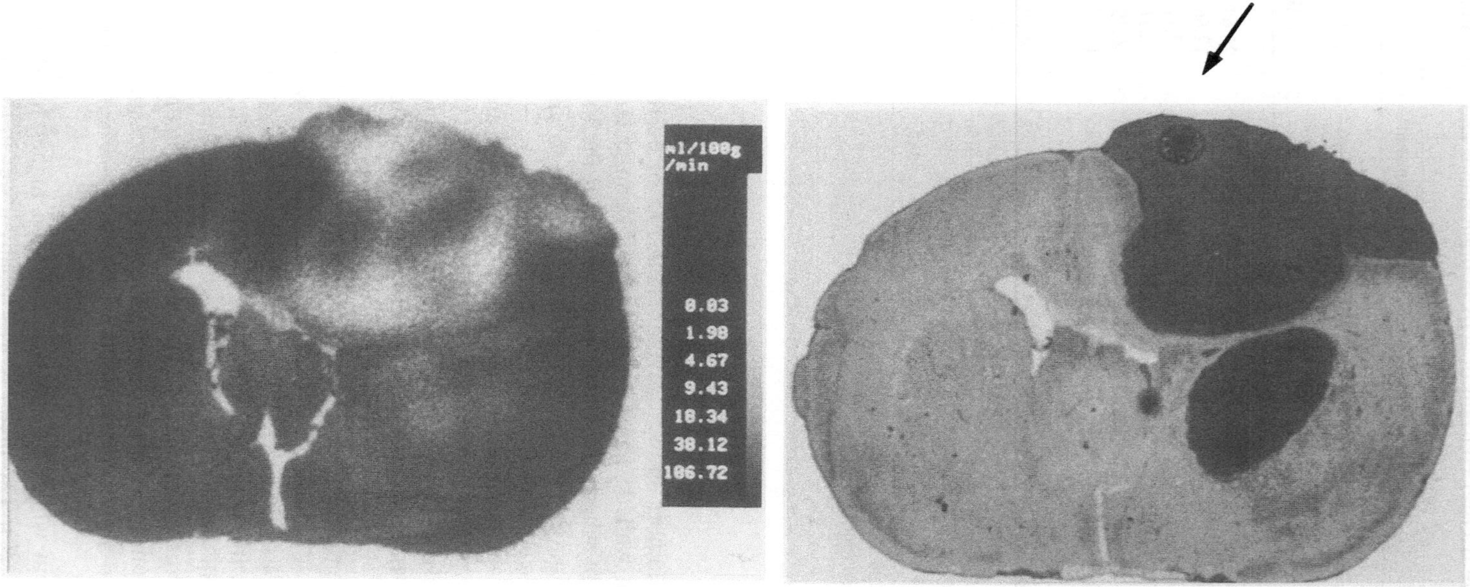

a

b

Fig. 1. **a** Digitized autoradiographic image of blood flow (F) of a section with the maximum cross-sectional area of the tumor (non-irradiated animal No. 1). **b** Digitized image of the adjacent histological section. The tumor has a lower F than that in the cerebral cortices. Note a local variation in F within the tumor. Necrotic focus (*arrow* in **b**) has a low F, but otherwise the local variation in F does not correlate with histological features

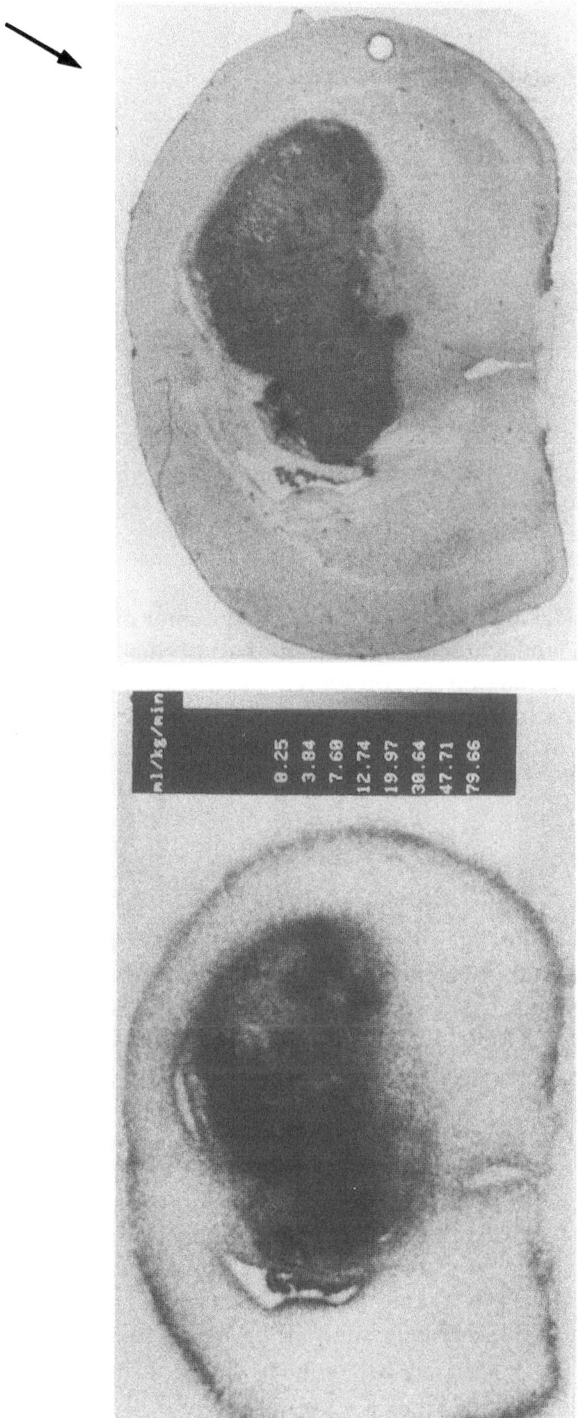

Fig. 2. a Digitized autoradiographic image of the blood-to-tissue transfer constant (K) of a section with the maximum cross-sectional area of the tumor (non-irradiated animal No. 1). **b** Digitized image of the adjacent histological section. The tumor has a higher K than that in the normal cortices. Note a local variation in K within the tumor. Necrotic focus (*arrow* in **b**) has a low K, but otherwise the local variation in K does not correlate with histological features

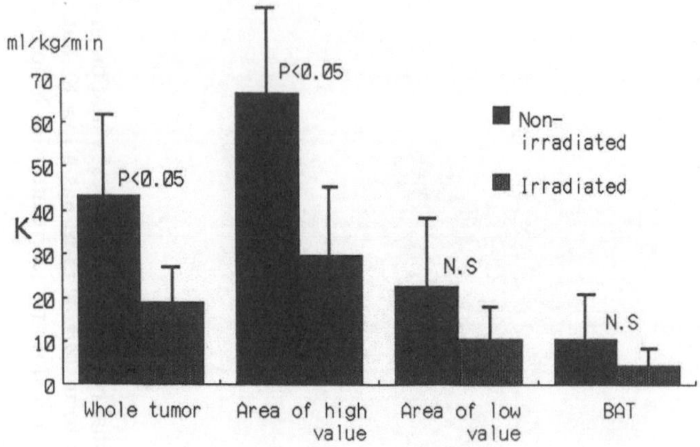

Fig. 3. Comparison in the blood-to-tissue transfer constant (*K*) between the non-irradiated and irradiated animals. Values are average means and +S.D. *BAT*, brain adjacent to tumor; *N.S.*, not significant

whole tumor (Table 2). The averaged mean K in whole tumor of the irradiated animals showed a 56% reduction compared to that of the non-irradiated animals; this significant reduction is considered mainly dependent upon a reduction of K in the area of high value (Table 2, Fig. 3). No difference was observed in the averaged mean K in the BAT between the two groups of animals (Table 2, Fig. 3).

Discussion

This preliminary study demonstrated that 20 Gy irradiation of transplanted 9 L glioma results in a significant reduction of K for AIB in vital tumor areas 2 days after irradiation, without changing any histological features. The relation of AIB transfer constant (K) to the extraction fraction (E), blood flow (F), the fraction of blood involved in exchange (V_f), and permeability-surface area product (PS) is discussed by Blasberg et al. [2]. E, defined as K/FV_f, is a function of both vascular permeability (PS) and blood flow (F), and the value of E indicates the relative importance of these two transport processes. Briefly, when E is less than 0.1, K reflects vascular permeability, and when E is approaching 1.0, K reflects blood flow rather than permeability. Because AIB is mainly distributed in plasma, V_f is considered to be approximately 0.5; 0.74, as suggested by Spence et al. [4]. Taking these V_f values and averaged means of F and K of whole tumor in the present study, E of AIB is roughly estimated to be 0.17 or 0.11 for the non-irradiated tumors, and 0.13 or 0.09 for the irradiated tumors. Because these estimated Es are sufficiently low, Ks are more likely to reflect PS rather than F in the both non-irradiated and irradiated tumors. Our results show that F is not reduced significantly 2 days following

20 Gy irradiation. Therefore, it is concluded that the reduction of K for AIB was probably due to irradiation effects on the tumor capillary endothelium, causing a decrease in permeability and/or surface area.

Properties of AIB such as low molecular weight, high water solubility, and very slow passage across the blood-brain barrier are shared by some chemotherapeutic drugs in clinical use for brain tumors. Our results suggest that at a certain time following radiotherapy, the delivery of this kind of drugs to a brain tumor may be decreased.

References

1. Sakurada O, Kennedy C, Jehle J, Brown JD, Carbin GL, Sokoloff L (1978) Measurements of local cerebral blood flow with iodo {^{14}C} anti-pyrine. Am J Physiol 234:H59–H66
2. Blasberg RG, Molnar P, Groothuis D, Patlak C, Owens E, Fenstermacher J (1984) Concurrent measurements of blood flow and transcapillary transport in Avian sarcoma virus-induced experimental brain tumors: Implication for chemotherapy. J Pharmacol Exp Ther 231:724–735
3. Blasberg RG, Fenstermacher JD, Patlak CS (1983) Transport of alpha-aminoisobutyric acid across brain capillary and cellular membranes. J Cereb Blood Flow Metab 3:8–32
4. Spence AM, Graham MM, O'Gorman LA, Muzi M, Abott GL, Lewellen TK (1987) Regional blood-to-tissue transport in an irradiated rat glioma model. Radiat Res 111:225–236

Superoxide Dismutase Activity in Experimental Brain Tumors — Determination by Electron Spin Resonance Spectrometry Using the Spin Trap Method

Yukio Ikeda[1], Shozo Nakazawa[1], and Masako Yamada[2]

Introduction

It has been reported that oxygen-free radicals may be related to inflammation, carcinogenesis, immunity, trauma, ischemia, and aging [1]. The mechanisms of the therapeutic effect of radiation and some chemotherapeutic agents may be also mediated by oxygen-free radicals. Radiosensitivity and the cytotoxicity of chemotherapeutic agents are supposed to be associated with the status of endogenous oxygen-free radical scavengers in tumor tissues. A general characteristic of the tumor cell has been reported to be a diminished amount of superoxide dismutase (SOD) coupled with superoxide radical production [2]. We investigated SOD activity in experimental rat brain tumors and normal rat brains by electron spin resonance spectrometry (ESR) with the spin trapping method.

Materials and Methods

Experimental brain tumors were produced in 16 male Fischer 344 rats (Charles River Japan Inc.) 5–7 weeks old by the injection of a 10 µl suspension of 1×10^7 viable 9L glioma cells into the left frontoparietal lobe of the rat brain. Experimental subcutaneous tumors were produced in 14 rats by the injection of a 0.1 cc suspension of 1×10^7 viable 9L glioma cells into the animal's back. The rats were killed at 3 weeks after tumor implantation.

Determination of SOD activity was performed by ESR using 5,5-dimethlyl-1-pyrroline-1-oxide (DMPO) as a spin trap. Fifty microliters 2 mM hypoxanthine, 35 µl 5.5 mM diethylenetriaminepentaacetic acid (DETAPAC), 50 µl dialyzed SOD fraction of human plasma, 15 µl DMPO, and 50 µl xanthine oxidase were put into a test tube and mixed by an automatic mixer. Then, the solution was placed in a special flatt cell and DMPO-O_2, and the spin adduct was analyzed

---

[1] Department of Neurosurgery, Nippon Medical School, Bunkyo-ku, Tokyo, 113 Japan
[2] ESR Application Laboratory, JEOL Ltd., Akishima-ku, Tokyo, 196 Japan

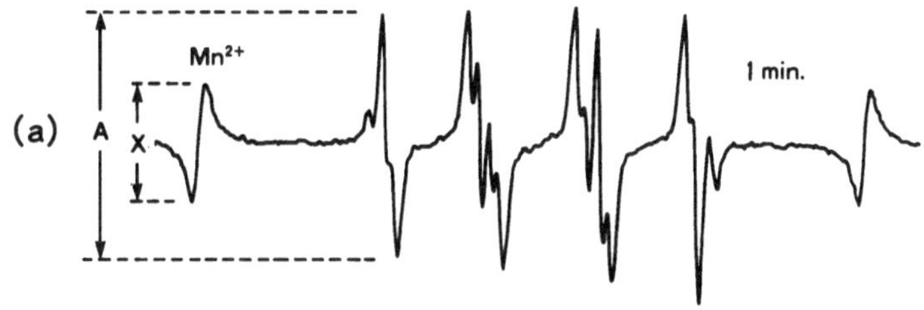

ESR spectrum of DMPO-O_2^- spin adduct produced by xanthine oxidase.
Relative signal intensity is expressed in the following equation :

$$\frac{\text{signal intensity (A)}}{Mn^{2+}\text{ marker intensity (X)}}$$

Fig. 1. Determination of superoxide dismutase activity by electron spin resonance spectrometry using the spin trap method

by ESR (Fig. 1). A standard curve was made using 0.8–100 unit/ml SOD, and manganese oxide was used as an internal standard [3]. DMPO, hypoxanthine, xanthine oxidase, DETAPAC, and SOD (bovine erythrocyte) were obtained from the Sigma Chemical Company.

Results

The SOD activity was 444.10 ± 45.42 U/gm.wet tissue (mean ± standard error of the means) in 9 samples of normal brain tissues. It was 294.85 ± 35.91 U/gm.wet tissue in 16 brain tumor tissues, and 96.92 ± 13.75, 112.02 ± 13.49,

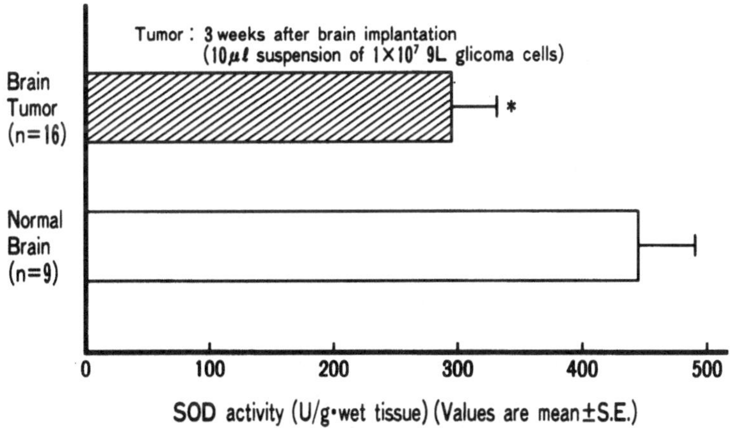

Symbols indicate a significant difference from the normal brain at the level of :
*P<0.05

Fig. 2. Superoxide dismutase (SOD) activity in 9 L glioma

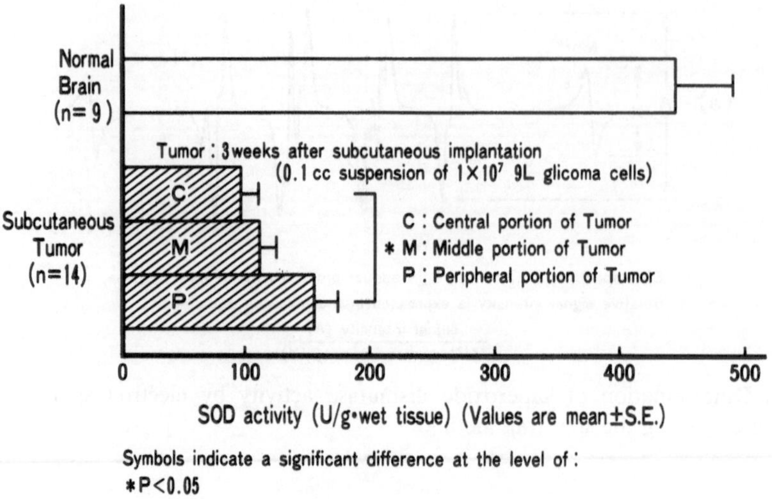

Fig. 3. Superoxide dismutase (SOD) activity in 9 L glioma

and 155.08 ± 19.02 U/gm.wet tissue in the central, middle and peripheral portions, respectively, of 14 subcutaneous tumor tissues. The SOD activity was significantly lower in brain tumors and subcutaneous tumors than in normal brains ($P < 0.05$) (Fig. 2). In the subcutaneous tumor, the SOD activity was lower in the central portion of the tumor than in its peripheral portion ($P < 0.05$) (Fig. 3).

Discussion

SOD is thought to be essential for life in aerobic cells and to provide a defense against the potentially damaging reactivity of the superoxide radicals [4]. Two forms of SOD have been found to date. A copper and zinc-containing form (CuZnSOD) is largely found in the cytosol, and a manganese-containing form (MnSOD) is largely found in the matrix of mitochondria. Diminished amounts of MnSOD have been found in all of the malignant tumors and lowered amounts of CuZnSOD also have been found in many [2]. Recent studies have shown that tumors have the capacity to produce superoxide radicals [2,5]. Oberley et al. [6] emphasized that a general characteristic of the tumor cell is a diminished amount of MnSOD and CuZnSOD coupled with superoxide production, and that the addition of SOD to tumor cells would cause cessation of cell division. They also suggested that the loss of the enzymatic activity of SOD in cancer cells leads to changes in key subcellular structures because of the presence of oxygen-derived radicals, and that cancer cells with a high glycolytic rate are associated with a low level of MnSOD and significant mitochondrial damage. Sun et al. [7] have demonstrated a decrease in all of the antioxidant enzymes, such as MnSOD, catalase, and glutathione peroxidase, except for Cu-Zn SOD, in mouse liver cells in culture. The diminished activity of these enzymes should render these tumor cells more sensitive to both superoxide radical and hydrogen peroxide compared to their normal cell counterparts. Our data indicated that SOD activity was significantly lower in subcutaneous larger 9 L glioma tumors than in normal rat brains and 9 L glioma brain tumors.

In the subcutaneous large 9 L glioma tumors, SOD activity was lower in the central portion of the tumor than in its peripheral portion. Halliwell and Gutteridge [8] postulate that areas within a large tumor mass often have a poor blood supply, and the low SOD activity could merely be a consequence of anoxia. This report was in agreement with our preliminary data on SOD activity in subcutaneous 9 L glioma tumors.

In conclusion, knowledge of this relationship between SOD activity and brain tumors may offer a new insight into the treatment of malignant brain tumors.

References

1. Ikeda Y, Long DM (1990) The molecular basis of brain injury and brain edema: The role of oxygen free radicals. Neurosurgery 27:1–11
2. Oberley LW, Buettner GR (1979) Role of superoxide dismutase in cancer: A review. Cancer Res 39:1141–1149
3. Hiramatsu M, Kohno M (1987) Determination of superoxide dismutase activity by electron spin resonance spectrometry using the spin trap method. JEOL NEWS 23:7–9
4. Fridovich I (1978) The biology of oxygen radicals. Science 201:875–880
5. Bize IB, Oberley LW, Morris HP (1980) Superoxide dismutase and superoxide radical in Morris hepatomas. Cancer Res 40:3686–3693
6. Oberley LW, Leuthauser SWHC, Buettner GR, Sorenson JRJ, Oberley TD, Bize IB (1982) The use of superoxide dismutase in the treatment of cancer. In: Autor AP (ed) Pathology of oxygen. Academic New York, pp 207–221
7. Sun Yi, Oberley LW, Elwell JH, Sierra-Rivera E (1989) Antioxidant enzyme activities in normal and transformed mouse liver cells. Int J Cancer 44:1028–1033
8. Halliwell B, Gutteridge JMC (1984) Review article. Oxygen toxicity, oxygen radicals, transition metals and disease. Biochem J 219:1–14

Studies of Active Oxygen Species in Brain Tumors

MASAHIRO KURISAKA[1], KUNIHIRO NAKAI[1], MAKOTO ARIMITSU[1], KOREAKI MORI[1], and YUKIE NIWA[2]

Introduction

Many factors, such as viral infection, irradiation, chemical substances, and others, are present as promoters of cancer. These factors act upon deoxynucleic acid (DNA) of normal cells and thereby induce cancer [1,2]. Among these factors, viruses act directly on the DNA, but radiation beams and chemical agents create a large amount of active oxygen species in the cytoplasm of the cells and the surplus active oxygen species produce the cancer due to their effect on DNA. We measured superoxide dismutase (SOD) [3], catalase, and lipidperoxidase in brain tumors, gliosis, and normal brain tissue, which were obtained by lobectomy with removal of the tumor. We compared the active oxygen species, and the anti-oxidization enzyme in malignant and benign brain tumors in order to determine the differences in metabolism or the mechanism of tumor growth in such tumors.

Materials and Methods

The cases in this study included 7 malignant and 3 benign tumors (Table 1). The tumors were grouped into 4 glioblastoma, 1 anaplastic astrocytoma, 2 metastatic tumors and 3 meningioma. The patients' ages ranged from 18 to 71 years, with an average of 55 years. The male to female ratio was 2:3; however, in the cases of malignant tumor the ratio was 4:3. Frontal or temporal lobectomy was done with removal of the tumor when the glioblastoma or anaplastic astrocytoma was localized in the frontal or temporal lobe. Samples were selected from a part of the tumor tissue, gliosis, and normal gray and white matter. In the other tumor cases, a specimen was chosen from the tumor and from the gliosis, which were diagnosed by frozen sections during the operation. The samples were kept at a temperature of −20°C as soon as possible after removal of the tissues. SOD was counted by the cytochrome C method and the

[1] Department of Neurosurgery, Kochi Medical School, Nangoku, 783 Japan
[2] Niwa Immunological Institute, 4-4 Asahi-cho, Tosashimizu, 787-03 Japan

Table 1. Case list of brain tumors

Case	Age (years)	Sex	Histological diagnosis	Site of lesion
1.	71	Male	Glioblastoma	Rt. frontal
2.	72	Male	Glioblastoma	Rt. parietal
3.	60	Female	Glioblastoma	Lt. frontal
4.	18	Male	Anaplastic astrocytoma	Rt. temporal
5.	44	Male	Glioblastoma	Lt. frontal
6.	67	Male	Malignant fibrous histiocytoma	Lt. parietal
7.	67	Female	Lymphoma	Rt. temporal
8.	62	Female	Meningioma	Tentrial
9.	65	Female	Meningioma	Falx
10.	74	Female	Meningioma	Sphenoidal ridge

modified Yagi's method was used for measurement of lipidperoxidase; catalase was measured by the routine method.

Results

The value of lipidperoxidase (nmol/g · tissue) was found to be 1.21 ± 0.3 in malignant tumor tissue, 2.83 ± 1.12 in gliosis, 1.75 ± 0.66 in normal white matter, and 5.85 ± 3.32 in normal gray matter. However, it was 0.74 ± 0.26 in benign brain tumor. Higher values of lipidperoxidase were demonstrated in malignant than in benign tumor, but the difference was not significant ($P < 0.01$). Other than tumor tissues, the lipidperoxidase value was highest in gray matter, higher in gliosis, and lower in white matter without any significant

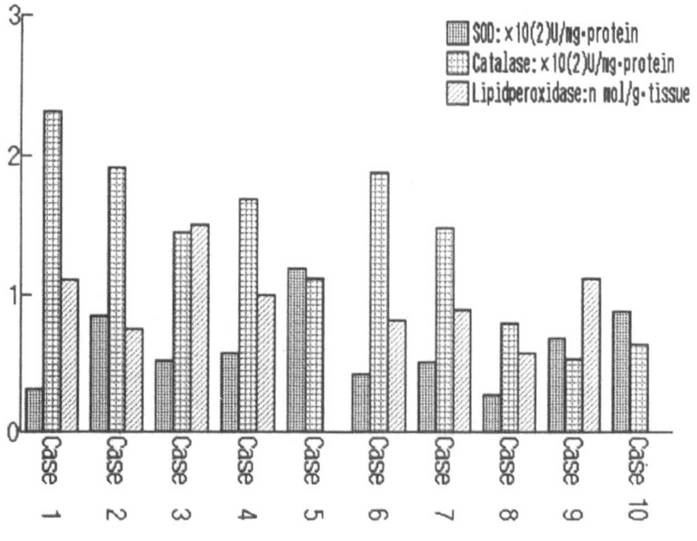

Fig. 1. Active oxygen species in brain tumors

Table 2. Results of measurement of active oxygen species and its scavengers

	Tissue	SOD ($\times 10^2$ U/mg · protein)	Catalase ($\times 10^2$ U/mg · protein)	Lipidperoxidase (nmol/g · tissue)
Case 1	Tumor	0.32	2.32	1.10
	Gliosis	0.57	1.94	1.73
	White matter	0.85	1.36	2.41
	Gray matter	0.72	1.28	7.60
Case 2	Tumor	0.85	1.91	0.75
	Gliosis	0.94	1.75	3.02
	White matter	0.93	1.04	2.79
	Gray matter	1.47	1.05	4.95
Case 3	Tumor	0.52	1.45	1.50
	Gliosis	0.68	0.80	3.95
	White matter	—	—	—
	Gray matter	0.33	0.83	8.27
Case 4	Tumor	0.58	1.68	0.99
	Gliosis	0.51	1.21	3.22
Case 5	Tumor	1.19	1.11	—
	Gliosis	0.67	1.32	2.76
Case 6	Tumor	0.42	1.88	0.81
	Gliosis	0.71	1.65	1.72
Case 7	Tumor	0.51	1.48	0.89
	White matter	0.68	0.93	1.09
	Gray matter	0.33	0.75	1.53
Case 8	Tumor	0.28	0.79	0.58
Case 9	Tumor	0.68	0.53	1.11
Case 10	Tumor	0.88	0.64	—

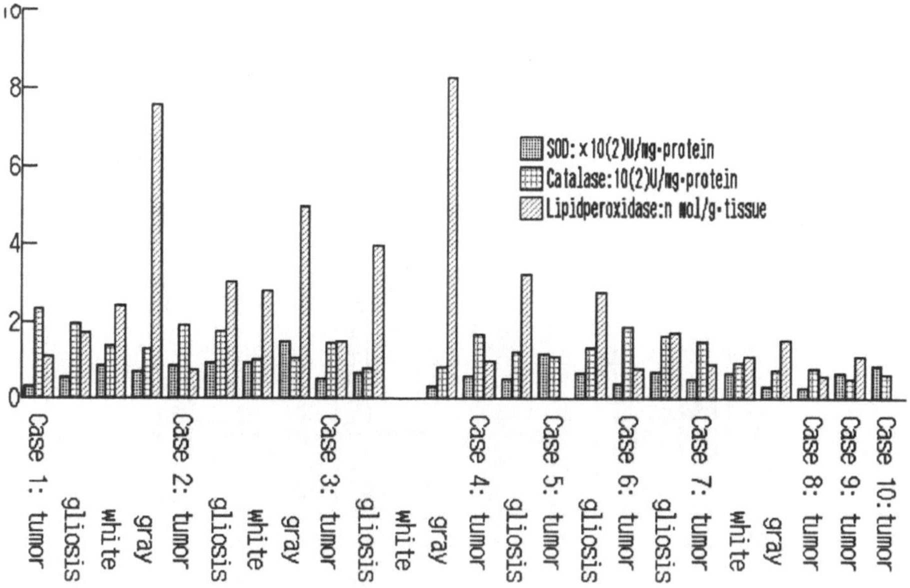

Fig. 2. Active oxygen species in tumor and other tissues

differences ($P < 0.01$) (Table 2). Catalase (×100 U/mg · protein) was 1.72 ± 0.61 in malignant tumors, 1.37 ± 0.57 in gliosis, 1.64 ± 0.72 in white matter, 1.00 ± 0.25 in gray matter, and 0.66 ± 0.13 in benign tumors. A higher value of catalase was revealed in malignant tumors than in benign tumors (Fig. 1) with a statistical significance ($P < 0.01$). Other than tumor tissues, catalase increased mostly in gliosis, moderately in white matter, and slightly in gray matter without any statistical significance ($P < 0.01$). The catalase value in tumor tissues was higher in malignant tumor, higher than 100 U/mg · p, and lower than 100 U/mg · p in benign tumor. Measured data of each case are shown in Table 2 and Fig. 2. The SOD (×100 U/mg · protein) value was 0.76 ± 0.43 in malignant tumor, 0.73 ± 0.22 in gliosis, 0.78 ± 0.15 in white matter, 0.87 ± 0.59 in gray matter, and 0.58 ± 0.30 in benign tumor. A higher value of SOD was obtained in malignant than in benign tumor, but with no statistical significance ($P < 0.01$). The SOD value was higher in normal brain tissue. Other than tumor tissues, the SOD value was highest in normal gray matter, and higher in white matter and gliosis (Fig. 2).

Discussion

It has been recently considered that the intracytoplasmic activation of oxygen and free radicals may promote the expression of tumor [1,4]. This especially applies to · OH and lipidperoxidase which are produced by the Haber Weiss reaction of the Fenton type with H_2O_2 and O_2^- being related to the promotion of tumor [5]. The active oxygen causes damage to the DNA and the cells may die if the damage is too great. However, even if mild damage of active oxygen is repeated to the cells, the double strand of DNA will be broken and a gene conversion or defect and/or transposition of chromosome will be revealed in the cells [2,5]. These phenomena suggest the possibility that active oxygen species promote the expression of tumor. In the few kinds of experimental cancer which were produced by irradiation or administration of chemical agents in animals, acceleration of the promoter was confirmed to be inhibited by anti oxidization agents and SOD [6]. A quantitative analysis of the active oxygen species and anti-oxydization agents in the tumor tissues has not yet been sufficiently studied. There is no published report on any quantitative analysis of SOD, catalase, and lipidperoxidase in human brain tumors. However, there are a number of reports on experimental cancers, and the lower value of SOD was confirmed in such tumor tissues [4,6–9]. Oberley et al. [4] suggested that the gene of Mn-SOD and cancer gene may promote the tumor growth in these experimental cancers. The reduced SOD in the tumor tissue was considered to be the result of reduction of SOD production and/or of decrease of the receptive capacity of SOD in each tumor cell. In these tumor cells, the activity of SOD is reduced, and this causes dysfunction of respiration of the mitochondria due to production of energy change to the anaerobic metabolism [10]. It is well known that the metabolism in tumor cells is anaerobic, so the value of O_2^- is considered to be low and H_2O_2 may be reduced as a result. For these reasons, catalase which converts H_2O_2 to H_2O and O was rarely used, and large amounts of catalase remained in the tumor tissues. The lipidperoxidase value was lower in tumor tissue than in the other tissues because of a lower content of O_2^- and/or of lipid in the tumor tissue, and the highest value was found in gray matter which has a higher content of these substances.

Conclusion

1. The catalase value was higher in malignant brain tumor than in benign tumor, and its borderline was 100 U/mg protein.
2. There was no significant difference in SOD and lipidperoxidase between malignant and benign tumor tissues.
3. The highest SOD content was revealed in gray matter, the second highest was in white matter, there was a lower value in gliosis, and the lowest appeared in tumors. However, catalase and lipidperoxidase were reversed, and higher values were obtained as follows: tumor > gliosis > white matter > gray matter.
4. Superoxide might be low in tumor tissue and its scavenger may also be reduced. These results might stimulate tumor growth.
5. Reduction of superoxide and its scavenger might depend upon anaerobic metabolism in tumor tissues.

References

1. Birnboim HC (1982) DNA strand blockage in human leukocytes exposed to a tumor promoter, phorbol myristate acetate. Science 215:1247–1249
2. Michelson AM (1982) Oxygen radicals. Agents Actions [Suppl] 11:179–210
3. McCord JM, Fridovich I (1969) Superoxide dismutase: An enzymic function for erythrocuprein (hemocuprein). J Biol Chem 244:6049–6055
4. Oberley LW, Oberley TD (1984) The role of superoxide dismutase and gene amplification in carcinogenesis. J Theor Biol 106:403–422
5. Imray JA, Chin SM, Linn S (1988) Toxic DNA damage by hydrogen peroxide through the Fenton reaction in vivo and in vitro. Science 240:640–642
6. Balansky RM, Blagoeva PM, Mircheva ZI, Stoitchev I, Chernozemski I (1986) The effect of antioxidants on MNNG-induced stomach carcinogenesis in rats. Cancer Res Clin Oncol 112:272–277
7. Bize IB, Oberley LW (1980) Superoxide dismutase and superoxide radical in Morris hepatomas. J Theor Biol 40:3686–3693
8. Bozzi A, Mavelli I, Agro AF, Atrom R, Wolf AM, Mondovi B, Rotilio G (1976) Enzyme defense against reactive oxygen derivatives. II. Erythrocyte and tumor cells. Mol Cell Biochem 10(1):11–17
9. Decuyper-Debergh D, Piette J, Jassonge-Lion M, Van de Vorst A (1986) Singlet oxygen mutagenicity induced in the lac operon. Arch Int Physiol Biochim 94(5):S35–43
10. Swaroop A, Ramasarma T (1981) Inhibition of H_2O_2 generation in rat liver mitochondria by radical quenchers and phonolic compounds. Biochem J 194:657–665

The Relationship Between Nucleolar Organizer Regions and Hormone-Producing Activity in Pituitary Adenoma

TAKASHI MATSUHISA, TOMOHIDE MAESHIRO, MINORU NAKAGAWA, HIDEAKI SHIGEMATSU, KAZUYUKI TSUNO, KENGO MATSUMOTO, TOMOHISA FURUTA, and AKIRA NISHIMOTO[1]

Introduction

Nucleolar organizer regions (NORs) are loops of DNA which contain ribosomal RNA genes. Recently the number of NORs has been reported to be a marker of histological malignancy [1] or proliferative potential of the tumor cell [2–5]. Fundamentally, however, NORs contribute to protein synthesis. In this study, the relationship between the number or the size of NORs and hormone-producing activity was examined in pituitary adenoma.

Materials and Methods

1. Tissues

Surgical specimens obtained from 42 patients with pituitary adenoma were used in this study. The patients were 16 males and 26 females and the mean age was 45.9 years, ranging from 14 to 74 years. This series included 14 prolactin (PRL)-secreting adenomas, 10 growth hormone (GH)-secreting adenomas, 4 adreno-corticotrophic hormone (ACTH)-secreting adenomas, 4 luteinizing hormone-follicle stimulating hormone (LH-FSH)-secreting adenomas, and 10 non-functioning (NON) adenomas.

2. Silver Staining of NORs

The surgical specimens were fixed in 10% formalin and embedded in paraffin wax. Sections 6 µm thick were dewaxed and hydrated. Two-percent gelatin in 1% formic acid solution was mixed in 1:2 volumes ratio with 50% aqueous silver nitrate solution. This solution was poured over the sections and left for 30 min. The sections were then washed, dehydrated, and mounted. No counterstain was performed.

---

[1] Department of Neurological Surgery, Okayama University Medical School, Okayama, 700 Japan

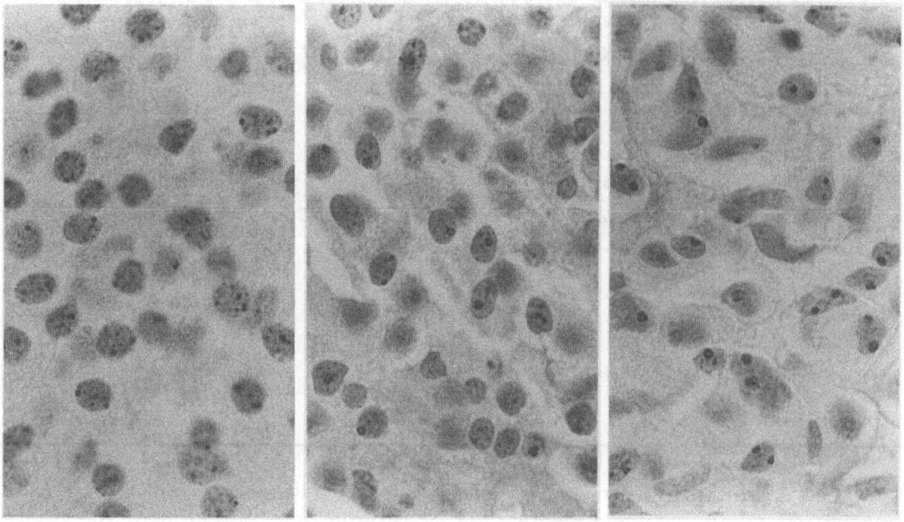

Type I **Type II** **Type III**

Fig. 1. The types of NOR size

3. Evaluation of NORs

The number of NORs was counted in each nucleus under oil immersion at a magnification of × 1000. The NOR number was defined as the mean number of NORs per nucleus in 200 cells. According to the size of NORs, the pituitary adenomas were classified into the 3 types as follows: type I included the adenomas which contained exclusively small NORs in their nuclei. Type II carried a mixture of small and large NORs, and Type III only large NORs (Fig. 1).

4. Hormone-Producing Activity

The ratio of hormone level in the serum to adenoma volume (H/V) was calculated as the index of hormone-producing activity in PRL-secreting adenomas. The relationship between H/V and NOR number or size was investigated.

Results

The mean NOR numbers (± standard deviation) were 2.83 (±0.88) for PRL-secreting adenomas, 2.42 (±0.66) for GH-secreting adenomas, 3.75 (±1.66) for ACTH-secreting adenomas, 4.78 (±0.91) for LH-FSH-secreting adenomas, and 3.99 (±1.45) for NON adenomas. There were significant differences in mean NOR numbers between PRL- and LH-FSH-secreting adenomas and between GH- and LH-FSH-secreting adenomas and NON adenomas. There was a significant correlation between H/V and the NOR number in PRL-

Table 1. The types of NOR size in pituitary adenoma

Adenomas	No.	I	II	III
PRL	14	7	4	3
GH	10	1	5	4
ACTH	4	2	2	0
LH-FSH	4	3	1	0
NON	10	8	1	1

secreting adenomas (R = 0.665, $P < 0.01$) (Fig. 2). The relationship between the types of NOR size and adenoma groups is presented in Table 1. NON adenomas contained a significantly higher number of Type I than the functioning adenomas. There was a tendency for H/V of Type I to be higher than those of both Type II and Type III in PRL-secreting adenomas (Fig. 3), but there were no significant differences between them.

Discussion

NORs are the loops of DNA which contain the gene coding the ribosomal RNA, and are closely associated with argyrophlic proteins which can be visualized by silver staining. The number of NORs is considered to reflect the cellular activity and proliferative potential because ribosomal RNAs contribute to the regulation of cellular protein synthesis [1]. Recently silver staining of NORs has been applied to estimate the proliferative potentials of tumor cells [2–5], but, to our knowledge, there has been no report on the relationship between the hormone-producing activity and the number or the size of NORs.

Pituitary adenoma is a benign tumor and the proliferative potential of this tumor was reported to be low [6,7]. In this study, however, the mean NOR number of each adenoma was relatively high, compared with those of other benign tumors which were investigated in our laboratory. For example, mean NOR numbers were 2.66 for meningiomas and 1.63 for craniopharyngiomas (unpublished data). It was suggested that the NOR number reflected the hormone-producing activity rather than the proliferative potential in functioning adenomas.

The means of NOR numbers were significantly different in individual adenoma groups. The NOR numbers of LH-FSH-secreting and NON adenomas tended to be higher than those of PRL- and GH-secreting adenomas. The higher NOR number of LH-FSH-secreting adenomas was considered to indicate the higher hormone-producing activity.

In PRL-secreting adenomas, there was a significant correlation between the NOR number and the hormone-producing activity (Fig. 2).

Concerning the size of NORs, there was a tendency for the NORs of NON adenomas to be smaller and scattered in the nucleus than those of functioning

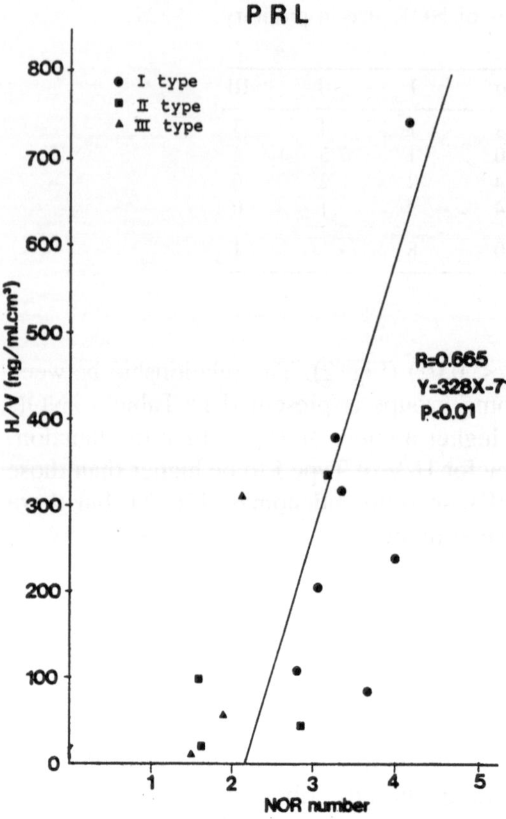

Fig. 2. The relationship between NOR number and H/V in PRL-secreting adenoma

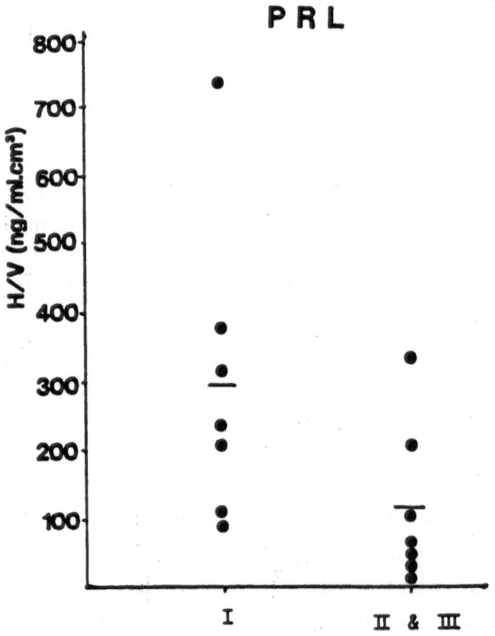

Fig. 3. The relationship between the types of NOR size and H/V in PRL-secreting adenoma

adenomas (Table 1). In PRL-secreting adenomas, the NORs tended to become smaller as the hormone-producing activity increased (Fig. 3).

These results indicate that the NOR number is closely related with the hormone-producing activity in PRL-secreting adenomas, and that the NORs of these adenomas become smaller in size and increase in number as the hormone-producing activities increase.

References

1. Crocker J, Nar P (1987) Nucleolar organizer regions in lymphomas. J Pathol 151:111–118
2. Dervan PA, Gilmartin LG, Loftus BM, Carney DN (1989) Breast carcinoma kinetics. Argyrophilic nucleolar organizer region counts correlate with Ki-67 scores. Am J Clin Pathol 92:401–407
3. Orita T, Kajiwara K, Nishizaki, T, Ikeda N, Kamiryo T, Aoki H (1990) Nucleolar organizer regions in meningioma. Neurosurgery 26:43–46
4. Kajiwara K, Nishizaki T, Orita T, Nakayama H, Aoki H, Ito H (1990) Silver colloid staining technique for analysis of glioma malignancy. J Neurosurg 73:113–117
5. Hara A, Hirayama H, Sakai N, Yamada H, Tanaka T, Mori H (1990) Correlation between nucleolar organizer region staining and Ki-67 immunostaining in human gliomas. Surg Neurol 33:320–324
6. Nagashima T, Murovic JA, Hoshino T, Wilson CB, Dearmond SJ (1986) The proliferative potential of human pituitary tumors in situ. J Neurosurg 64:588–593
7. Knosp E, Kitz K, Perneczky A (1989) Proliferation activity in pituitary adenomas: Measurement by monoclonal antibody Ki-67. Neurosurgery 25:927–930

Section 3. Brain Tumor and Cytokines

The Interaction Between Cytokines and Growth Factors on the Growth of Glioma Cells

JUN YOSHIDA, TOSHIHIKO WAKABAYASHI, MASAAKI MIZUNO, HIROFUMI OYAMA, KYOKO NEHASHI, and KENICHIRO SUGITA[1]

Introduction

There are several cytokines and growth factors which are related to the autocrine or paracrine growth of human glioma cells. Platelet-derived growth factor (PDGF) [1], insulin-like growth factor-II (IGF-II) [2], tumor necrosis factor-α (TNF-α), interferon-β (IFN-β) [3], and transforming growth factor-β (TGF-β) [4] have been reported to be synthesized from human glioma cells and released by a variety of forms of induction; they are believed to stimulate or inhibit the growth of glioma cells themselves. On the other hand, IFN and TNF were proved to have a direct anti-proliferative activity against glioma cells in vitro [5–7] and in vivo [5,6], and both cytokines were used clinically for the treatment of patients with malignant glioma [5]. The high dose of $1–3 \times 10^6$ IFN-β or of $1–5 \times 10^5$ TNF-α is usually administered intravenously, intra-arterially, and/or intrathecally. The results show that a regression of tumor was definitely demonstrated in some cases, although the response rate was not very high, while a reversed progression of tumor was also encountered in a few cases. In order to analyze the mechanism of exogenously added cytokines on growth regulation of human glioma cells, we examined the effect of IFN-β and TNF-α on human glioma cell lines in vitro, and studied the interaction between the growth factors PDGF, IGF-II, and TGF-β.

Materials and Methods

Cell Lines

A human glioma cell line of U251-MG and its subline U251-MG-SF were used. The former was originally established by Pontén at Uppsala University, Sweden and the latter was established in our laboratory. U251-MG was cultured in a Dulbecco's modified Eagle's medium (DME-M) with 10% fetal

[1]Department of Neurosurgery, Nagoya University School of Medicine, Nagoya, 466 Japan

bovine serum (FBS), 100 μg/ml streptomycin, and 100 U/ml penicillin. The concentration of FBS was gradually decreased for metabolic recovery during more than 2 months and obtained a subline of U251-MG-SF, which was adapted and grew in a serum- and protein-free culture medium. This subline showed a similar morphology as the mother cell line of U251-MG and contained a glial fibrillary acidic protein in the cytoplasm. However, the growth rate of U251-MG-SF was decreased to 1/5–1/10 compared with U251-MG. In the condition medium of U251-MG-SF, 50–80 ng/ml IGF-II was constantly detected by enzyme immunoassay with a monoclonal antibody against IGF-II.

Cytokines and Growth Factors

Human TGF-β (purity 96%) isolated from human platelets was purchased from R and D Systems (Minneapolis, Wis., USA). Human PDGF (specific activity of 50,000 U/mg protein) isolated from human platelet was purchased from Biomedical Technologies Inc. (Stoughton, Mass., USA). Recombinant human TNF-α (PAC-4D) was obtained from Asahi Chemical Industry Co., Ltd. (Tokyo). The specific activity was 2.2×10^6 JRU/mg protein. HuIFN-β, induced from fibroblasts by Poly I:C and purified, was obtained from Toray Industries, Inc. (Tokyo). The specific activity was more than 1×10^7 IU/mg protein. Recombinant human IGF-II was obtained from Daiichi Seiyaku Co., Ltd. (Tokyo). The reactivity with a monoclonal antibody and binding activity to the receptor was identical with that of purified natural IGF-II.

Cellular Proliferation Assay

The effect of five growth factors on cellular proliferation and the interaction between the factors were determined in a U251-MG-SF cell line. Approximately 5×10^4 cells were seeded into 24 well microplates (Falcon #3524) containing 2 ml medium. After 3 days of culture in a 37°C CO_2 incubator, cells were exposed to PDGF (1, 3, 5 U/ml), IGF-II (1×10^2, 1×10^3 ng/ml), IFN-β (1×10^2, 1×10^3, 1×10^4 IU/ml), TNF-α (1×10^2, 1×10^3, 1×10^4 JRU/ml), or TGF-β (0.1, 1.0, 5.0 ng/ml). The plates were sacrified on the 5th day of additional incubation, and the cells were counted in a hemocytometer. The growth stimulation or inhibition by the factors was estimated as relative per cent viability, which was the cell number of tested well/cell number of control of well × 100.

Results

Effect of Each Cytokine and Growth Factor on the Growth of Glioma Cells

The dose responses of five cytokines on the growth of U251-MG-SF glioma cells were studied. PDGF and IGF-II stimulated the growth, while TNF-α, IFN-β and TGF-β inhibited it in a dose-dependent manner (Fig. 1a,b).

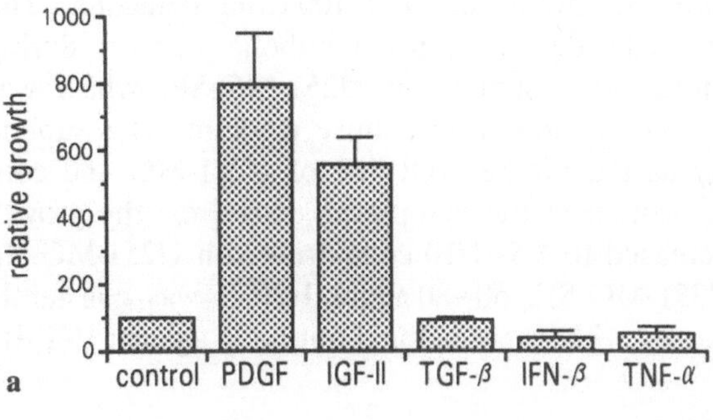

a

Fig. 1. a Growth stimulation and growth inhibition on the growth of U251-MG-SF glioma cells by PDGF (5 U/ml), IGF-II (1000 ng/ml), TGF-β (1 ng/ml), IFN-β (1000 IU/ml), and TNF-α (1000 JRU/ml). **b** Growth stimulation or inhibition in a dose-dependent manner

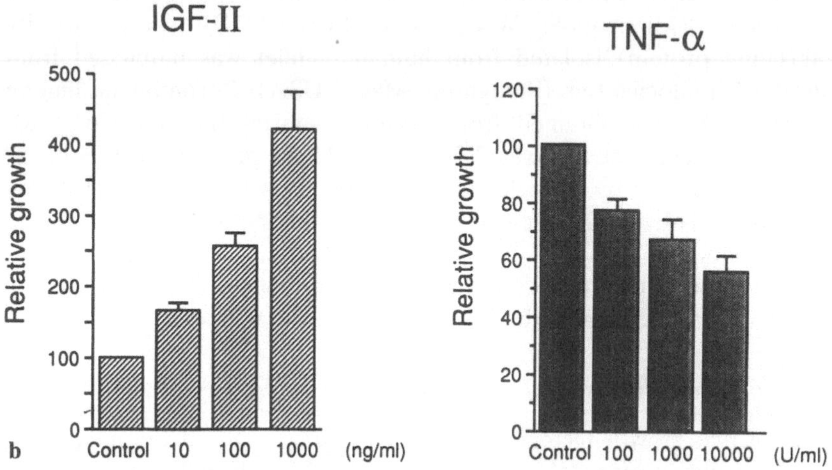

b

Interaction Between the Factors

The overall effect of positive (PDGF and IGF-II) and negative (TNF-α, IFN-β, and TGF-β) growth factors was dependent upon the combination used. The interaction between the factors could be classified into three types of action, synergistic, antagonistic, and paradoxical. Among the interactions between two negative growth factors, IFN-β vs TNF-α and IFN-β vs TGF-β were synergistic (Fig. 2a). The growth inhibition of glioma cells was augmented by the combination. Contrarily, the interaction between TNF-α vs TGF-β showed a paradoxical action in which the growth of U251-MG-SF was reversely increased in combination with these two growth inhibitors (Fig. 2b). Among the interactions between positive and negative growth factors, a sufficient dose of growth inhibitors overcame the growth-stimulating action of PDGF (antagonistic) (Fig. 2c), while the same dose of growth inhibitors reversely enhanced the growth-stimulating action of IGF-II (paradoxical).

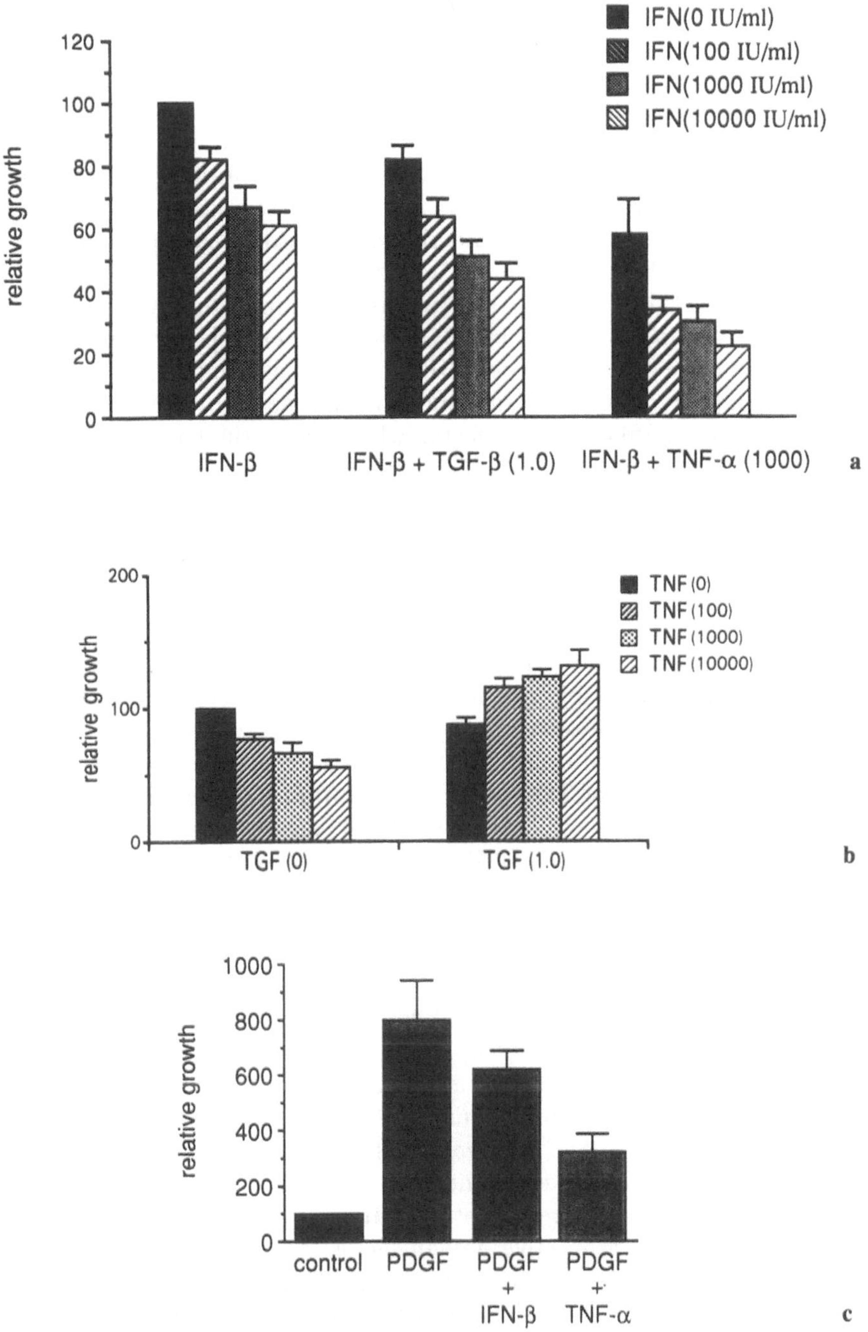

Fig. 2. **a** Synergistic action of IFN-β vs TGF-β and IFN-β vs TNF-α on the growth of U251-MG-SF glioma cells. **b** Paradoxical action of TGF-β vs TNF-α. **c** Antagonistic action of IFN-β and TNF-α against growth stimulation by PDGF

Discussion

The growth of a normal cell is largely regulated systemically by endocrine secretion of several polypeptide hormones and locally by paracrine secretion of polypeptide growth stimulators (positive growth factors) and inhibitors (negative growth factors). It has been suggested that uncontrolled growth of transformed or malignant cells results in part from the escape from exogenous growth control and gain of the autocrine mechanism of growth control by the secretion of growth stimulators [8]. Several growth stimulators were produced or expressed in glioma cells. Autocrine growth stimulation on the growth of glioma cells was first suggested in PDGF by Nister et al. [1] The autocrine loop of TGF-α and the over-expressed EGF receptor is also implied by the works of Rutka et al. [9] From our experimental data and the reports of Sara et al. [10], IGF-II may be another growth factor which has a similar autocrine growth mechanism of glioma cells. The IGF-II that stimulates the growth of glioma cells was produced from glioma cells themselves, and the IGF-II receptor was enhanced in glioblastoma. A breakdown of growth inhibitory regulation may be another mechanism for the overgrowth of malignant cells. Lack of endogenous growth inhibitors and/or abnormal responses of cells by exogenous growth inhibitors were implied. It has been established that TNF-α and the different classes of interferon exert an inhibitory effect on the growth of a variety of malignant cells. The inhibitory effect of TGF-β on the growth of certain types of malignant cells has also recently been demonstrated [11]. All of these three polypeptide factors were expressed in human glioma cells. Clark and Bressler reported the isolating of TGF-β-like activity from the extract of a U251-MG glioma cell line [4]. We and Larsson et al. [3] demonstrated IFN-β and TNF-α in the culture medium of U251-MG glioma cells by the superinduction with poly I:C, cycloheximide, and actinomycin D.

In the present experiments, we studied the effect of exogenously added purified cytokines and growth factors, those similar molecules which are endogenously secreted from glioma cells. We used a serum-free culture of U251-MG-SF cells that made it possible to characterize absolutely the in vitro effect of growth factors. To our knowledge, this is the first report demonstrating the interaction between these factors on the growth of human glioma cells maintained in a serum-free culture medium.

Our results indicate that the overall effect of growth factors is dependent upon the combination we used, and that the interaction between the factors could be classified into three types of actions, synergistic, antagonistic, and paradoxical. TNF-α, a negative growth factor to U251-MG-SF, reversely increased the cells in the presence of TGF-β. Three negative growth factors, TNF-α, IFN-β, and TGF-β enhanced the growth-stimulating action of IGF-II. These findings suggest that cytokine therapy with IFN and TNF-α for patients with malignant glioma must be given with caution. If IGF-II and/or TGF-β are secreted endogenously from glioma cells, intracranial glioma may be reversely increased by exogenously added cytokines of IFN-β and/or TNF-α.

Conclusion

In order to analyze the local growth regulation of glioma by autocrine and/or paracrine factors, we studied the effect of exogenously added cytokines or growth factors on the growth of glioma cells using a human glioma cell line, U251-MG-SF, which was adapted and grew in a serum-free culture medium. PDGF and IGF-II stimulated the growth, while IFN-β, TNF-α, and TGF-β inhibited it in a dose-dependent manner. The overall effect of positive and negative factors was dependent upon the combination used, and the interaction between the factors could be classified into three types of actions, synergistic, antagonistic, and paradoxical. Abnormal responses were induced by the combination of growth factors. TNF-α in the presence of TGF-β reversely stimulated growth, and IFN-β, TNF-α, and TGF-β enhanced the growth-stimulating action of IGF-II.

References

1. Nister M, Heldin CH, Westermark B (1986) Clonal variation of a platelet-derived growth factor-like protein and expression of corresponding receptors in a human malignant glioma. Cancer Res 46:332–340
2. Yoshida J, Inoue I, Mizuno M, Oyama H, Nehashi K, Sugita K (1989) Production of HuIFN-β and IGF-II from human glioma cell lines. Neurological Res (Japan) 2:159–164
3. Larsson I, Landstrom LE, Larner E, Lundgren E, Miorner H, Strannegard O (1987) Interferon production in glia and glioma cell lines. Infect Immun 22:786–789
4. Clark WC, Bressler J (1988) Transforming growth factor-b-like activity in tumors of the central nervous system. J Neurosurg 67:920–924
5. Yoshida J, Kato K, Wakabayashi T, Enomoto H, Inoue I, Kageyama N (1986) Antitumor activity of interferon-b against malignant glioma in combination with chemotherapeutic agent of nitrosourea (ACNU). In: Cantell K, Schellekens (eds) The biology of the interferon system. Martinus Nijhoff, Boston, pp 399–406
6. Enomoto H, Yoshida J, Kageyama N, Ueda R, Kato T, Ota (1986) Anti-tumor activity of human recombinant TNF against human malignant glioma cell lines and combination effect with HuIFN-β. Gan To Kakagu Ryoho (Jpn J Cancer Chemotherap) 13:1953–1961
7. Rutka J, Giblin JR, Berens ME, Bar-Shiva E, Tokuda K, McCulloch JR, Rosenblum ML, Eessalu TE, Aggarwal BB, Bodel WJ (1988) The effect of human recombinant tumor necrosis factor on glioma-derived cell lines: Cellular proliferation, cytotoxicity, morphological and radioreceptor studies. Int J Cancer 41:573–582
8. Sporn MB, Todaro GJ (1980) Autocrine secretion and malignant transformation of cells. New Engl J Med 303:878–880
9. Rutka J, Rosenblum ML, Stern R, Ralston HJ III, Dougherty D, Biblin J, DeArmond S (1989) Isolatiion and purification of growth factor with TGF-like activity from human malignant gliomas. J Neurosurg 71:875–883

10. Sara V, Prisell P, Sjogren B, Persson L, Boethhius J, Enberg G (1986) 32:229–234
11. Helseth E, Unsgaar G, Dalen A, Vik R (1988) The effect of type beta transformaing growth factor on proliferation and epidermal growth factor receptor expression in a human glioblastoma cell line. J Neurooncol 6:267–276

Interferon Effect on Cytotoxicity of Autologous Stimulated Lymphocytes from Patients with Malignant Glioma

KOICHI MIYAGI[1], JIRO MUKAWA[1], HISASHI KOGA[1], YASUSHI HIGA[1], SUSUMU NAKASONE[1], SUSUMU MEKARU[1], and MARYLOU INGRAM[2]

Introduction

Itoh et al. [1] demonstrated that the rIL-2-induced activated killer (AK) activity of peripheral blood lymphocytes (PBLs) was augmented when treated by recombinant inteferon γ (rIFNγ), and that the lymphocytes were also promoted in proliferation. A human brain tumor cell line (allogeneic) was used as one of the target cells for AK assay in their study. However, there has been no study of its action against autologous tumor cells. Ellis et al. [2] reported that natural killer (NK) cells, when activated by either rIFNα or γ, acquired lymphokine-activated killer (LAK) cytolytic activity and lysed NK-resistant cells. Inteferon (IFN)-induced LAK cytotoxicity reached a peak value 24 h after culture with IFNα (500 units/ml) and IFNγ (1000 units/ml). The question of whether or not IFN makes LAK cells cytotoxic against autologous glioma still remains unsolved. The present study was designed to elucidate this question.

Whereas LAK cells are derived from a minority population of peripheral blood lymphocytes that already bear surface receptors for IL-2, the autologous-stimulated lymphocyte (ASL) must be induced for the expression of such receptors by preliminary exposure to processed antigen or mitogen (PHA in Huntington Medical Research Institutes [3] and our protocol). Virtually all T lymphocytes respond to PHA, hence ASLs represent a broader spectrum of cells than do LAK cells. LAK cells and ASLs differ morphologically as well as serologically, and can also be distinguished on the basis of their cytotoxicity for certain widely used target cell lines [4–6].

Materials and Methods

Tumor cells from six out of eight patients were cultured. PBLs from these six patients (glioblastoma, 4; malignant astrocytoma, 1; ependymoma, 1), PBLs

[1] Department of Neurosurgery, University of the Ryukyus, School of Medicine, Okinawa, 903–01 Japan
[2] Experimental and Clinical Immunotherapy Laboratory, Huntington Medical Research Institutes (HMRI), Pasadena, CA, USA

from one major histocompatibility complex (MHC)-matched healthy brother of a patient with medulloblastoma and from one patient with a metastatic lesion (squamous cell carcinoma) were also cultured. The lymphocyte cultures were grown in RPMI-1640 containing 10% fetal bovine serum (FBS) and phytohemagglutinin-P (PHA-P) (5 μg/ml) after removing adherent cells. After 2 days, the cell count was adjusted to 5×10^5/ml and recombinant interleukin-2 (rIL-2) (100 units/ml) was added to the medium. On day 6, the medium was replaced with fresh medium supplemented with rIL-2. On day 8, the culture was divided into three equal parts which were cultured for 2 additional days in either the same medium (control), medium supplemented with 500 units/ml of rIFNγ (rIFNγ-SL), or medium supplemented with 500 units/ml HuIFNβ (HuIFNβ/SL). Cytotoxicity of these three types of stimulated lymphocytes (SLs) was examined in vitro against autologous or syngeneic tumor cells, K562 cells and Raji cells by 4-h chromium release assay at various effector-to-target ratios (2.5, 5, 10, 20, 40:1). Before the assay, the effector cells were washed and suspended in the medium with 10% FBS without lymphokine. Cytotoxicity (%) was calculated by the following formula: Cytotoxicity (%) = (Test release-spontaneous release) × 100/(maximum release-spontaneous release). The Wilcoxon rank sum test was used for statistical analysis. The rIL-2 and rIFNγ were kindly supplied by the Shionogi Pharmacy (Tokyo) and HuIFNβ from Toray (Tokyo). Subpopulations of lymphocytes (CD4, CD8, CD22, CD56 positive cell) were analyzed on a flow cytometer (Ortho Cytron).

In three cases of glioblastoma, adoptive immunotherapy was performed by injecting HuIFNβ-SLs into the tumor cavity via a ventricular access device (Pudenz-Schulte Medica) placed in the subgaleal space. Then, 4.91×10^8 HuIFNβ-SLs and 3.5×10^5 units rIL-2 in a cumulative dosage were injected in case 1, 8.68×10^8 HuIFNβ-SLs and 8.5×10^5 units rIL-2 in case 2, and 1.25×10^9 HuIFNβ-SLs and 2.7×10^5 units rIL-2 in case 3. The efficacy of this therapy was determined by comparing the tumor volumes on enhanced CT scans before and after the therapy. Complete response (CR) indicates no tumor mass in the enhancement, partial response (PR) more than 50% reduction, minor response (MR) 25%–50% reduction, and no change (NC) less than 25% of either increase or decrease. Progression of disease (PD) indicates 25% or more of an increase.

Results

A. Cytotoxicity in Three Types of SLs

The cytotoxicity in three types of SLs (case 1) against autologous tumor cells is given in Fig. 1. HuIFNβ-SL were more cytotoxic than rIFNγ-SL or control. The cytotoxicity is summarized in Table 1a. Cytotoxicity of HuIFNβ-SL was augmented in 3 out of 6 cases and reduced in 1 case compared with control. Stimulation by rIFNγ augmented the cytotoxicity of rIL-2 SL in 2 out of 6 cases.

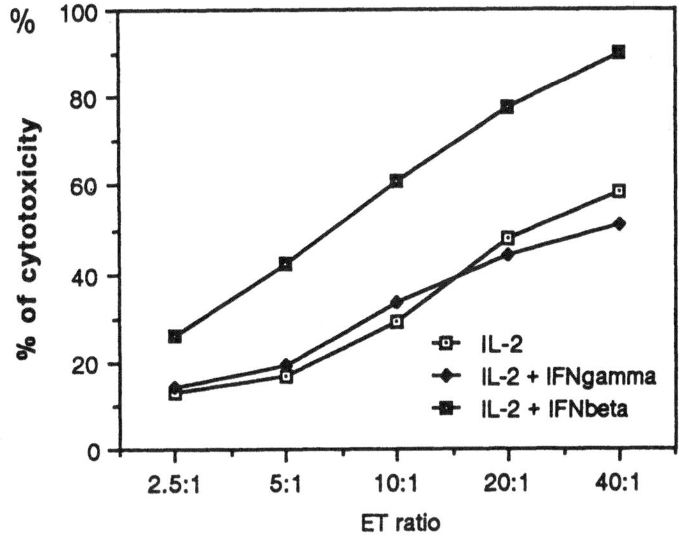

Fig. 1. Cytotoxicity of SL stimulated with or without IFN against autologous glioma cells (case 1)

The cytotoxicity against NK sensitive K562 cells is summarized in Table 1b. Compared with control, HuIFNβ-SL increased the activity in 4 out of 7 cases. Stimulation by rIFNγ inversely increased the activity of rIL-2 SLs in 2 and reduced it in 1 out of 7 cases.

The cytotoxicity against NK-resistant Raji cells is summarized in Table 1c. Stimulation by HuIFNβ increased the activity in 2 out of 7 cases, but reduced it in 4. In contrast, stimulation by rIFNγ increased the activity of rIL-2 SLs in 1 and decreased it in 1 out of the 7 cases.

As seen in Table 2, we could not predict cytotoxicity in three types of SLs against autologous tumor cells from data represented in K562 and Raji cells.

B. Flow Cytometric Analysis of Lymphocyte Subpopulation

Flow cytometric analysis of the subpopulation of lymphocyte subsets indicated that the percent of CD56-positive cells of HuIFNβ-SL decreased.

C. Clinical Results of Adoptive Immunotherapy Using HuIFNβ-SLs

Three cases of malignant glioma received adoptive immunotherapy with HuIFNβ-SL through a ventricular access device. These gliomas were reduced to 58.4%, 64.3%, and 42.8% of the pre-treatment volume (initial response), which correspond to MR, MR, and PR, respectively, in efficacy criteria.

Table 1. **a** The cytolytic activity in three types of effector cells was measured in a ^{51}Cr release assay (E/T ratio 20:1)

Case	Age (years)/Sex	Type of tumor	% Lysis against **autologous tumor cells** rIL-2 Only	rIL-2 + rIFNγ	rIL-2 + HuIFNβ
1	71/F	Glioblastoma	47.96	44.38	**77.36**
2	45/F	Glioblastoma	20.13	26.04	12.08
3	45/M	Glioblastoma	41.23	**67.81**	34.60
4	49/M	Ependymoma	1.76	5.01	**8.76**
7*	1/M	Medulloblastoma	77.15	74.84	*67.50**
8*	56/M	Squamous cell carcinoma	52.63	**68.63**	**63.63**

b The cytolytic activity in three types of effector cells was measured in a ^{51}Cr release assay

Case	Age (years)/Sex	Histological diagnosis	% Lysis against **K562** cells (E/T ratio 20:1) rIL-2 Only	rIL-2 + rIFNγ	rIL-2 + HuIFNβ
1	71/F	Glioblastoma	65.79	68.93	*67.86*
2	45/F	Glioblastoma	39.21	*47.44*	*75.79*
3	49/M	Glioblastoma	78.50	84.05	*94.77*
4	49/M	Ependymoma	24.01	15.18	22.43
5*	63/F	Glioblastoma*	37.75	*66.48*	*67.89*
6	65/F	Malig. astro.	27.92	33.96	25.96
7*	1/M	Medulloblastoma	78.45	*66.52**	75.82

c The cytolytic activity in three types of effector cells was measured in a ^{51}Cr release assay.

Case	Age (years)/Sex	Histological diagnosis	% Lysis of **Raji cell** (E/T ratio 20:1)		
			rIL-2 Only	rIL-2 + rIFNγ	rIL-2 + HuIFNβ
1	71/F	Glioblastoma	96.16	*94.44**	*83.53**
2	45/F	Glioblastoma	58.71	53.02	*47.88**
3	49/M	Glioblastoma	66.76	69.01	**79.55**
4	49/M	Ependymoma	0.00	1.48	1.97
5	63/F	Glioblastoma*	7.38	**25.83**	**38.37**
6	65/F	Malig. astro.	26.00	27.72	*24.34**
7*	1/M	Medulloblastoma	69.80	48.49	*41.39**

Percent cytotoxic activity based on data obtained from 4-hour chromium-release assay of three types of effector cell
Bold indicates cytotoxic activity greater than of SL significantly ($P < 0.05$)
Itlalic *indicates cytotoxic activity less than of SL significantly ($P < 0.05$)
The significance of differences in tumor burden between groups was determined by the Wilcoxon rank sum test. Two-sided P values were used in all experiments *5**, *8**: E/T ratio 40:1, and *7**: syngeneic SL was adopted
Glioblastoma*: This case was reported at first as malignant astrocytoma (*malig. astro.*) according to stereotaxic biopsy specimens. Recent surgical specimens revealed that the pathological result was glioblastoma

Table 2. a Summary of cytolytic activity in three types of effector cells against K562, Raji, and autologous tumor cell (E/T ratio)

Case#	Age (years)/sex	Type of tumor	Cytolytic activity against		
			K562	Raji	Autologous
1	71/F	Glioblastoma	β⇑	γ⇓,β⇓	β⇑
2	45/F	Glioblastoma	γ⇑,β⇑	β⇓	NS
3	45/M	Glioblastoma	β⇑	β⇑	γ⇑
4	49/M	Ependymoma	NS	NS	β⇑
*5	63/F	*Glioblastoma	γ⇑,β⇑	γ⇑,β⇑	ND
6	65/F	Malig. astro.	NS	β⇓	ND
*7	1/M	Medulloblastoma	γ⇓	β⇓	β⇓
*8	56/M	Squamous cell carcinoma	ND	ND	γ⇑,β⇑

b Summary of Table 2a

	Cytotoxic activity against		
	K562	Raji	Autologous tumor cell
SLs Stimulated with	$n = 7$	$n = 7$	$n = 6$
HuIFNβ	⇑4, ⇓0	⇑2, ⇓4	⇑3, ⇓1
rIFNγ	⇑2, ⇓1	⇑1, ⇓1	⇑2, ⇓0

γ, β indicate rIFNγ and HuIFNβ respectively

⇑ , ⇓ indicate increased cytotoxic activity and reduced cytotoxic activity respectively, compared with SL significantly ($P < 0.05$)

**5*, **8*: E/T ratio 40:1, and **7*: syngeneic SL were adopted

**Glioblastoma*, this case was reported at the 8th Nikko Brain Tumor conference as malignant astrocytoma based on the pathological results of stereotaxic biopsy specimens. The result of recent surgical specimens was the diagnosis of glioblastoma.

Malig. astro., malignant astrocytoma; *NS*, not significant; *ND*, not determined

Discussion

Since the LAK cell phenomenon was first described by Grimm et al. in 1982 [7], effective immunotherapy has been sought.

Itoh et al. [1] demonstrated that rIFNγ treatments of peripheral blood lymphocytes augmented rIL-2-induced AK activity and that cell proliferation was also promoted. However, there has been no report of cytotoxicity against autologous tumor cells. Brooks et al. [8] reported that IFNα and β induced NK activity of cytotoxic T lymphocytes (CTL), but IFNγ did not. Ochoa et al. [9] also reported that total LAK activity could be further enhanced by IFNβ or γ. Toledano et al. [10] reported that cytotoxicity of PBL induced by rIL-2 was not modified by rIFNγ. Sone et al. [11] reported that IFNβ reduced cytotoxicity of rIL-2 AK cells from the peripheral blood of healthy donors when Daudi cells were used as target cells, but IFNγ did not. In short, the effects of IFNs seem to be inconstant against NK and LAK activity.

In our experience, HuIFNβ-SL showed increased cytotoxicity against NK-sensitive target cells in 4 out of 7 cases. In contrast, cytotoxicity of HuIFNβ-SL against NK-resistant Raji cells was reduced in 4 cases and increased in 2, but rIFNγ had no consistent cytotoxic effect on NK-sensitive or -resistant cell.

although the influence of the difference between LAK cells and ASL should be considered [3], our results differ from Ochoa's and Itoh's conclusions but are similar to those of Brooks, Toledano, and Sone. Our data would suggest that IFNβ and γ have no enhancing cytotoxic effect of SLs on NK-resistant cells.

With respect to the cytotoxicity in the three types of SLs, our data revealed no positive correlation between autologous tumor cells and NK-sensitive K562 cells or NK-resistant Raji cells. These results suggest that increasing cytotoxic effect with HuIFNβ against autologous tumors (in 3 out of the 6 cases) is not due to acquired LAK or NK activity but is probably due to increasing CTL activity.

What will be the effects of systemic or focal administration of IFN on tumor resistance to host immune function if HuIFNβ can enhance the NK or CTL activity with rIL-2? There is no available information concerning HuIFNβ. Powell et al. [12] reported that IFNγ-treated K562 cells became relatively resistant to NK cell lysis. Gronberg et al. [13] reported that pretreatment of K562 and HHMS melanoma cells with IFNγ and Daudi cells with IFNα significantly reduced their susceptibility to LAK cells, which were generated in vitro in the presence of human recombinant IL-2 (100 units/ml).

It is possible that some IFNs decrease the host immune response of the patient with glioma and inhibit the immunotherapy for malignant glioma. Therefore, it must be stressed that IFNs should be used clinically only after clarifying the presence of such an adverse effect on the immune system.

Conclusions

When cultured with HuIFNβ SLs had increased cytotoxicity against autologous tumor cells in 3 out of 6 cases and decreased effectiveness in 1 case. When cultured with rIFNγ, SLs had increased cytotoxicity in 2 out of 6 cases. When cultured with HuIFNβ, SLs had increased cytotoxicity against NK-sensitive K562 cells in 4 out of 7 cases. In contrast, stimulation by rIFNγ revealed no consistent effect. Stimulation by HuIFNβ increased the activity of SL against NK-resistant Raji cells in 2, but reduced it in 4 out of 7 cases. Judging from the data of cytotoxicity on Raji and K562 cells, the cytotoxic enhancement of HuIFNβ against autologous glioma cells is mainly related to the increasing CTL activity.

References

1. Itoh K, Shiiba K, Shimizu Y, Suzuki R, Kumagai K (1985) Generation of activated killer (AK) cells by recombinant interleukin 2 (rIL 2) in collaboration with interferon-γ (IFNγ). J Immunol 134:3124–3129
2. Ellis TM, McKenzie RS, Simms PE, Helfrich BA, Fisher RI (1989) Induction of human lymphokine-activated killer cells by IFN-alpha and IFN-gamma. J Immunol 143:4282–4286

3. Ingram M, Buckwalter JG, Jacques S, Freshwater DB, Abts RM, Techy G, Miyagi K, Sheldon H, Rand RW, English LW (1990) Immunotherapy for recurrent malignant glioma: An interim report on survival. Neurol Res 12:265–273
4. Ingram M, Jacques S, Freshwater DB, Techy G, Sheldon H, Helsper JT (1987) Salvage immunotherapy of malignant glioma. Arch Surg 122:1483–1486
5. Kruse CA, Lillehei KO, Johnson SD, McCleary EL, Moor GE, Mitchell DH, Waldrop S, Mierau GW (1989). Two preparations of interleukin-2 activated lymphocytes used for adoptive immunotherapy of primary glioma. Cancer 64:1629–1637
6. Grimm EA, Ramsey KM, Mazumder A, Wilson DJ, Djeu JY, Rosenberg SA (1983) Lymphokine-activated killer cell phenomenon. J Exp Med 157:884–897
7. Grimm EA, Mazumder A, Zhang HZ, Rosenberg SA (1982) The lymphokine activated killer cell phenomenon: Lysis of NK resistant fresh solid tumor cells by IL-2 activated autologous human peripheral blood lymphocytes. J Exp Med 155:1823–1841
8. Brooks C, Holschen M, Urdal D (1985) Natural killer activity in cloned cytotoxic T lymphocytes: Regulation by interleukin 2, interferon, and specific antigen. J Immunol 135:1145–1152
9. Ochoa AC, Hasz DE, Rezonzew R, Anderson PM, Bach FH (1989) Lymphokine-activated killer activity in long-term cultures with anti-CD3 plus interleukin 2: Identification and isolation of effector subsets. Cancer Res 49:963–968
10. Toledano M, Mathiot C, Michon J, Andreu G, Lando D, Brandely M, Fridman WH (1989) Interferon-gamma (IFN-gamma) and interleukin-2 in the generation of lymphokine-activated killer cell cytotoxicity—IFN-gamma-induced suppressive activity. Cancer Immunol Immunother 30:57–64
11. Sone S, Utsugi T, Nii A, Ogura T (1988) Differential effects of recombinant interferons alpha, beta, and gamma on induction of human lymphokine (IL-2)-activated killer activity. Cancer Inst 80:425–431
12. Powell J, Stone J, Chan WC, Yang ZD, Leatherbury A, Sell KW, Wiktor-Jedrzejczak W, Ahmed-Ansari A (1989) Interferon-gamma-treated K562 target cells distinguish functional NK cells from lymphokine-activated killer (LAK) cells. Cell Immunol 118:250–264
13. Gronberg A, Ferm M, Tsai L, Kiessling R (1989) Interferon is able to reduce tumor cell susceptibility to human lymphokine-activated killer (LAK) cells. Cell Immunol 118:10–21

IL-2-Induced Signal Transduction in an Oligodendroglioma Line

YUTAKA OKAMOTO[3], SEIJIRO MINAMOTO[1], KEIJI SHIMIZU[2], TORU HAYAKAWA[2], and TADATSUGU TANIGUCHI[1]

Introduction

Recently, many reports have indicated that glial cells in the central nervous system (CNS) respond to immunoregulatory cytokines [1–3]. Furthermore, it has been shown that some of the cytokines are produced locally in the brain [1,3–5]. The role of interleukin-2 (IL-2) in the CNS has been documented by a number of studies in which IL-2 has been shown to stimulate proliferation of neonatal rat oligodendrocytes and human glioblastoma cell clones at relatively high concentrations (5–50 nM) [6,7]. These observations suggest a potential role of IL-2 in the CNS and raise the issue as to whether the IL-2 signal is transduced in these cells by the same IL-2 receptors (IL-2R) in the immune system.

Materials and Methods

Cell Culture

The human oligodendroglioma cell clone, ONS-21-C2 [8], was maintained in Dulbecco's modified Eagle's medium (DMEM) supplemented with 10% fetal bovine serum, 100 μg kanamysin per ml, and 0.03% glutamine.

Construction of the Expression Plasmid and Transfection to ONS-21-C2 Cells

Constraction of the plasmids was carried out essentially following the usual procedures [9]. To constract pdKCRβ, the HhaI fragment containing the entire coding region of the human IL-2Rβ was inserted into BamHI-cleaved pdKCR containing the simian virus 40 early promoter [10]. The resulting plasmid, pdKCRβ, was introduced together with the neomycin-resistance gene,

[1] Institute for Molecular and Cellular Biology, Osaka University, Osaka, 565 Japan
[2] Department of Neurosurgery, Osaka University Medical School, Osaka, 553 Japan
[3] Department of Neurosurgery, Hanwa Memorial Hospital, Osaka, 558 Japan

pSTneoβ [11] into ONS-21-C2 cells by the calcium phosphate precipitation method. The neomycin-resistant clones were selected in the above-described medium containing G418 (1 mg/ml), as described.

Assay for IL-2-Induced Cell Proliferation

The proliferative response of cells to IL-2 was monitored by [^{3}H]thymidine incorporation. Cells suspended in DMEM containing 1% fetal bovine serum were seeded into 96-well flat-bottom microtiter plates at a density of 3×10^3 cells per well. After a 24-h incubation period, various concentrations of recombinant IL-2 were added to those cultures in the presence or absence of monoclonal antibodies against the human IL-2R α(anti-Tac [12], 1:50 dilution of sacites fluid) or IL-2Rβ (Mik-β1 [13], 1:50 dilution of ascites fluid). On day 3, cells were incubated with [^{3}H]thymidine (37kBq) per well for 18 h. [14]

General Procedures

DNA transfection, Scatchard plot analysis, and IL-2 internalization assays were carried out following the procedures as previously described [15,16].

Results

To investigate the function of IL-2R, the expression plasmid pdKCRβ was introduced into the cloned cell line ONS-21-C2 to selectively amplify the expression of IL-2Rβ. Two out of eleven G418-resistant clones, C2β-3 and C2β-6, expressed IL-2Rβ as judged by flow cytometry. S1 mapping analysis of the mRNA expressed in C2β-3 and C2β-6 revealed that IL-2Rβ-specific RNA was derived from the transfected cDNA, but not from the endogenous IL-2Rβ gene, without affecting other phenotypic properties of the cells, such as MBP^+, $GalCer^+$, and $GFAP^-$ (data not shown).

The IL-2-binding studies were performed with ^{125}I-labeled recombinant human IL-2. The following binding profiles were obtained by Scatchard analysis: clones C2β-6 and C2β-3 displayed 1.7×10^3 and 1.3×10^3 IL-2-binding sites per cell with estimated Kd values of 2.2 and 1.7 nM, respectively (Fig. 1). In contrast, IL-2 binding was undetectable in both the parental ONS-21-C2 cells and in the IL-2Rβ-negative, G418-resistant clones. It has been shown that both intermediate- and high-affinity IL-2 receptors expressed in lymphoid cells can internalize the bound IL-2. The IL-2R expressed in clones C2β-6 and C2β-3 was also capable of internalizing bound IL-2 (Fig. 2). The proliferative response of the IL-2Rβ-expressing clones to IL-2 was monitored by the [^{3}H]thymidine incorporation. IL-2 enhanced [^{3}H]thymidine incorporation by the C2β-6 and C2β-3 cells, but not by the parental ONS-21-C2 cells at IL-2 concentration above 1 nM (Fig. 3). All other G418-resistant transformant clones that do not express IL-2Rβ did not show a proliferative response to IL-2. There was no indication of any induction of endogenous IL-2Rα and IL-2Rβ genes by

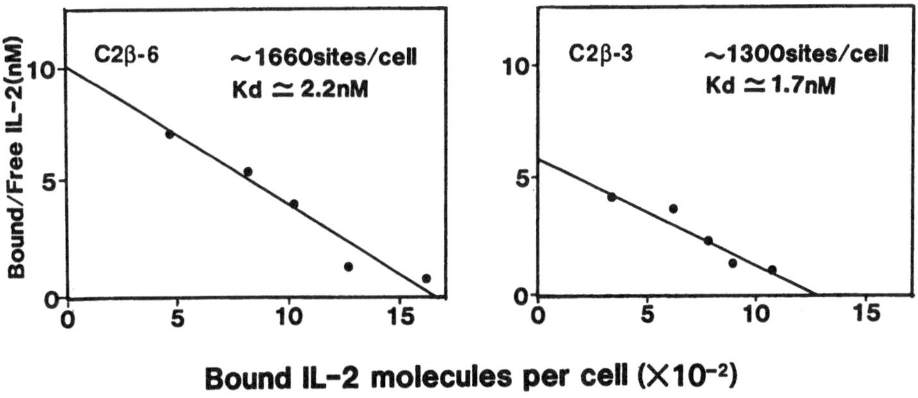

Fig. 1. Scatchard analysis of ^{125}I-labeled IL-2 binding to clones C2β-6 and C2β-3. The number of IL-2 binding sites per cell and receptor affinity (Kd) were determined by computer-assisted analysis of IL-2 binding data

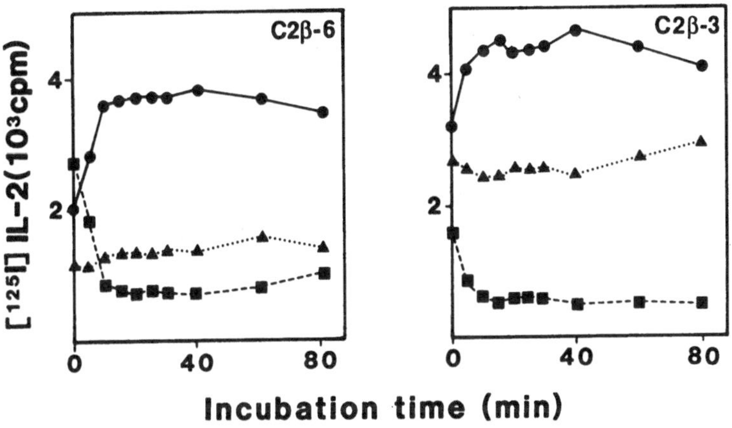

Fig. 2. IL-2 internalization in clones C2β-6 and C2β-3. Cells (5×10^7) were treated with ^{125}I-labeled IL-2 (5nM) at 4 °C for 2 h. The cells were suspended in the culture medium (37 °C) and the kinetics of IL-2 internalization were examined. At each time point, radioactivity in the cell supernatent was measured (▲). The cells were then resuspended in pH 4 buffer and centrifuged through a layer of oil. The radioactivity in the cell pellet was measured in order to determine the level of pH 4-resistant, internalized IL-2 (●). The radioactivity in the supernatant was measured in order to determine the amount of cell surface-bound IL-2 dissociated in the pH4 buffer (■)

IL-2 as judged by S1 mapping analysis of mRNA from IL-2-stimulated C2β-3 and C2β-6 cells (results not shown). Additionally, proliferative responses to IL-2 detected in C2β-6 and C2β-3 cells were strongly inhibited by the Mik-β1 antibody raised against IL-2Rβ but not by anti-Tac antibody. The IL-2 response in the C2β-3 and C2β-6 cells was most likely due to the IL-2R derived from the transfected cDNA.

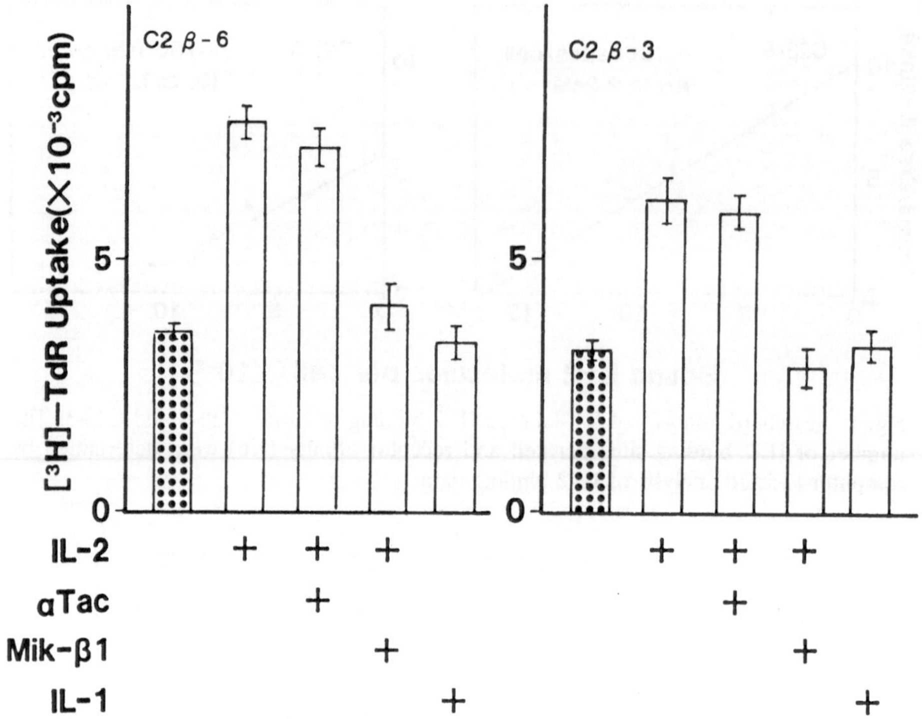

Fig. 3. Cells were cultured for 72 h with or without recombinant human IL-2 (10 nM) in the presence or absence of Mik-β1 (anti-IL-2Rβ), anti-Tac (anti-IL-2Rα). Results represent mean ±SD of triplicated samples

Discussion

Very little is known at present about the nature and function of the receptors in cytokine-mediated signal transduction in the CNS. The present study demonstrated that the cDNA-directed human IL-2R in the human oligodendroglioma cell line ONS-21-C2, unlike IL-2R expressed in a fibroblast cell line, behaves similarly to the IL-2R in lymphoid cells. It binds IL-2 with intermediate affinity, internalizes IL-2, and transduces growth signals. These findings thus give us further insight into the function of the IL-2R, by demonstrating that the same receptor for IL-2 can function in both lymphocytes and cells of CNS origin. It would be interesting to examine whether or not the IL-2Rβ-expressing transformant clones derived from ONS-21-C2 cells can be made responsive to IL-2 at low concentrations by coexpression of IL-2Rβ cDNA. Induction of the IL-2Rα by IL-2 via the IL-2Rβ has been documented in T cells as well as in the IL-2-responsive, GalCer$^+$ glioblastoma cell line [7]. However, we have not dectected IL-2Rα induction by IL-2 in either the parental ONS-21 cells or in the IL-2Rβ-expressing transformants, nor have we seen significant induction of MBP by IL-2, which has been reported previously in neonatal rat oligodendrocytes [17]. Presumably, such discrepancies are due to differences in the cell types and the degree of maturation. Our findings indicate that IL-2-mediated growth in oligodendrocytes, as reported previously, may occur by a similar or identical mechanism, as described here. Further investigation of the IL-2 system operating in neural cells may be of value in understanding the mechanism involved in the control of the CNS.

References

1. Fontana A, Grob PJ (1984) Lymphokines and the brain. Springer Semin Immunopathol 7:375–386
2. Frei K, Bodmer S, Schwerdel C, Fontana A (1986) Astrocytes-derived interleukin 3 as a growth factor for microglia cells and peritoneal macrophages. J Immunol 137:3521–5327
3. Merrill JE (1987) Macroglia: Neural cells responsive to lymphokines and growth factors. Immunol Today 8:146–150
4. Heiter E, Ayala J, Denefle P, Bousseau A, Rouget P, Mallat M, Prochiants A (1988) Brain macrophages synthesize interluekin-1 and interleukin-2 mRNA in vitro. J Neurosci Res 21:391–397
5. Farrar WL, Vinocour M, Hill JM (1989) In situ hybridization histochemistry localization of interleukin-3 mRNA in mouse brain. Blood 73:137–140
6. Benveniste EN, Merrill JE (1986) Stimulation of oligodendroglial proliferation and maturation by interleukin-2. Nature 321:610–613
7. Benveniste EN, Tozawa H, Gasson JC, Quan S, Golde DW, Merrill JE (1988) Response of human glioblastoma cells to recombinant interleukin-2. J Neuroimmunol 17:301–314
8. Okamoto Y, Minamoto S, Shimizu K, Mogami H, Taniguchi T (1990) Interleukin 2 receptor chain expressed in an oligodendroglioma line binds interleukin 2 and delivers growth signal. Proc Natl Acad Sci USA 87:6584–6588
9. Sambrook J, Fritsch EF, Maniatis T (1989) Molecular cloning: A laboratory manual 2nd edn. Cold Spring Harbor, New York
10. Fukunaga R, Sokawa Y, Nagata S (1984) Constitutive production of human interferons by mouse cells with bovine papillomavirus as a vector. Proc Natl Acad Sci USA 81:5086–5090
11. Katoh K, Takahashi Y, Hayashi S, Kondoh H (1987) Improved mammalian vectors for high expresson of G418 resistance. Cell Struct Funct 12:575–580
12. Uchiyama T, Broder S, Waldmann TA (1981) A monoclonal antibody (anti-Tac) reactive with activated and functionally mature human T cells. J Immunol 126:1393–1397
13. Tsudo M, Kitamura F, Miyasaka M (1989) Characterization of the interleukin 2 receptor β chain using three distict monoclonal antibodies. Proc Natl Acad Sci USA 86:1982–1986
14. Okamoto Y, Shimizu K, Tamura K, Miyao Y, Yamada M, Tsuda N, Matsui Y, Mogami H (1988) Effects of phenytoin on cell-mediated immunity. Cancer Immunol immunother 26:176–179
15. Hatakeyama M, Tsudo M, Minamoto S, Kono T, Doi T, Miyata T, Miyasaka M, Taniguchi T (1989) Interleukin-2 receptorβ chain gene: Generation of three receptor forms by cloned human α and β chain cDNAs. Science 244:551–556

16. Fujita T, Sakakibara J, Sudo Y, Miyamoto M, Kimura Y, Taniguchi T (1988) Evidence for a nuclear factor(s), IRF-1, mediating induction and silencing properties to human INF-β gene regulatory elements. EMBO J 11: 3397–3405
17. Benveniste ET, Herman PK, Whitaker JN (1987) Myelin Basic protein-specific RNA levels in interleukin-2-stimulated oligodedrocytes. J Neurochem 49:1274–1279

Acute Effects of the Human Recombinant Tumor Necrosis Factor (rTNF) on the Cerebral Vasculature of the Rat in Both Normal Brain and an Experimental Glioma Model

Goro Kido[1], Saburo Nakamura[1], Takashi Tsubokawa[1], Randall E. Merchant[2], and Harold F. Young[2]

Introduction

Since its isolation by Carswell et al. in 1975 [1] as the agent responsible for hemorrhagic necrosis of sarcoma, the tumor necrosis factor (TNF-α) has been implicated in a variety of physiological activities. Studies in animal models and humans have shown that at least one of the cytokine's antitumor actions is mediated through these inflammatory mechanisms, leading to hemorrhagic necrosis of tumors [2]. The successful cloning of TNF-α DNA in 1985 [3] and production of recombinant TNF-α (rTNF-α) was followed by an increase in research to more clearly define the specific actions of the cytokine. *In vitro*, rTNF-α was shown to increase neutrophil adherence to endothelial cells, induce an adhesion-dependent migration of neutrophils through endothelial monolayers, enhance endothelial susceptibility to neutrophil-mediated killing, and stimulate neutrophil respiratory burst and degranulation [4,5]. The mechanism of TNF-α's action, therefore, is thought to be through neutrophils which, when stimulated by TNF-α, release H_2O_2, resulting in the production of tissue-damaging oxygen radicals [6]. TNF-α may also be directly cytotoxic for tumor cells through stimulation of the production of oxygen radicals in the cells themselves [7].

In a phase I study, Kimura and colleagues [8] first investigated the potential of rTNF-α as an anti-cancer therapy in 33 patients with carcinoma of the lung, breast, colon, or liver. Although no anti-tumor effect was seen, the authors established that the maximum tolerable dose was 10^6 U by intravenous (IV) injection per day. As part of a series of preclinical studies aimed at establishing dosage levels that would have limited toxicity to normal brain but are therapeutic for glioma, the present study examined rTNF-α's effect on the vasculature of normal brain and that of malignant gliomas in rats following a single or multiple systemic injection(s) of high-dose human rTNF-α.

[1] Department of Neurological Surgery, School of Medicine, Nihon University, Itabashi-Ku, Tokyo, 173 Japan
[2] Department of Surgery, Division of Neurosurgery, Medical College of Virginia, Virginia Commonwealth University Richmond, VA, USA

Materials and Methods

Animals

Female Fischer 344 rats (Harlan) weighing 140 g–160 g (n = 42) were used.

Tumor

A Rous sarcoma virus-induced rat glioma cell line, RT-2, syngeneic for Fischer 344 rats was used.

Cytokine

Lyophilized human rTNF-α was provided by the Cetus Corporation (Emeryville, CA). Purity was >99% as determined by sodium dodecyl sulfate-polyacrylamide gel electrophoresis (SDS-PAGE) technique, with a specific activity of 24 × 10^6 U/mg protein and an endotoxin content of 0.02 ng/ml by Limulus Amebocvte Lysate (LAL) assay. Recombinant TNF-α in a bulking agent of 1% mannitol was reconstituted with sterile, endotoxin-free H_2O. The sterile TNF-α excipient (TNF-E) was composed of 1% mannitol (Sigma) in sterile, endotoxin-free H_2O.

Glioma Models

Under pentobarbital anesthesia (40 mg/kg, IP), 30 Fischer 344 rats received a stereotaxic inoculation of 10^4 syngeneic RT-2 glioma cells into the right parietal lobe. By 7 days post-inoculation, a single well-vascularized lesion developed at the injection site. By 10 days, the tumor volume increased and prominent neovascularization occurred within the tumor and the peritumoral margins. Animals began dying from their tumors on days 14 post-inoculation and nearly all succumbed by day 17.

Experimental Design

Twelve normal rats were divided into two groups, half receiving 10^6 U human rTNF-α (in 0.2 ml H_2O) and half receiving an equal volume of TNF-E through the femoral vein. The second group was similarly subdivided, with half receiving multiple injections of 5 × 10^5 U rTNF-α each and half receiving multiple injections of TNF-E through a cannula implanted in the jugular vein over 3 consecutive days.

The 30 tumor-bearing rats were divided as above. Single injection models received either 10^6 U rTNF-α or TNF-E on day 3, 7, or 10 post-tumor inoculation. The second group of rats received 5 × 10^5 U rTNF-α or TNF-E for 3 days beginning on day 7, 10, or 12 post-tumor inoculation.

For all animals, 24 h following the final rTNF-α or TNF-E injection, Type VI horseradish peroxidase (HRP) (0.1 mg HRP/g body wt) was administered IV, and the rats were perfused 1 h later with a buffered fixative containing 2%

paraformaldehyde and 2.5% glutaraldehyde. Vibratome sections of the brain were evaluated for HRP extravasation by reaction with tetramethylbenzidine for light microscopy and diaminobenzidine for electron microscopy (EM). The remaining brain sections were stained with hematoxylin and eosin.

Results

Normal Rats

Examination of brains from normal rats 24 h post-rTNF-α injection revealed no pathological effects, although histological examination of the small intestines from the same animals indicated flattened villi and hemorrhage of vessels within the lamina propria accompanied by infiltration of neutrophils. Injections of TNF-E caused no demonstrable histopathological effects.

Glioma Models

Three days after tumor inoculation, HRP extravasation was limited to the immediate vicinity of the tumor injection site, where only discrete areas of tumor cells were observed. There was no evidence of neovascularization, and vessels in the surrounding edematous neuropil remained impermeable to HRP. Single IV injections of either rTNF-α or TNF-E caused no demonstrable increase in HRP extravasation than in non-injected controls.

At 7 days post-tumor inoculation, HRP extravasated into the untreated tumor, within the white matter surrounding the tumor, and in the corpus callosum. Numerous mitotic figures and neovascularization were observed as glioma foci coalesced to form a single mass. A single IV injection of rTNF-α resulted in greater amount of HRP reaction product within the tumor site even though there was no evidence of hemorrhagic necrosis nor was there a difference in the number of the newly formed vessels. Histopathological profiles and blood-brain barrier (BBB) permeability in TNF-E injected rats were identical to controls.

In 10-day glioma models. extravasated HRP exceeded in extent that which was seen in 7-day tumor models, but was still contained within the ipsilateral hemisphere (Fig. 1a). Tumors after 10 days showed an increase in mass and displayed a high degree of neovascularization both within the tumor and in the adjacent neuropil (Fig. 1b). After a single rTNF-α injection, HRP extravasation extended via the corpus callosum into the contralateral hemisphere (Fig. 2a). Histologically, hemorrhagic necrosis was prominent within the tumor, accompanied by leukocytic adherence to neovasculature and pericapillary halos around vessels of the corpus callosum (Fig. 2b,3a–b). The extravascular presence of HRP was confirmed upon EM examination. TNF-E-treated rat models possessed tumors similar to those of uninjected controls.

Following three daily rTNF-α injections begun on day 7 post-tumor inoculation, extravasated HRP extended along the corpus callosum into the contra-

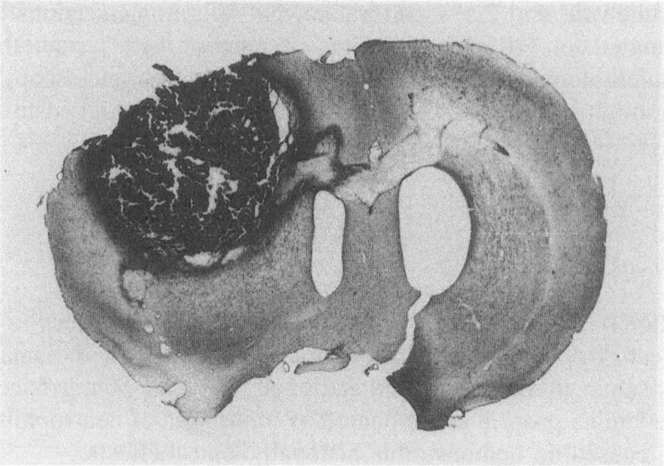

a

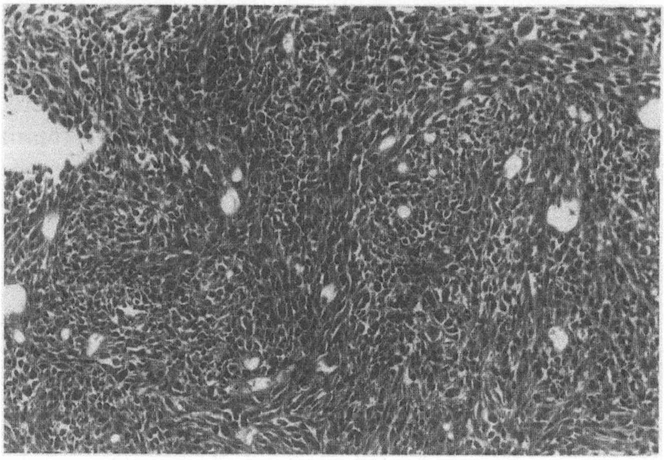

b

Fig. 1. 10-Day glioma model, uninjected control. **a** HRP extravation exceeds that seen in controls, but remains within the ipsilateral hemisphere, × 11.5. **b** The individual foci have coalesced into a single mass that displays a high degree of neovascularization both within the tumor and adjacent neuropil. No areas of necrosis are seen, × 50

lateral hemisphere. These was also widespread hemorrhagic necrosis within the tumor and vascular damage in the surrounding neuropil with accompanying neutrophil adherence and infiltration. These observations mimicked those seen in 10-day glioma models receiving a single injection of 10^6 U rTNF-α. Differences between controls and TNF-E models were insignificant.

In vehicle controls 15 days following tumor inoculation, HRP extended from the tumor into the contralateral hemisphere. At this late stage of tumor development, the glioma occupied most of the right hemisphere. In animals receiving three daily injections of either 5×10^5 U rTNF-α or TNF-E beginning on day 12 post-tumor inoculation, the HRP reaction product extended from

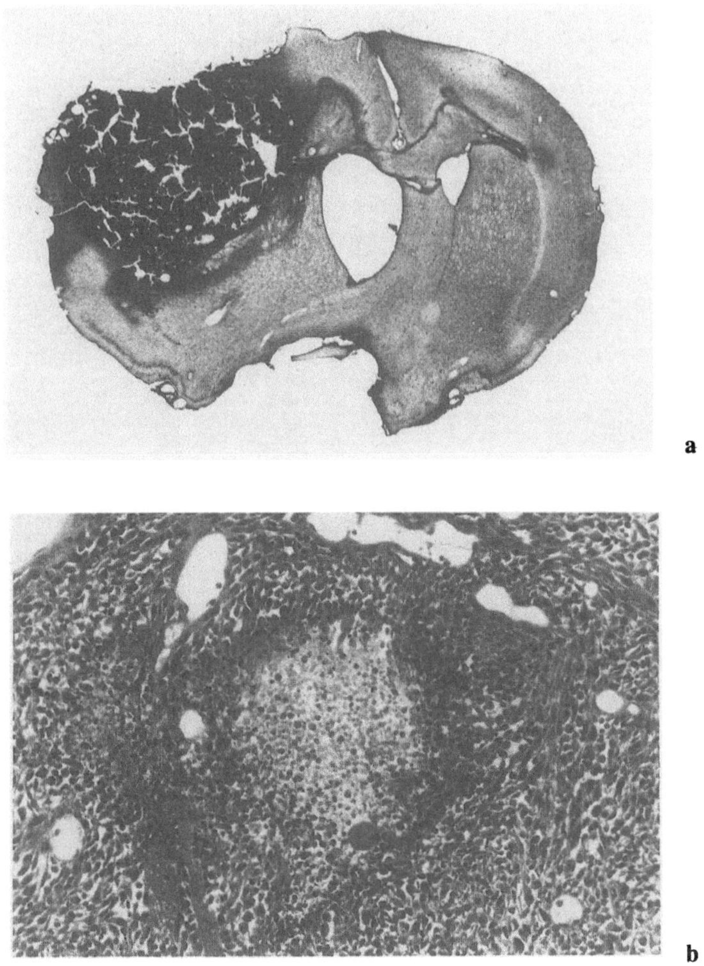

Fig. 2. 10-Day glioma model, single IV rTNF-α infusion. **a** Extravasated HRP extends via the corpus callosum to the contralateral hemisphere, × 11.5. **b** Large areas of hemorrhagic necrosis are prominent within the tumor, × 50

the tumor into the contralateral hemisphere via the corpus callosum. Areas of hemorrhagic necrosis in the rTNF-α recipients, however, were greater in both size and number than in those which were given TNF-E. In models receiving rTNF-α, profiles of tumor vessels were irregular and showed adherent neutrophils, but no leukocytic cuffing.

Discussion

We selected maximally tolerable single or multiple rTNF-α dosages for normal rats and those with glioma. These dosages were defined as causing damage to

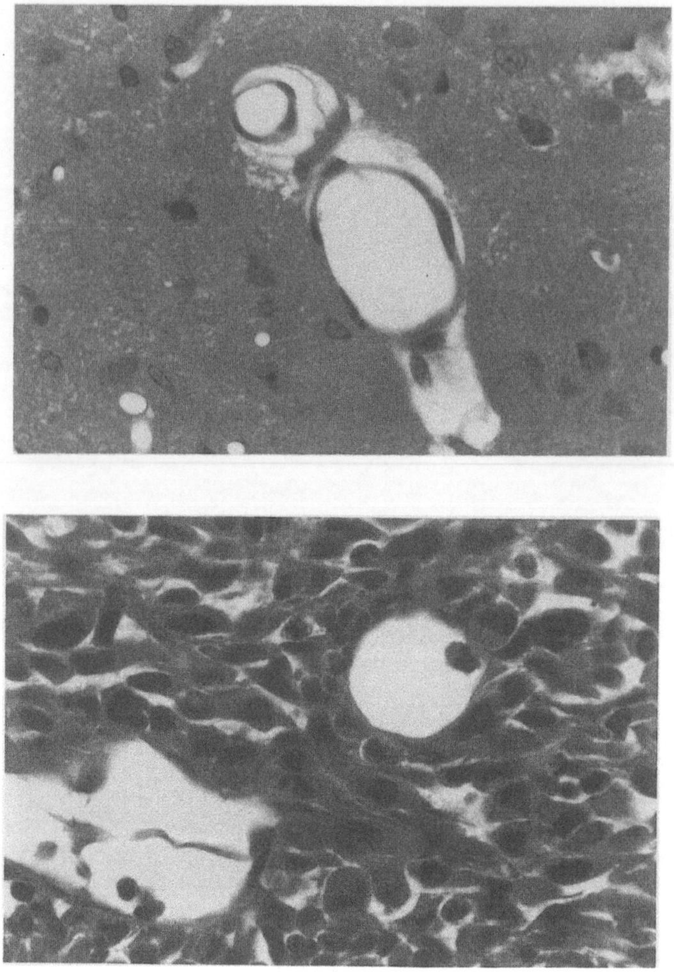

a

b

Fig. 3. 10-Day glioma model, single IV rTNF-α infusion. **a** Along the route of HRP extravasation, halos surround capillaries within the corpus callosum, × 200. **b** Leukocytes adhered to the endothelium of newly-formed vessels, × 200.

the small intestine in the form of hemorrhagic enterocolitis which was evidenced clinically as a diarrheic, bloody stool. Microscopically, the small intestines showed flattening of the villi and hemorrhage within the lamina propria in a manner which has been reported elsewhere [9].

In the RT-2 rat glioma model, we observed no neovascularization, and accordingly, no breach of the BBB over that seen in TNF-E-treated or untreated control rats until 7 days after tumor inoculation, when the tumor formed one cohesive mass. Hemorrhagic necrosis apparently induced by rTNF-α was first seen in 10-day glioma models, characterized by extensive infiltration of bloody components. Neutrophils and monocytes also adhered to vessel walls. In 10-, 13-and 15-day tumor models, which had received daily rTNF-α infusions over a 3-day period, had a similar histopathology consisting of widespread HRP extravasation throughout both hemispheres, areas of hemorrhagic necrosis, neutrophil adherence to vasculature, and infiltration of neutrophils throughout the lesion.

Although recent *in vitro* studies on rTNF-α's effect on murine spinal cord explants have revealed that cytokine can damage myelin and is cytotoxic for oligodendrocytes [10], in the present study, we saw no adverse effects on normal brains at the dosages used. This discrepancy is not surprising since embryonic tissue may have greater susceptibility to rTNF-α-mediated damage and also, because ours was an *in vivo* study, protective mechanisms may have come into play against some of the deleterious effects of rTNF-α. Alternatively, in normal animals, entry of rTNF-α into the central nervous system (CNS) could have been blocked by the BBB as the barrier remained impermeable to HRP following rTNF-α injection(s). Within the tumor mass, but not in the surrounding edematous neuropil, blood vessels are composed of endothelium which is fenestrated and held together by fewer intercellular junctions, both of which factors apparently contribute to the increased permeability to tracers in the gliomas. It has been suggested that susceptibility of TNF-α's effects may be related to the degree of adhesion between cells. For example, Fletcher and coworkers showed that hamster ovary cell lines, which normally display a high degree of intercellular contact through junctions and are normally resistant to the effects of rTNF-α, become rTNF-α-sensitive when those gap junctions are disrupted [9]. Vascular damage observed in this and other *in vivo* studies was usually confined to vessels of high permeability such as those found in the small intestines, while vessels with tight intercellullar junctions, such as those that form the BBB, are generally unaffected. The reduced adhesion between endothelial cells of neovascularized tumors would, therefore, be more susceptible to rTNF-α-mediated damage and resultant hemorrhagic necrosis of surrounding tumor. Tumor necrosis is most likely secondary to rTNF-α-induced hemorrhage rather than to a direct effect of rTNF-α, since RT-2 cells are unaffected by rTNF-α *in vitro* (unpublished data).

A persistent observation in rTNF-α-injected glioma models was the adhesion of neutrophils to the tumor vasculature and infiltration of neutrophils into the tumor. This finding is consistent with studies citing a neutrophil accumulation in other tumors following rTNF-α injection [3]. It is likely that neutrophils accumulated in the tumor as a result of chemoattraction and hemorrhage, and this may have played a role in tissue damage, since activated neutrophils produce and release hydrogen peroxide and proteases [7]. Additionally, hypoxic conditions caused by vessel damage could potentiate the production of oxygen radicals within the tumor.

Conclusion

Our results suggest that systemic administration of rTNF-α at a maximally tolerable dosage may have some therapeutic benefit for glioma since cytokine caused no detectable morphologic evidence of damage to normal brain parenchyma and its vasculature. In addition, in glioma models, cytokine caused more BBB permeability in and around the tumor, increased neutrophilic infiltration into the area of the glioma, and caused hemorrhagic necrosis of newly-formed vessels within the tumor. Recombinant TNF-α's preferetial actions against glioma are due largely to the difference in susceptibility between blood vessels of normal brain and those of glioma; it is likely that rTNF-α targets glioma vasculature as a result of this difference. Employing the glioma model we have described, future studies will examine rTNF-α's impact on survival using various dosages, treatment schedules, and routes of administration in hopes of uncovering the cytokine's mechanism of action and elucidating whether it may be potentially efficacious in the treatment of glioma.

References

1. Carswell EA, Old LJ, Kassel RL, Green S, Fiore N, Williamson B (1975) An endotoxin-induced serum factor that causes necrosis of tumors. Proc Nat Acad Sci USA 72:3666–3670
2. Asher A, Mule JJ, Reichert CM, Shiloni E, Rosenberg SA (1987) Studies on the anti-tumor efficacy of systemically administered recombinant tumor necrosis factor against several murine tumors *in vivo*. J Immunol 138:963–974
3. Shirai T, Tamaguchi H, Ito H, Todd CW, Wallance B (1985) Cloning and expression in *Escherichia coli* of the gene for human tumor necrosis factor. Nature 313:803–806
4. Moser R, Schleiffenbaum B, Groscurth P, Fehr J (1989) Interleukin 1 and tumor necrosis factor stimulate human vascular endothelial cells to promote transendothelial neutrophil passage. J Clin Invest 83:444–455
5. Varani J, Bendelow MJ, Sealey DE, Kunkel SL, Gannon DE, Ryan US, Ward PA (1988) Tumor necrosis factor enhances susceptibility of vascular endothelial cells to neutrophil-mediated killing. Lab Invest 59:292–295
6. Shau H (1988) Characteristics and mechanism of neutrophil-mediated cytostasis induced by tumor necrosis factor. J Immunol 141:234–240
7. Neal ML, Fiera RA, Matthews N (1988) Involvement of phospholipase A_2 activation in tumor cell killing by tumor necrosis factor. Immunology 64:81–85
8. Kimura K, Taguchi T, Urushizaki I, Ohno R, Abe O, Furue H, Hattori T, Ichihashi I, Inoguchi K, Majima H, Niitani H, Ota K, Saito T, Suga S (1987) The A-TNF Cooperative Study Group: Phase I study of recombinant human tumor necrosis factor. Cancer Chemother Pharmacol 20:223–229
9. Flectcher WH, Shiu WW, Ishada TA, Haviland DL, Ware CF (1987) Resistance to the cytolytic action of lymphotoxin and tumor necrosis factor coincides with the presence of gap junctions uniting target cells. J Immunol 139:956–962
10. Selmaji KW, Raine CS (1988) Tumor necrosis factor mediates myelin and oligodendro-cyte damage in vitro. Ann Neurol 23:339–346

PDGF-Related Proteins in Human Brain Tumors

TAKAHARU NAKAMURA, IWAO TAKESHITA, and MASASHI FUKUI[1]

Introduction

The platelet-derived growth factor (PDGF) is one of the well known mitogenic factors for glial cells and connective tissue cells [1–3]. It is suggested that PDGF-related protein has an autocrinic effect and participates in malignant neoplastic transformation [4–6]. The mRNA expression of A and B chains was detected in some glioma cells [7]. It was reported that meningiomas expressed both PDGF and its receptor [8]. Expression of the PDGF-related proteins in the various types of brain tumors has not yet been estimated. We have detected 17 kilodalton (kd) PDGF-related proteins in glioma cells [9], and obtained rabbit antibody against glioma-derived PDGF-related protein, with which we studied the presence of PDGF-related proteins in various cultured human cells and brain tumors.

Materials and Methods

1. Cell Culture

The established human glioma cell lines, U251MG [10], NP-1 [11], and NP-2 [11] were used in this study. To obtain cultured meningioma cells, surgically resected meningioma tissue was dissected, trypsinized, filtered through two sheets of gauze, and cultured. All cultures were maintained in 10-cm petri dishes at 37°C in humidifed air containing 5% CO_2.

2. Preparation of Rabbit Antibody Against 17 kd PDGF-Related Protein

The U251MG cells were homogenized in phosphate buffered saline (PBS) and centrifuged. The supernatant mixed with the sample buffer A[0.5M Tris HCl pH 6.8, 3% sodium laurylsulfate (SDS), 10% glycerin], was applied to 15% polyacrilamide gel and electrophoresed (SDS-PAGE). At the end of elec-

[1] Department of Neurosurgery, Neurological Institute, Faculty of Medicine, Kyushu University, Fukuoka, 812 Japan

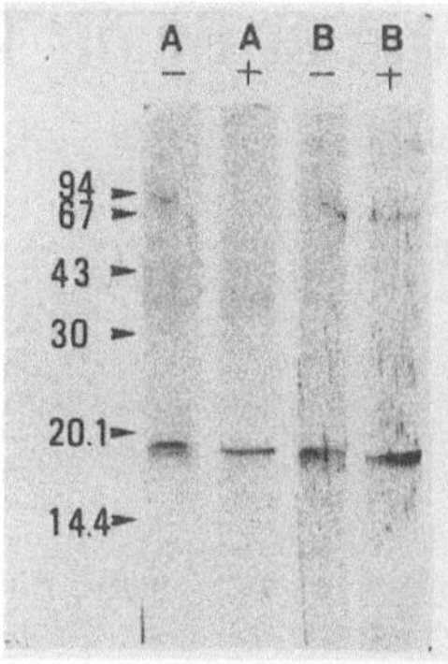

Fig. 1

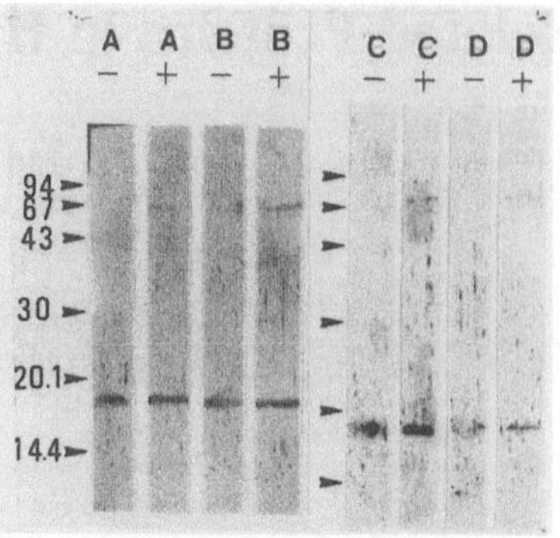

Fig. 2

Fig. 1. Western blotting of U251MG cells reacted with anti-PDGF-antibody (*A*) and purified rabbit IgG (*B*). −: nonreduced condition, +: reduced condition

Fig. 2. Western blotting of NP-1 (*A*), NP-2 (*B*) and cultured meningioma cells (*C,D*) reacted with purified rabbit IgG

trophoresis, the protein at the 17 kd band was eluted and immunized to rabbit. After three immunizations, the rabbit was bled and the whole IgG was obtained through the Protein-A cellulofine column. To purify the monospecific IgG against 17 kd PDGF-related protein, we employed the method of Beckerle [12]. We confirmed that the affinity purified rabbit IgG recognized the 17 kd PDGF-related protein of U251MG in the same manner as a monoclonal anti-PDGF antibody [13] did (Fig. 1).

3. PDGF-Related Proteins in Cultured Cells

The cultured cells were detached by a silicone policeman, homogenized in PBS, and centrifuged. The samples were adjusted to the same protein concentrations and mixed with sample buffer A or sample buffer B [sample buffer A supplemented with 10% 2-mercaptoethanol (2ME), 10 mM dithiothreitol (DTT) and 6 M urea], and subjected to SDS-PAGE. After electrophoresis, the proteins were transblotted to nitrocellulose membrane. A lane for marker proteins was stained with amido-black. The other part of the membrane was incubated with 5% nonfat milk in 0.01 M Tris HCl pH 8.0 with 0.15 M NaCl and 0.05% Tween 20 (TBST) for 1 h. The membrane was incubated with the immunoaffinity purified rabbit IgG, then incubated with alkaline phosphatase conjugated anti-rabbit IgG (Promega, USA) at room temperature, and colorized. Between each reaction, the membrane was rinsed 3 times for 10 min each in TBST.

4. PDGF-Related Proteins in Brain Tumor Tissues

The brain tumor tissues were obtained at surgery and stored at −80°C until use. The total of 20 specimens included 1 astrocytoma, 2 glioblastomas, 1 mixed oligo-astrocytoma, 1 gliosarcoma, 2 medulloblastomas, 4 meningiomas, 3 neurinomas, 4 neurocytomas, 1 metastatic adenocarcinoma, and 1 hypothalamic hamartoma. Each tumor tissue was dissected and washed 3 times in 0.17 M Tris HCl pH 7.65 with 0.83% (w/v) NH_4Cl for disrupting erythrocytes. The samples were homogenized in PBS and analyzed as described above. The proliferative activity of some tumor samples were examined in vivo by uptake of bromodeoxyuridine (BrdU) [14].

Results

1. The Expression of PDGF-Related Proteins in Cultured Cells

The established cell lines from malignant gliomas and short-term cultures from meningiomas all contained 17 kd PDGF-related protein, which was detected under both nonreduced and reduced conditions (Fig. 2). The staining intensity of the 17 kd band was almost equal in each glioma cell line. The staining intensity of the 17 kd band was different in the two meningioma cell lines (Fig. 2C,D).

2. PDGF-Related Proteins in Brain Tumors

The results are shown in Table 1. The 92 kd and 17 kd bands were detected under a non-reduced condition, and the 56 kd and 17 kd bands were recognized

Table 1. PDGF-related proteins in brain tumor tissues

Histology	Age (years)	Sex	Non-R		R		BrdU
			92	17	56	17	L.I.
Glioblastoma	61	F	++	+	−	+	3.9
Glioblastoma	67	F	++	+	+	+	ND
Gliosarcoma	66	M	++	+	+	+	7.6
Astrocytoma	61	M	+	+	−	+	ND
M.O.Astrocytoma	26	F	++	+	+	+	ND
Medulloblastoma	10	M	++	+	+	+	5.2
Medulloblastoma	28	M	++	+	+	+	16.2
Metastatic tumor	54	M	+	+	+	+	ND
Meningioma	38	F	++	+	+	−	0.2
Meningioma	52	M	++	+	+	+	0.4
Meningioma	70	F	++	+	+	+	0.1
Meningioma	73	F	++	+	+	+	0.1
Neurinoma	15	F	++	+	+	+	0.1
Neurinoma	32	F	++	+	+	+	ND
Neurinoma	41	F	++	+	+	+	ND
Neurocytoma	7	F	+	+	+	+	ND
Neurocytoma	19	F	+	+	+	+	ND
Neurocytoma	35	F	++	+	+	+	ND
Neurocytoma	45	F	+	+	+	+	ND
H. Hamartoma	7/12	F	+	+	−	+	ND

Non-R, non-reduced; *R*, reduced; *BrdU*, bromodyoxyuridine, *M.O.*, mixed oligo-, *H.*, hypothalamic; *ND*, not done under a reduced condition in brain tumors (Fig. 3). In the glioma tissues, such as astrocytoma (grade II), mixed oligo-astrocytoma and glioblastoma, all expressed PDGF-related proteins. The other brain tumors, meningioma, neurinomas, neurocytomas, medulloblastomas, and metastatic adenocarcinoma, contained the PDGF-related proteins as in the gliomas. The hypothalamic hamartoma also contained PDGF-related proteins but the bands at high molecular weight, 92 kd and 56 kd, were somewhat thinner than those of the other tumors.

In PDGF-related proteins of all brain tumors, the 92 kd protein was stained most intensely. The expressions of PDGF-related proteins in brain tumors were not correlated with the BrdU labeling indexes of tumor cells (Table 1).

Discussion

It has been suggested that PDGF or PDGF-related protein acts on the cells in an autocrinic fashion [4,7,15,16]. In brain tumors, the autocrinic effect of PDGF was suggested in glioblastoma [4] and meningioma [8], although the PDGF pathway in an autocrine loop has not been elucidated. Furthermore, the correlation between the expression of the PDGF-related protein and the grade of malignancy of brain tumors is still unclear.

Using the monospecific rabbit antibody to a native 17 kd PDGF monomer, we analyzed PDGF-related proteins in cultured brain tumor cells and tumor tissues. All established human glioma cell lines studied here had a nearly similar amount of 17 kd PDGF-related protein, while cultured meningiomas cells showed different amounts.

The presence of a 17 kd monomer in cultured cells under a nonreduced condition has not been evidenced [7]. We detected the intracellular 17 kd monomer in all brain tumors examined, and this might be due to the engaged

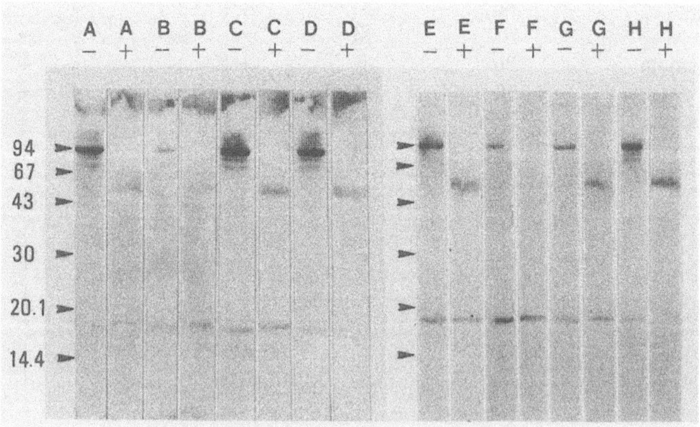

Fig. 3. Western blotting of brain tumor tissues reacted with purified rabbit IgG. *A*, glioblastoma; *B*, hypothalamic hamartoma; *C,D,E*, neurinoma; *F*, astrocytoma; *G*, neurocytoma; *H*, meningioma

antibodies, which we obtained by immunizing the monomer extracted from cultured cells.

In all brain tumor extracts, the PDGF-related proteins were detected at 92 kd and 17 kd under a nonreduced condition, and at 56 kd and 17 kd under a reduced condition. The most intensely stained one was the 92 kd protein in all brain tumors except in the hypothalamic hamartoma. Our previous data suggested that the PDGF-related protein is produced and stored as a 17 kd monomer intracellularly, and preserved as a 92 kd form extracellularly. The 92 kd form may degrade to 56 kd or about 30 kd dimer or 17 kd monomer. Highly malignant brain tumors, such as glioblastoma and medulloblastoma, showed a high uptake of BrdU, while benign ones, such as meningioma, neurocytoma, and neurinoma, showed a low uptake of BrdU. The BrdU incorporation is well correlated to proliferative activities of tumors [14]. Because of an almost equal amount of PDGF in malignant and benign tumors, PDGF may play key roles for sustaining neoplastic properties.

Conclusions

The antibody we produced reacted not only with the monomer but also with high molecular forms of PDGF. The 17 kd monomer of the PDGF-related protein was detected intracellularly, and a high molecular weight form of 92 kd was detected extracellularly. These facts applied to all of the kinds of brain tumors examined. The expression of PDGF-related proteins did not correlate with the grade of malignancy of brain tumors which were estimated by uptake of bromodeoxyuridine.

References

1. Heldin C-H, Westermark B, Wasteson Å (1979) Platelet-derived growth factor: Purification and partial characterization. Proc Natl Acad Sci USA 76:3722–3726
2. Ross R, Raines EW, Bowen-Pope DF (1986) The biology of platelet-derived growth factor. Cell 46:155–169
3. Westermark B, Wasteson Å (1976) A platelet factor stimulating human normal glial cells. Exp Cell Res 78:170–174
4. Hermansson M, Nistér M, Betsholtz C, Heldin C-H, Westermark B, Funa K (1988) Endothelial cell hyperplasia in human glioblastoma: Coexpression of mRNA for platelet-derived growth factor (PDGF) B chain and PDGF receptor suggests autocrine growth stimulation. Proc Natl Acad Sci USA 85:7748–7752
5. Heldin C-H, Betsholtz C, Johnsson A, Westermark B (1986) Role of PDGF-like growth factors in malignant transformation. Cancer Rev. 2:34–47
6. Sporn MB, Roberts AB (1985) Autocrine growth factors and cancer. Nature 313:745–747
7. Betsholtz C, Johnsson A, Heldin C-H, Westermark B, Lind P, Urdea MS, Eddy R, Shows TB, Philpot K, Mellor AL, Knott TJ, Scott J (1986) cDNA sequence and chromosomal localization of human platelet-derived growth factor A-chain and its expression in tumour cell lines. Nature 320:695–699

8. Maxwell M, Galanopoulos T, Hedley-Whyte ET, Black PM, Antoniades HN (1990) Human meningiomas co-express platelet-derived growth factor (PDGF) and PDGF-receptor genes and their protein products. Int J Cancer 46:16–21
9. Nakamura T, Takeshita I, Fukui M (1989) PDGF-related proteins in human gliomas. Neuroimmunolog Res 2:150–154
10. Ponten J, Westermark B (1978) Properties of human malignant glioma cells in vitro. Med Biol 56:184–193
11. Yamazaki K (1982) Tumorigenicity of established human glioma cell lines in lasat and nude mice—in relation to differentiation and anaplasia of glioma cells—(in Japanese with an English summary). Neuropathol. 3:29–38
12. Beckerle MC (1986) Identification of a new protein localized at sites of cell substrate adhesion. J Cell Biol 103:1679–1687
13. Shiraishi T, Morimoto S, Itoh K, Sato H, Onishi T, Ogihara T (1989) Radioimmunoassay of human platelet-derived growth factor using monoclonal antibody toward a synthetic 73–97 fragment of its B-chain. Clin Chim Acta 184:65–74
14. Fukui M, Iwaki T, Sawa H, Inoue T, Takeshita I, Kitamura K (1986) Proliferative activity of meningiomas as evaluated by bromodeoxyuridine uptake examination. Acta Neurochir (Wien) 81:135–141
15. Huang JS, Huang SS, Deuel TF (1984) Transforming protein of simian sarcoma virus stimulates autocrine growth of ssv-transformed cells through PDGF cell-surface receptors. Cell 39:79–87
16. Keating MT, Williams LT (1988) Autocrine stimulation of intracellular PDGF receptors in v-sis-transformed cells. Science 239:914–916

Measuring the Effect of PDGF on Fibroblasts Using Glioma Cell Lines

NOBUSADA SHINOURA, TATSUYA KONDOU, and MASUMI YOSHIOKA[1]

Introduction

The platelet-derived growth factor (PDGF) was first identified as having a potent growth-promoting activity in bovin serum, followed by evidence of this activity over glia, smooth muscle cell, and fibroblasts. Purification of PDGF revealed a heterodimeric glycoprotein composed of two basic polypeptide chains, A and B, in a disulfide linkage. Many PDGF-like growth factors, called cellular PDGF (PDGFc), were found without platelets, and were composed of AA, AB, and BB. We investigated PDGFc using 4 cell lines and, in this paper, we describe the existence of PDGF (AA, BB) in tumor cell lines and the effects of PDGF (AA, BB) on the fibroblasts and on the secretion of PDGF from the tumor cell lines.

Materials and Methods

Cell culture

We took the NMCG-1 cell line from a 40-year-old female patient with an astrocytoma grade III, and the NMCG-2 from a 36-year-old male patient with an astrocytoma grade III. The other 2 cell lines used were C6 (derived from rat glioma) and U-251 (derived from human glioma). NMCG-1 is easy to proliferate and could be stained by glial fibrillary acidic protein (GFAP) and neuron-specific enolase (NSE), but not by S-100. NMCG-2 is difficult to proliferate and is now frozen.

Growth stimulation with fetal bovine serum (FBS). The fibroblasts in the microplate (20000/well) were incubated for 3 days in Dulbecco's modified Eagles's medium (DMEM) with FBS (0%–50%) and stimulated for 2 days by a medium of 3 tumor cell lines (C6, NMCG-1, and NMCG-2) which were incubated using the same method. The cell count of the fibroblasts was measured on the 5th and 7th days and was compared with the control.

---

[1]National Medical Center, Shinjuku-ku, Tokyo, 162 Japan

Immunohistochemistry. Three tumor cell lines (C6, NMCG-1, and U-251) were incubated with the medium of cosmedium without FBS and fixed on the slide glass by two methods. In the first method they were centrifuged at 2000 cpm for 5 min, frozen, cut by cryostat, and dry-fixed. They were then stained with anti-PDGF (AA, BB) by the immunofluorescence and the avidin-biotin complex (ABC) methods using a Vecstasin kit.

Assay for growth-promoting activity (stimulation of PDGF-AA and -BB on the fibroblasts. Mitogenic activity was determined by measuring the thymidine incorporation. Fibroblasts were plated in 96-well microplates in DMEM containing 10% FBS. The starting cell density was 8000 cells/well. After 3–4 days, when the cultures appeared confluent, the spent medium was removed and replaced with 0.2 ml DMEM containing 1% FBS. After 24 h, the medium was replaced with DMEM containing PDGF-AA and -BB. After 16 h, the medium was replaced with DMEM containing 2.5 μCi/ml 3H-thymidine. The cells were washed 3 times with DMEM. Using 0.25% trypsin with cold trichloroacetic acid (TCA), Triton X, and 95% ethanol, the cells were filtrated with a glass filter and counted in a scintillation counter. The fibroblasts were stimulated by PDGF-AA and -BB and were counted. The starting cell density was 2000 cells/well. On the next day, the spent medium was removed and replaced with 1% FBS. After 2 days, the medium was replaced with DMEM containing PDGF-AA and -BB. After 2 more days, the cells were trypsinized and counted. Thymidine incorporation was also determined in the same way and stimulated by PDGF-AA and -BB at the same time.

The medium of 3 tumor cell lines (C6, NMCG-1, U-251) was concentrated fourfold with Mizubutorikum (ATT, Tokyo). Thymidine incorporation was then determined in the same way and stimulated by the concentrated medium with and without anti-PDGF (50 μg/ml)

Results

1. The cell count of fibroblasts stimulated by C6, NMCG-1 and NMCG-2 increased (Fig. 1).
2. All cell lines (C6, NMCG-1, U251) could be stained with PDGF-AA and -BB by immunofluorescence (IF) and the ABC method (Fig. 2).
3. Mitogenic activity increased stimulation by PDGF-AA and -BB in comparison with the control (Fig. 3). The maximum response was achieved with 10 ng/ml PDGF-AA and 100 ng/ml PDGF-BB, and the maximum value of PDGF-BB was more than that of PDGF-AA. The maximum number of cell counts achieved by the stimulation of PDGF-AA and PDGF-BB was also the same concentration as that with the thymidine incorporation (Fig. 4). Mitogenic activity stimulated by both PDGF-AA and PDGF-BB at the concentrations of 1, 10, 100, and 1000 ng/ml was completely depressed.
4. The conditioned medium of tumor cell lines which were concentrated four-

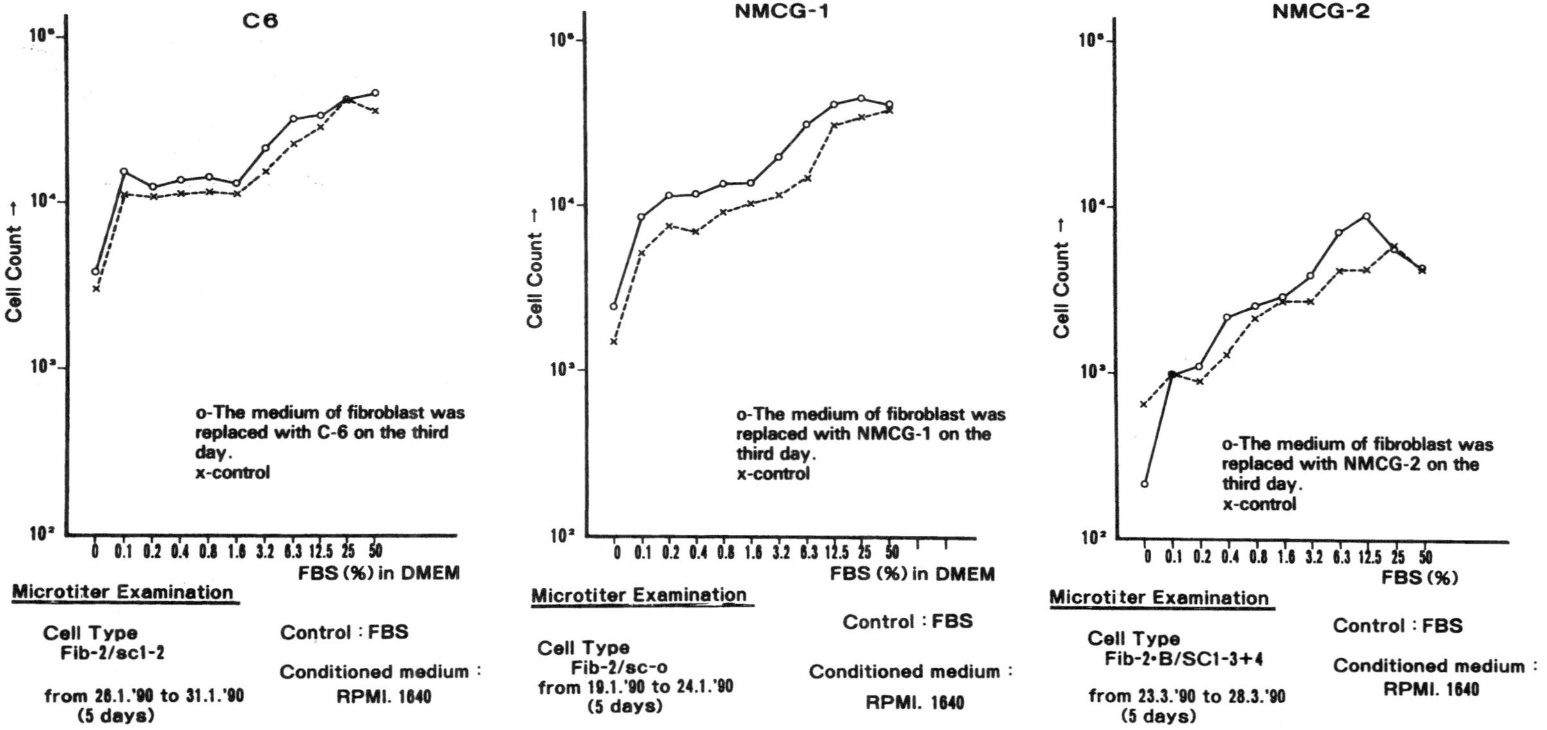

Fig. 1. All 3-cell lines increased cell count of the fibroblast. The *horizontal line* shows density of a FBS and the *vertical line* cell count by logarithm. *Left* C6, *middle* NMCG-1, *right* NMCG-2

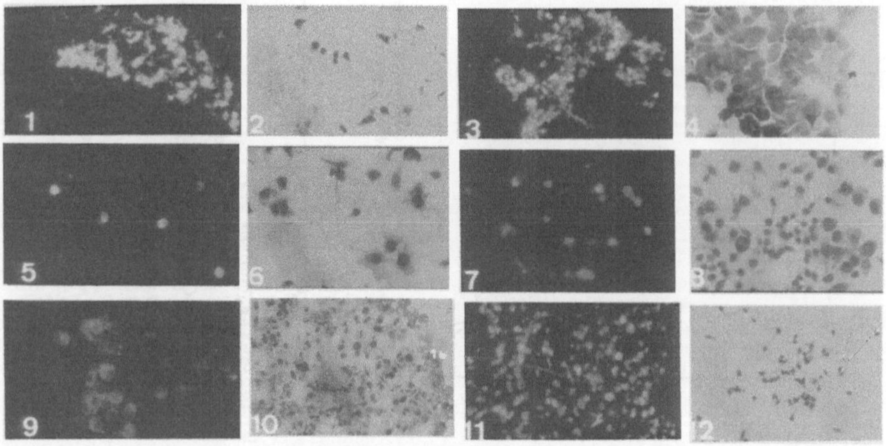

Fig. 2. All 3 cell lines were stained with PDGF-AA and -BB according to IF and ABC methods. *1*, C6 was stained with PDGF-AA according to the IF method; *2*, C6, AA, ABC; *3*, C6, BB, IF; *4*, C6, BB, ABC; *5*, NMCG-1, AA, IF; *6*, NMCG-1, AA, ABC; *7*, NMCG-1, BB, IF; *8*, NMCG-1, BB, ABC; *9*, U-251, AA, IF; *10*, U-251, AA, ABC; *11*, U-251, BB, IF; *12*, U-251, BB, ABC

fold produced a dramatic increase in DNA synthesis in response to NMCG-1, a moderate increase in response to U-251, and no increase in response to C-6 (Fig. 5). The neutralizing antibodies (anti-PDGF) effectively blocked the growth-enhancing effect of the conditioned medium of NMCG-1 and U-251. On the other hand, the neutralizing antibodies of PDGF-AA and PDGF-BB effectively produced the growth-enhancing effect of the conditioned medium of NMCG-1 and U-251 (Fig. 6).

Discussion

In 1971, Balk [1] found that the use of heat-inactivated serum, rather than heat-inactivated plasma, resulted in the rapid cell division of both normal and transformed cells in the same low-calcium medium. He thought that there were some mitogenic factors absent from plasma but present in the serum during its preparation from blood. In 1974, Kohler and Lipton [2], Ross et al. [3] and Westermark and Westeson [4] found the growth factor derived from platelets which promoted the growth of Balb/c3T3 cells, smooth muscle cells, and glia cells. In 1975, Antoniades et al. [5] isolated from whole human serum a basic polypeptide that stimulated DNA synthesis and cell division in confluent populations of mouse Balb/c-3T3 cells. The PDGF molecule is constructed as a dimer of A and B chains [6]. However, there are many PDGF-like proteins which consist of AA, AB, and BB and those are secreted by macrophages [7], rat aortic smooth muscle cells [8], developing human placenta [9], tumor cell lines (e.g., U-2 osteosarcoma [10] lines) and others. We investigated the

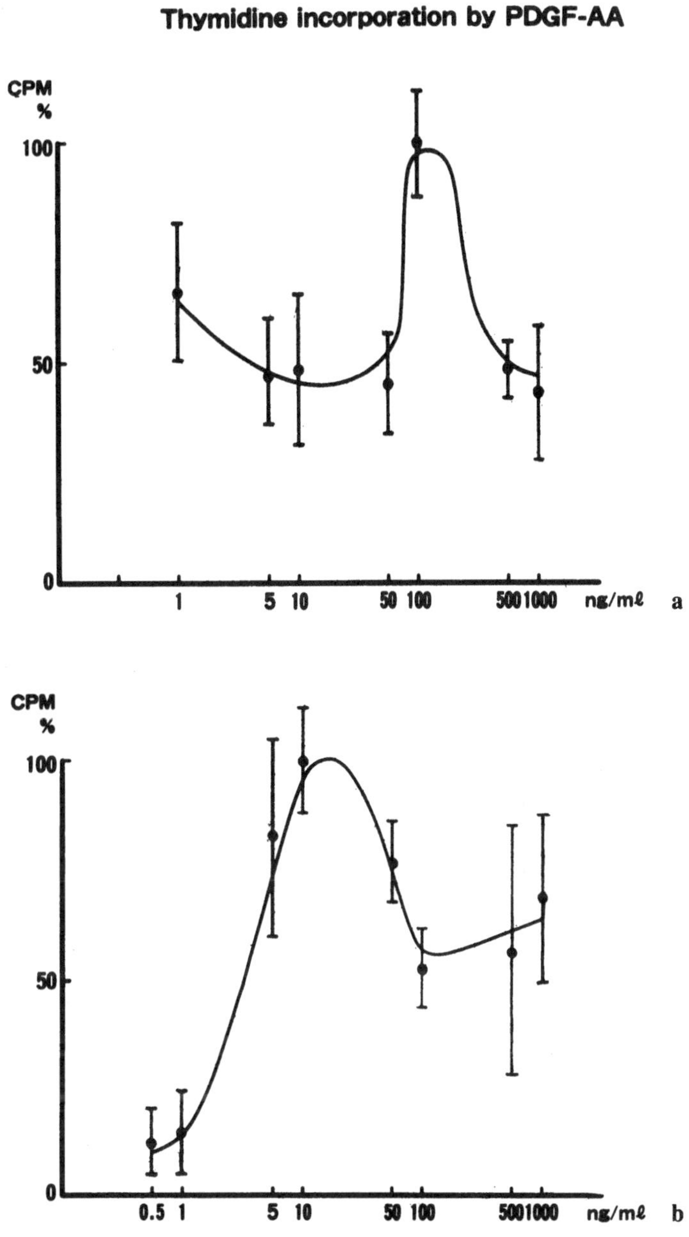

Fig. 3. Thymidine incorporation of a fibroblast was measured with **a** PDGF-AA and **b** PDGF-BB. For each kind of measurement the activity of unstimulated cultures (basal) was subtracted from that of the stimulated ones and the data are expressed as a percentage of the maximal value. The maximal value was at 100 ng/ml PDGF-AA and 10 ng/ml PDGF-BB

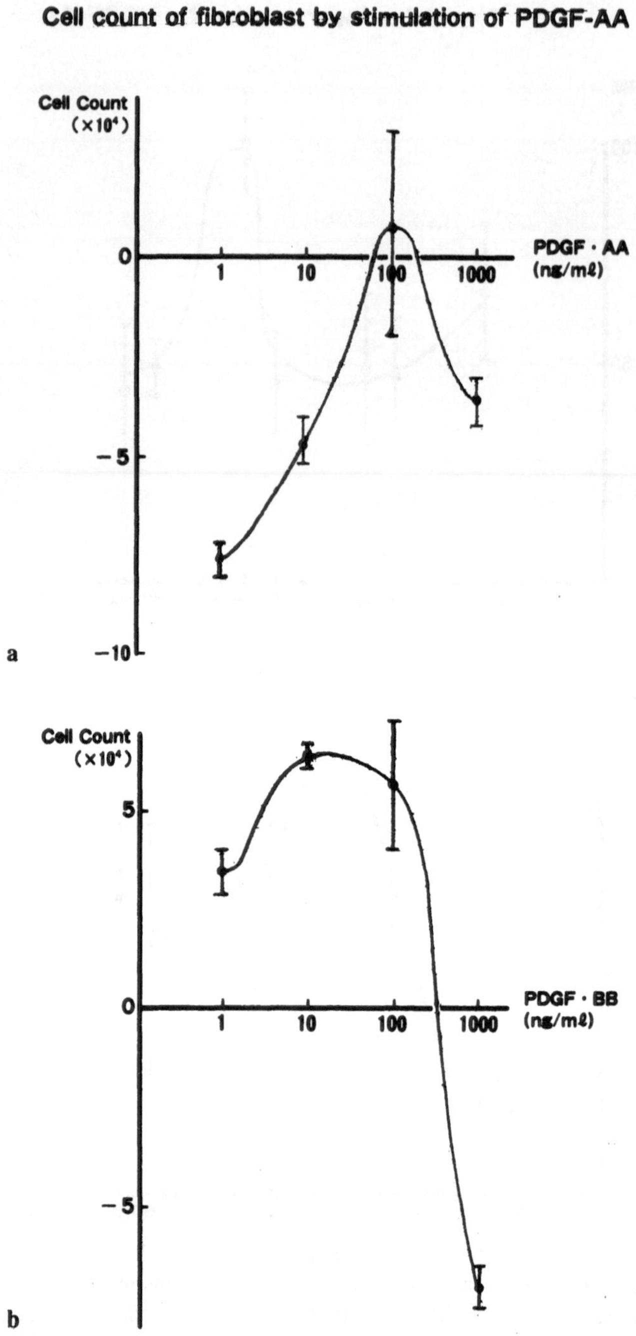

Fig. 4. Cell count of fibroblast was measured by the stimulation of **a** PDGF-AA and **b** -BB. The peak of the cell count was the same value as the thymidine incorporation.

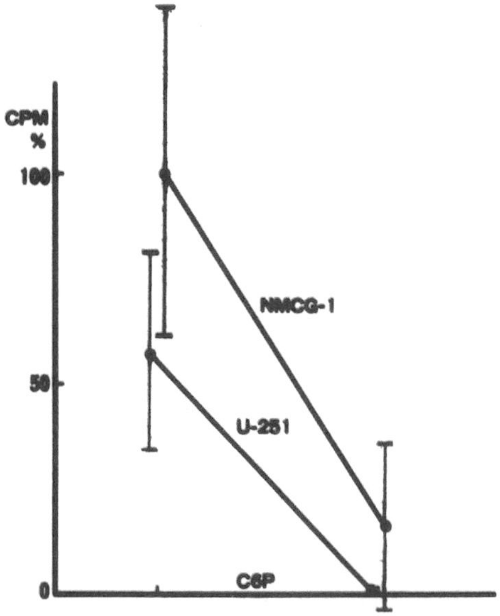

Fig. 5. The medium of NMCG-1 and U-251 had a mitogenic activity over the fibroblast when they were concentrated fourfold. For each kind of measurement the activity of unstimulated cultures (basal) was subtracted from that of the stimulated ones and the data are expressed as a percentage of the maximal value. The mitogenic activity of NMCG-1 and U-251 was suppressed by anti-PDGF (50 µg/ml)

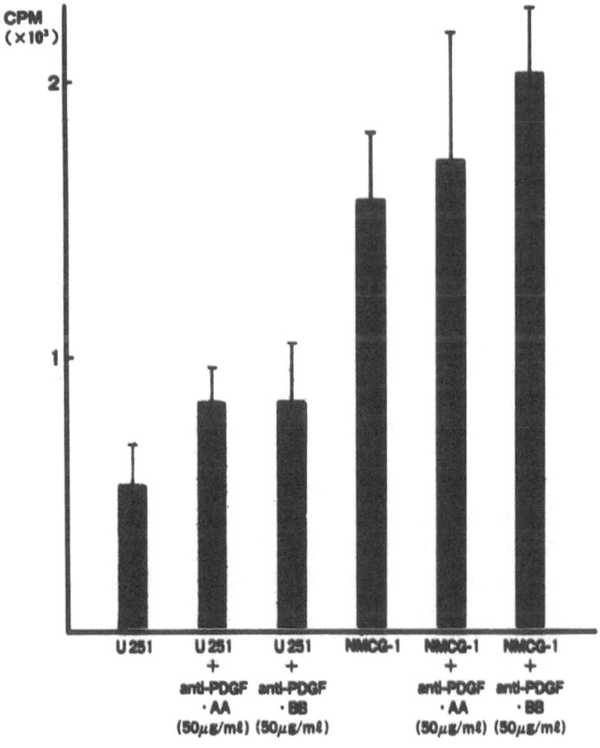

Fig. 6. The mitogenic activity of NMCG-1 and U-251 was increased with the stimulation of anti-PDGF-AA and -BB at the same time

existence of PDGF-AA and PDGF-BB in the tumor cell lines by the ABC and immunofluorescence methods and confirmed its existence in the cell lines of C-6, U-251, and NMCG-1. We also investigated the effect of PDGF-AA and PDGF-BB on mitogenesis in fibroblasts. The maximum responses were achieved at about 100 ng/ml PDGF-AA and at about 10 ng/ml PDGF-BB, respectively. The effect of maximum concentration of PDGF-BB on thymidine incorporation was greater than that of PDGF-AA. What is the effect of the sub-type of PDGF combined with another sub-type of PDGF on DNA synthesis? The aspect of functional differences between PDGF and GDGF-1, which is structurally a PDGF-A chain homodimer, is an antagonistic effect of GDGF-1 on PDGF-induced chemotaxis and, under certain conditions, on PDGF-induced actin reorganization [11]. When GDGF-1 was added to PDGF, no significant change in the PDGF-induced ^{3}H-thymidine incorporation was seen. However, when PDGF-AA and PDGF-BB were added together at various concentrations, ^{3}H-thymidine incorporation was completely suppressed. Perhaps the tumor cell lines (U-251 and NMCG-1) secreted different amounts of PDGF-AA and PDGF-BB. When PDGF-AA and PDGF-BB existed at the same time in the medium, ^{3}H-thymidine incorporation on fibroblasts was suppressed. Therefore, when anti-PDGF-AA or anti-PDGF-BB was added into the medium of the tumor cell lines, ^{3}H-thymidine incorporation increased.

Conclusion

One of the most important factors which was secreted by glioma cell lines and which promoted the growth of fibroblasts was proved to be PDGF.

References

1. Balk SD (1971) Calcium as a regulator of the proliferation of normal, but not of transformed, chicken fibroblasts in a plasma-containing medium Proc Natl Acad Sci USA 68:271–275
2. Kohler N, Lipton A (1971) Platelets as a source of fibroblast growth-promoting activity Exp Cell Res 98:297–301
3. Ross R, Glomset J, Kariya B, Harker L (1974) A platelet-dependent serum factor that stimulates the proliferation of arterial smooth muscle cells in vitro. Proc Natl Acad Sci USA 71:1207–1210
4. Westermark B, Westeson A (1976) A platelet factor stimulating human normal glial cells. Exp Cell Res 98:170–174
5. Antoniades, HN, Stathkos D, Scher CD (1975) Isolation of a cationic polypeptide from human serum that stimulates proliferation of 3T3 cells. Proc Natl Acad Sci USA 72:2635–2639
6. Johnsson A, Heldin CH, Westermark B, Wasteson A (1982) Platelet-derived growth factor Identification of constituent polypeptide chains. Biochem Biophys Res Commun 104:66–74

7. Shimokado K, Raines EW, Medtes DK, Barrett TB, Benditt EP, Ross R (1985) A significant part of macrophage-derived growth factor consists of at least two forms of PDGF. Cell 43:277–286
8. Seifert RA, Schwartz SM, Bowen-Pope DF (1984) Developmentally regulated production of platelet-derived growth factor-like molecules. Nature 311:669–671
9. Goustin AS, Betsholts C, Pfeifer-Ohlsson S, Persson H, Rydnert J, Bywater M, Holmgren G, Heldin CH, Westermark B, Ohosson R (1985) Co-expression of the *sis* and *myc* proto-oncogenes in developing human placenta suggests autocrine control of trophoblast growth. Cell 41:301–312
10. Heldin CH, Johnsson A, Wennergren S, Warnstedt C, Betsholtz C, Westermark C (1986) A human osteosarcoma cell line secretes a growth factor structurally related to a homodimer of PDGF-A chains. Nature 319:511–514
11. Nister M, Hammacher A, Mellstrom K, Siegbahn A, Ronnstrand L, Westermark K, Heldin CH (1988) A glioma-derived PDGF-A chain homodimer has differnet functional activities from a PDGF-AB heterodimer purified from human platelets. Cell 52:791–799

Section 4. Drug Resistance of Brain Tumor

Potentiation of 3-(4-Amino-2-Methyl-5-Pyrimidinyl) Methyl-1-(2-Chloroethyl)-Nitrosourea Cytotoxicity in Resistant Human Glioma Cell by Pretreatment with 5-(3-Methyl-1-Triazeno) Imidazole-4-Carboxamide

Toshimitsu Aida, Hiroshi Abe, Kouichi Tokuda, and Shinji Sugimoto[1]

Introduction

In our previous studies, we reported the results that O^6-alkylguanine DNA alkyltransferase (O^6-AT) plays an important role in determining the cellular resistance to treatment with chloroethylnitrosourea (CENU) [1–3]. The mechanism of cellular resistance has not been fully understood, but it is clear that O^6-AT repairs O^6-chloroethylguanine before it can rearrange to form the DNA interstrand cross-link [4–5], and this results in cellular resistance to the cytotoxic effects of CENUs. O^6-AT also prevents the induction of sister chromatid exchanges (SCEs) by CENUs, since the increased induction of SCEs is due to higher levels of DNA interstrand cross-links [1,2,6]. The reduction of O^6-AT activity in tumor cells which are resistant to CENUs may be used to improve the clinical effectiveness of CENUs, since this activity protects the cytotoxic effects of these agents. This has been approached by pretreatment with a monofunctional methylating agent [2,7,8]. 5-(3-dimethyl-1-triazeno) imidazole-4-carboxamide (DTIC) is a chemotherapeutic agent used primarily to treat malignant melanoma, sarcoma, and lymphoma. DTIC requires metabolic activation through oxidative N-demethylation leading to the formation of the N-demethyl derivative, 5-(3-methyl-1-triazeno) imidazole-4-carboxamide (MTIC), a potent alkylating agent. Recently, MTIC has been shown to alkylate DNA in the O^6 of guanine and to be more cytotoxic in O^6-AT deficient cells (Mer^-) than in O^6-AT proficient cells (Mer^+) [9,10]. We investigated the effect of pretreatment with MTIC on cytotoxicity and the induction of SCEs in a resistant human glioma cell line treated with 3-(4-amino-2-methyl-5-primidinyl) methyl-1-(2-chloroethyl)-nitrosourea (ACNU) to overcome the cellular resistance to ACNU.

[1] Department of Neurosurgery, Hokkaido University, Sapporo, 060 Japan

Materials and Methods

Cell Lines

The human glioma cell lines SF-188 and SF-126 were provided by Dr. M.L. Rosenblum (San Francisco, Calif.). These lines were subcultured in Eagle's minimum essentials medium with 10% fetal bovine serum.

Drugs

MTIC was synthesized by preparing the diazo derivative (DZC) of 5-aminoimidazole-4-carboxamide (AICA) and reacting this with methylamine in dimethyl sulfoxide (DMSO). Immediately before use, MTIC was dissolved in DMSO, and ACNU was dissolved in sterile water.

Drug Treatment and Assay of Colony-Forming Efficiency (CFE)

Cells were placed in $25\,cm^2$ tissue culture flasks in 5 ml medium approximately 48 h before drug treatment. The cells were treated for 1 h with various concentrations of ACNU. For the combination studies, SF-188 cells were treated with MTIC for 1 h, washed with phosphate buffered saline (PBS), and treated for 1 h with ACNU. After drug treatment, the cultures were incubated for the CFE assay. Details of the CFE assay procedure have been described elsewhere [1].

SCE Assay

SF-188 cells ($1.0–1.5 \times 10^6$) were seeded into $75\,cm^2$ flasks. Two days later, the cells were treated for 1 h with various concentrations of either MTIC or ACNU. For the combination studies, the cells were treated with MTIC for 1 h, washed with PBS, and treated with ACNU for 1 h. The medium was replaced with fresh medium containing bromodeoxyuridine, 10 µmol/1, and the cells were incubated for two replication cycles (48 h). The mitotic cells were accumulated by treatment with 0.04 µg/ml of colcemid for 4 h and dislodged by shaking the flasks. The medium was poured off and the mitotic cells were collected by centrifugation at 1000 rpm for 5 min. The pellet was treated with 2.0 ml 0.05 M KCL for 8–10 min, fixed twice with glacial acetic acid and methanol (1:3), and the methaphase chromosomes were spread on glass microscope slides. The method of Perry and Wolff was used for differential staining of sister chromatids. For each experiment, the frequency of SCEs was determined in 15–30 metaphase cells.

Results

The cytotoxic effects of MTIC on SF-188 cells are shown in Fig. 1. Although low doses of MTIC were not very toxic, cellular survival decreased with

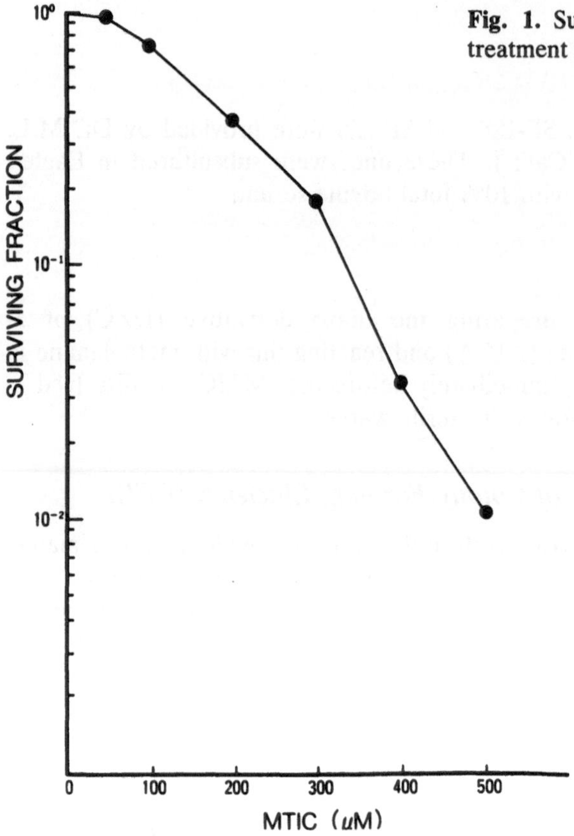

Fig. 1. Survival curves for SF-188 after treatment for 1 h with MTIC

increasing doses of MTIC. Treatment for 1 h with 100 μM MTIC reduced cellular survival by 25%, whereas 350 μM MTIC produced a 1 log cell kill.

SF-188 cells were highly resistant to the cytotoxic effects of ACNU (Table 1). A concentration of 108 μM was needed to produce a 1 log cell kill. SF-126 cells were sensitive, with 90% of the cells killed after a 1 h treatment with 13 μM ACNU. Measured as the ratio of concentrations needed to produce a 1 log cell kill, SF-188 cells were 8.3 times more resistant to the cytotoxic effects of ACNU than were SF-126 cells. Pretreatment of SF-188 cells with 100,200 and 300 μ MTIC for 1 h potentiated the cytotoxicity 108 μM ACNU by 1.3-, 2.8-, and 5.4-fold, respectively. Since 400 μM MTIC potentiated ACNU cytotoxicity by ninefold, SF-188 cells became as sensitive as SF-126 cells.

The induction of SCEs by ACNU treatment with or without pretreatment with MTIC is shown in Table 2. SF-188 cells were highly resistant to the induction of SCEs by ACNU; treatment with 10 μM ACNU induced only 11–13 SCEs per metaphase. The potentiation of ACNU-induced SCEs by MTIC was dose-dependent. Pretreatment with 100 and 200 μM MTIC induced 15–18 and 27–28 more SCEs/cell, respectively, than were expected on the basis of additivity.

Table 1. Potentiation of ACNU-induced cytotoxicity in SF-188 cells by pretreatment with MTIC

Cell line	Pretreatment	Treatment	LD_{10} (μM)	LD_{10} (No treatment) / LD_{10} (Pretreatment)
126	None	ACNU	13	
188	None	ACNU	108	
188	100 μM MTIC	ACNU	85	1.3
188	200 μM MTIC	ACNU	38	2.8
188	300 μM MTIC	ACNU	20	5.4
188	400 μM MTIC	ACNU	12	9.0

Table 2. Induction of SCEs in SF-188 cells treated with ACNU or ACNU and MTIC

Treatment (μM)	Experiment	Total SCEs /cell	Induced SCEs /cell	Expected SCEs /cell	Induced-expected
Control	1	7.7 ± 1.5			
	2	6.2 ± 0.9			
	3	6.8 ± 1.4			
MTIC (100)	1	14.4 ± 2.0	6.7		
	2	12.8 ± 1.7	6.6		
	3	13.5 ± 2.3	6.7		
MTIC (200)	1	19.9 ± 2.1	12.2		
	2	24.4 ± 3.5	18.2		
	3	20.2 ± 2.1	13.4		
ACNU (10)	1	19.7 ± 2.5	12.0		
	2	19.6 ± 2.3	13.4		
	3	17.4 ± 1.8	10.6		
MTIC (100) + ACNU (10)	1	41.2 ± 3.0	34.5	18.7	15.8
	2	41.3 ± 2.8	35.1	20.0	15.1
	3	42.4 ± 2.6	35.6	16.7	18.4
MTIC (200) + ACNU (10)	1	59.3 ± 4.5	51.6	24.2	27.4
	2	65.5 ± 5.3	59.3	31.6	28.0
	3	57.3 ± 4.7	50.5	24.4	26.6

Induced SCEs, total number of SCEs/cell in treatment groups minus untreated control value; *expected SCEs/cell*, sum of SCEs expected from treatment with each drug

Discussion

SF-188 cells are very resistant to cytotoxic effects of ACNU, compared with SF-126 cells, and have five-fold higher levels of O^6-AT [1]. In a previous study [2], we treated SF-188 cells with various concentrations of N-methyl-N-nitrosourea (MNU) to reduce the cellular level of O^6-AT. Pretreatment with MNU, in which concentrations depleted O^6-AT, potentiated the cytotoxicity of 1,3-bis(2-chloroethyl)-1-nitrosourea (BCNU) and the inhibition of SCEs in SF-188 cells. However, the combination of MNU and CENUs can not be placed into clinical trials since MNU is a potent carcinogen. Therefore, in seeking a less dangerous way in which to deplete the O^6-AT, we treated SF-188 cells with various concentrations of MTIC. In the concentrations used in this study, MTIC was minimally cytotoxic. However, pretreatment with MTIC increased the cytotoxicity of ACNU in a dose-dependent manner. Pretreatment with 400 μM MTIC potentiated ACNU cytotoxicity by nine-fold, and the cells became as sensitive as SF-126 cells.

SF-188 cells are very resistant to the induction of SCEs by ACNU [1]. In this study, MTIC potentiated the cytotoxic effects of ACNU and resulted in a dose-dependent increase in the number of SCEs. We have reported that a comparison of the induction of SCEs by mono- and bifunctional nitrosoureas indicated that the DNA interstrand cross-links formed by CENUs are the DNA alkylation products responsible for SCE induction by these agents [11]. These studies suggest that the increased induction of SCEs is due to the increased formation of DNA interstrand cross-links.

We are presently measuring the inhibition of O^6-AT in SF-188 cells treated with MNU. The premature data show that treatment of SF-188 cells with 300 μM MTIC inhibited O^6-AT activity by 40%. This result suggests that inactivation of O^6-AT by removal of O^6-methylguanine formed by MTIC treatment of SF-188 cells disturbs the repair of the O^6-chloroethylguanine, resulting in an increased level of DNA interstrand cross-links, which, in turn, leads to the increases in cytotoxicity and the induction of SCEs. This model is supported by the results of Zlotogorski and Erickson, who have shown that pretreatment of resistant cells with N-methyl-N′-nitro-N-nitrosoguanidine results in an increased level of DNA interstrand cross-links after treatment with CENUs [7]. In a previous study of five human glioma cell lines [1], the cellular resistance to the cytotoxic effects of CENUs varies from three- to eight-fold, depending upon the agents. Since the relative magnitude of resistance to CENUs is low, a clinical regimen that utilizes DTIC pretreatment prior to exposure to CENUs may be useful in overcoming the resistance of human malignant gliomas to killing by these antitumor agents.

Acknowledgements. We thank Dr. W.J. Bodell for his kind advice, and Miss M. Sudou for excellent technical assistance. This work was supported in part by a Grant-in-Aid from the Ministry of Education, Science and Culture, Japan.

References

1. Aida T, Bodell WJ (1987) Cellular resistance to chloroethylnitrosoureas, nitrogen mustard, and cis-diamminedichloroplatinum (II) in human glial-derived cell lines. Cancer Res 47:1361–1366
2. Aida T, Cheitlin RA, Bodell WJ (1987) Inhibition of O^6-alkylguanine DNA alkyltransferase activity potentiates cytotoxicity and induction of SCEs in human glioma cells resistant to 1,3-bis(2-chloroethyl)-1-nitrosourea. Carcinogenesis 8:1219–1223

3. Bodell WJ, Aida T, Berger MS, Rosenblum ML (1986) Increased repair of O^6-alkylguanine DNA adducts in glioma-derived human cells resistant to the cytotoxic and cytogenetic effects of 1,3-bis(2-chloroethyl)-1-nitrosourea. Carcinogenasis 7:879–883
4. Smith DG, Brent TP (1989) Response of cultured human cell lines from rhabdomyosarcoma xenografts to treatment with chloroethylnitrosoureas. Cancer Res 49:883–886
5. Robins P, Harris AL, Goldsmith I, Lindall T (1983) Cross-linking of DNA induced by chloroethylnitrosourea is prevented by O^6-methylguanine DNA methyltransferase. Nucleic Acids Res 11:7743–7758
6. Tokuda K, Bodell WJ (1988) Cytotoxicity and induction of sister chromatid exchanges in human and rodent brain tumor cells treated with alkylating agents. Cancer Res 48:3100–3105
7. Zlotogorski C, Erickson LC (1984) Pretreatment of human colon tumor cells with DNA methylating agents inhibits their ability to repair chloroethylmonoadducts. Carcinogenesis 5:83–87
8. Futsher BW, Micetith KC, Barres DM, Fisher RI, Erickson LC (1989) Inhibition of a specific DNA repair system and nitrosurea cytotoxicity in resistant human cells. Cancer Commun 1:65–73
9. Catapano CV, Broggini, Erba E, Ponti M, Mariani L, Citti L, D'Incalci M (1987) In vitro and in vivo methazolastone-induced DNA damage and repair in L-1210 leukemia sensitive and resistant to chloroethylnitrosoureas. Cancer Res 47:4884–4889
10. Lunn JM, Harris AL (1988) Cytotoxicity of 5-(3-methyl-1-triazono)imidazole-4-carboxamide (MTIC) on Mer^+, Mer^+Rem^- and Mer^- cell lines: Differential potentiation by 3-acetanidobenzamide. Br J Cancer 57:54–58
11. Bodell WJ, Aida T, Rusmussen J (1985) Comparison of sister chromatid exchange induction caused by nitrosoureas that alkylate or alkylate and crosslink DNA. Mutat Res 149:95–100

Potentiation of VP-16 Cytotoxicity by Dipyridamole in Malignant Glioma Cells

Takanori Ohnishi, Hiromitsu Iwasaki, Norio Arita, Shoju Hiraga, and Toru Hayakawa[1]

Introduction

VP-16 (etoposide) has been currently used for the treatment of malignant gliomas not only as a chemotherapeutic agent for induction of initial remission but also as a drug for the long-term treatment after remission of the tumors. When VP-16 is used for the latter purpose, however, two major problems should be solved in order to obtain a successful result with this drug. One is to overcome VP-16-resistant cells which may appear in the course of the treatment, and the other is to develop a new mode to treat G_0/G_1 cells which predominate after intensive treatment of the tumors. These cells make VP-16 cytotoxicity less effective due to the lower amount of DNA topoisomerase II, a target of VP-16 [1].

Dipyridamole (DPM), a drug described clinically as a vasodilator and an antiplatelet agent, is a potent inhibitor of membrane nucleoside transport [2,3] and has been noted to enhance the cytotoxic effect of antimetabolites, such as methotrexate [4] and 5-FU [5] *in vitro*. Furthermore, it has been reported that DPM increases VP-16 cytotoxicity both in rat hepatoma cells and in VP-16-resistant human leukemia cells by inhibiting the efflux of VP-16 [6]. In the present study, we report a synergic effect of DPM with VP-16 in the cytotoxicity against both VP-16-sensitive and -resistant human glioma cells. We also compare the effect of the calcium entry blocker, diltiazem (DTZ), combined with VP-16 to that of DPM.

Materials and Methods

Drugs

Dipyridamole was provided by Boehringer Ingelheim Japan Co. (Tokyo) and diltiazem was provided by Tanabe Pharmaceutical Co. (Osaka, Japan). VP-16 was obtained from Nippon Kayaku Co. (Tokyo).

[1] Department of Neurosurgery, Osaka University Medical School, Osaka, 553 Japan

Cell Culture

Two human glioblastoma cell lines, T98G and U373MG, were purchased from American Type Culture Collection. VP-16-resistant cells (U373MG/R) were produced in our laboratory from U373MG by spontaneous mutation. All cells were grown as a monolayer in Eagle's minimum essential medium (MEM) containing 10% fetal bovine serum, 1% sodium pyruvate, and 1% non-essential amino acid.

Cytotoxicity Assay

Inhibition of cell growth was determined by MTT [(3–4,5-dimethylthiazol-2-yl)-2,5-diphenyltetrazolium bromide] assay [7]. Cells were seeded in a 96-well microtiter plate (Falcon Labware) at 10,000 cells/well for T98G cells and at 15,000 cells/well for U373MG and U373MG/R cells, and incubated for 24 h at 37°C in a humidified 5% CO_2 atmosphere. The cells were then exposed to various concentrations of (a) VP-16 alone, (b) VP-16 and DPM, and (c) VP-16 and DTZ for 48 h. After exchanging to a culture medium without the drugs, MTT (Sigma, St. Louis, MO.) (50 µg per 100 µl medium) was added to each well and the plates were incubated at 37°C for 4 h. Acid isopropanol (100 µl 0.04 N HCl in isopropanol) was added to all wells and mixed thoroughly to dissolve the dark blue crystals. The plates were then read on a microplate reader (MTP-120, Corona) at a test wave length of 570 nm and a reference wave length of 630 nm. To obtain a relation between the number of cells and the optical density of MTT formazan which was formed, the number of viable cells was also determined in all cell lines by the dye exclusion method using 0.05% nigrossin.

Treatment with Dibutyryl cAMP, Aminophylline, and MY5445

In order to examine an action mechanism of the synergic effect of DPM with VP-16, the cells were treated with cAMP agonists, dibutyryladenosine 3′:5′ cyclic monophosphate (dibutyryl cAMP) (Sigma), aminophylline (Sigma), and cGMP phosphodiesterase inhibitor (MY5445) (kindly provided by Dr. I Sakuma, Hokkaido University School of Medicine), which were combined with VP-16.

Flow Cytometric Analysis

Three glioma cell lines were plated in culture flasks and incubated for 24 h at 37°C in a humidified atmosphere. The cells were exposed to various concentrations of DPM for 48 h and then were pulse-labeled with 10 µM BrdU for 30 min. After washing twice with phosphate buffered saline (PBS), the cells were harvested with 0.125% trypsin and fixed with 70% cold ethanol for 30 min. The cells were treated with 4 N HCl for 20 min and then neutrized with 0.1 M sodium tetraborate. After centrifugation (1500 × g, 30 s), 0.5% Tween

20 in PBS was added to the cell pellets and the cells were centrifuged again. The cells were then incubated with anti-BrdU-FITC (Becton Dickinson, Japan) at 37°C for 30 min. The cells were washed twice with PBS and treated with 20 μg/ml propidium iodide (Sigma) at 4°C for 20 min. The cells were passed through a 50 μm nylon mesh and analyzed by FACS III (Becton Dickinson).

Results

Inhibition of Cell Growth

When the cytotoxic effect of VP-16 combined with DPM or DTZ against glioma cells was assessed using the MTT assay, VP-16 inhibited the cell growth in a dose-dependent manner. The optical density, which represents the amount of MTT formazan which was generated, was directly proportional to the number of cells counted by the dye exclusion method in the range from 5,000 to 1×10^5 cells in all three glioma cell lines. In the present study, IC_{50} was defined as 50% reduction of absorbance in the MTT assay. DPM (1, 2.5, or 5 μg/ml) alone did not affect cell growth, but these doses enhanced the cytotoxicity of VP-16 in a dose-dependent manner in all cell lines (Fig. 1). On the other hand, DTZ at any dose tested did not increase the cytotoxicity of VP-16 in these glioma cells (Fig. 1). The results of IC_{50}s determined by MTT assay are shown in Fig. 2. DPM (2.5, 5 μg/ml) significantly decreased IC_{50} of VP-16 in all cell lines. In U373MG/R cells, 5 μg/ml DPM combined with VP-16 reduced IC_{50} about nine-fold lower than VP-16 alone.

Effects of cAMP or cGMP Agonists Combined with VP-16

Neither cAMP agonists, dibutyryl cAMP and aminophylline, nor cGMP agonist, MY5445, enhanced the cytotoxicity of VP-16 in any cell line when they were used in combination with VP-16.

Effects of DPM on Cell Turnover

Results of the distribution of glioma cells in cell cycle after the treatment with or without DPM are summarized in Table 1. DPM (5, 10 μg/ml) increased the number of cells in S-phase in a dose-dependent manner in all of the glioma cell lines.

Discussion

We demonstrated that the non-toxic level of DPM (5 μg/ml) markedly enhanced the cytotoxicity of VP-16 against human malignant glioma cells *in vitro*. This synergic effect of DPM was also seen in VP-16-resistant glioma cells (U373MG/R). On the other hand, DTZ did not significantly increase the

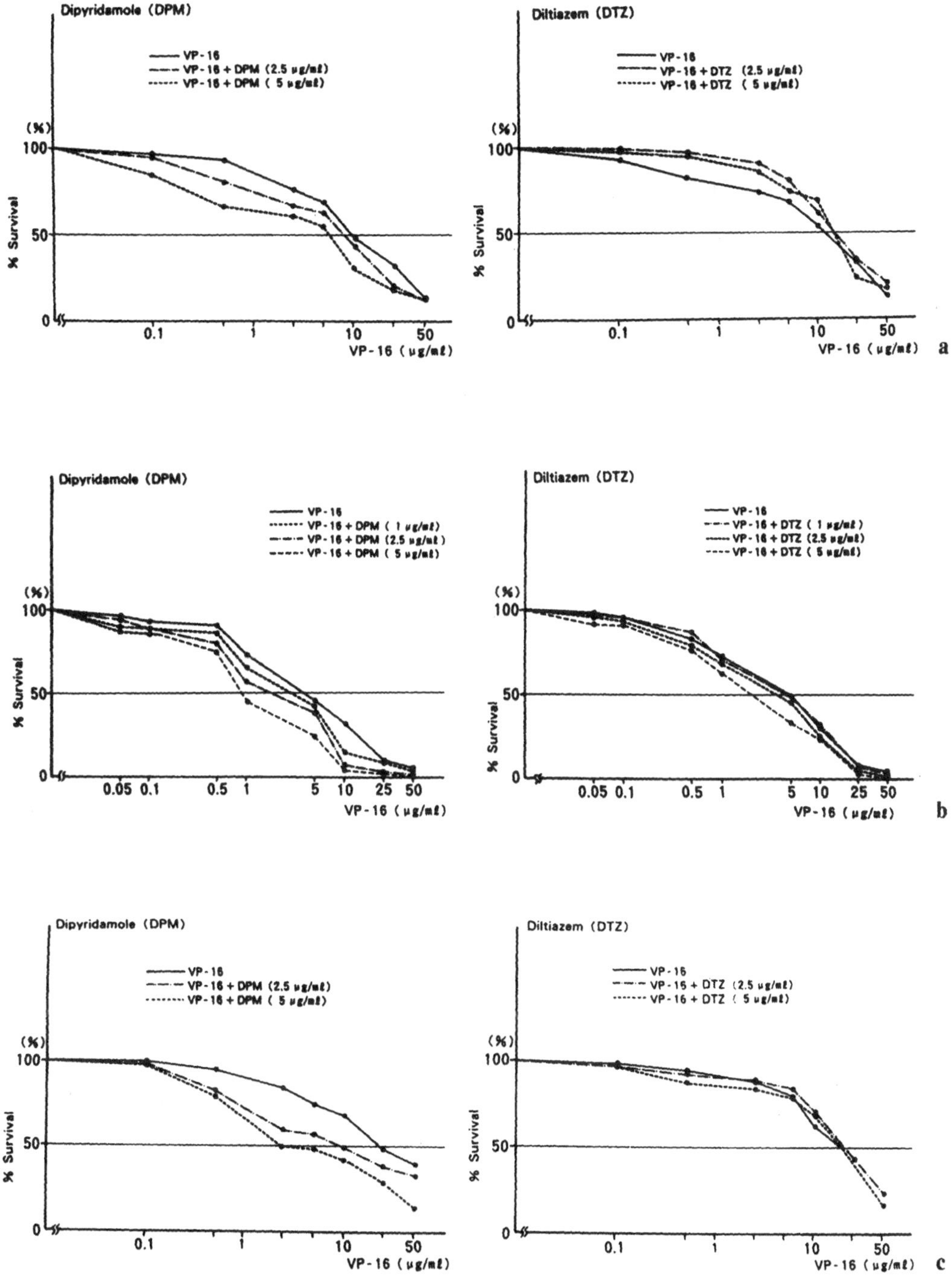

Fig. 1. Inhibition of cell growth by VP-16 combined with dipyridamole (DPM) or diltiazem (DTZ). The cytotoxicity of drugs was determined by MTT assay. **a** T98G cells, **b** U373MG cells, **c** U373MG/R cells

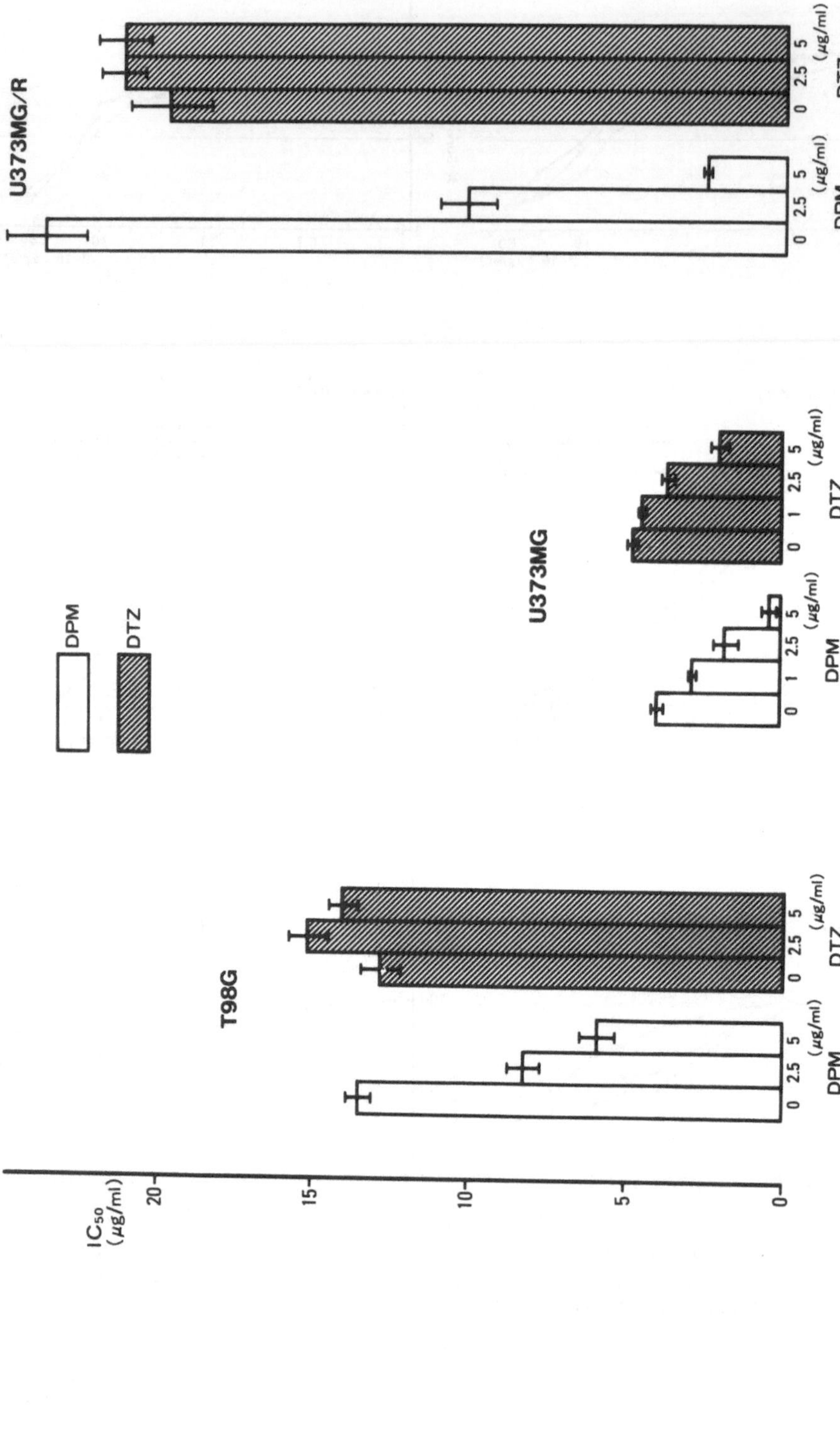

Fig. 2. Effects of dipyridamole (DPM) or diltiazem (DTZ) combined with VP-16 on cytotoxicity against human glioma cell lines, which are shown by IC_{50}s calculated from optical density. *Bars* show means ±SD for five experiments

Table 1. Effect of dipyridamole (DPM) on cell turnover in human malignant glioma cells

Cell line/ DPM (μg/ml)		Cell turnover (%)		
		G_0/G_1	S	G_2M
T98G	0	46.7 ± 3.7	28.4 ± 1.3	15.5 ± 1.2
	5	47.1 ± 1.9	31.9 ± 1.5	12.3 ± 1.2
	10	48.9 ± 2.4	31.5 ± 1.8	14.3 ± 0.8
U373MG	0	28.7 ± 0.4	35.7 ± 0.3	15.9 ± 0.4
	5	29.0 ± 1.5	40.2 ± 0.5*	15.3 ± 0.3
	10	27.7 ± 0.3	43.1 ± 0.2*	14.4 ± 0.1
U373MG/R	0	28.4 ± 0.6	37.5 ± 0.2	16.9 ± 0.4
	5	29.4 ± 0.7	41.1 ± 0.5*	15.9 ± 0.2
	10	35.3 ± 3.0	41.0 ± 0.8*	13.7 ± 1.6

Values are shown as means ±SD for triplicate experiments
*significantly different from each control (0 μg/ml of DPM) at $P < 0.001$

cytotoxic activity of VP-16 in any glioma cell line when it was used at concentration within 5 μg/ml. The ineffectiveness of DTZ on the augmentation of VP-16 cytotoxicity in these cells may suggest that the drug-resistance in U373MG/R cells does not relate to the development of multidrug resistance gene products [8]. Actually, immunohistochemistry disclosed that an expression of P-glycoprotein in U373MG/R cells was not so markedly different from that in U373MG cells (data not shown).

In relation to the mechanism of the synergic effect of DPM, we investigated effects of cAMP and cGMP agonists, both of which represent pharmacological properties of DPM, on VP-16 cytotoxicity against glioma cells. The increased level of cAMP or cGMP, however, did not affect the cytotoxic activity of VP-16, although the concentration of MY5445 (cGMP phosphodiesterase inhibitor) used in the experiment was relatively low because it was extremely difficult to obtain the drug in a water-soluble form.

The possible mechanisms of the synergism between VP-16 and DPM include (a) inhibition of nucleoside salvage by DPM, (b) increased uptake of VP-16 by DPM, and (c) increased number of proliferating cells by DPM. DPM is an inhibitor of membrane nucleoside transport in various cultured cells [2,3], and this property has been utilized to enhance the cytostatic action of antimetabolites by preventing nucleoside salvage [4,5,9,10]. Although it is unknown whether the inhibition of nucleoside salvage by DPM is also operative in the case of VP-16, blockade of nucleoside transport by DPM might not influence the cytotoxic effect of VP-16 significantly because *de novo* synthesis of nucleosides is not inhibited by VP-16. It is possible that DPM might increase the intracellular accumulation of VP-16 in these glioma cells. It has been reported that DPM increased adriamycin uptake without influencing the efflux [11]. On the other hand, Ikegami et al. [6] described that DPM enhanced the intracellular level of VP-16 in rat hepatoma cells by inhibiting the efflux of VP-16. In a preliminary study, we could not demonstrate an increased level of intracellular concentration of VP-16 by the addition of DPM (data not shown). Further studies related to the drug uptake, however, would be required to clarify the exact mechanism of DPM synergism with VP-16 in glioma cells.

It is well known that VP-16 stimulates the formation of DNA topoisomerase II-DNA cleavage complexes, which is responsible for the cytotoxicity of the drug [12,13]. That is, it is suggested that the intracellular target of VP-16 is the nuclear enzyme, DNA topoisomerase II [1,14]. Furthermore, it has been demonstrated that proliferating cells have a much higher activity of topoisomerase II than quiescent cells [15]. In the present study, we showed that DPM increased the number of glioma cells in a proliferating pool of cell cycle in a dose-dependent manner. The effect of DPM was observed not only in VP-16-sensitive cells but also in VP-16-resistant cells. This indicates that the synergic effect of DPM with VP-16 in the cytotoxicity against glioma cells may be due to an increase in proliferating cells induced by DPM, thus increasing enzyme activity of DNA topoisomerase II.

A combination of VP-16 with DPM may present much more effective chemotherapy in the long-term management of patients with malignant gliomas. To examine *in vivo* synergic effects of DPM with VP-16 is a future study.

Conclusion

Dipyridamole (DPM) (1–5 μg/ml) enhanced the cytotoxicity of VP-16 against human malignant glioma cells *in vitro* in a dose-dependent manner. On the other hand, the calcium entry blocker, diltiazem, did not increase VP-16 cytotoxicity on malignant glioma cells when it was used at a concentration within 5 μg/ml. DPM also augmented the activity of VP-16 in VP-16-resistant glioma cells. Flow cytometric studies demonstrated that the synergic effect of DPM with VP-16 in the cytotoxicity against glioma cells might be the consequence of an increased number of cells in proliferating pools.

References

1. Long BH, Musial ST, Brattain MG (1985) Single and double strand DNA breakage and repair in human lung adenocarcinoma cells exposed to etoposide and teniposide. Cancer Res 45:3106–3112
2. Paterson ARP, Lau EY, Dahlig E, Cass CE (1980) A common basis for inhibition of nucleoside transport by dipyridamole and nitrobenzylthioinosine. Mol Pharmacol 18:40–44
3. Aronow B, Ullman B (1986) Role of the nucleoside transport function in the transport and salvage of purine nucleobases. J Biol Chem 261:2014–2019
4. Nelson JA, Drake S (1984) Potentiation of methotrexate toxicity by dipyridamole. Cancer Res 44:2493–2496
5. Grem JL, Fischer PH (1985) Augmentation of 5-fluorouracil cytotoxicity in human colon cancer cells by dipyridamole. Cancer Res 45:2967–2972

6. Ikegami T, Kubota N, Matsui K, Funabiki T, Shuin T (1989) Enhance effect of etoposide by dipyridamole (abstract). Proc Jpn Cancer Assoc 48:30
7. Mosmann T (1983) Rapid colorimetric assay for cellular growth and survival: Application to proliferation and cytotoxicity assays. J Immunol Methods 65:55–63
8. Gros P, Croop J, Housman D (1986) Mammalian multidrug resistance gene: Complete cDNA sequence indicates strong homology to bacterial transport proteins. Cell 47:371–380
9. Zhen Y, Lui MS, Weber G (1983) Effects of acivicin and dipyridamole on hepatoma 3924A cells. Cancer Res 43:1616–1619
10. Chan TCK, Howell SB (1985) Mechanism of synergy between N-phosphoacetyl-L-aspartate and dipyridamole in a human ovarian carcinoma cell line. Cancer Res 45:3598–3604
11. Kusumoto H, Maehara Y, Anai H, Kusumoto T, Sugimachi K (1988) Potentiation of adriamycin cytotoxicity by dipyridamole against HeLa cells in vitro and sarcoma 180 cells in vivo. Cancer Res 48:1208–1212
12. Yang L, Rowe TC, Liu LF (1985) Identification of DNA topoisomerase II as an intracellular target of antitumor epipodophyllotoxins in simian virus 40-infected monkey cells. Cancer Res 45:5872–5876
13. Wang JC (1987) Recent studies of DNA topoisomerases. Biochem Biophys Acta 909:1–9
14. Liu LF, Rowe TC, Yang L, Tewey KM, Chen GL (1983) Cleavage of DNA by mammalian DNA topoisomerase II. J Biol Chem 258:15365–15370
15. Sullivan DM, Glisson BS, Hodges PK, Smallwood-Kentro S, Ross WE (1986) Proliferation dependence of topoisomerase II-mediated drug action. Biochemistry 25:2248–2256

The Role of O^6-Alkylguanine-DNA Alkyltransferase in Glioma in Resistance to Chloroethylnitrosoureas

TAKUHIRO HOTTA[1], TOHRU UOZUMI[1], KATSUZO KIYA[1], KAORU KURISU[1], TAKASHI MIKAMI[1], HIDENORI OGASAWARA[1], KAZUHIKO SUGIYAMA[1], YUJI SAITOH[2], KANJI ISHIZAKI[3], and MITSUO IKENAGA[3]

Introduction

Chloroethylnitrosoureas (CENUs) have been commonly used as chemotherapy for malignant gliomas [1]. Based on the anticipated cytotoxic mechanisms of these agents, the results of a number of studies using cultured tumor cells have confirmed that a DNA repair enzyme, O^6-alkylguanine-DNA alkyltransferase (AGT), affects the susceptibility of human tumor cells to CENUs [2,3]. A similar finding was also noted in rat and human glioma cell lines [4,5]. However, little is known about the contribution of AGT to the resistance to CENUs in clinically observed malignant gliomas. In this study, we investigated to what degree AGT influenced the mechanism of acquired resistance to CENUs in rat brain tumor cells, and evaluated the significance of this DNA repair enzyme in clinical resistance to CENUs by analyzing AGT activity measured in human malignant glioma surgical specimens.

Materials and Methods

Cell Cultures

The cell strains used in this study were 9L and C6 rat brain tumor cells. 9LR1, 9LR3, and 9LR12 are ACNU-resistant cells established from the 9L cell by means of repetitious ACNU treatments. All cultures were maintained in Dulbecco's modified Eagle's medium (DMEM, Nissui Co., Tokyo) with 10% fetal bovine serum.

Reagents

1-(4-amino-2-methyl-5-pyrimidinyl) methyl-3-(2-chloroethyl)-3-nitrosourea hydrochloride (ACNU) and O^6-methylguanine (O^6-mG) were obtained from

[1] Department of Neurosurgery, Hiroshima University School of Medicine, Hiroshima, 734 Japan
[2] Department of Neurosurgery, Koseiren Onomichi Sogo Hospital, Onomichi, Hiroshima, 722 Japan
[3] Radiation Biology Center, Kyoto University, Kyoto, 606 Japan

Sankyo Co., Tokyo, and methyl 6-[3-(2-chloroethyl)-3-nitrosoureido]-6-deoxy-α-D-gluco-pyranoside (MCNU) from Tokyo-Tanabe Drug Co., Tokyo.

Treatment of Cultures

The surviving fractions were calculated from the number of colonies formed after incubation for 12 days following a 60-min treatment with ACNU or MCNU. For AGT assay, 2–8 × 10^7 cells were collected and stored at –80 °C. O^6-mG was dissolved in acid water and adjusted to appropriate pH, 7.2–7.4 with 1 N NaOH. The cell cultures were incubated in a medium containing 0.4 mM O^6-mG for 24 h, and collected for the survival and AGT assays. The treatment of the 9L and 9LR12 cells with ACNU was conducted for 60 min in serum-free DMEM. The cells were harvested for 0, 12, 24, and 24 hours, and then AGT was measured.

Assay of AGT Activity

The assay for AGT activity in extracts from cells and tissues was performed as previously described [6]. The AGT activity of each cell strain or excised tumor was determined by measuring the radioactivity which was transferred from the substrate DNA containing methyl-[^{3}H]-labeled O^6-methylguanine.

Clinical Subjects

The total of 57 surgical specimens which could be histologically diagnosed were: 24 anaplastic astrocytomas, 18 glioblastomas, 11 brain tumors (except for malignant gliomas), and 4 normal brain tissues excised for the extirpation of deep-seated tumors.

Results

Investigation of the Rat Brain Tumor Cells

The results of the survival assay to CENUs and AGT activity of the cultured cells are shown in Table 1. A high correlation was observed between the degree of resistance to each drug and AGT activity. The effects of O^6-mG on AGT activity and on cellular sensitivity to ACNU are shown in Table 2. Pretreatment with 0.4 mM O^6-mG significantly reduced AGT activity of the ACNU-resistant cells to levels ranging from 18.4 % to 44.9 % of that of non-treated cells. We observed a 1.69- to 2.64-fold augmentation of sensitivity from the evaluation of IC37 in the resistant cells due to the treatment. Figure 1 shows the regeneration of AGT after ACNU treatment with 1 μg/ml for the 9L cell and with 40 μg/ml for the 9LR12 cell. These sublethal doses were confirmed in other experiments (not shown here) to imbue each cell with the same minimal cytotoxity, respectively. AGT activity had recovered to the approxi-

Table 1. Sensitivity to ACNU or MCNU presented as IC37 and O^6-alkylguanine-DNA alkyltransferase (*AGT*) activity of each rat brain tumor cell line. Each surviving fraction was obtained from a colony-forming assay. *IC37* means the dose at which survival was 37%. Alkyltransferase activity was measured by the method described in [6]. Data are presented as the means ± standard deviations

	IC37 (μg/ml)		AGT Activity
	ACNU	MCNU	(pmoles/mg protein)
9L	2.17 ± 0.24	3.95 ± 0.24	0.158 ± 0.043
C6	18.00 ± 1.77	13.62 ± 0.59	0.232 ± 0.046
9LR1	21.63 ± 2.05	25.80 ± 2.00	0.647 ± 0.122
9LR3	45.33 ± 1.59	66.20 ± 1.10	0.837 ± 0.339
9LR12	54.50 ± 3.51	58.10 ± 1.70	0.901 ± 0.392

Table 2. Effects of O^6-methylguanine (O^6-mG) on O^6-alkylguanine-DNA alkyltransferase (*AGT*) activity and on cell survivals to *ACNU* in the rat brain tumor cell lines. Cultures were treated or not treated for 24 h with 0.4 mM O^6-methylguanine. Data are presented as the means ± standard deviations

	AGT Activity (pmoles/mg)		IC37 to ACNU (μg/ml)	
	O^6-mG(−)	O^6-mg(+)	O^6-mG(−)	O^6-mg(+)
9L	0.158 ± 0.043	0.071 ± 0.016	2.17 ± 0.024	2.33 ± 0.33
9LR1	0.647 ± 0.122	0.177 ± 0.018	21.60 ± 2.50	8.17 ± 3.00
9LR3	0.837 ± 0.339	0.154 ± 0.021	45.30 ± 1.60	26.80 ± 6.31
9LR12	0.901 ± 0.392	0.238 ± 0.025	54.50 ± 3.50	25.63 ± 6.41

mate value of the basal activity in the 9LR12 cell within 24 h after exposure, whereas it was not yet recovered in the 9L cell within the same period ($P < 0.001$).

Clinical Investigations

In normal brain tissues and brain tumors except for malignant gliomas, all specimens had more than 0.1 pmoles/mg protein AGT. On the other hand, among 42 malignant gliomas 7 samples (16.7 %) had the low AGT activity of less than 0.1 pmoles/mg protein (Fig. 2). The results of remission-induction therapy, including CENUs, for glioblastomas were effective (complete or partial response) in 3 out of 8 patients in whom tumoral AGT activity was lower than 0.2 pmoles/mg protein , whereas no effective results were seen in five patients with AGT activities equal to or higher than 0.2 pmoles/mg protein. In three patients investigated before and after the therapy, including CENUs, no significant change in AGT activity was observed.

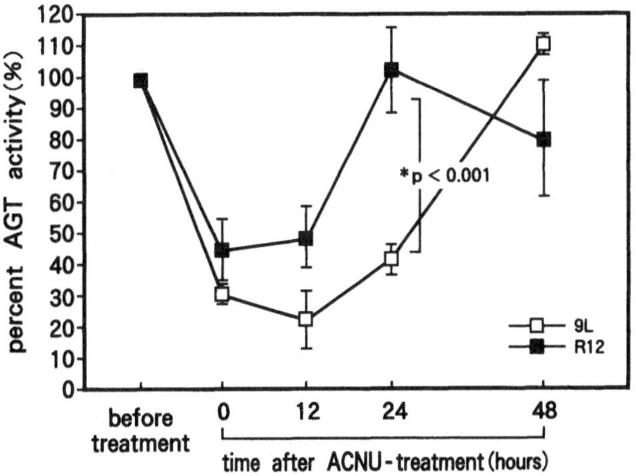

Fig. 1. Regeneration of O^6-alkylguanine-DNA alkyltransferase (*AGT*) after ACNU treatment. The dose used for ACNU was 1.0 µg/ml for the 9L cell and 40 µg/ml for the 9LR12 cell. After a 60-min treatment with ACNU, the cells were incubated for indicated periods, and then alkyltransferase activity was measured. *Points*, duplicate data; *bars*, standard deviations

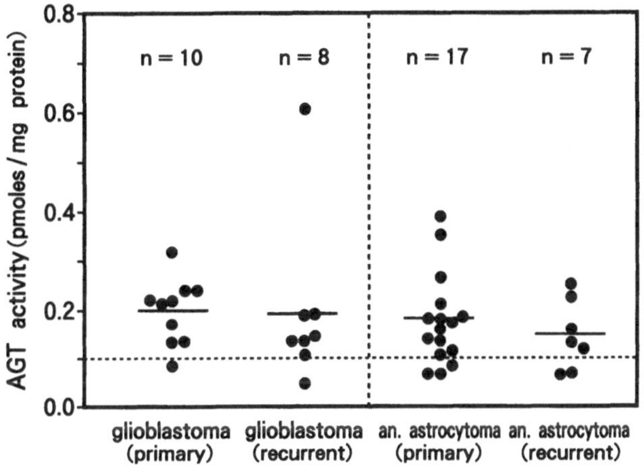

Fig. 2. O^6-alkylguanine-DNA alkyltransferase (*AGT*) activity of 42 malignant gliomas surgical specimens. The term '*primary*' means being excised at the first operation before other adjuvant therapy. *Bars* indicate means of data within each group

Discussion

In our experiments using rat brain tumor cell lines, we observed an exact correlation between AGT activity and the degree of resistance to toxicity of CENUs. It is known that the reduction of AGT activity observed following the treatment with a reagent consuming this enzyme, such as O^6-mG, leads to an increase of sensitivity to CENUs [7,8]. We observed this result in all three resistant cell lines studied, although there were discrepancies among them in the magnitudes of AGT decrease and sensitivity increase. It is suggested that factors other than static AGT activity may play roles in the mechanism of resistance to CENUs. The existence of individual differences in the regeneration after a depletion of AGT was stressed [9]. The regeneration of AGT within 24 h after ACNU exposure was significantly slower in the 9L cell than in the 9LR12 cell. Such differences in the rate of AGT regeneration may have relevance to CENU-resistance as has been previously suggested [10].

AGT activity in human gliomas has been generally reported to be low [11]. In our clinical study, however, there were wide variations in AGT activity between individuals. In preliminary studies of glioblastomas, tumors possessing higher AGT activity tended to be less responsive to therapy, including CENUs. From our results, in general, it was unlikely that systemic administration of CENUs would directly affect the intrinsic AGT activity in the human body. Since cDNA for the human AGT has been cloned [12], it is expected that a more precise delineation of the mechanism by which AGT activity affects sensitivity to CENUs will be developed.

Conclusions

In the acquired resistance to CENUs of rat brain tumor cells, not only the static level of AGT but also the capacity to recover this enzyme was thought to be important. Although it was suggested in the clinical study that AGT was important in constitutional resistance to CENUs, no evidence that this enzyme was closely associated with acquired resistance has been observed.

References

1. Takakura K, Abe H, Tanaka R, Kitamura K, Miwa T, Takeuchi K, Yamamoto S, Kageyama N, Handa H, Mogami H, Nishimoto A, Uozumi T, Matsutani M, Nomura K (1986) Effect of ACNU and radiotherapy on malignant glioma. J Neurosurg 64:53–57
2. Tsujimura T, Zhang YP, Fujio C, Chang HR, Watatani M, Ishizaki K, Kitamura H, Ikenaga M (1987) O^6-methylguanine methyltransferase activity and sensitivity of Japanese tumor cell strains to 1-(4-amino-2-methyl-5-pyrimidinyl)methyl-3-(2-chloroethyl)-3-nitrosourea hydrochloride. Jpn J Cancer Res 78:1207–1215
3. Smith DG, Brent TP (1989) Response of cultured human cell lines from rhabdomyosarcoma xenografts to treatment with chloroethylnitrosoureas. Cancer Res 49:883–886
4. Bodell WJ, Aida T, Berger MS, Rosenblum ML (1986) Increased repair of O^6-alkylguanine DNA adducts in glioma-derived human cells resistant to the cytotoxic and cytogenetic effects of 1,3-bis(2-chloroethyl)-1-nitrosourea. Carcinogenesis (Lond) 7:879–883

5. Aida T, Bodell WJ (1987) Cellular resistance to chloroethylnitrosoureas, nitrogen mustard, and cis-diamminedichloroplatinum (II) in human glial-derived cell lines. Cancer Res 47:1361–1366
6. Ikenaga M, Tsujimura T, Chang HR, Fujio C, Zhang YP, Ishizaki K, Kataoka H, Shima A (1987) Comparative analysis of O^6-methylguanine methyltransferase activity and cellular sensitivity to alkylating agents in cell strains derived from a variety of animal species. Mutat Res 184:161–168
7. Yarosh DB, Hurst-Calderone S, Babich MA, Day RS III (1986) Inactivation of O^6-methylguanine-DNA methyltransferase and sensitization of human tumor cells to killing by chloroethylnitrosourea by O^6-methylguanine as a free base. Cancer Res 46:1663–1668
8. Gerson SL, Trey JE, Miller K (1988) Potentiation of nitrosourea cytotoxicity in human leukemic cells by inactivation of O^6-alkylguanine-DNA alkyltransferase. Cancer Res 48:1521–1527
9. Gerson SL (1988) Regeneration of O^6-alkylguanine-DNA alkyltransferase in human lymphocytes after nitrosourea exposure. Cancer Res 48:5368–5373
10. Pegg AE (1990) Mammalian O^6-alkylguanine-DNA alkyltransferase: Regulation and importance in response to alkylating carcinogenic and therapeutic agents. Cancer Res 50:6119–6129
11. Wiestler O, Kleihues P, Pegg AE (1984) O^6-alkylguanine-DNA alkytransferase activity in human brain and brain tumors. Carcinogenesis (Lond) 5:121–124
12. Tano K, Shiota S, Collier J, Foote RS, Mitra S (1990) Isolation and structural characterization of a cDNA clone encoding the human DNA repair protein for O^6-alkylguanine. Proc Natl Acad Sci USA 87:686–690

O^6-Methylguanine-DNA Methyltransferase (O^6-MT) Activity as an Index of Drug Responsiveness to Antitumor Chloroethylnitrosoureas in Xenografted Brain Tumors

Katsuyoshi Mineura, Naoyuki Kuwahara, Katsuo Watanabe, and Masayoshi Kowada[1]

Introduction

The synthesized chloroethylnitrosoureas (CENUs), 1-(4-amino-2-methyl-5-pyrimidinyl)methyl-3-(2-chloroethyl)-3-nitrosourea hydrochloride (ACNU), and methyl-6-[3-(2-chloroethyl)-3-nitrosoureido]-6-deoxy-α-D-glucopyranoside (MCNU), have been among the antitumor agents widely used for the treatment of malignant brain tumors [1]. Methods for monitoring responsiveness of brain tumors to CENUs on the basis of a cell-killing mechanism have been needed to enhance therapeutic effectiveness. It is well documented that a DNA repair enzyme O^6-methylguanine-DNA methyltransferase (O^6-MT), identical to the term O^6-alkylguanine-DNA alkyltransferase, eliminates the O^6-methylguanine induced by CENUs and reflects the cellular resistance to CENUs in cultured cell strains and xenografted tumors [2–5]. Further in vivo work was warranted to establish a chemosensitivity index of O^6-MT activity. In the present paper, we test the relationship of O^6-MT activity and responsiveness to CENUs in xenografted brain tumors.

Materials and Methods

1. Cell Strains and Culture

The cell strains used in the present experiment were rat glioma cell lines (9L, C6) and HeLa S_3 cells as a representative methylation repair positive (Mer^+) phenotype. All cell strains were maintained in Eagle's minimal essential medium (MEM, Flow Lab, McLean, Va.) supplemented with 10% (vol/vol) fetal bovine serum, penicillin G (50 units/ml), streptomycine (50 μg/ml), and fungizone (2.5 μg/ml). Cells were grown under a humidified 5% atmosphere at 37°C, and yielded in logarithmic growth after trypsinization.

[1] Neurosurgical Service, Akita University Hospital, Akita, 010 Japan

2. *Xenografts and Treatment*

Female nude mice, 6–7 weeks old, weighing 21 ~ 23 g with a BALB/c genetic background were purchased from Nihon Clea Co. (Osaka, Japan). They were maintained in a specific pathogen-free room. About 5×10^6 cells of three strains were inoculated subcutaneously into the back and flank of the animal; xenografted tumors were measured repeatedly with calipers. The tumor volume was calculated as a prolate spheroid from the following equation: $4/3\pi \times a/2 \times (b/2)^2$, when a and b are measured as the maximum length and width at a right angle, respectively.

When the tumor reached a size of 50–50 mm^3, mice harboring xenografts were treated intraperitoneally with a single dose of ACNU (25 mg/kg), MCNU (25 mg/kg), bleomycin (BLM, 400 mg/kg), and *cis*-diamminedichloroplatinum (II) (CDDP, 3 mg/kg). The given doses of each agent were determined as comparable doses which give 10% survival of clonogenic cells. ACNU treatment included two different doses of 25 and 50 mg/kg. Non-treated control mice received an equal volume of saline. Each treated group and control group consisted of 5–15 animals. Tumor volumes were measured repeatedly during the 40 days after the treatment. Doubling time, maximum inhibition rate, and disappearance rate of each tumor strain were compared among treated and control groups for evaluation of therapeutic effectiveness.

3. *O^6-MT Assay*

For quantitative measurement of O^6-MT enzymic activity, the xenografts of three non-treated mice were excised 30 days after inoculation, and kept frozen at −80°C until assay.

The tissues were cut into pieces on a dry ice block and dissolved in Buffer C as described elsewhere in detail [5]. The chopped tissues were homogenized by a Polytron PT-10 (Kinematica, Switzerland) and a Potter-Elvehjem homogenizer. Then, the homogenate was sonicated at 4°C three times for 30 s bursts and 30 s intervals with a Bioruptor (UCD-1303, CosmoBio, Tokyo). The lysate was then spun with a centrifuge (Tomy MR-150, Tokyo) at 15000 rpm for 10 min. The supernatant was collected as a crude protein extract.

The crude protein extracts from tissues were reacted in vitro with the substrate DNA containing methyl-^3H-labeled ^6O-methylguanine, as described previously [5]. The O^6-MT activity of each tumor tissue was determined by measuring the radioactivity which was transferred from the substrate DNA to an acid-insoluble protein fraction in the extracts.

Results

1. *Antitumor Drug Sensitivity of Tumor Xenografts*

A summary of antitumor effects of four chemotherapeutic agents is shown in Table 1. Figures 1 and 2 illustrate changes in tumor growth for each tumor

Table 1. Antitumor effect of chemotherapeutic agents and O^6-MT activity in xenografted tumors

Cell	O^6-MT (fmol/mg)	Agent (mg/kg)	Doubling time (days)*	Inhibition rate (max. %)	Disappearance of tumors
9L	15	Control	6 ± 2	0	0/10
		ACNU (25)	ND	93	5/15
		ACNU (50)	ND	99	7/10
		MCNU (25)	35 ± 2	96	1/5
		BLM (400)	5 ± 2	19	0/5
		CDDP (3)	9 ± 4	36	0/5
C6	131	Control	4 ± 1	0	0/10
		ACNU (25)	5 ± 1	45	0/15
		ACNU (50)	10 ± 2	69	0/10
		MCNU (25)	7 ± 2	45	0/5
		BLM (400)	7 ± 2	50	0/5
		CDDP (3)	7 ± 3	59	0/5
HeLa	341	Control	5 ± 1	0	0/7
S3		ACNU (25)	4 ± 3	17	0/10
		ACNU (50)	5 ± 2	23	0/10
		MCNU (25)	5 ± 3	14	0/5
		BLM (400)	10 ± 7	59	0/5
		CDDP (3)	16 ± 6	70	0/5

*mean ± S.D., ND: not determined
Inhibition rate was calculated as the maximum percentage regression to tumor volumes of non-treated groups.

xenograft implanted on nude mice following treatment at various concentrations of the antitumor agents.

The 9L tumors were most sensitive to ACNU and MCNU. A moderate dose of ACNU (25 mg/kg) inhibited the semi-exponential growth of 9L tumors during some periods, and caused the disappearance of tumors in 5 out of 15 tumors (33%). A high dose of ACNU (50 mg/kg) decreased tumor size, and showed complete remission in 7 our of 10 tumors (70%). The maximum inhibition rate of 9L tumor growth at doses of 50 mg/kg and 25 mg/kg was 99% on the 22th post-treatment day and 93% on the 24th day, respectively. MCNU (25 mg/kg) as well as ACNU retarded growth of 9L tumors soon after the termination treatment.

The C6 tumors responded marginally to ACNU or MCNU. The maximum inhibition rate of C6 tumors was 45% at a dose of 25 mg/kg (ACNU, MCNU) and 69% at a dose of 50 mg/kg (ACNU). Shortly after a transient delay of growth, the tumors continuously increased in size. In contrast, the growth pattern of HeLa S3 tumors after ACNU or MCNU treatment at any doses used for the present study was similar to that of non-treated controls. In HeLa S3 tumors, ACNU (50 mg/kg) showed only a 23% growth inhibition rate.

BLM and CDDP inhibited tumor growth of each tumor to some extent; however, they did not completely eradicate the tumors. The maximum inhibition rate for BLM or CDDP showed a relation with the previous results of sensitivity using the colony formation assay [5].

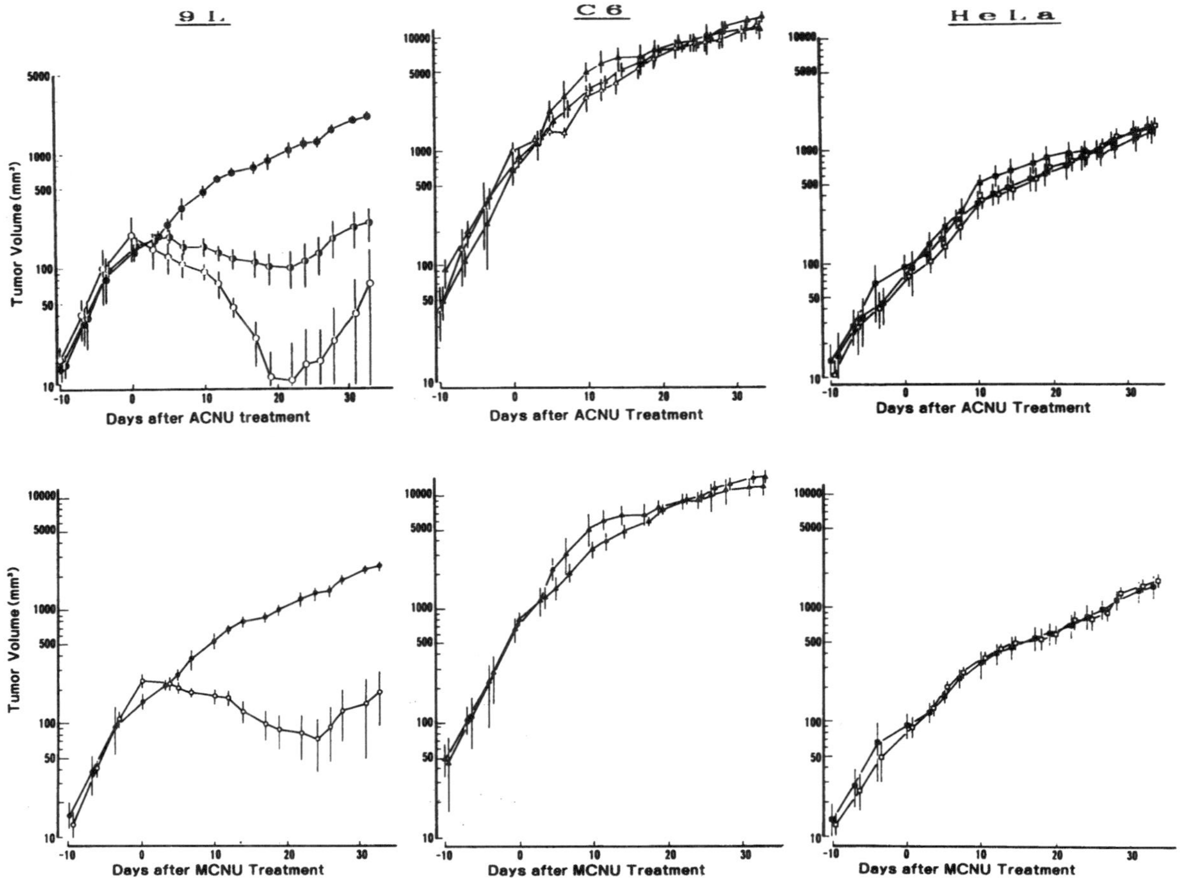

Fig. 1. The growth curves for each tumor transplanted into nude mice after ACNU (*top*) or MCNU treatment (*bottom*). The 9L tumors strongly responded to ACNU or MCNU with increasing doses; the other C6 and HeLa S3 tumors showed marginal retardation after the treatment. *Symbols* and *bars*, which represent the mean and standard deviation of at least two independent experiments including 5–15 nude mice, were plotted on a logarithmic scale of volume. *Non-treated control group*: ● 9L, ▲ C6, ■ HeLa S3; *ACNU-treated group*: ○△□ 25 mg/kg, ○△□ 50 mg/kg; *MCNU-treated group*: ○△□ 25 mg/kg

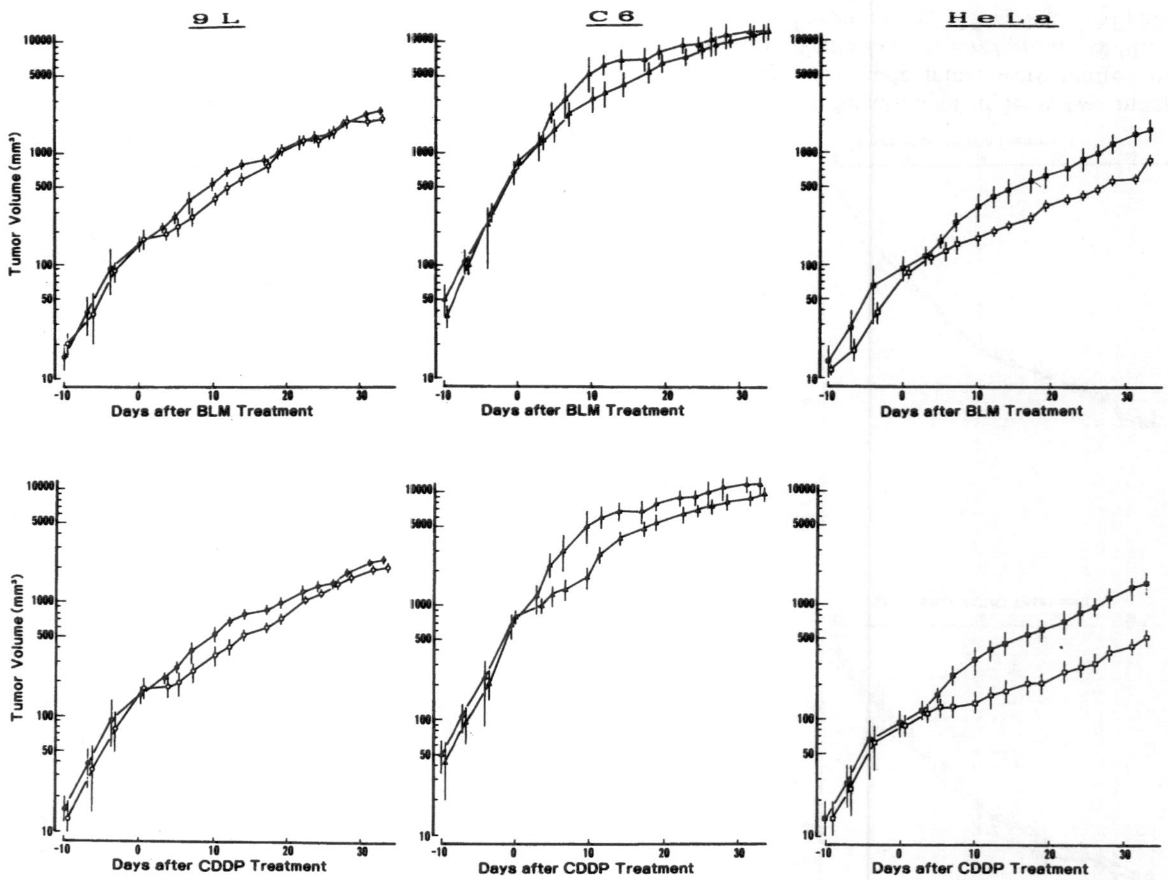

Fig. 2. The growth curves for each tumor transplanted into nude mice after BLM (*top*) or CDDP treatment (*bottom*). All species of tumors showed a slight decrease in size after the treatment. *Symbols* and *bar* represent the mean and standard deviation. *Non-treated control group*: ● 9L, ▲ C6, ■ HeLa S3; *BLM-treated group*: ○△□ 400 mg/kg; *CDDP-treated group*: ○△□ 3 mg/kg

2. *O^6-MT Activity of Tumor Xenografts*

The O^6-MT activity of xenografted tumors is summarized in Table 1. The O^6-MT activity was expressed as fmols of ^3H-methyl transferred per mg protein by at-least linear regression analysis. The mean activity of the HeLa S3 tumors was 341 fmol/mg, the C6 tumors 131 fmol/mg, and the 9L tumors 15 fmol/mg.

Discussion

Methods for selecting active antitumor agents in the chemotherapy of brain tumors include the incorporation of ^3H-thymidine measuring DNA synthesis rate of tumor cells and the in vitro colony-formation assay implying the ratio of clonogenic cells. The number of sensitivity tests based upon different cell-killing mechanisms specific to different agents remains scarce.

CENUs are among the antitumor agents used in the chemotherapy for malignant gliomas, mainly because of blood-brain barrier (BBB) permeability and of cell-cycle non-specific agents. Clinical results of the CENU treatment in gliomas clarified a marginally therapeutic benefit [1].

CENUs produce biological effectiveness through alkylation at the O^6-position of guanine, resulting in cross-link formation. The O^6-MT enzyme is responsible for repair of O^6-methylguanine-DNA. In a previous report, 9L cultured cells indicative of a low O^6-MT activity were defined as having a methylation repair negative (Mer^-) phenotype, while C6 cells showing a high activity possessed a Mer^+ type [5]. We also demonstrated that the effectiveness of CENUs in clonogenic tumor cells varied among tumor cell species and related well with O^6-MT activity [5].

The O^6-MT activity of xenografted tumor tissues indicated a lower level than that of respective cultured cells. This disparity can be influenced by heterogenous components, including stromal tissues and small foci of necroses in xenografts. Nevertheless, the tumors which responded poorly to ACNU or MCNU exhibited the higher O^6-MT values, and the O^6-MT activities can be compared among the three cell strain tumors. This indicates that drug sensitivity to the CENUs, such as ACNU and MCNU, is greatly attributable to differences in the biological activity of O^6-MT.

The assay using O^6-MT activity can directly determine the chemosensitivity to CENUs in in vivo experimental brain tumors and human tumor specimens [6], and creates the possibility of selective chemotherapy protocols to enhance the specific killing of repair-deficient brain tumors.

Summary

We tested the correlation between enzymatic activity of O^6-methylguanine-DNA methyltransferase (O^6-MT) and responsiveness to antitumor chloroethylnitrosoureas (CENUs) in xenografted brain tumors. The 9L tumors with a low

O^6-MT activity responded well to ACNU or MCNU treatment. In contrast, C6 tumors with a high O^6-MT activity continued to grow after chemotherapy of ACNU or MCNU, as was seen in methylation repair positive (Mer^+) HeLa S3 tumors. These data indicate that O^6-MT activity is promising in evaluating responsiveness to CENUs in the chemotherapy of brain tumors.

Acknowledgment. This work was supported in part by a Grant-in-Aid for Scientific Research from the Ministry of Education, Science and Culture, Japan.

References

1. Takakura K, Abe H, Tanaka R, Kitamura K, Miwa T, Takeuchi K, Yamamoto S, Kageyama N, Handa H, Mogami H, Nishimoto A, Uozumi T, Matsutani M, Nomura K (1986) Effects of ACNU and radiotherapy on malignant glioma. J Neurosurg 64:53–57
2. Scudiero DA, Meyer SA, Clatterbuck BE, Mattern MR, Ziolkowski CHJ (1984) Sensitivity of human cell strains having different abilities to repair O6-methylguanine in DNA to inactivation by alkylating agents including chloroethylnitrosoureas. Cancer Res 44; 2467–2474
3. Ikenaga M, Tsujimura T, Chang HR, Fujio C, Zhang YP, Ishizaki K, Kataoka H, Shima A (1987) Comparative analysis of O^6-methylguanine methyltransferase activity and cellular sensitivity to alkylating agents in cell strains derived from a variety of animal species. Mutat Res 184:161–168
4. Fujio C, Chang HR, Tsujimura T, Ishizaki K, Kitamura H, Ikenaga M (1989) Hypersensitivity of human tumor xenografts laking O6-alkylguanine-DNA alkyltransferase to the antitumor agent 1-(4-amino-2-methyl-5-pyrimidinyl)methyl-3-(2-chloroethyl)-3-nitrosourea. Carcinogenesis 10:351–356
5. Mineura K, Fushimi S, Kowada M, Isowa G, Ishizaki K, Ikenaga M (1990) Linkage between O^6-methylguanine-DNA-methyltransferase activity and cellular resistance to antitumor nitrosoureas in cultured rat brain tumor cell strains. Acta Neurochir (Wien) 103:62–66
6. Mineura K, Kuwahara N, Kowada M (to be published) Clinical implication of selective nitrosourea treatment for cerebral gliomas with respect to O^6-methylguanine-DNA methyltransferase activity. J Neurooncol

Cytokinetic Resistance of Malignant Glioma Cells: Antineoplastic Agents During Maintenance Therapy

Shoju Hiraga, Norio Arita, Takanori Ohnishi, Takuyu Taki, and Toru Hayakawa[1]

Introduction

Maintenance chemotherapy cannot be simply a prolonged induction treatment. One of the important biological differences present during remission from untreated malignant gliomas is within cell kinetics. No definitive evidence concerning this phenomenon of human gliomas has been obtained, but it is thought that the tumors contain a large fraction of non-cycling cells during remission. Chemotherapeutic failure results from many factors, including drug resistance and poor accessibility of drugs. In this report, we examined decreased sensitivity to drugs due to changes of the cell fraction, i.e., cytokinetic resistance, for further understanding of maintenance chemotherapy against malignant gliomas [1]. For this purpose, we tested the effectiveness of etoposide (VP-16), one of the cell cycle-specific agents, against the T98G glioblastoma cell line which possesses a unique biological character of being arrested in the G_0 or G_1 phase when deprived of serum [2–4].

Materials and Methods

Cell

The human glioma cell line T98G was obtained from ATCC (Rockville, Md) and the cells were grown in Eagle's minimum essential medium containing 10% fetal bovine serum, 1% sodium pyruvate, and 1% nonessential amino acid at 37°C in a humidified incubator with an atmosphere of 5% CO_2 and 95% air. Cells were seeded in 96-well plates with an initial cell density of 1.5×10^4 per well and allowed to grow for 24 h.

Cell synchronization

The T98G cell line has been proven to be quiescent and stays in the G_0 or G_1 phase when deprived of serum [4]. For G_0 or G_1 synchronization, exponentially growing cells were cultured in a serum-free medium for 72 h. For partial S

[1] Department of Neurosurgery, Osaka University Medical School, Osaka, 553 Japan

phase synchronization, thymidine (2.5 mM) and/or hydroxyurea (2 mM) were used, and the cells were maintained for 24 h. The effect of these procedures on cell viability was checked and proven to be non-cytotoxic (data not shown).

Treatment with VP-16

After synchronization, cells were exposed to VP-16 (Nippon Kayaku, Tokyo) at a concentration of 0.25–80 µg/ml for 12, 24, or 48 h. The cells were refed with fresh medium after drug contact and allowed to regrow for another 48 h. In some experiments, VP-16 treatment started 9 or 12 h after cell synchronization was released.

Cytotoxic Assay

To test the inhibitory effect of VP-16 against T98G cells, MTT [(3–4, 5-dimethylthiazol-2-yl)-2, 5-diphenyltetrazolium bromide] assay was used. For this procedure, the medium was removed and 100 µl fresh medium and 10 µl MTT dye (Sigma chemical, 5 mg/ml in 0.1 M phosphate buffered saline [PBS] stock solution) were added to each well. The cells were incubated with MTT for 4 h, after which blue formazan crystals were dissolved in 0.04 N HCl in 2-propanol (100 µl per well). Within 15 min each plate was read on a microplate reader (MTP-120, Corona) with a test wave length of 570 nm and a reference wave length of 630 nm. To obtain a dose response curve, a concentration of VP-16 was plotted on the abscissa against percent optical density to a drug-free reference on the ordinate. The IC_{50} (the drug concentration resulting in 50% inhibition of MTT dye formation) was estimated directly from semilogarithmic dose-response curves [5].

Flow cytometric Analysis

Flow cytometric analysis was performed to assess cell synchronization. Cells (1.0×10^6 initial concentration) were plated and cultured in 75 cm^2 flask for 24 h. Cell synchronization was performed in the same manner as described above. The cells were 30-min pulse labeled with 10 µM 5-bromodyoxyuridine (BrdU), and then trypsinized, collected, and fixed in cold 70% ethanol for 30 min. The cells were treated with 4 N HCl for 20 min and neutralized with 0.1 M sodium tetraborate. The cells were centrifuged (1,000 × g, 30 s) and washed in PBS containing 0.5% Tween 20. They were then incubated in PBS with 20 µl FITC-labeled anti-BrdU antibody (Becton Dickinson) for 30 min and excess antibody was washed in PBS. The cells were resuspended in 1.0 ml PBS and propidium iodide (20 µg per cell) was added. Single cell suspension was obtained using 50 µm nylon mesh. Fluorescence intensity from 1.0×10^4 cells was measured on a flow cytometer FAC III (Becton Dickinson) and recorded on a data file. The cell kinetic pattern of the cell cycle for each synchronization experiment was generated using a computer Consort 30 interface [6].

Results

Cytotoxic Assay

A standard curve representing the semilogarithmic cell number on the abscissa and the optical density on the ordinate was bi-linear, i.e., composed of the lower slope at the low cell concentration (less than 0.5×10^4/well) and the higher slope at the higher cell concentration. Our experiments were performed at the higher cell concentration. From the resultant curve, a decrease by half of optical density meant at least more than 60% decrease of actual cell number in any concentration, and the cell number decreased to 10% particularly in the low cell concentration state. Therefore, IC_{50} by MTT assay underestimates actual drug effect, but never overestimates it.

Flow cytometry and VP-16 Treatment in G_1 Synchronization

The cell fractions in each phase were 55%, 31%, and 14% in G_0 or G_1, S, and G_2-M, respectively, for cells cultured in the medium containing 10% serum for 24 h. The flow cytometric patterns of G_1 arrested cells and serum-added cells are illustrated in Fig. 1a. The G_1 fraction was 85% when cells were cultured in the serum-free medium for 72 h. The G_1 fraction decreased to 72% 12 h after addition of serum. The cells moved into the proliferative cycle 24 h after addition of serum, and the fraction was 29%, 48%, and 23% in G_0 or G_1, S, and G_2-M, respectively (Fig. 1a). The VP-16 dose response curves of G_1-synchronized, or synchronized and then serum-added cells are demonstrated in Fig. 1b. The IC_{50}s of control cells exposed to VP-16 for 12, 24, or 48 h were 80, 20, or 5.5 μg/ml, respectively. The drug exposure time was 24 h in G_1 synchronized cells. The IC_{50} of cells in serum-free medium was over 80 μg/ml. Simultaneous addition of VP-16 and serum changed the cell sensitivity in the higher drug concentration, but IC_{50} was still over 80 μg/ml. IC_{50} decreased to 12 μg/ml when VP-16 treatment was initiated 12 h after serum addition (Fig. 1b).

Flow cytometry and VP-16 Treatment in S Synchronization

In cells treated by hydroxyurea, the S fraction was increased to 63%. G_1 and G_2-M fractions were 32% and 5%, respectively. Twelve hours after cell proliferation resumed, the fraction was changed to 15%, 62%, and 22% for S, G_1, and G_2-M, respectively (Fig. 2a). IC_{50} of cell synchronized by hydroxyurea was 9 μg/ml (24 h exposure). When cells were allowed to resume proliferation, IC_{50} was lowered to 5 μg/ml (24 h exposure) (Fig. 2b).

Double S-phase synchronization using thymidine and hydroxyurea increased the S fraction to 70%. This fraction decreased to 11% 12 h after synchronization was released (Fig. 3a). The IC_{50} for 24 h exposure was 2.5 μg/ml (Fig. 3b). The IC_{50} of the double synchronized cells for 12 h (one-half of the usual drug exposure time) treatment was 10 μg/ml. Tumor cell sensitivity of VP-16

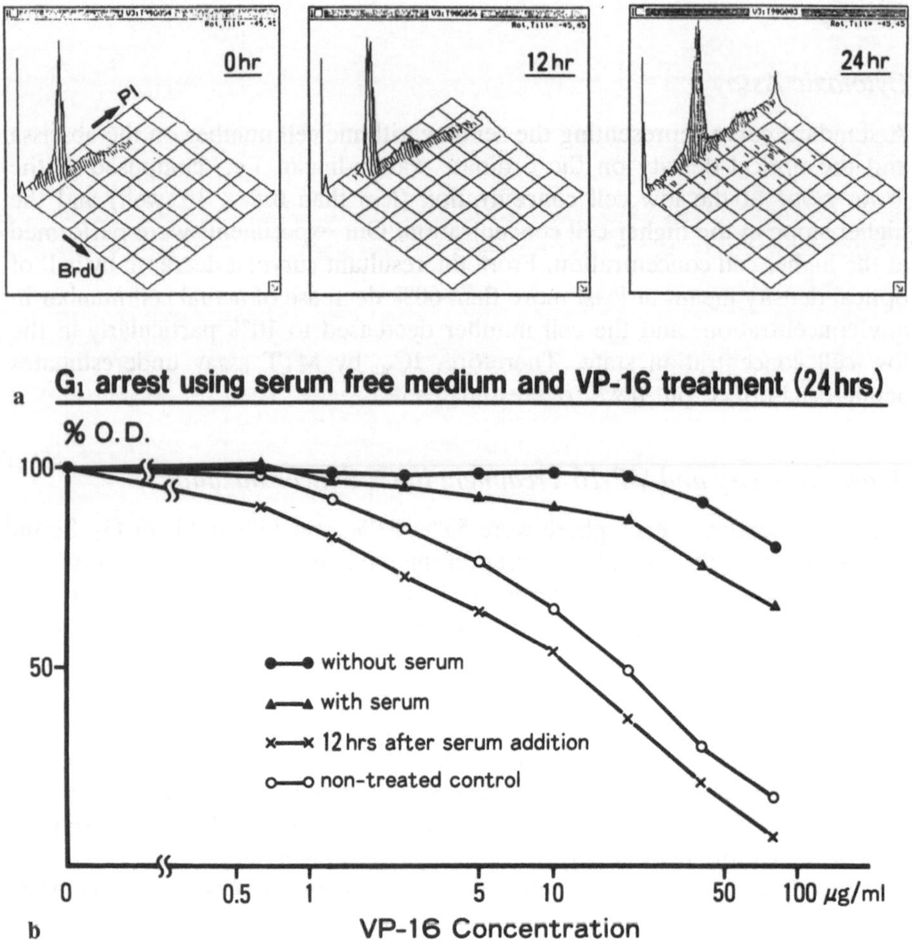

Fig. 1. **a** Flow cytometric patterns of T98G cells; growth arrested cells in 72 h serum-free medium (*left*), 12 h and 24 h after serum addition (*middle* and *right*). **b** VP-16 dose-response curve of G_1 arrested cells and regrowing cells after serum addition (24 h treatment)

decreased when treatment started 9 h and 12 h after synchronization. The IC_{50} values for those cells were 35 μg/ml and more than 80 μg/ml, respectively (Fig. 3b).

Discussion

It is well recognized that the major intracellular target compound of VP-16 is an intracellular DNA topoisomerase II. VP-16 stimulated the formation of DNA topoisomerase II-DNA cleavage complexes, which resulted in in-

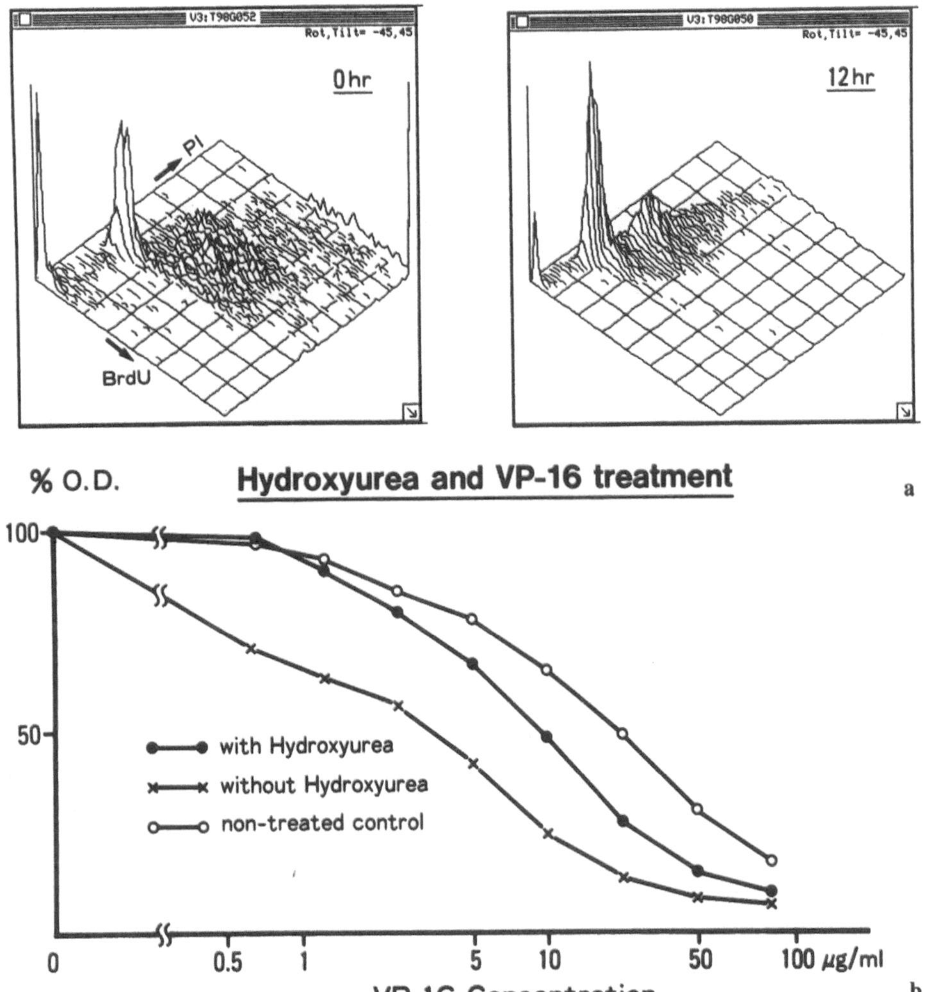

Fig. 2. a Flow cytometric pattern of S-synchronized cells using hydroxyurea (*left*) and cells 12 h after synchronization (*right*). **b** VP-16 dose-response curve of S-synchronized cells (24 h treatment); VP-16 treatment was performed to cells in the medium with hydroxyurea (*S arrested* ●) without hydroxyurea (*regrowing after S synchronization* ×)

complete DNA synthesis and cell death. Enzyme activity and content of DNA topoisomerase II is remarkably increased in the late S and G_2-M phases therefore, the cytocidal effects of VP-16 depend upon cell kinetic patterns [3,7]. The more the cells proliferate rapidly, the more the cell-killing effects increase and become time- and dose-dependent. Our numerical results coincided with the theoretical pattern and suggested the usefulness of VP-16 treatment for rapidly growing glioma cells. The most effective results were exhibited from cell synchronization in the S phase (Fig. 2). The double synchro-

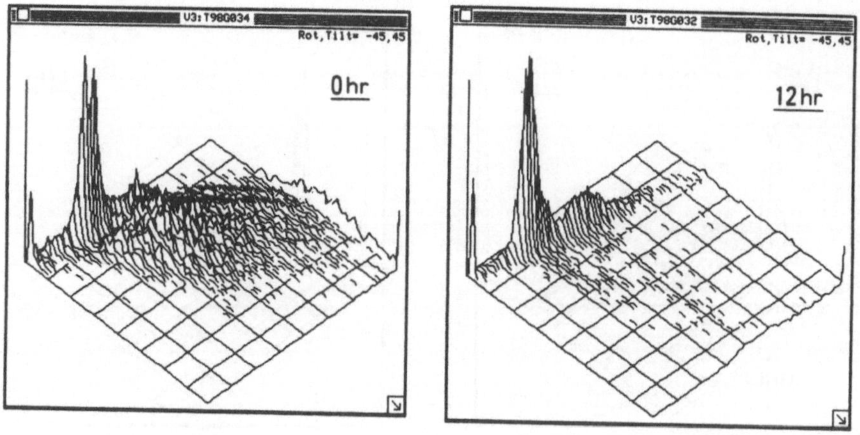

a

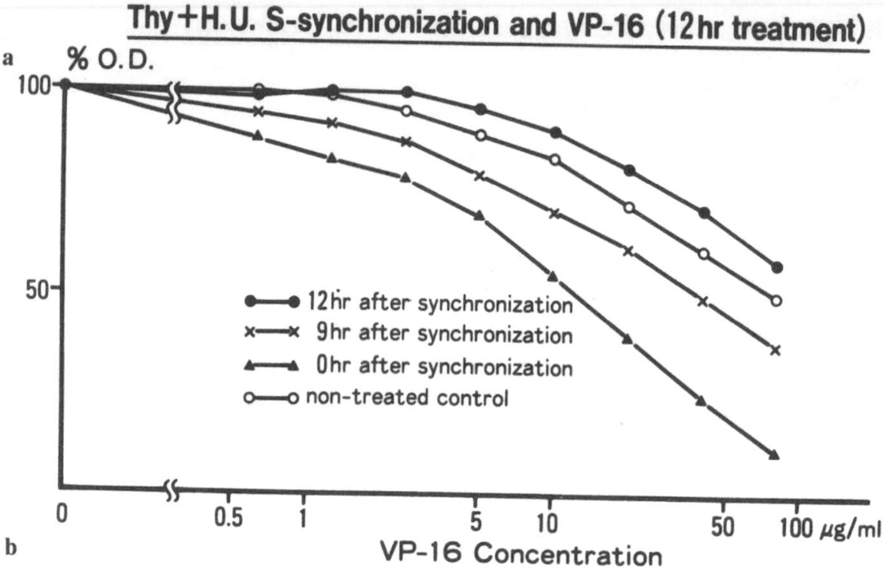

b

Fig. 3. a Flow cytometric patterns of cells with double-S synchronization technique (*left*) and 12 h after (*right*). **b** VP-16 dose-response curves (12 h after treatment). Cells were treated *0 h* ▲, *9 h* ×, or *12 h* ● after the synchronization

nization technique decreased IC_{50} to 2.5 μg/ml. Although it has not yet been developed in vivo, S-phase synchronization may provide the possibility of low-dose chemotherapy without any side effects.

It is postulated that the tumor cells are quiescent and nonproliferative in remission. Those cells are mostly diploid and stay in the G_0 or G_1 phase. Since T98 glioma cells remain in G_1 or G_0 in a serum-free medium, the cell line may be used as a model of assessing chemotherapeutic effects of VP-16 on nonproliferative cells. VP-16 exposure to those cells demonstrated extremely increased IC_{50} (more than 80 μg/ml). The G_0 or G_1 cells became slightly sensitive but were still refractory to concomitantly given VP-16 and serum. When the cells were contacted with VP-16 12 h after serum addition, IC_{50} decreased to a smaller value than the non-treated control (12 µg/ml). Probably these cells synchronously entered into the S or G_2-M phase 12 h afterwards.

The results described above indicated the following: first, cells are essentially resistant to VP-16 when they are in a non-proliferative phase. This phenomenon is called "cytokinetic resistance" to the cell cycle phase of specific drugs such as VP-16 [1]. VP-16 is not suitable for killing quiescent tumor cells. Second, there may be some cells which were either in or were moving into the growth cycle even in remission, and VP-16 is effective to those cells and suppress the tumor regrowth. However, the fraction of those cells may be small and the actual antineoplastic effect non-beneficial. Third, it took more than 12 h before the T98G cells entered S and G_2-M (Fig. 3a). The period before growth resumption may be different in each tumor. Some method enforcing a resting cell to get into a growth cycle should be designed. However, if VP-16 treatment is performed when most cells have already entered into G_1 after S synchronization, the cytotoxic effect would not be expected since the cells become resistant compared with nontreated controls (Fig. 3b). These facts suggested that the timing of drug administration should be taken into account in attempting cell recruitment therapy.

Conclusion

We have to consider cytokinetic resistance along with tumor drug resistance when we chose cell cycle phase-specific agents for maintenance therapy, since it is assumed that most of the tumor cells in the patients with remission stayed in the G_0 or G_1 phase and not in the proliferative state. Administration of VP-16 may be effective for patients with a progressive tumor, but not with a quiescent tumor in which case another drug should be selected.

Acknowledgement. This work was supported in part from a Grant-in-Aid (No. 2-14) from the Ministry of Welfare, Japan.

References

1. Finlay GJ, Wilson WR, Baguley BC (1987) Cytokinetic factors in drug resistance of Lewis lung carcinoma: Comparison of cells freshly isolated from tumours with cells from exponential and plateau-phase clusters. Br J Cancer 56:755–762
2. Long BH, Musial ST, Brattain MG (1985) Single and double strand DNA breakage and repair in human lung adenocarcinoma cells exposed to etoposide and teniposide. Cancer Res 45:3106–3112
3. Issel BF, Crook ST (1979) Etoposide (VP-16-213). Cancer Treat Rev 6:107–124
4. Stein GH (1979) T98G: An anchorage-independent human tumor cell line that exhibits stationary phase G1 arrest *in vitro*. J Cell Physiol 99:43–54

5. Mosmann T (1983) Rapid colorimetric assay for cellular growth and survival: Application of proliferation and cytotoxic assays. J Immunol Methods 65:55–63
6. Dolbeare F, Gratzner H, Pallavicini MG, et al. (1983) Flow cytometric measurement of total DNA content and incorporated bromodeoxyuridine. Proc Natl Acad Sci (USA) 80:5573–5577
7. Wang JC (1987) Recent studies of DNA topoisomerases. Biochem Biophys Acta 909:1–9

Quantitative Analysis of Glutathione S-Transferase in Human Brain Tumors, C6 Rat Glioma Cells, and Drug Resistant C6 Cells

YOSHIHITO MATSUMOTO, NOBORU SASAOKA, TAKAHIRO TSUCHIDA, TAKASHI FUJIWARA, and TAKASHI OHMOTO[1]

Introduction

Cellular detoxification of exogenous toxins, antibiotics, carcinogens, and anticancer agents involves detoxifying enzymes, such as superoxide dismutase, catalase, glutathione peroxidase, and glutathione S-transferase. Glutathione S-transferases (GST; enzymal code (EC) 2.5.1.18) compromise a group of abundant and widely distributed catalytic and binding proteins that facilitate the conjugation of glutathione (GSH) with the electrophilic center of a large spectrum of hydrophobic molecules. Multiple GST isozymes in mammalian tissues arise from dimeric combinations of a number of distinct subunits grouped into three major classes, α, μ, and π [1]. GST, a π-class enzyme, has been found overexpressed in human malignant tumor tissues [2], suggesting that it may be a good tumor marker. GST is also reported to be elevated in an Adriamycin-induced multidrug resistant human breast cancer cell line (MCF-7) [3] as well as in some alkylating agent resistant cell lines [4]. Despite these reports indicating GST to possibly have a critical role in carcinogenesis and anticancer drug resistance, little is known of the role of GST in brain tumors. We report the GST activities of human brain tumors, C6 rat glioma cells, and drug resistant cells.

Materials and Methods

Tissues and Cells

In this study, we used 27 samples of brain tumor (5 glioblastomas multiforme, 5 grade II or III astrocytomas, 1 medulloblastoma, 1 malignant lymphoma, 1 yolk sac tumor, 8 meningiomas, 3 neurinomas, and 3 metastatic tumors) and 8 normal brains. All of the tissues were stored at −70°C until they were used.

The rat glioma C6 cell line was cultured in a minimal essential medium (MEM) containing 10% newborn calf serum. The 1-(4-amino-2-methyl-5-pyrimidinyl)-methyl-3-(2-chloroethyl)-3-nitrosourea hydrochloride (ACNU) and vincristine (VCR) resistant cell lines (C6/ACNU, C6/VCR) were isolated

[1] Department of Neurological Surgery, Kagawa Medical School, 761-07 Japan

from C6 cells in the selection medium with increasing concentrations of ACNU and VCR, and maintained in an MEM containing 30 μg/ml ACNU and 0.2 μg/ml VCR.

BSO Treatment

To deplete GSH in rat glioma cells, buthionine sulfoximine (BSO) was added to flasks of cells to give a final concentration of 20 μM. After 24 h, the cells were harvested and used for GST assay. This BSO exposure produced no toxicity in either wild-type or resistant cells.

Assay for Drug-Sensitivity of C6, C6/ACNU, and C6/VCR Cells

ACNU, VCR, and cisplantin (CDDP) sensitivities of the cells were studied by methyl thiazolyl tetrazolium dye reduction (MTT) assay [5]. The relative resistance of C6, C6/ACNU, and C6/VCR cells compared with C6 cells without drugs was calculated from survival rates at peak plasma concentrations (PPC) of the drugs [5].

Quantitative Assay of Total GST Activity

Specimens of 100 mg tissue or cells were homegenized with 2 ml 10 mM potassium phosphate buffer pH 7.0 containing 1.4 mM 2-mercaptoethanol. The total homogenate was centrifuged at 4°C at 27,000 g for 40 min to obtain the supernatant for the GST assay. Total GST activity was determined by the method of Habig [6]. The assay mixture (2.5 ml) contained 100 μl supernatant, 1 mM GSH, and 1 mM 1-chloro-2,4-dinitrobenzene (CDNB) as the substrate. The rate of conjugate formation was monitored at 340 nm. One unit of GST activity was defined as the amount required to catalyze the conjugation of 1 nmol of CDNB to GSH per min at 25°C. Protein content was determined using a Bio-Rad protein assay kit.

Results

C6/ACNU cells did not show cross resistance or sensitivity to VCR and CDDP. C6/VCR cells showed a cross resistance to ACNU and CDDP (Table 1).

The total GST activity was 92.6 ± 25.1 units (mean ± standard deviation) in 8 samples of normal brain tissue, 126.1 ± 58.8 units in 5 grade II or III astrocytomas, (153.9 ± 63.3 units in 3 grade II astrocytomas and 84.4 ± 2.7 units in 2 grade III astrocytomas), 66.2 ± 29.3 in 5 glioblastomas 94.7 ± 47.7 units in 3 metastatic tumors, 301.8 ± 114.1 units in 8 meningiomas, and 212.8 ± 90.4 units in 3 neurinomas (Fig. 1). Differences in GST activity between glioblastomas and meningiomas, grade II or III astrocytomas and meningiomas, and in normal brain tissues and meningiomas were statistically signficant

Table 1. Relative resistance of C6, C6/ACNU and C6/VCR to drugs (determined by MTT assay)

	Relative resistance to:		
Cell line	ACNU	CCR	CDDP
C6	1.00	1.00	1.00
C6/ACNU	1.50	1.19	0.96
C6/VCR	1.40	1.63	2.08

The relative resistance of cells, compared with C6 cells without drugs, was calculated from their survival rates at peak plasma concentration of drugs

($P < 0.01$). The differences between normal brain tissues and benign tumors (meningiomas and neurinomas) and gliomas and benign tumors were also statistically significant ($P < 0.05$). One each of medulloblastoma (case 11), malignant lymphoma (case 12) and yolk sac tumor (case 13) showed low GST activity: 46.8, 100.8, and 71.5 units, respectively (Table 2).

The total GST activity of C6, C6/ACNU, and C6/VCR cells is shown in Fig. 2. C6/ACNU cells exhibited 1.5-fold higher and C6/VCR cells exhibited 2.2-

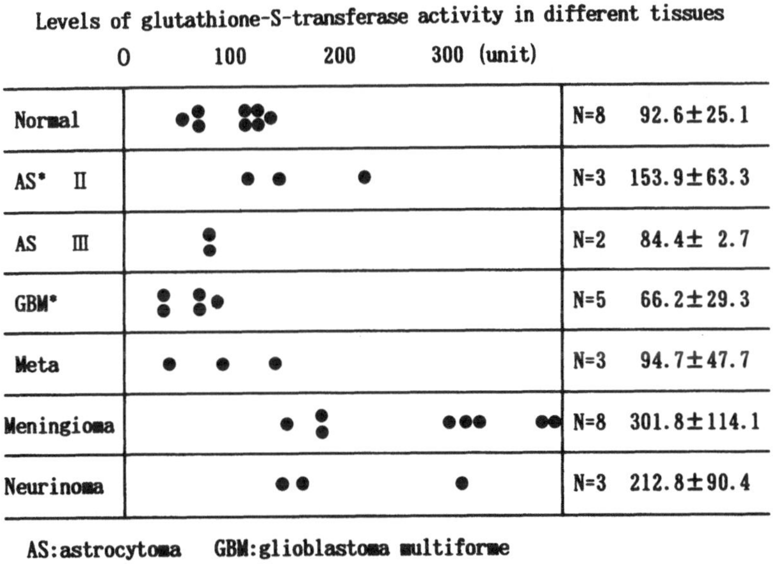

Levels of glutathione-S-transferase activity in different tissues
0
100
200
300 (unit)
Normal
N=8 92.6±25.1
AS* II
N=3 153.9±63.3
AS III
N=2 84.4± 2.7
GBM*
N=5 66.2±29.3
Meta
N=3 94.7±47.7
Meningioma
N=8 301.8±114.1
Neurinoma
N=3 212.8±90.4
AS:astrocytoma GBM:glioblastoma multiforme

Fig. 1. Levels of glutathione S-transferase (GST) activity in different tissues. Differences of the GST activity between glioblastomas and meningiomas, grade II and III astrocytomas and meningiomas, normal brain tissues, and meningiomas were statistically significant ($P < 0.01$). Differences between normal brain tissues and benign tumors (meningiomas and neurinomas), gliomas and benign tumors were also statistically significant ($P < 0.05$)

Table 2. GST levels in 35 samples

Case No.	Histological diagnosis	GST Levels (units*)
1	Low grade astrocytoma	135.9
2	Low grade astrocytoma	224.3
3	Low grade astrocytoma	101.5
4	High grade astrocytoma	86.3
5	High grade astrocytoma	82.5
6	Glioblastoma multiforme	32.4
7	Glioblastoma multiforme	102.6
8	Glioblastoma multiforme	40.0
9	Glioblastoma multiforme	79.8
10	Glioblastoma multiforme	76.0
11	Medulloblastoma	46.8
12	Malignant lymphoma	100.8
13	Yolk sac tumor	71.5
14	Metastatic tumor (adenocarcinoma)	141.0
15	Metastatic tumor (adenocarcinoma)	45.7
16	Metastatic tumor (squamous cell carcinoma)	97.4
17	Meningioma	190.7
18	Meningioma	312.0
19	Meningioma	335.8
20	Meningioma	487.5
21	Meningioma	158.4
22	Meningioma	357.4
23	Meningioma	189.3
24	Meningioma	383.6
25	Neurinoma	316.5
26	Neurinoma	150.8
27	Neurinoma	171.2
28	Normal brain tissue	128.4
29	Normal brain tissue	83.8
30	Normal brain tissue	82.8
31	Normal brain tissue	73.4
32	Normal brain tissue	104.7
33	Normal brain tissue	115.6
34	Normal brain tissue	106.9
35	Normal brain tissue	57.6

*1 unit activity is defined as the amount required to catalyze the conjugation of 1 nmol CDNB per min at 25°C

fold higher GST activity than that in C6 cells. However, there was no difference between the wild-type and the BSO-pretreated GSH-deplected cells.

Discussion

Radiation and certain chemotherapeutic agents exert their effects via the generation of free radicals, such as hydroxy or hydroxyperoxy radicals. These radicals are highly reactive, but can readily be intercepted by GST and/or

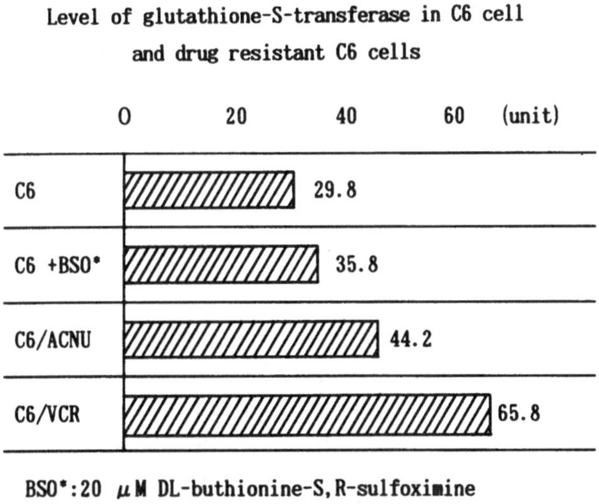

Fig. 2. Level of glutathione-S-transferase (GST) in C6 cell and drug resistant C6 cells

GSH. Some brain tumors are drug sensitive, while others are drug resistant. Niitsu et al. [2], showed elevated serum GST-π levels in patients with various gastrointestinal malignancies, including gastric, esophageal, colonic, pancreatic, hepatocellular, and biliary tract cancers. The mean serum GST-π levels in patients with stomach cancer at Stage III or IV were significantly higher than those at Stage I or II, indicating that this marker, similar to many other markers, reflects the tumor burden. From our data, gliomas, thought to be relatively drug sensitive and radiosensitive, showed low GST activity. GST activity was extremely low especially in glioblastomas. In contrast, meningiomas and neurinomas, considered to be drug resistant and radioresistant, had high GST activity. The difference in GST activity between gliomas and benign tumors (meningiomas and neurinomas) was statistically significant ($P < 0.01$). Other malignant and drug-sensitive tumors, such as medulloblastoma (case 11), malignant lymphoma (case 12), and yolk sac tumor (case 13) expressed low GST activity. These data suggest that a low level of GST activity reflects chemosensitivity and radiosensitivity of brain tumor tissues.

Kudo et al. [7] reported that brain tumors sensitive to radiotherapy and chemotherapy had low levels of GSH. Some reports show that depletion of intracellular GSH levels by pretreatment with BSO alters the response of several tumor cells to alkylating agents [8]. In C6 cells pretreated with BSO, GST activity was not affected (Fig. 2). Thus, BSO may inhibit GSH synthesis, and the level of GSH may not be correlated to GST activity.

Recently, it was reported that drug resistance to nitrogen mustards in Chinese hamster overy cells is associated with increased GST-α activity as well as mRNA overexpression [9]. Similar results were reported for rat Walker 256 chlorambucil-resistant cells [10]. In contrast, overexpression of GST-μ was demonstrated in nitrosouea-resistant 9L rat gliosarcoma cells [11,12]. From this study, overall GST activity slightly but significantly increased in C6/ACNU cells, and C6/VCR cells consistently exhibited from 2.0- to 2.4-fold higher GST activity than did C6 cells. C6/ACNU cells did not show cross resistance and were sensitive to VCR and CDDP. C6/VCR cells showed cross resistance to ACNU and CDDP (Table 1). Thus, enhanced GST activity may be involved in ACNU and VCR resistance and may be related to factors involved in the multidrug resistance of C6/VCR. Previous reports suggest that multidrug resistance is caused by decreased intracellular drug concentration as a result of increased drug efflux from cells, which is closely associated with the 170 kd glycoprotein, P-glycoprotein (P-gp) [13]. Yoshimura et al. showed that a fluorescent basic dye, rhodamine-6G, was accumulated less in multidrug resistance cells than in drug-sensitive cells, and that this was due to the active efflux of the dye by P-gp from the cells (unpublished data). By this method, we found the accumulation of R-6G in C6/VCR cells to be less than 40% of that in C6 cells, and the accumulation of R-6G to be similar in C6/ACNU cells and C6 cells (data not shown). Based on these results, a possible mechanism is proposed for multidrug resistance of C6/VCR, including both decreased drugs uptake and increased inactivation of drugs by GST. In the case of C6/ACNU cells, increased inactivation of ACNU by GST may be responsible for chemosensitivity. Taken together, GST activity may serve as a novel marker to predict the sensitivity of brain tumors to chemotherapy while resistance to the drug will be reflected by elevation of GST activity.

References

1. Mannervik B, Alin P, Guthenberg C (1985) Identification of three classes of cytosolic glutathione transferase common to several mammalian species: Correlation between structural data and enzymatic properties. Proc Natl Acad Sci USA 82:7292–7206
2. Niitsu Y, Takahasi Y, Saito T (1989) Serum glutathione S-transferase-π as a tumor marker for gastrointestinal malignancies. Cancer 63:317–323
3. Sinha BK, Katki AG, Batist G (1987) Differential formation of hydroxyl radicals by Adriamycin in sensitive and resistant MCF-7 human breast tumor cells: Implications for the mechanism of action. Biochemistry 26:3776–3781
4. Margie L, Kenneth D (1987) Identification of a glutathione S-transferase associated with microsomes of tumor cells resistant to nitrogen mustards. Biochem Pharmacol 38:1915–1921
5. Sasaoka N (1990) Chemosensitivity assays for malignant gliomas (in Japanese). Gan To Kagaku Ryoho (Jpn J Cancer Chemotherap) 17:2247–2252
6. Habig W, Pabst M, Jakoby W (1974) Glutathione S-transferases. J Biol Chem 249:7130–7139
7. Kudo H, Mio T, Kokunai T (1990) Quantitative analysis of glutathione in human brain tumors. J Neurosurg 72:610–615
8. Russo A, Carmichael J, Friedman N, DeGraff W (1986) The role of intracellular glutathione in antineoplastic chemotherapy. Int J Radiat Oncol Biol Phys 12:1347–1354

9. Lewis AD, Hickson ID, Robson CN (1988) Amplification and increased expression of alpha class glutathione S-transferase encoding genes associated with resistance to nitrogen mustard. Proc Natl Acad Sci USA 85:8511–8515
10. Buller AL, Clapper ML, Tew KD (1987) Glutathione S-transferases in nitrogen mustard-resistant and -sensitive cell lines. Mol Phamacol 31:575–578
11. Evans CG, Bodell WJ, Tokuda K (1987) Glutathione and related enzymes in rat brain tumor cell resistance to 1,3-bis(2-chloroethyl)-1-nitrosourea and nitrogen mustard. Cancer Res 47:2525–2530
12. Smith MT, Evance CG, Mannervik B (1989) Denitrosation of 1,3-bis(2-chloroethyl)-1-nitrosourea by class mu glutathione transferase and its role in cellular resistance in rat brain tumor cells. Cancer Res 49:2621–2625
13. Pearce HL, Safa AR, Bach NJ (1989) Essential features of the P-glycoprotein pharmacophore as defined by a series of reserpine analogs that modulate multidrug resistance. Proc Natl Acad Sci USA 86:5128–5132

Glutathione S-Transferase Placental Form in Human and Rat Gliomas and Its Possible Role in Drug Resistance

Akira Hara, Noboru Sakai, Shuji Niikawa, Hiroshi Hirayama, Hiromu Yamada, Takuji Tanaka, and Hideki Mori[1]

Introduction

Glutathione S-transferases (GSTs) are an important family of the detoxifying enzymes catalyzing the conjugation of glutathione to a wide variety of hydrophobic electrophilic substances [1]. GSTs have various isoenzymes which have been studied extensively in rats [2]. The isozyme, rat placental form (GST-P) has been shown to be a marker for preneoplastic or neoplastic lesions in chemical hepatocarcinogenesis [3], GST-P is well recognized to exist in normal rat astrocytes, and is regarded as a major form of isozymes expressed in rat brain [4]. GST-P is expressed in GST-P-negative rat glioma cells after induction of benign transformation by dibutyryladenosine 3′,5′-cyclic monophosphate [5]. The human placental form of GST (GST-π), which is closely related to GST-P immunologically, is also contained in normal human astrocytes. It may be that the GST-π or GST-P contained in normal astrocytes is concerned with the detoxifying function against xenobiotics for the protection of neurons from their toxic effects. We have already demonstrated the expression of GST-π in human gliomas [6].

In the present study, the expression and localization of GST-π in human gliomas and GST-P in N-ethyl-N-nitrosourea (ENU)-induced rat gliomas and their preneoplastic lesions were investigated immunohistochemically, and the pattern of expression of both enzymes was compared. Induction of GST-P in a rat glioma cell line was also examined by treatment with the ACNU that is an anti-cancer drug. The molecular weight of GST-P and GST-π in rat and human glioma cell lines was investigated by Western blotting.

Materials and Methods

Human Gliomas

A total of 31 gliomas and 6 cerebral white matters specimens as normal controls were used. The histological diagnosis of the gliomas was based on the

[1] Departments of Neurosurgery and Pathology, Gifu University School of Medicine, Gifu, 500 Japan

WHO classification. Gliomas examined in this study were as follows: benign astrocytomas grade II (5 cases), anaplastic astrocytomas grade III (10 cases), and glioblastomas grade IV (16 cases). All tissues were fixed in 10% formalin, embedded in paraffin, and cut into 3 µm-thick sections.

ENU-Induced Glial Lesions of Rats

For induction of gliomas and their preneoplastic lesions, ENU at a dose of 50 mg/kg was injected into pregnant female Wister rats via a tail vein at the 16th day of gestation according to the method by Koestner et al. [7]. A total of 70 offsprings were obtained. To follow the process of the histogenesis of gliomas, they were sacrificed sequentially at 6 (6 rats), 9 (10 rats), 12 (10 rats), and 17 weeks (10 rats) of age. The remaining animals were killed when they showed progressive neurological signs or weight loss after 17 weeks from birth. From ENU-treated rats, 29 early neoplastic proliferation (ENP), 18 microtumors, 6 oligodendrogliomas, 6 astrocytomas, 18 mixed gliomas, 30 anaplastic gliomas, and 3 glioblastomas were obtained and examined for the expression of GST-P. Tumors and preneoplastic lesions of glial origin were diagnosed according to the criteria described by Koestner et al. [7]. As for the preneoplastic lesions, ENP was recognized as abnormal glial proliferation within a 300 µm diameter, and microtumors showed destructive features, although their sizes were still less than 500 µm in diameter.

Immunohistochemical Staining

Anti human GST-π antibody (rabbit immunogloblin) was purchased from Bioprep Co., Dublin, Ireland. Anti-rat GST-P antibody was kindly provided by Dr. K. Sato. Immunoreactivities for GST-π in human gliomas and those for GST-P in rat gliomas and their preneoplastic lesions were graded as follows: GST-π negative (−), positive (+), and strongly positive (++); GST-P negative (−), weakly positive (±), positive (+), and strongly positive (++). The intensity of GST-P positivity in normal rat glia cells is defined as positive (+).

Induction of GST in a Rat Glioma Cell Line

Rat T9 glioma cells, which were derived from a glioma induced by N-methyl N-nitrosourea in a CD Fisher rat, was used for induction of GST-P by treatment with ACNU. At 2 and 4 days after seeding, 2 µg/ml ACNU was added to the medium. On day 6 after seeding, immunohistochemistry for GST-P was performed.

Western Blot Analysis for GST-P and GST-π

Normal rat white brain matter and a rat glioma cell line which was established from ENU-induced rat glioma in our laboratory were used for GST-P immunoblotting. Normal human white brain matter obtained at autopsy and a human glioma cell line established by our colleague were used for GST-π immunoblotting.

Results

In both human and rat gliomas, the intensity of the immunostaining for GST-π or GST-P in malignant gliomas was much higher than that of benign glioma (Fig. 1A–D, Tables 1, 2). The positive staining reaction in malignant human and rat gliomas was remarkable, especially in gemistocytes and giant cells. Significantly, glioblastomas had a number of strongly positive cells. Many astrocytomas and components of astrocytoma in mixed gliomas of ENU-treated rats showed positive or weakly positive GST-P expression. In the preneoplastic lesions, however, most ENP in ENU-treated rats showed negative or weakly positive GST-P expression, whereas surrounding normal astrocytes still had positive GST-P expression. ENU-induced rat oligodendrogliomas showed no GST-P expression.

The T9 glioma cells without treatment of ACNU showed no response for GST-P immunohistochemistry (Fig. 1E). On the contrary, T9 cells treated with ACNU had strong positivity for GST-P (Fig. 1F).

Western blot analysis demonstrated that normal rat white brain matter and rat glioma cells had GST-P in the same molecular weight (24 kd), and that normal human white brain matter and human glioma cells also had GST-π in the same molecular weight (24 kd) (Fig. 2).

Discussion

The results of the present study demonstrated that clear expression of the enzymes was present in both human and ENU-induced rat gliomas, and that the intensity of the immunostaining reaction as well as the staining pattern of the enzymes correlated with the histological grades of neoplasms. The finding that the advancement of the histological grade was associated with the increase of intensity on immunostaining reaction for GST-π and GST-P appeared to be important. In the ENU-treated rat, ENP showed negative or weakly positive

Table 1. Immunostaining reaction of GST-π in human gliomas

Histological types	No. of cases	No. of cases with negative or positive response		
		Negative (−)	Positive (+)	Strongly positive (++)
Normal brain	6	0	6	0
Gliomas				
Benign gliomas	5	0	5	0
Anaplastic gliomas	10	0	4	6
Glioblastoma multiforme	16	0	2	14

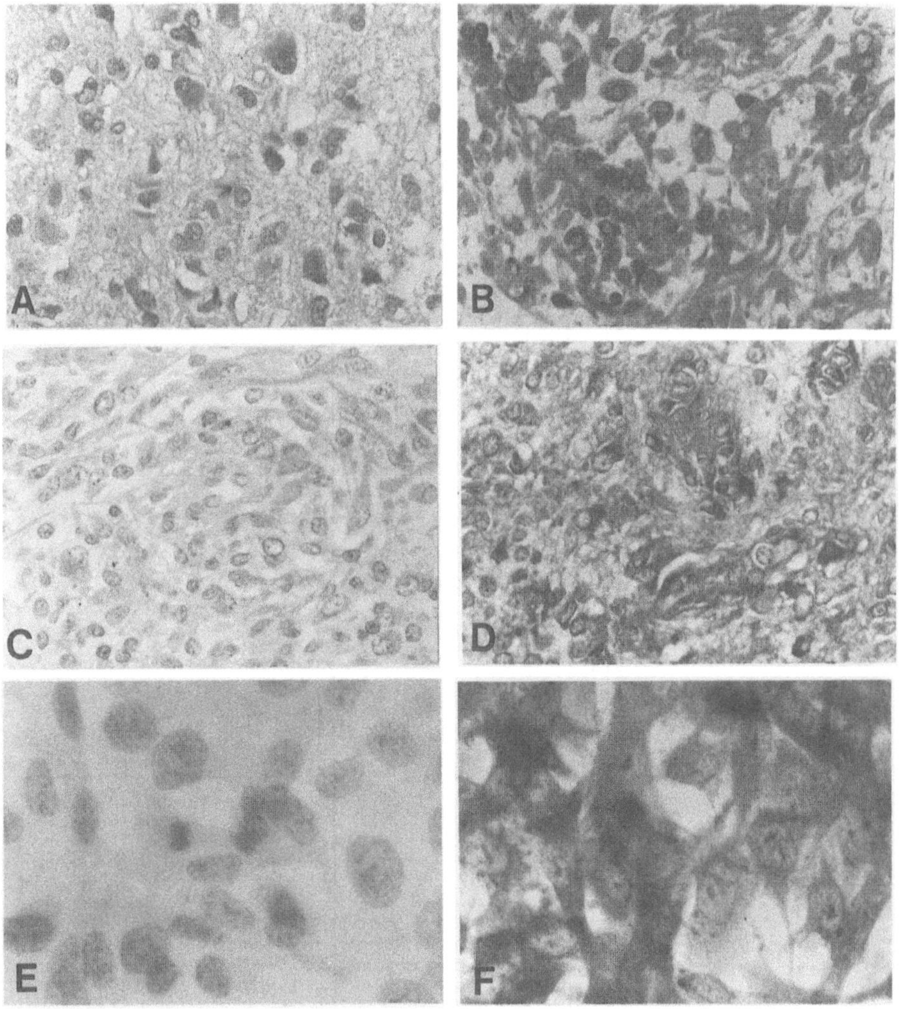

Fig. 1. Human benign astrocytoma. Some tumor cells with relatively enriched cytoplasm have positive staining reaction recognized diffusely in their cytoplasm. Finely fibrous glial processes in the background are weakly positive. GST-π immunostaining and counterstaining with hematoxylin, × 200. **B** Human glioblastoma multiforme. The strongly positive staining reaction is seen in anaplastic gemistocytes. GST-π immunostaining and counterstaining with hematoxylin, × 200. **C** Rat benign mixed glioma has weakly positive expression of GST-P in the finely fibrous glial processes. Tumor cells with relatively enriched cytoplasm have positive staining reaction for GST-P in their cytoplasm. GST-P immunostaining and counterstaining with hematoxylin, × 200. **D** Rat glioblastoma multiforme has strongly positive expression of GST-P. GST-P immunostaining and counterstaining with hematoxylin, × 200. **E** Control T9 glioma cells do not show any positive reaction for GST-P. GST-P immunostaining and counterstaining with hematoxylin, × 400. **F** T9 glioma cells exposed to ACNU show strong reactivity of GST-P. GST-P immunostaining and counterstaining with hematoxylin, × 400

Table 2. Histological types of rat brain lesions of glial origin and immunohistochemical reactivities for GST-P

	Immunostaining response				
Histological types of lesions	Negative (−)	Weakly positive (±)	Positive (+)	Strongly positive (++)	Total No. of tumors
ENP	11	15	3	0	29
Microtumor	2	5	11	0	18
Oligodendroglioma	6	0	0	0	6
Astrocytoma	0	2	3	1	6
Mixed glioma	0	6	12	0	18
Anaplastic glioma	0	0	6	24	30
Glioblastoma	0	0	0	3	3

ENP, early neoplastic proliferation

The intensity of GST-P positivity in normal rat glia cells is defined as positive (+)

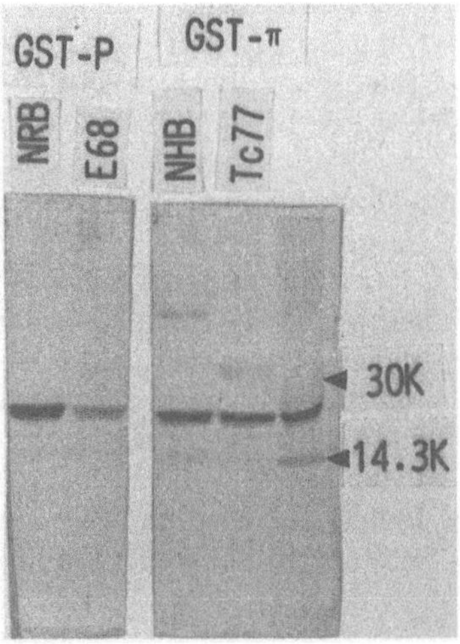

Fig. 2. Immunoblotting of cytosolic protein (105000 g supernatant; 20 μg protein) from normal white matter and glioma cells of rat and human. Specific immunoblotting reaction with the anti-GST-P or anti-GST-π antibody is demonstrated. *Marker proteins 30* and *14.3* kd are shown. *NRB* normal rat white matter, *E68* rat glioma cell line, *NHB* normal human white matter, *Tc77* human glioma cell line

expression of GST-P, compared with surrounding normal astrocytes. ENP is considered to be the first step of malignant change of gliomas. This finding suggested that astrocytes lost the expression of the detoxifying enzyme when they were in the first step of atypical change. However, neoplastic astrocytes in gliomas showed re-expression of GST-P according to the advancement of their malignancy. Subsequently, malignant gliomas began to have a more strongly positive expression of GST-P than did normal astrocytes. Recently, correlations between the expression of GSTs and anti-cancer drug resistance have been reported [8]. The intensity of the expression of GST-π in human gliomas thus may be concerned with the sensitivity for anti-cancer drug treatment. The results of the present study clarified that transformed cells still have the enzyme that is originally present in normal glia cells and possess a possible detoxifying function. Moreover, the finding that the T9 glioma cell exposed to ACNU showed strong expression of GST-P suggested that the glioma cells had a detoxifying function against ACNU treatment. The enzyme in neoplastic glia cells may also have the role of a protecting mechanism against xenobiotics, including anti-cancer drugs.

References

1. Jakoby WB (1978) The glutathione S-transferases: A group of multi-functional detoxification proteins. Adv Enzymol 46:383–414
2. Mannervik B, Jensson H (1982) Binary combinations of four protein subunits with different catalytic specificities explain the relationship between six basic glutathione S-transferases in rat liver cytosol. J Biol Chem 257:9909–9912
3. Satoh K, Kitahara A, Soma Y, et al. (1985) Purification, induction, and distribution of placental glutathione transferase: A new marker enzyme for preneoplastic cells in the rat chemical hepatocarcinogenesis. Proc Natl Acad Sci USA 82:3964–3968

4. Tsuchida S, Izumi T, Shimizu T, et al. (1987) Purification of a new acidic glutathione S-transferase, GST-Yn_1Yn_1, with a high leukotriene-C4 synthase activity from rat brain. Eur J Biochem 170:159–164
5. Hara A, Sakai N, Yamada H, et al. (1989) Induction of glutathione S-transferase, placental type in T9 glioma cells by dibutyryladenosine 3′,5′-cyclic monophosphate and modification of its expression by naturally occurring isothiocyanates. Acta Neuropathol 79:144–148
6. Hara A, Yamada H, Sakai N, et al. (1990) Immunohistochemical demonstration of the placental form of glutathione S-transferase, a detoxifying enzyme in human gliomas. Cancer 66: 2563–2568
7. Koestner A, Swenberg JA, Wechsler W (1971) Transplacental production with ethylnitrosourea of neoplasms of the nervous system in Spraque-Dawley rats. Am J Pathol 63:37–56
8. Buller AL, Clapper ML, Tew KD (1987) Glutathione S-transferases in nitrogen mustard -resistant and -sensitive cell lines. Molec Pharmacol 34:2583–2586

Electrophoretical Analysis of DNA Topoisomerase I and II Expressions in Human Malignant Gliomas

Takahiro Tsuchida, Yoshihito Matsumoto, Noboru Sasaoka, Takashi Fujiwara, Takashi Ohmoto[1], Benjamin S. Carson[2], and Peter C. Phillips[3]

Introduction

DNA topoisomerases have been reported to play an important role in DNA replication and transcription [1]. They have been classified into two types of enzyme, topoisomerase I (Topo I) and topoisomerase II (Topo II). Topo I acts on single strand DNA in an adenosine triphosphate (ATP)-independent manner while Topo II acts on double strand DNA in the presence of ATP [2]. Topoisomerases appear to be essential for cell proliferation.

Recently, it has been reported that Topo II activity increased in the tumor cell line resistant to nitrogen mustard [3]. This suggests that Topo II is involved in the mechanism of chemoresistance of tumor cells.

There are some cancer chemotherapeutic agents which show cytotoxicity on tumor cells by inhibiting topoisomerases. Camptothecin is a specific inhibitor for Topo I, and VP-16 and VM-26 are specific inhibitors for Topo II [2]. Sklansky et al. [4] used VM-26 for 19 patients with malignant glioma, and 11 of them showed good responses to VM-26. It is interesting to note that 6 of the 11 patients showing good response to VM-26 had shown resistance to prior nitrosourea chemotherapy.

Topo I and Topo II expressions in the malignant glioma were electrophoretically analyzed as a preliminary study for evaluating the clinical effect of topoisomerase inhibitors on the treatment of malignant glioma.

Materials and Methods

Normal human cerebrum and brain tumor tissues were obtained from surgical biopsy specimens. The tissues were homogenized, sonicated, and then centrifuged. The supernatant was collected and lyophilized. The protein concentration of each sample was measured by a BCA protein assay kit (Pierce), and

[1] Department of Neurological Surgery, Kagawa Medical School, Kita-gun, Kagawa, 761-07 Japan
[2] Department of Neurosurgery, The Johns Hopkins Hospital
[3] Department of Pediatric Neurology, The Johns Hopkins Hospital

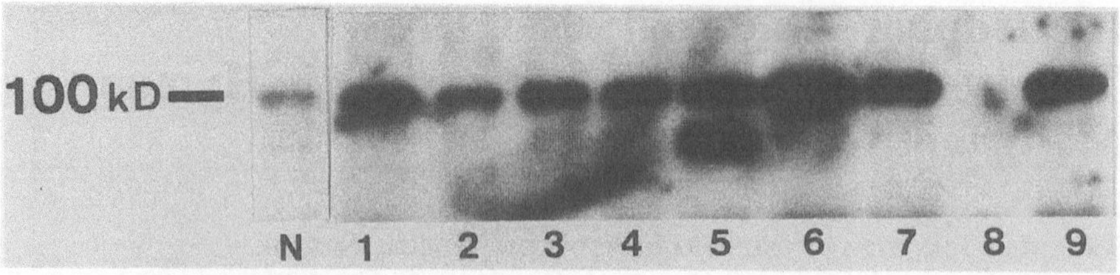

Fig. 1. Immunoblotting of Topoisomerase I, *N*, Normal human cerebrum; *lanes 1–9*, human malignant gliomas

DNA values were analyzed by the method of Labarca and Paigen [5]. Samples were reconstituted in the electrophoresis sample buffer (4 M urea, 2% SDS, 62.5 mM Tris-HCl, 1 mM EDTA, pH 6.8) and applied to 0.1% SDS polyacrylamide gel electrophoresis (SDS-PAGE, 5%–15% gradient gel). The samples containing 5 ng DNA in each lane were transferred from the gel onto the nitrocellulose membrane. The blots were dried and then separately incubated overnight with anti-Topo I rabbit serum (1:2000) or with anti-Topo II rabbit serum (1:2000) (a generous gift from Dr. Scott Kaufmann, The Johns Hopkins Hospital), respectively. The both blots were then incubated with ^{125}I-labeled anti-rabbit IgG goat Ig (10 μCi/blot) for 90 min, followed by autoradiography for 1 week.

Results

Topo I

Eight out of the 9 examined patients with malignant gliomas showed positive bands for Topo I on the blot. The degree of the expression in the positive cases was stronger than that of the normal human cerebrum (Fig. 1).

Topo II

Eight out of 10 patients with malignant gliomas showed positive bands for Topo II. In 5 out of the 8 positive cases, the degree of expression of Topo II was stronger than that of the normal human cerebrum (Fig. 2).

Discussion

Radiation therapy and chemotherapy have been widely attempted for patients with malignant glioma. Generally, nitrosoureas have been used for treating these tunmors. However, the clinical efficacy of this drug on malignant gliomas is not always satisfactory, even if a toxic dose is administered [6].

Topo I and Topo II, which are essential for cellular DNA replication, have received attention, because they have proved to be intracelluar targets of some

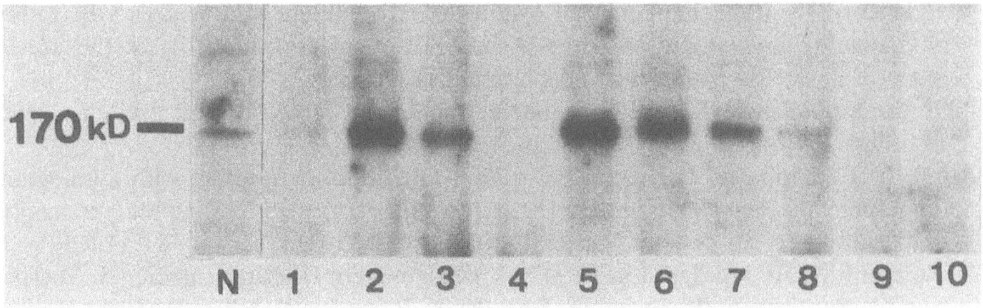

Fig. 2. Immunoblotting of Topoisomerase II, *N*, Normal human cerebrum; *lanes 1–10*, human malignant gliomas

chemotherapeutic drugs [2]. Camptothecin is a specific inhibitor for Topo I, and Adriamycin, Actinomycin D, VP-16, and VM-26 are known Topo II poisons. These drugs stabilize topoisomerase-DNA complex, and consequently cause DNA fragmentation. It seems that topoisomerase poison is a potential cancer agent possessing a distinct action from nitrosourea.

Sklansky et al. [4] used VM-26, one of the Topo II poisons, for 19 patients with malignant glioma. Seven of these patients had had a history of prior chemotherapy using BCNU and CCNU. Interestingly, 6 out of the 7 patients responded well to VM-26. Tan et al. [3] reported elevated Topo II activity in nitrogen mustard-resistant tumor cells. This phenomenon may occur in malignant glioma cells resistant to alkylating agents including nitrosourea. Potmesil et al. [7] reported that low levels of Topo II reflected the decreased sensitivity of tumor cells to Topo II poisons. It appears that the efficacy of Topo II poisons is predictable by Topo II activity in the tumor cells.

The clinical effect of Topo I poisons, such as camptothecin, on patients with malignant glioma is still unknown. However, the action of Topo I poisons on Topo I is similar to that of Topo II poisons. The former stabilizes the DNA-Topo I cleavable complex, and the latter stabilizes the DNA-Topo II cleavable complex [2,8–10]. Therefore, Topo I activity in the glioma tissue may also reflect their sensitivity to Topo I poisons.

From this study, most of the malignant gliomas proved to have relatively high Topo I and Topo II activities. Our results suggest that Topo I and Topo II poisons are potentially promising drugs for the treatment of malignant glioma.

References

1. Kuenzle CC (1985) Enzymology of DNA replication and repair in the brain. Brain Res Rev 10:231–245
2. Liu LF (1989) DNA Topoisomerase poisons as antitumor drugs. Annu Rev Biochem 58:351–375
3. Tan KB, Mattern MR, Boyce RA, Schein PS (1987) Elevated DNA Topoisomerase II activity in nitrogen mustard-resistant human cells. Proc Natl Acad Sci USA 84:7668–7671

4. Sklansky BD, Mann-Kaplan RS, Reynold AF, Rosenblum ML, Walker MD (1974) 4′-dementhyl-epipodophyllotoxin-β-D-thenylidene-glucoside (PTG) in the treatment of malignant intracranial neoplasms. Cancer 33:460–467
5. Labarca C, Paigen K (1980) A simple, rapid, and DNA assay procedure. Anal Biochem 102:344–352
6. Wolff SN, Phillips GL, Herzig GP (1987) High-dose carmustine with autologous bone marrow transplantation for the adjuvant treatment of high-grade gliomas of the central nervous system. Cancer Treat Rep 71:183–185
7. Potmesil M, Hsiang YH, Liu LF, Bank B, Grossberg H, Kirschenbaum S, Forlenzar TJ, Penziner A, Kanganis D, Knowles K, Traganos F, Silber R (1988) Resistance of human leukemic and normal lymphocytes to drug-induced DNA cleavage and low levels of DNA Topoisomerase II. Cancer Res 48:3537–3543
8. Hertzberg RP, Caranfa MJ, Hecht SM (1989) On the mechanism of Topoisomerase I inhibition by camptothecin: Evidence for binding to an enzyme-DNA complex. Biochemistry 28:4629–4638
9. Hsiang YH, Liu LF, Wall ME, Wani MC, Nicholas AW, Manikumar G, Kirschenbaum S, Silber R, Potmesil M (1989) DNA Topoisomerase I-mediated DNA cleavage and cytotoxicity of camptothecin analogues. Cancer Res 49:4385–4389
10. Ling YH, Andersson BS, Nelson JA (1990) DNA Topoisomerase I as a site of action for 10-hydroxycamptothecin in human promyelocytic leukemia cells. Cancer Biochem Biophys 11:23–30

Section 5. Oncogene and Anti-Oncogene of Brain Tumor

Allele Loss on Chromosome 10 in Human Glioblastomas

SHUICHI IZUMOTO[1], NORIO ARITA[1], TAKANORI OHNISHI[1], SYOUJU HIRAGA[1], TAKUYU TAKI[1], MASAYUKI YAMAMOTO[2], TETSURO MIKI[3], SIN-ICHIRO TAKAI[4], and TORU HAYAKAWA[1]

Introduction

Recently, specific chromosomal deletions have been reported to be associated with many human malignancies. It is now thought that loss of constant genetic loci can be taken as evidence of recessive tumor suppressor genes involved in the genesis of human cancers. In this report, allelic deletions on chromosome 10 were studied in human malignant gliomas by using restriction fragment length polymorphisms (RFLPs) analyisis.

Materials and Methods

For RFLPs analysis, DNA samples were prepared from the tumor tissue and peripheral blood leukocytes of 22 patients with malignant gliomas (13 glioblastomas, 7 anaplastic astrocytomas, and 2 medulloblastomas). The tumor tissue obtained by surgery was frozen at −70°C until it was used. Isolation of high molecular weight DNA, digestion of restriction endonucleases (Toyobo, Osaka), agarose gel (0.8%) electrophoresis, Southern transfer to nylon membrane, hybridization with probes, and autoradiography were performed by using the standard methods [1,2]. DNA samples (10 μg) were hybridized with four polymorphic markers mapped to chromosome 10. The loci (location) of probes used were FNRB (10p11.2), RBP3 (10q11.2), D10S4 (10q22–q23), and D10S20 (10q21–q26), respectively (Fig. 1). DNA was digested by HinfI for FNRB BglII for RBP3, SacI for D10S4, and HindIII for D10S20, respectively. Probes were radiolabeled with ^{32}P by multiprime DNA labelling system [3] (Amersham, London). The histopathological diagnosis of each tumor was made according to the WHO classification system of brain tumors in the tissue adjacent to the sample from which the DNA was extracted.

[1]Department of Neurosurgery, [2]2nd Department of Surgery, [3]Department of Medicine and Geriatrics, and [4]Department of Medical Genetics, Biomedical Research Center, Osaka University Medical School, Osaka, 553 Japan

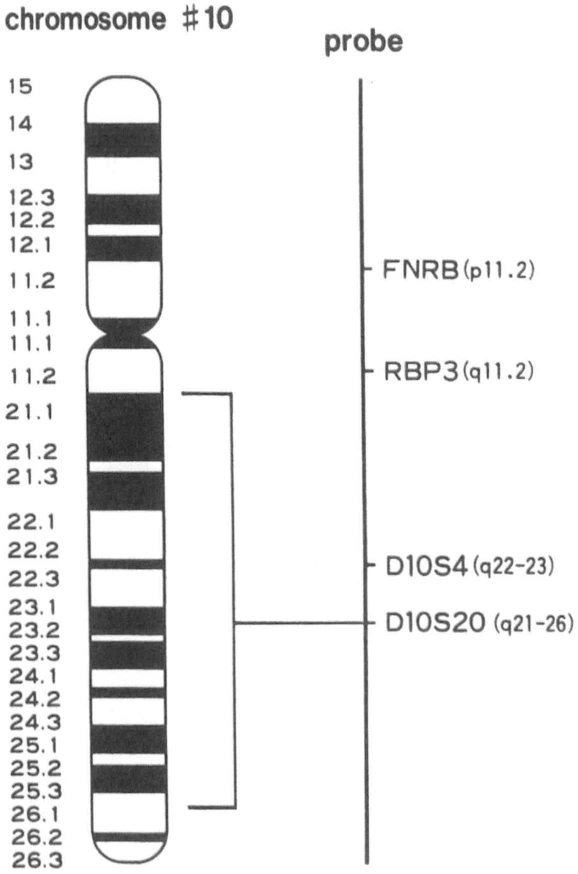

Fig. 1. Loci of 4 polymorphic markers used on chromosome 10

Results

Table I shows the summary of the RFLPs analysis in 22 malignant gliomas. No loss of constitutional heterozygosity was observed in either the 7 anaplastic astrocytomas or 2 medulloblastomas.

Of the 13 patients with glioblastomas, 11 were informative. Among these 11 tumors, 6 (55%) showed loss of constitutional heterozygosity. In the locus of FNRB, 8 cases were informative and loss of heterozygosity was seen in 2 tumors. In the locus of RBP3, 2 cases were informative, but both tumors maintained constitutional heterozygosity. In the locus of D10S4, 6 cases were informative and loss of heterozygosity was seen in 4 tumors. In the locus of D10S20, 7 cases were informative and loss of heterozygosity was seen in 5 cases. An example of an autoradiogram that showed allele loss on chromosome 10 in the tumor is shown in Fig. 2. Figure 3 is a diagram of allele loss pattern on chromosome 10 among 6 glioblastomas. Two tumors seem to have a large

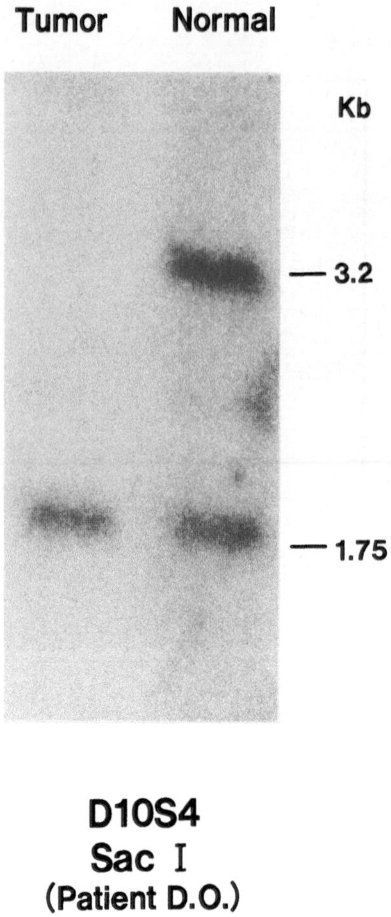

Fig. 2. RFLP analysis on chromosome 10. Southern hybridization of a probe at a locus of D10S4 to tumor and leukocytes (normal) DNA from a patient with glioblastoma. Two alelles are present in the normal DNA, but only one is seen in the tumor DNA

Table 1. Loss of heterozygosity in GB, AIII and MB at loci on chromosome 10

		Patients tested	Heterozygous patients	Loss of heterozygosity
GB *n* = 13	FNRB	13	8	2
	RBP3	7	2	0
	D10S4	13	6	4
	D10S24	13	7	5
AIII *n* = 7	FNRB	5	3	0
	RBP3	3	0	0
	D10S4	4	2	0
	D10S24	5	2	0
MB *n* = 2	FNRB	2	2	0
	RBP3	1	0	0
	D10S4	1	0	0
	D10S20	2	1	0

GB, Glioblastoma; *AIII* Anaplastic astrocytoma; *MB*, Medulloblastoma

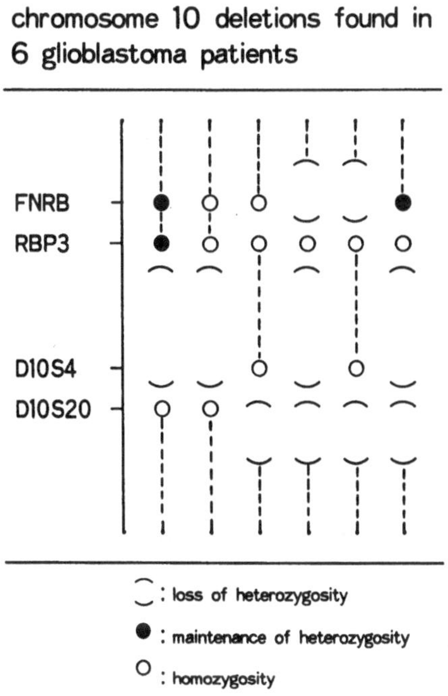

Fig. 3. A diagram of allele loss pattern on chromosome 10 found among 6 glioblastomas., loss of heterozygosity; ●, maintenance of heterozygosity; ○, homozygosity

deletion extending from FNRB to D10S4. In another 2 tumors, constitutional heterozygosity was maintained on the loci of both FNRB and RBP3.

Discussion

Tumor suppressor genes are suggested to be involved when specific chromosome loci are consistently lost in a particular tumor. Cytogenetic analysis in human malignant gliomas demonstrated that losses of chromosome 10 were present in 60% of the tumors [4]. Molecular genetic studies with RFLPs in gliomas was first reported by James et al. [5] They found losses of constitutional heterozygosity on chromosome 10 loci in 97% of glioblastomas. Table 2 summarizes the results of similar studies reported since then [5–8]. The frequency of allelic deletion on chromosome 10 was different in each report, and

Table 2. Loss of heterozygosity on chromosome 10 in malignant gliomas

	GB	AA	No. of probes
James [5]	28/29 (97%)	0/22 (0%)	3
Fujimoto [6]	10/13 (77%)	—	4
Fults [7]	17/32 (53%)	2/13 (15%)	13
Watanabe [8]	4/7 (57%)	—	4
Our present series	6/11 (55%)	0/7 (0%)	4

GB, glioblastoma; *AA*, anaplastic astrocytoma

ranged between 53% and 97%. A common important finding was the fact that constitutional heterozygosity on chromosome 10 loci was maintained in anaplastic astrocytomas, although in one report, it was lost in 15% of the tumor. The smallest common region of loss of heterozygosity in our study lies between the loci of RBP3 and D10S4. In a recent report concerning allelo-type analysis of human astrocytomas, loci on chromosomes 10 and 17p were revealed to be frequently lost [9]. RFLPs analysis, using polymorphic markers on chromosome 17, revealed that loss of heterozygosity was shown in both anaplastic astrocytomas and glioblastomas with an equal frequency of 40%. Lower-grade astrocytomas often relapse as glioblastomas after the first treatment. Both of these clinical experiences and molecular genetic studies suggest that two recessive oncogenes on chromosomes 10 and 17p may be involved in the tumorigenesis and/or progression of astrocytic lineage.

We have not thus far obtained evidence which suggests any significant correlation between allelic loss and clinical features. However, we believe that molecular genetic approaches will provide further understanding of the glial tumor.

Conclusion

Normal and tumor DNA samples were studied by RFLPs analysis using polymorphic markers on chromosome 10 in patients with malignant gliomas. In 11 informative cases out of 13 glioblastomas, 6 (55%) showed loss of constitutional heterozygosity. In 7 anaplastic astrocytomas and 2 medulloblastomas, constitutional heterozygosity was maintained in all tumors. These results indicate that a recessive gene related to the genesis of glioblastomas is located on chromosome 10.

Acknowledgement. This work was supported in part from a Grant-in-Aid (No. 2–14) from the Ministry of Welfare, Japan.

References

1. Barker D, Schafer M, White R (1984) Restriction sites containing CpG show a higher frequency of polymorphism in human DNA. Cell 36:131–138
2. Cavenee WK, Dryja TP, Philips RA, Benedict WF, Godbout R, Gallie BL, Murphree AL, Strong LC, White R (1984) Isolation and regional localization of DNA segments revealing polymorphic loci from human chromosome 13. Am J Hum Genet 36:10–24
3. Freiberg AP, Vogelstein B (1984) A technique for radiolabeling DNA restriction endonuclease fragments to high specific activity. Anal Biochem 137:266–267
4. Bigner SH, Mark J, Burger PC, Mahaley MS Jr, Bullard DE, Muhlbaier LH, Bigner DD (1988) Specific chromosomal abnormalities in malignant human gliomas. Cancer Res 88:405–411

5. James CD, Carlbom E, Dumanski JP, Hansen M, Nordenskjold M, Collins VP, Cavenee WK (1988) Clonal genomic alterations in glioma malignancy stages. Cancer Res 48:5546–5551
6. Fujimoto M, Fults DW, Thomas GA, Nakamura Y, Heibrun MP, White R, Story JL, Naylor SL, Kagan-Hallet KS, Sheridan PJ (1989) Loss of heterozygosity on chromosome 10 in human glioblastoma multiforme. Genomics 4:210–214
7. Fults DF, Tippets RH, Thomas GA, Nakamura Y, White R (1989) Loss of heterozygosity for loci on chromosome 17p in human malignant astrocytoma. Cancer Res 49:6572–6577
8. Watanabe K, Nagai M, Wakai S, Arai T, Kawashima K (1990) Loss of constitutional heterozygosity in chromosome 10 in human glioblastoma. Acta Neuropathol 80:251–254
9. Fults D, Pedone CA, Thomas GA, White R (1990) Allelotype of human malignant astrocytoma. Cancer Res 50:5784–5789

Loss of Heterozygosity of Chromosomes 10 and 17 in Human Malignant Astrocytomas

Kouichi Tokuda[1], Miri Fujita[2], Kazuo Nagashima[2], Hiroshi Abe[1], Toshimitsu Aida[1], Shinji Sugimoto[1], Yutaka Sawamura[1], and Mitsuhiro Tada[1]

Introduction

Astrocytomas are the most common tumors of the human central nervous system. Tumors of this type can be classified into four histopathologic grades of malignancy according to Kernohan [1]. Glioblastoma (astrocytoma grade IV) is always lethal despite surgery, radiotherapy, and/or chemotherapy. Low-grade or anaplastic astrocytomas vary in their response to treatment. However, a recurrent tumor is often less well differentiated, suggesting that astrocytoma can be a progressive disease. It is now believed that the genes responsible for tumorigenesis are recessive oncogenes.

Inactivation of both copies of a recessive oncogene may contribute to tumorigenesis. In the present study, we analyzed astrocytomas of various malignancy grades by using polymorphic DNA markers to search for loss of chromosomal regions that contain recessive oncogenes. We used DNA markers that detect restriction fragment length polymorphisms (RFLPs) at specific chromosome loci in order to compare the genotypes of constitutional DNA and tumor DNA by means of the Southern transfer analysis.

Materials and Methods

Human Tissue Samples

Human glioma samples were obtained from 10 patients with an age range of 11–71 years. All of the tumors were removed surgically before irradiation and/or chemotherapy, and fresh specimens were frozen before DNA was isolated. Peripheral venous blood was obtained prior to surgery.

The histopathologic grading of astrocytomas was based on the classification of Kernohan [1].

Departments of [1]Neurosurgery and [2]Pathology, University of Hokkaido School of Medicine, Sapporo, 060 Japan

DNA Isolation

Tissue samples were homogenized in lysis buffer containing 0.5% SDS, 0.1 M NaCl, 40 mM Tris-Cl (pH 8.0), and 20 mM EDTA. The viscous cell lysate was digested with proteinase K at 37°C overnight. Lysates were then extracted twice with phenol and once with chloroform before precipitation of high molecular weight DNA with sodium acetate and ethanol. Clumps of precipitated DNA were removed and dissolved in a TE buffer (10 mM Tris-Cl, pH 8.0, 1 mM EDTA) and then quantified spectrophotometrically.

Blood samples were treated in the same manner after incubation of whole blood with a lysis buffer (10 mM Tris-HCl, pH 7.6, 5 mM magnesium chloride, 10 mM NaCl) at 4°C and pelleting of the nuclear fraction.

Southern Transfer Analysis

Genomic DNA (10 µg) from peripheral blood leukocytes and tumor tissue was digested to completion with restriction enzymes and separated by electrophoresis on 0.8% agarose gels. The DNA fragments were alkali-denatured in the gels and transferred to nylon membranes. DNA probes (25 ng each) were labeled to high specific radioactivity (more than 10^8 cpm/µg) with ^{32}P, according to the random oligonucleotide priming technique.

DNA Markers

The following DNA markers and restriction enzymes were used in RFLP analysis: p5-1 (D1OS1), Bgl II, Taq I; pHUK-1 (UK), BamH I; OS-2 (D10S20), Hind III, Taq I; pYNZ 22.1 (D17S30), Msp I, Taq I, Pst I; pYNH37.3 (D17S28), Msp I, Taq I, and pMCT35.1 (D17S31), Msp I.

Results

A comparison of constitutional and tumor genotypes at various loci on chromosomes 10 and 17 was performed for DNA samples from 10 cases of astrocytoma grades II, III, and IV (1 astrocytoma grade II, 3 atrocytomas grade III, and 6 astrocytomas grade IV [glioblastomas]). Five of the 10 patients (50%) showed loss of constitutional heterozygosity for loci on the p arm of chromosome 17. Loss of heterozygosity for loci on chromosome 17 was found in 2 of the 4 patients with astrocytomas grades II and III (50%) and in 3 of the 6 patients with astrocytoma grade IV (50%). This loss of constitutional heterozygosity for loci on chromosome 17 was found with equal frequency in both astrocytoma grades II and III and glioblastoma multiforme (grade IV).

Four of the 6 glioblastomas showed loss of constitutional heterozygosity for loci on chromosome 10 (67%). The four remaining tumors of lower grades (II and III) did not show a loss of alleles at any of the chromosome 10 loci examined.

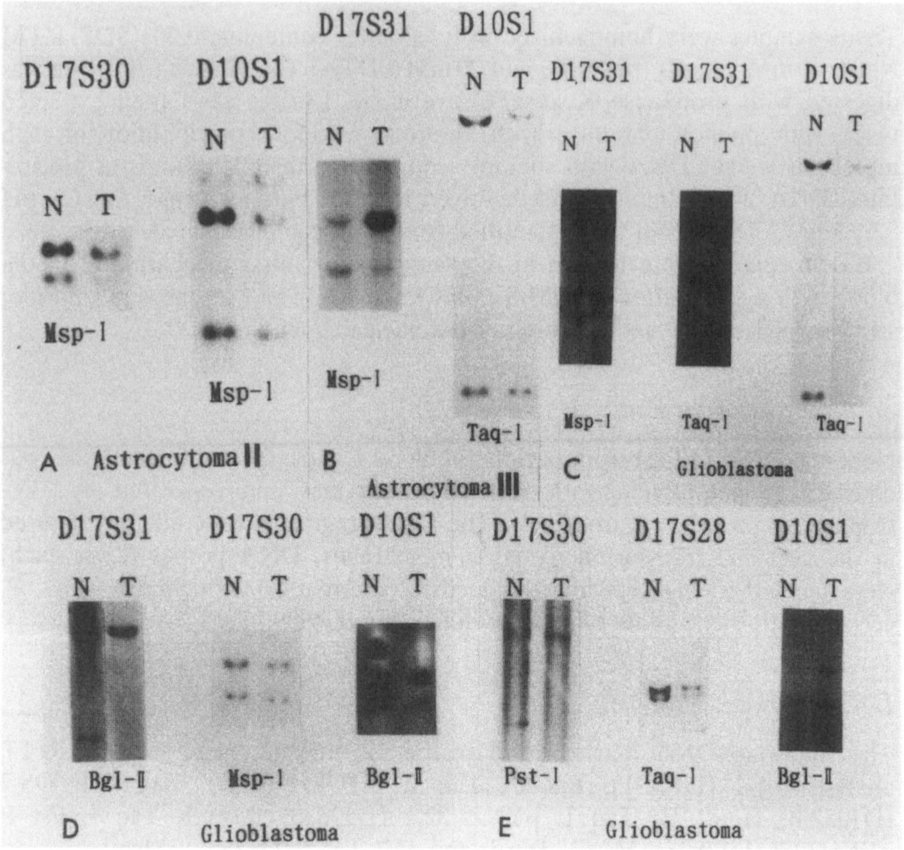

Fig. 1. Specific loss of heterozygosity at loci on the short arm of chromosome 17 and/or on the long arm of chromosome 10 in astrocytoma tumor tissue. DNA from tumor and normal tissue (peripheral leukocytes) was analyzed with polymorphic DNA markers as described. *N*, DNA from normal tissue (peripheral leukocytes); *T*, astrocytoma tumor tissue; *Astrocytoma II*, *III*, astrocytoma grades II and III

Discussion

We found that the loss of constitutional heterozygosity for loci on the p arm of chromosome 17 occurred in a significant proportion of patients with astrocytoma grades II and III and glioblastoma multiforme. This finding suggests that a tumor suppressor gene which is important in the development of astrocytoma may be present on 17p. Recently, Fults et al. reported that loss of constitutional heterozygosity for loci on chromosome 17 was found with equal frequency in patients with anaplastic astrocytoma and in patients with glioblastoma [2]. Their mapping data revealed a region of loss on chromosome 17p between physical loci p11.2 and p ter. The nuclear protein p53, which is coded by a gene that maps to p13.1 of chromosome 17, is believed to be the protein product of a tumor suppressor gene [3]. Baker et al. have recently shown that a greater than 75% of colorectal cancers are associated with deletions on chromosome 17p, including the region from 17 p12 to 17 p13.3 which contains the gene coding for p53 [3]. Sequence analysis of the coding region of the remaining allele for p53 in 4 glioblastomas and 10 colon carcinomas showed point mutations in a highly conserved region of the p53-encoding gene [4].

Thus, the p53-encoding gene not only may be associated with tumorigenesis of colon carcinoma, but also may be the target of chromosome 17p deletions in astrocytomas.

James et al. observed a loss of constitutional heterozygosity for loci on chromosome 10 in 28 out of 29 tumors classified histologically as glioblastoma, no similar losses were observed in any of 22 gliomas of lower malignancy grade [5]. Our results support the finding of this study by James. The formation of glioblastoma may involve multiple genetic hits. Loss of an astrocytoma tumor suppressor gene on chromosome 17p (probably p53) is involved in an early stage in the development of astrocytoma. Additional independent genetic events, such as loss of other tumor suppressor genes on chromosome 10, may lead to dedifferentiation of lower-grade tumors into more malignant for ms.

We have shown that tumor DNA from patients with astrocytoma grades II and III frequently exhibits loss of heterozygosity for certain loci on chromosome 17. Loss of heterozygosity for loci on chromosomes 10 and 17 is common in patients with glioblastoma multiforme. These findings support a model of progression of glioblastoma which is characterized by the clonal expansion of an earlier-stage precursor.

References

1. Zulch, KJ (1979) Histological typing of tumors of the central nervous system. Public Health Pap No. 21
2. Fults D, Tippets RH, Thomas GA, Nakamura Y, White R (1989) Loss of heterozygosity for loci on chromosome 17p in human malignant astrocytoma. Cancer Res 49:6572–6577
3. Baker SJ, Fearon ER, Nigro JM, Hamilton SK, Preisinger AC, Jessup JM, Vantuinen P, Ledbetter DH, Baker DF, Nakamura Y, White R, Vogelstein B (1989) Chromosome 17 deletions and p53 gene mutations in colorectal carcinomas. Science 244:217–221
4. Nigro JM, Baker SJ, Preisinger AC, Jessup JM, Hostetter R, Cleary K, Bigner SH, Davidson N, Baylin S, Devilee P, Glover T, Collins FS, Weston A, Modali R, Harris C, Vogelstein B (1989) Mutations in the p53 gene occur in diverse human tumor types. Nature 342:705–708
5. James CD, Carlbom EC, Dumanski JP, Hansen M, Nordenskjold M, Collins VP, Cavenee WK (1988) Clonal genomic alterations in glioma malignancy stages. Cancer Res 48:5546–5551

6. El-Azouzi M, Chung RY, Farmer GE, Martuza RL, Black PM, Rouleau GA, Hettlich C, Hedley-White ET, Zervas NT, Panagopoulos K, Nakamura Y, Gusella JF, Seizinger BR (1989) Loss of distinct regions on the short arm of chromosome 17 associated with tumorigenesis of human astrocytomas. Proc Natl Acad Sci USA 86:7186–7190

Detection of p53 Gene Mutations in Human Brain Tumors by Single-strand Conformation Polymorphism Analysis of Polymerase Chain Reaction Products

SHOJI MASHIYAMA[1], TAKAMASA KAYAMA[1], RYUICHI KATAKURA[1], TAKASHI YOSHIMOTO[1], YOSHINORI MURAKAMI[2], TAKAO SEKIYA[2], and KENSHI HAYASHI[2]

Introduction

The normal (wild-type) p53 product acts as a suppressor of transformation [1], while mutated p53 proteins may inactivate the wild-type p53 function resulting in cell transformation [2]. Mutations of the p53 gene have been found in conjunction with chromosome 17p allelic deletions in many human tumors [3,4].

Various DNA sequence alterations have been found in tumors, including point mutations, amplifications, rearrangements, and losses of genes. Point mutations can not be detected by restriction fragment length polymorphism (RFLP) using Southern hybridization unless the nucleotide substitution occurs in the recognition sequence of restriction endonuclease or if the insertion or deletion of DNA is sufficiently large. We have developed a simple and sensitive method for the detection of structural alterations of DNA including point mutations, i.e., single-strand conformation polymorphism (SSCP) analysis of DNA fragments obtained by the polymerase chain reaction (PCR) [5] (PCR-SSCP analysis) [6,7]. Recently, we have improved this technique by reducing the consumption of primers and radioisotopes, making it suitable for screening many DNA samples [8]. In the present study, we examined 45 brain tumors (41 primary and 4 metastatic) by this technique and detected mobility shifts in 6 of them. The DNA fragments of these 6 tumors were then amplified by the asymmetric polymerase chain reaction (PCR) method [9] and sequenced. The results showed that 4 of them had single-base substitutions, and the other 2 had deletions of 1 and 8 bases, respectively.

Materials and Methods

Tumor Specimens and DNA Isolation

Specimens of brain tumors were obtained at operations for the removal of tumors or by biopsy at the Division of Neurosurgery, Institute of Brain

[1] Division of Neurosurgery, Institute of Brain Diseases, Tohoku University School of Medicine, Sendai, 980 Japan
[2] Oncogene Division, National Cancer Center Research Institute, Chuo-ku, Tokyo, 104 Japan

Diseases, Tohoku University School of Medicine, Sendai, Japan, between 1985 and 1989. The specimens of primary brain tumors consisted of 6 low-grade astrocytomas, 3 anaplastic astrocytomas, 10 glioblastomas, 3 medulloblastomas, 2 ependymomas, 8 meningiomas, 2 neurinomas, 2 pituitary adenomas, 2 chordomas, and 1 specimen each of ganglioma, chondroma, and hemangioblastoma. The metastatic brain tumors were from lung, breast, renal, and colon cancers. High molecular weight DNA was prepared from surgical specimens by the method of Blin and Stafford [10].

PCR-SSCP Analysis

Oligonucleotide primers were synthesized by the phosphoroamidite method in a 380B DNA synthesizer (Applied Biosystems) and purified with Oligonucleotide Purification Cartridges (Applied Biosystems). Nucleotide sequence of the p53 gene was obtained from Buchman et al. [11]. The names and lengths of the amplified DNA fragments are indicated in Fig. 1. Genomic DNAs (50 ng) were subjected to PCR using $5'$-^{32}P oligonucleotides as primers. Thirty cycles of the reaction at 94°C for 20 s and at 60°C for 2 min were performed in a Gene ATAQ Controller (Pharmacia LKB). The amplified and labeled DNA fragments were subjected to electrophoresis at 40 W for 1–4 h in 5% non-denaturing polyacrylamide gel with or without 10% glycerol at room temperature. Autoradiograms were prepared as described previously [6,7].

Direct DNA Sequencing

Abnormal bands detected by SSCP analysis were eluted from the gel and amplified by the asymmetric PCR method [9]. The products were sequenced with $5'$-^{32}P oligonucleotides as primers and a Sequenase II kit. The primers used for amplification were also used for most fragments in the sequencing reaction. Three internal primers (P1–P3) were used for sequencing exons 5 and 8 (Fig. 1).

Results

PCR-SSCP Analysis of the p53 Gene

The regions indicated in Fig. 1 were amplified using 7 sets of primers. In some samples, PCR-SSCP analyses of fragments containing E4, E5, E7, and E8–9 showed mobility shifts, while those containing E6, E10, and E11 did not. Representative results of PCR-SSCP analyses are shown in Fig. 2. The bands in lanes 3 and 9 of the figure show mobility shifts relative to those of the other samples. Normal bands were not detected in these two cases, indicating loss of normal allele. The weak normal band seen in lane 3 was probably due to the presence of normal cells.

Mobility shifts were detected in six samples, and loss of normal allele was observed in all of these cases.

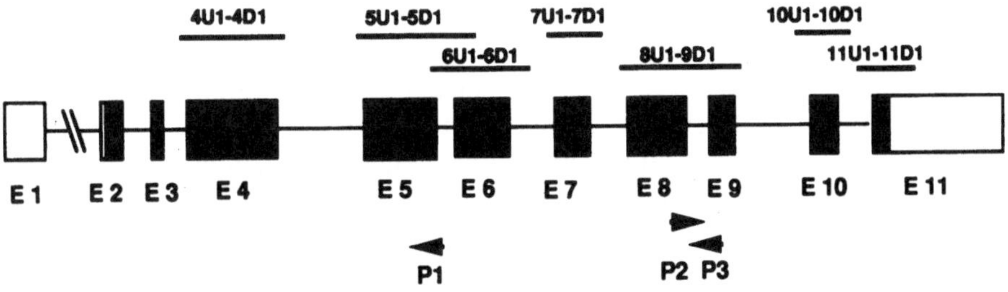

Name	4U1-4D1	5U1-5D1	6U1-6D1	7U1-7D1	8U1-9D1	10U1-10D1	11U1-11D1
Codon included	33-125	126-201	179-224	225-261	262-331	332-367	368-393
Length (bp)	293	325	236	139	330	139	202

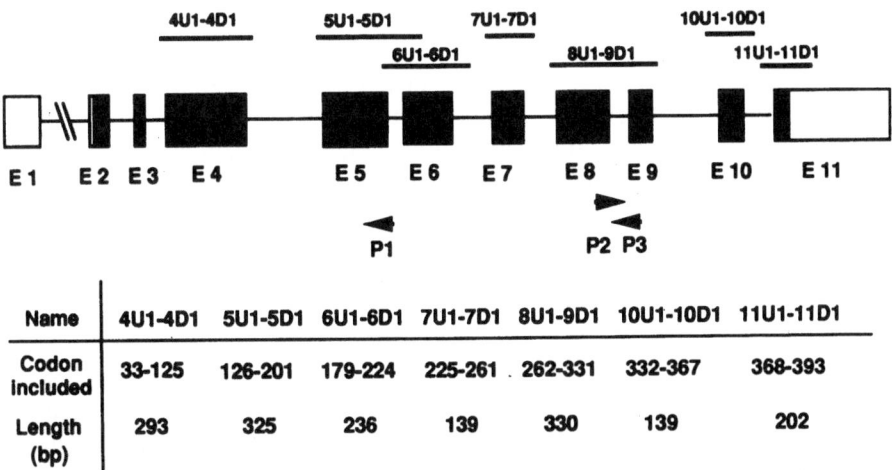

Fig. 1. Amplified DNA fragments of the p53 gene. Names, lengths and codons included in the fragments are indicated. *E1–E11* are exons of the p53 gene. *Open boxes* indicate non-coding exons and *solid boxes* indicate coding exons. *Arrowheads* under the exons (P1–P3) indicate the internal primers used for sequencing

Direct DNA Sequencing

To determine the nucleotide aberrations detected by mobility shifts of single-stranded DNA fragments, we subjected the DNA samples that showed mobility shifts to direct sequencing by the asymmetric PCR method [9]. When it was difficult to determine the nucleotide sequence alterations because of the length

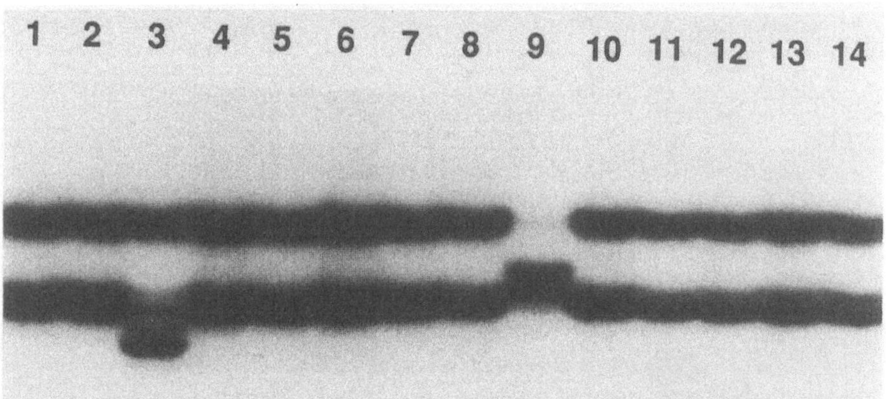

Fig. 2. Representative results of SSCP analysis of the p53 gene. *Lanes 3* and *9* showed mobility shifts. The *bands* of normal alleles in lanes 3 and 9 are weak or not detectable, indicating loss of normal allele. Electrophoresis was carried out at 40W for 3.5h in 5% non-denaturing polyacrylamide gel (5mm per lane) containing 10% glycerol at room temperature

of the amplified DNA fragments, we synthesized internal primers of the middle parts of the amplified fragments. We found that six cases of mobility shift detected by SSCP analysis were due to nucleotide sequence alterations (Table 1). An example of sequence determination is shown in Fig. 3.

In all, four single nucleotide substitutions and two deletions causing frame shifts were found. Five of the six nucleotide alterations detected were located within conserved regions of this gene [12].

Discussion

The effectiveness of PCR-SSCP analysis for detecting point mutations of the *ras* gene has been reported [13]. In this study, we used this analysis for analysis of the p53 gene in surgical specimens of brain tumors, and detected sequence alterations due not only to point mutations but also to deletions of 1 and 8 nucleotides, respectively. We examined details of these DNA sequence alterations by direct sequencing of the DNAs [9].

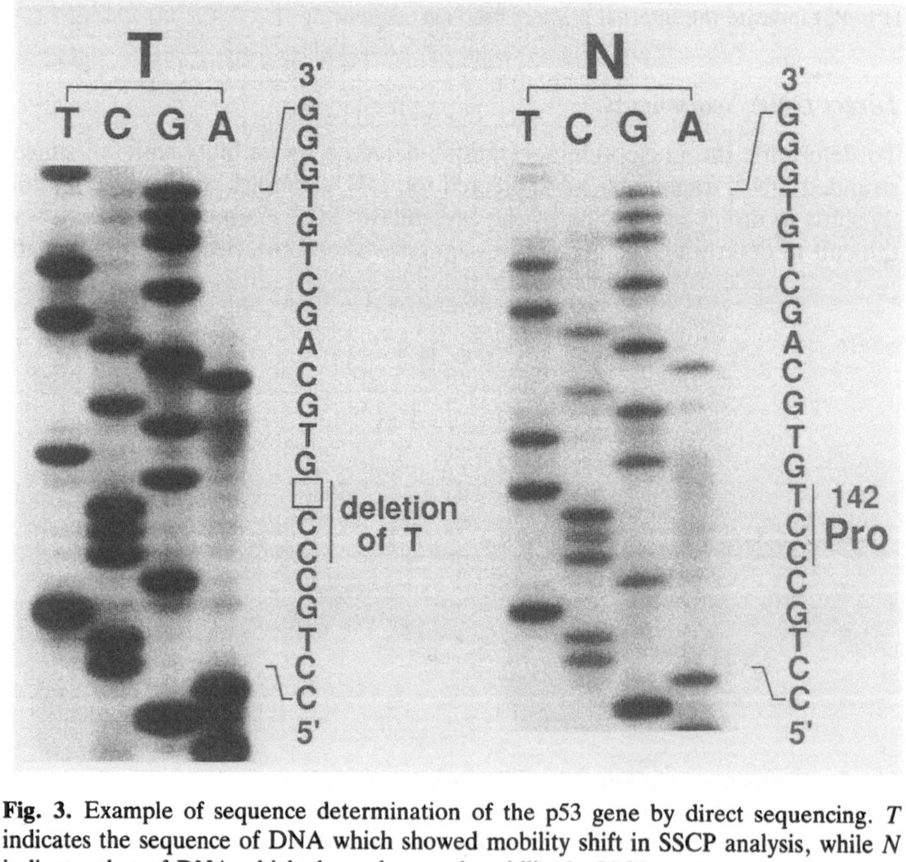

Fig. 3. Example of sequence determination of the p53 gene by direct sequencing. *T* indicates the sequence of DNA which showed mobility shift in SSCP analysis, while *N* indicates that of DNA which showed normal mobility in SSCP-analysis. In this case, a single base deletion (T) was detected, resulting in frame shift

Table 1. *p53* Gene mutations in human brain tumors

Case	Pathological identification	Codon	Mutation	
			Nucleotide	Amino acid
		Primary		
1	Anaplastic astrocytoma	142	Deletion of T	Frame shift
2	Meningioma	175	CGC → GGC	Arg → Gly
3	Glioblastoma multiforme	248	CGG → TGG	Arg → Trp
4	Anaplastic astrocytoma	271	GAG → AAG	Glu → Lys
5	Colon carcinoma	87–90	Deletion of 8 bp	Frame shift
6	Lung carcinoma	239	AAC → GAC	Asn → Asp

In some conditions, the p53 gene is thought to behave as a recessive oncogene or tumor suppressor [1]. There are many reports of p53 gene mutations in human cancer [3,4,14–16]. Mutation of the p53 gene is the most frequently identified genetic change in human lung and colorectal cancers [4,14,16]. This may be because the mutations inactivate the tumor suppressor function of the wild-type p53 gene [14]. Mulligan et al. [15] also reported frequent inactivation of p53 in rhabdomyosarcomas and osteosarcomas. Mutations in the p53 gene of brain tumors have been reported by Nigro et al. [3]. In four of the five cases they examined, the sequence alterations were point mutations. In four of the six cases detected in the present study, the DNA sequence alterations were also single-base substitutions, while in the other two they were deletions of 1 and 8 base-pairs, which caused frame shifts. In all of our six cases, the nucleotide sequence alterations changed the amino acid sequences. The mutations in five of the six cases were clustered in highly conserved regions of the p53 gene [12]. The frequency of p53 mutations in the primary brain tumors examined was 9.8%, which appeared to be significant, but was not as high as those in colorectal and lung cancers [4,14,16].

Acknowledgements. This work was supported in part by a grant-in-aid from the Ministry of Health and Welfare for a comprehensive 10-year strategy for cancer control (Japan), a grant from the Ministry of Science, Education and Culture of Japan, and a grant from the Special Coordination Fund of the Science and Technology Agency of Japan. Shoji Mashiyama was a recipient of a Research Resident Fellowship from the Foundation for Promotion of Cancer Research.

References

1. Finlay CA, Hinds PW, Levine AJ (1989) The p53 proto-oncogene can act as a suppressor of transformation. Cell 57:1083–1093
2. Hinds P, Finlay C, Levine AJ (1989) Mutation is required to activate the p53 gene for cooperation with the *ras* oncogene and transformation. J Virol 63:739–746

3. Nigro JM, Baker SJ, Preisinger AC, Jessup JM, Hostetter R, Cleary K, Binger SH, Davidson N, Baylin S, Devilee P, Glover T, Collins FS, Weston A, Modari R, Harris CC, Vogelstein B (1989) Mutations in the p53 gene occur in diverse human tumour types. Nature 342:705–708
4. Takahashi T, Nau MM, Chiba I, Birrer MJ, Rosenberg RK, Vinocour M, Levitt M, Pass H, Gazdar AF, Minna JD (1989) A frequent target for genetic abnormalities in lung cancer. Science 246:491–494
5. Saiki RK, Gelfand DH, Stoffel S, Scharf SJ, Higuchi R, Horn GT, Mullis KB, Erlich HA (1988) Primer-detected enzymatic amplification of DNA with a thermostable DNA polymerase. Science 239:487–491
6. Orita M, Iwahana H, Kanazawa H, Hayashi K, Sekiya T (1989) Detection of polymorphisms of human DNA by gel electrophoresis as single-strand conformation polymorphisms. Proc Natl Acad Sci USA 86:2766–2770
7. Orita M, Suzuki Y, Sekiya T, Hayashi K (1989) Rapid and sensitive detection of point mutations and DNA polymorphisms using polymerase chain reaction. Genomics 5:874–879
8. Mashiyama S, Sekiya T, Hayashi K (1991) Screening of multiple DNA samples for detection of sequence changes. Technique (in press)
9. Suzuki Y, Sekiya T, Hayashi K (to be published) Single allele-PCR: A method for amplification and sequence determination of a single component among a mixture of sequence variants. Anal Biochem
10. Blin N, Stafford DW (1976) A general method for isolation of high molecular weight DNA from eukaryotes. Nucleic Acids Res 3:2303–2308
11. Buchman VL, Chumakov PM, Ninkina NN, Samarina OP, Georgiev GP (1988) A variation in the structure of the protein-coding region of the human p53 gene. Gene 70:245–252
12. Soussi T, Caron de Fromentel C, May P (1990) Structural aspects of the p53 protein in relation to gene evolution. Oncogene 5:945–952
13. Suzuki Y, Orita M, Shiraishi M, Hayashi K, Sekiya T (1990) Detection of *ras* gene mutations in human lung cancers by single-strand conformation polymorphism analysis of polymerase chain reaction products. Oncogene 5:1037–1043
14. Baker SJ, Fearon ER, Nigro JM, Hamilton SR, Preisinger AC, Jessup JM, vanTuinen P, Ledbetter DH, Barker DF, Nakamura Y, White R, Vogelstein B (1989) Chromosome 17 deletions and p53 gene mutations in colorectal carcinomas. Science 224:217–221
15. Mulligan LM, Matlashewski GJ, Scrable HJ, Cavenee WK (1990) Mechanisms of p53 loss in human sarcomas. Proc Natl Acad Sci USA 87:5863–5867
16. Rodrigues NR, Rowan A, Smith MEF, Kerr IB, Bodmer WF, Gannon JV, Lane DP (1990) p53 mutations in colorectal cancer. Proc Natl Acad Sci USA 87:7555–7559

An Analysis of Genetic Alterations of the p53 Gene in Human Glioma

Kouzou Fukuyama[1], Mamoru Oh-uchida[2], Toshihiro Mineta[1], Nobuaki Momozaki[1], Katsuji Hori[2], and Kazuo Tabuchi[1]

Introduction

Restriction fragment length polymorphisms (RFLPs) analysis of human glioma tissue has revealed frequent loss of heterozygosity on the long arm of the chromosome 10 [1] as well as the short arm of the chromosome 17 [2,3]. It has recently been thought that certain tumor suppressor genes are located on chromosomes 10 and 17. The p53 gene is located on 17p13.1, which is often deleted in various human tumors such as those of colorectal cancer, breast cancer, lung cancer, and osteosarcoma [4]. Detailed study of the p53 gene revealed that the remaining allele contained mutations particularly in the region conserved throughout the species [4]. It is reported that the product of a mutant-type p53 gene has a prolonged half-life and contains a cellular transforming activity. The p53 gene product acts in a dimer and the mutant-type p53 gene product inactivates the wild-type p53 gene product by binding to it [5]. While the mutant-type p53 gene causes cell immortalization in combination with the activated *ras* gene, the wild-type p53 gene product supresses normal somatic cell transformation. Thus, the genetic alterations of the p53 gene are thought to contribute to the tumorigenetic process in various type of cells, with the p53 gene being a putative tumor suppressor gene. Recent studies revealed that the p53 gene product may be acting as a transcriptional activator for some other genes [6,7]. This fact may well explain the diversity of tumor types which result from mutations in the p53 gene.

Having found that the p53 gene products expressed in glioma cell lines had prolonged half-lives, we attempted to investigate the genetic alterations of the p53 gene of gliomas by Southern and Northern blot hybridization and polymerase chain reaction-single strand conformation polymorphism (PCR-SSCP) analyses [8]. Furthermore, we investigated the alterations of the p53 gene in formalin-fixed surgical specimens of glioma in order to directly disclose the role of the p53 gene in human glioma.

Departments of [1]Neurosurgery and [2]Biochemistry, Saga Medical School, Saga, 849 Japan

Materials and Methods

Cell Lines

Seven established human glioma cell lines (U87MG, T98G, 118MG, A172, U251MG, U373MG, and KMG4) were used in this study. The cells were cultured in modified Eagle's medium (MEM) containing 10% fetal bovine serum (FBS) at 37°C in a humidified atmosphere of 5% CO_2.

DNA and RNA Isolations and Hybridization

High molecular DNA was extracted from 1% NP-40-treated nuclear fraction of each cell line, and total RNA was extracted from its soluble fraction using the hot phenol method [9]. Each 10 µg DNA was digested completely with a restriction enzyme (*Eco*RI, *Bam*HI, *Hin*dIII, or *Bgl*II), fractionated by gel electrophoresis, transferred to a nlylon membrane in 25 mM sodium phosphate, and hybridized with a human-p53-cDNA probe radiolabeled by a random oligonucleotide primer. Each 20 µg RNA was denatured with 6.3% formaldehyde and 50% formamide, electrophoresed on a 1.5% agarose gel containing 6.6% formaldehyde, transferred to a nylon membrane, and hybridized with the same probe used for Southern blot hybridization.

PCR-SSCP Analysis

Oligonucleotides were synthesized as primers according to the nucleotide sequence of the introns just anterior and posterior to exons 5, 7, and 8 of the p53 gene (P5A: 5′-TTCGAATTCCTGCAGTACTCCCCTG, P5B: 5′-TAGGATCCGCCCCAGCTCACC, P7A: 5′-GTTGAATTCTAGGTTTTCTCTGAC, P7B: 5′-CAAGTGGATCCTGACCTGGAGTCTTC, P8A: 5′-CGGAATTCCCTATCCTGAGTAGTGG, and P8B 5′-ATGGATCCTGCTTGCTTGCTTACCTCGC). Genomic DNA (1 µg) was used in 30 µl PCR reaction consisting of 30 cycles at 94°C (1 min) 62°C (2 min), and 72°C (2 min). The PCR reaction contains 1.5 mM $MgCl_2$, 10 mM Tris-HCl, 50 mM KCl, 0.25 U Taq polymerase, 200 µM of each deoxynucleotide (dNTP) and 1 µM of each pair of ^{32}P-labeled primers. The products were diluted 100-fold in 95% formamide dye, denatured at 95°C, and then loaded onto 5% polyacrylamide gel (40 × 20 × 0.03 cm) containing 10% glycerol. Electrophoresis was performed at 4°C under a constant power of 15 W.

PCR from Formaline-fixed Tissue

Three slices of 10 µm tissue samples were cut from the paraffin block, deparaffinized three times with 300 µl xylene, and then washed three times with 300 µl 70% ethanol. After centrifugation, the pellet was dissolved in 300 µl proteinase K solution (100 µg/ml) and incubated for 24–48 h. DNA was extracted with phenol/chloroform, precipitated with 70% ethanol, dissolved in 50 µl RNase solution (10 μg/ml), and incubated for 1 h. Phenol/chloroform extraction and ethanol precipitation were repeated and the pellet was finally dissolved in 50 μl 1 mM tris-HCl/1 mM EDTA solution.

Results

Southern and Northern Blot Hybridization Analyses

Fifteen kilobase (kb) DNA fragments by *Eco*RI digestion, which covered nearly 80% of the p53 gene locus, were detected in every cell line (Fig. 1). DNA fragments of 7 kb and 2.5 kb by *Hin*dIII digestion and 7.8 kb DNA fragments by *Bam*HI digestion were also detected. T98G showed smaller *Bgl*II digested fragments than that of the normal control. This may be due to a known polymorphism in the first intron of the p53 gene [10]. Other coding

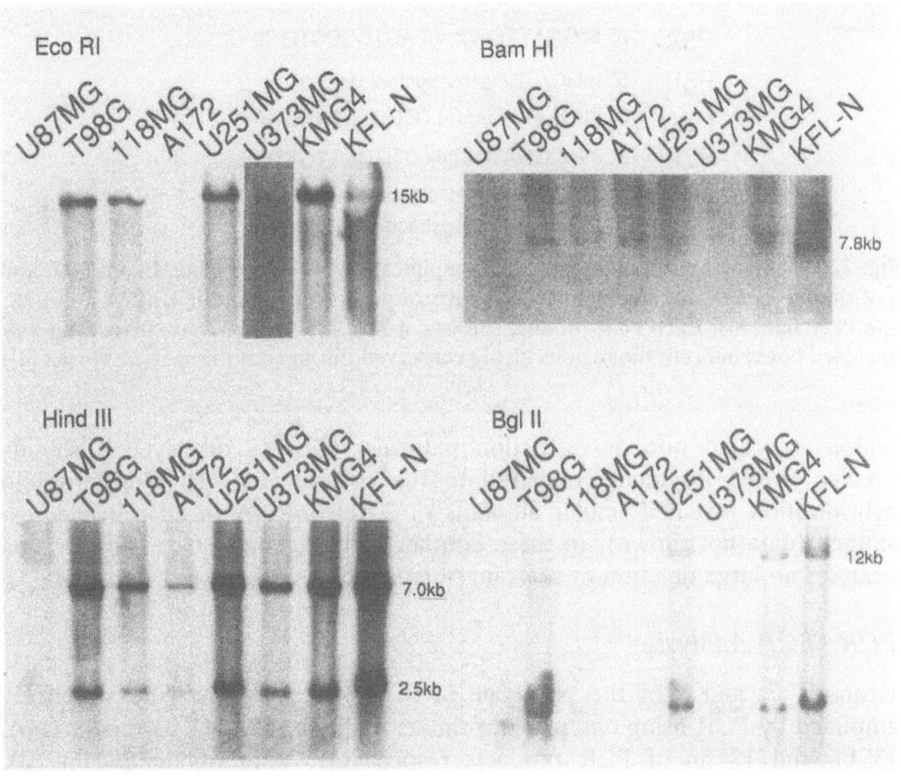

Fig. 1. Southern blot hybridization of DNA from glioma cells. Human p53 cDNA (2.2 kb *Bam*HI fragment) in a php53 B clone provided from American Type Culture Collection (ATCC) is used as a probe. Each *lane* contains 10 μg of completely digested DNA. *KFL-N* is the control DNA derived from normal human lymphcytes. *T98G* shows smaller *Bgl*II DNA fragment due to known rearrangement in the first intron of the p53 gene

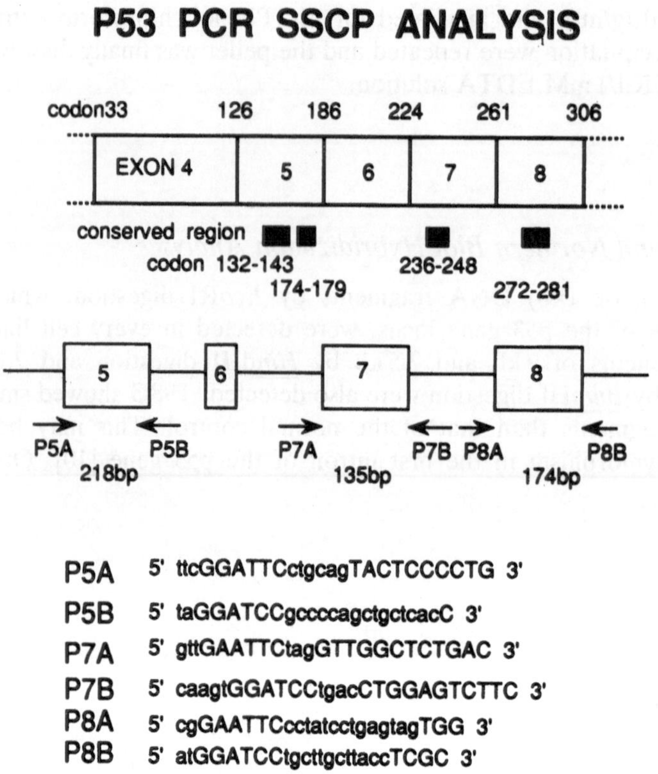

Fig. 2. Schematic representation of PCR amplification of the p53 gene. Exons 5, 7, and 8 of the p53 gene were amplified using 3 pairs of primers, P5A and P5B, P7A and P7B, and P8A and P8B. Each PCR product consists of 218, 135, and 174 base pairs. The *four opacified boxes* indicate the regions highly conserved throughout the species. (From [4])

regions revealed normal restriction patterns. U87MG displayed a slightly smaller *Eco*RI fragment compared to the control (Fig. 1). Northern blot hybridization revealed similar amounts of 2.8 kb mRNA in all cell lines examined (data not shown). In these Southern and Northern blot hybridization analyses no large deletion or rearrangement in the p53 gene was detected.

PCR-SSCP Analysis

Exons 5, 7, and 8 of the p53 gene of 7 glioma cell lines were selectively amplified by PCR using one pair of primers for each, and 215 base pairs (bp), 135 bp and 174 bp of PCR products respectively, were obtained. (Fig. 2). Following heat denaturation, these PCR products were located onto polyacrylamide gel electrophoresis. Altered mobility of the DNA fragments, which was due to a conformational change resulting from nucleotide substitution, was observed for T98G in exon 7 and for U251MG and U373MG in exon 8 (Fig. 3). These changes were considered to reflect point mutation or common polymorphisms of amino acid coding sequences.

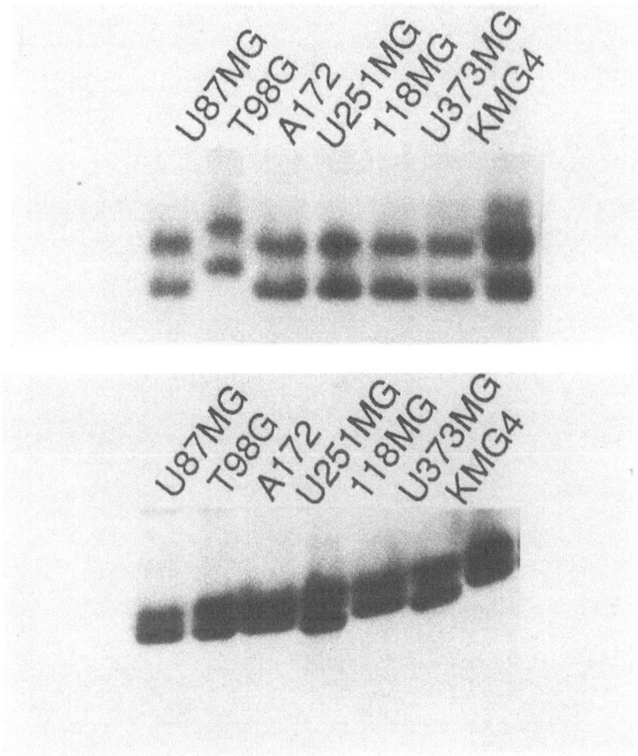

Fig. 3. PCR-SSCP analysis of exons 7 and 8 of the p53 gene in glioma cells. Radiolabeled PCR products were denatured and each strand was separated by polyacrylamide gel electrophoresis. *T98G* in exon 7, and *U251MG* and *U373MG* in exon 8 show altered mobility, indicating substitution of DNA sequences

DNA was extracted from 20 formalin-fixed surgical specimens of glioma (as described above) and used as templates of PCR. Two surgical specimens, 1 medulloblastoma (Fig. 4) and 1 glioma (data not shown), showed nucleotide substitutions in exon 8.

Discussion

Neither large deletion nor rearrangement of the p53 gene was detected in the glioma cell lines examined. However, 3 out of 7 cell lines showed polymorphisms in either exon 7 or 8 in which mutations were reported in other diverse types of tumors. At present, we are uncertain as to whether or not these genetic changes in coding sequences of the p53 gene are responsible for glial tumorigenesis. The fact that the products of these altered p53 gene had pro-

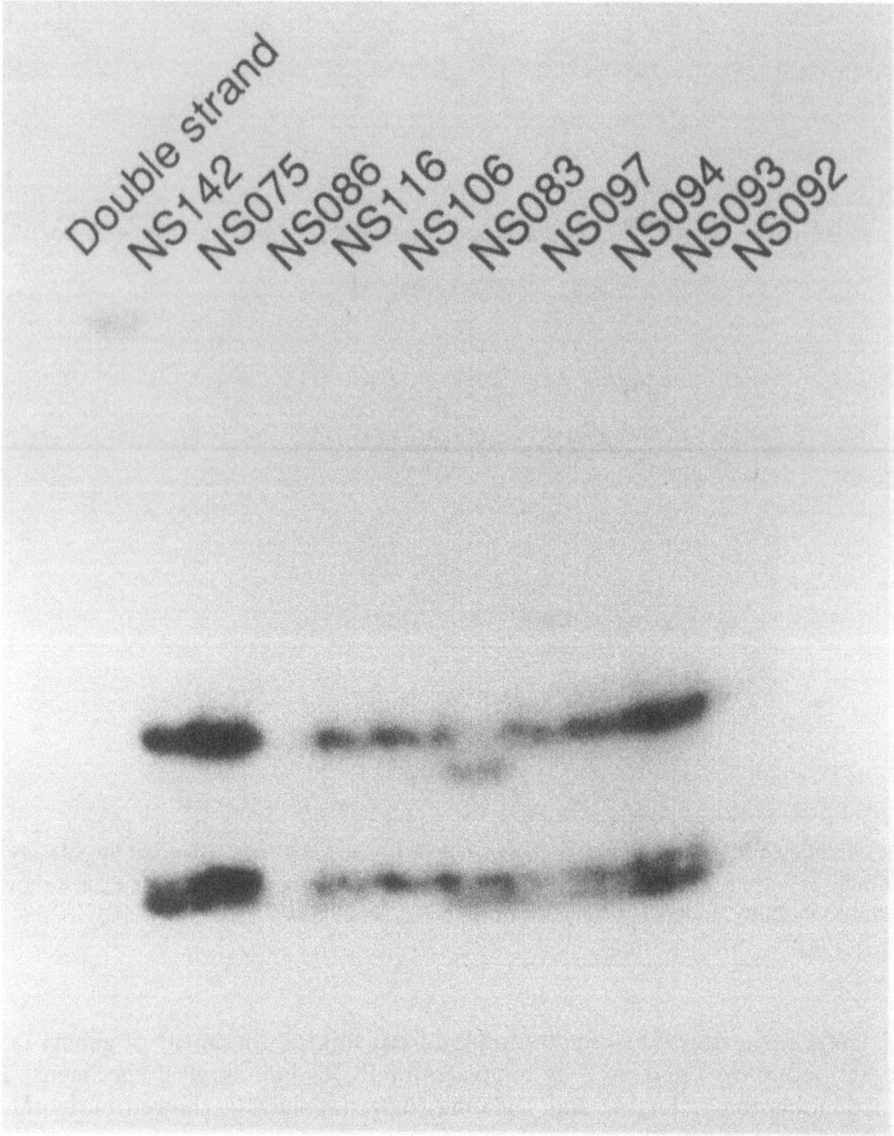

Fig. 4. PCR-SSCP analysis of exon 8 of the p53 gene in glioma tissue. DNA was prepared from a paraffin-embedded tissue sample and used as a PCR template. *NS083*, a case of medulloblastoma, shows altered mobility

longed half-lives indicates that these alterations may contribute to tumorigenesis of glial tumors.

Currently, it is not clear whether these genetic alterations of the p53 gene are secondary consequences in established glioma cell lines or a primary genetic characteristic of glioma. In this study, we could detect the nucleotide substitutions not only in glioma cell lines but also in surgical specimens. This fact suggests that the mutation of p53 gene is a primary genetic characteristic of certain glial tumors. The PCR-SSCP analysis is applicapable to a paraffin-embedded formaline-fixed tissue as a source of template DNA. Although only 2 out of 20 surgical specimens examined showed polymorphism in the hot region of the p53 gene, the possibility remains that it is present in other coding regions.

In summary, certain gliomas had mutations in the p53 gene, indicating that it may contribute to the tumorigenesis or development of glial tumors. The products of a mutated p53 gene may loose its native function, such as that of a transcriptional activator, and thus fail to trans-activate other tumor suppressor genes or trans-repress some oncogenes.

Conclusions

1. No large deletions or rearrangements of the p53 gene were detected by Southern and Northern blot analyses in 7 established glioma cell lines.
2. In 3 out of 7 glioma cell lines, PCR-SSCP analysis revealed nucleotide substitutions in either exon 7 or 8 of the p53 gene. These alterations were thought to be responsible for a tumorigenetic process or development of glial tumors.
3. PCR-SSCP analysis was applicapable to formaline-fixed tissues. Two surgical specimens of glioma were found to contain nucleotide substitution in exon 8 of the p53 gene.

Summary

We investigated the p53 gene and gene product in human glioma. Immunocytochemical evaluation of the p53 gene product in human glioma cell lines showed nuclear positivity. Because of the short half-life of the wild-type p53 gene product, it is rarely detected in normal cells. Therefore, the p53 gene product immunocytochemically detected in glioma was thought to be a mutant-type. Although Southern blot and Northern blot analyses revealed no definite alterations in the p53 gene, PCR-SSCP (polymerase chain reaction—single strand confromation polymorphism) analysis disclosed nucleotide substitution in 3 out of 7 cell lines in either exon 7 or 8 of the p53 gene, which were generally conserved throughout the species. It is uncertain whether these substitutions are responsible for cell immortalization or are common polymorphisms. We assumed these genetic alterations in the coding sequence of the p53 gene to be quite consistent mutations, because their products showed a prolonged half-life and a constantly positive immunocytochemical staining in the nucleus. PCR-SSCP analysis can detect genetic alterations, even in the paraffin-embedded formalin-fixed specimens, with higher specificity and sensitivity within a few days, and thus a significant number of samples can be processed for evaluation. We demonstrated nucleotide substitutions in 2 out of 20 formalin-fixed surgical specimens of glioma.

References

1. Fujimoto M, Fults DW, Thomas GA, Nakamura Y, Heilbrun, MP, White R, Story JL, Naylor SL, Kagan-Hallet KS, Sheridan PJ (1989) Loss of hetrozygosity on chromosome 10 in human glioblastoma multiforme. Genomics 4:210–214
2. James CD, Carlbom E, Nordenskjold M, Collons VP, Cavenee WK (1989) Mitotic recombination of chromosome 17 in astrocytomas. Proc Natl Acad Sci USA 86:2858–2862
3. E1-Azouzi M, Chung RY, Farmer GE, Martuza RL, Black PM, Rouleau GA, Hettlich C, Hedley-Whyte ET, Zervas NT, Panagopoulos K, Nakamura Y, Gusella JF, Seizinger BR (1989) Loss of distinct regions on the short arm of chromosome 17 associated with tumorigenesis of human astrocytomas. Proc Natl Acad Sci USA 86:7186–7190
4. Nigro JM, Baker SJ, Preisinger AC, Jessup, JM, Hostetter R, Cleary K, Bigner SH, Davidson N, Baylin S, Devilee P, Glover T, Collins FS, Weston A, Medali R, Harris CC, Vogelstein B (1989) Mutations in the p53 gene occur in diverse human tumor types. Nature 342:705–708
5. Levine AL, Momand J (1990) Tumor suppressor genes: The p53 and retinoblastoma sensitivity genes and gene products. Biochim Biophys Acta 1032:119–136
6. Field S, Jang SK (1990) Presence of potent transcription activating sequence in the p53 protein. Science 249:1046–1049
7. Raycroft L, Wu H, Lozano G (1990) Transcriptional activation by wildtype but not transforming mutant of the p53 anti-oncogene. Science 249:1049–1051
8. Orita M, Iwahara K, Kanazawa H, Hayashi K, Sekiya T (1989) Detection of polymorphisms of human DNA by gel electrophresis as single-strand conformation polymorphisms. Proc Natl Acad Sci USA 86:2766–2770
9. Sambrook J, Fritsch EF, Maniatis T (1989) Molecular cloning, 2nd edn. Cold Spring Harbor, New York
10. Buchman VL, Chumakov PM, Ninkina NN, Samarina OP, Georgiev GP (1988) A variation in the structure of the protein-coding region of human p53 gene. Gene 70:245–252

The Expression and Structure of p53 Gene Products in Cultured Glioma Cells

TOSHIHIRO MINETA, KOUZOU FUKUYAMA, TETSUYA SHIRAISHI, and KAZUO TABUCHI[1]

Introduction

Previous studies have demonstrated that the allelic deletions of the short arm of chromosome 17 (17p) and the long arm of 10 (10q) are closely associated with tumorigenesis of human malignant gliomas [1,2]. While the allelic deletion in chromosome 10q appears to occur in a relatively late phase associated with the transition from a less malignant to a more malignant state [3], the deletion in chromosome 17p seems to be an early event associated with the occurrence of neoplastic glial cells, suggesting that anti-oncogenes or tumor suppressor genes are important in the development of human gliomas. However, the role of anti-oncogenes in human gliomas has not been studied in detail. Recent studies have demonstrated that the cellular protein p53, which is encoded on chromosome 17p13.1, may function as a suppressor of neoplastic growth and may play an important role in the pathogenesis of human malignant tumors. The p53 protein was first identified through its interaction with the large T antigen of simian virus 40 (SV 40) [4], and had been thought to be a dominant oncogene enabling full transformation of vertebrate somatic cells in combination with an activated *ras* gene [5]. However, it has recently been shown that the p53 protein observed in the neoplastic cells is entirely mutant and that the wild type p53 suppresses normal cells from transforming [6], which means that the p53 protein may act as a tumor suppressor, like the product of the retinoblastoma susceptibility gene. The investigations on p53 gene have been focused on genetic abnormalities of breast, lung, bone, and colorectal tumors [7–10]. In light of these associations of the p53 gene with neoplasia, we have investigated the structure and expression of p53 protein in cultured glioma cells. The expression of the p53 protein was initially studied using immunohistochemical techniques. Electrophoresis was then performed in order to investigate the biochemical structure of p53 protein expressed in glioma cells.

[1] Department of Neurosurgery, Saga Medical School, Saga, 849 Japan

Materials and Methods

Cell Lines

Seven established human glioma cell lines U251-MG, U373-MG, T98G, U118-MG, U87-MG (American Type Culture Collection, Rockville, Md.), A172 (Japan Cancer Research Bank, Tokyo) and KMG4 (Kindly donated by Dr. Y. Ushio of Kumamato University, Kumamato, Japan), were used in this study. These glioma cells were grown in modified Eagle's medium (MEM) supplemented with 10% fetal bovine serum (FBS) at 37°C in a humidified atmosphere of 5% CO_2.

Monoclonal Antibody Reagents

Two anti-p53 monoclonal antibody (MoAb) reagents were used in this study: MoAb p53 (ab-1) (Oncogene Sci., Inc. Manhasset, N.Y.), which reacts with p53 of a broad range of mammalian species including human, was used for immunoprecipitation, and MoAb p53 (ab-2) (Oncogene), which reacts with p53 of human cellular origin, was used for immunohistochemistry.

Immunohistochemistry

The streptavidin-biotin-peroxidase complex (SAB) technique was employed for staining. Subconfluent monolayers of cells were fixed in absolute methanol and air dried. Cells were then incubated for 30 min in 0.3% H_2O_2 in methanol and washed in phosphate-buffered saline (PBS). MoAb p53 (ab-2) was applied for 30 min as primary antibody, and this was followed by washing the cells in PBS. Subsequently, SAB reagents (BioGenex Laboratories, San Ramon, Calif.) and diaminobenzidine hydrogen peroxide substrate were applied.

Immunoprecipitation and Electrophoresis

For metabolic labeling, subconfluent cells were grown for 3 h in MEM with 125 µCi/ml ^{35}S-methionine. Then, the cells were lysed in 150 mM NaCl, 50 mM

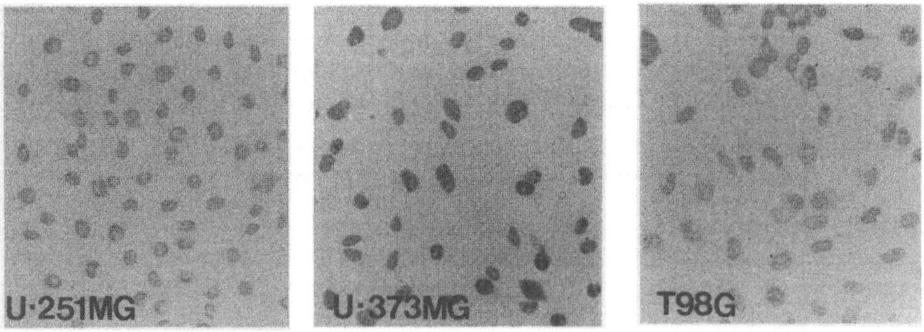

Fig. 1. Immunohistochemical studies of human glioma cells with p53 antibodies

Tris (pH 7.5), 1% NP-40, 1% sodium deoxycholate, and 1 mM phenyl methyl sulfonyl fluoride for 30 min on ice. The cell extract was centrifuged and the pellet was discarded. The extract was preabsorbed with Protein A-Sepharose, MoAb p53 (ab-1) was added, and the mixture was left overnight at 4°C on a roating wheel. Protein A-Sepharose beads were added and the incubation was continued for 30 min. The beads were then washed four times in 150 mM NaCl, 50 mM EDTA, 50 mM Tris (pH 7.4), and 0.05% NP-40, 0.02% sodium azide. The immunoprecipitates were directly resuspended in a protein sample buffer, heated at 70°C for 10 min, and subjected to sodium dodecyl sulfate polyacrylamide gel electrophoresis (SDS-PAGE) using 10% polyacrylamide slab gels.

Pulse-Chase Analysis

Plates (10 cm) containing equivalent numbers of cells from the cell line under investigation were labeled with ^{35}S-methionine for 90 min. Following the labeling, the radioactive medium was removed, and the cells were washed twice with MEM plus 10% FBS. The cells were then recultured with 10 ml MEM plus 10% FBS for specific periods of time. At the end of the specified chase period, cells were lysed and subjected to immunoprecipitation and SDS-PAGE analysis.

Results

First we studied p53 protein expression in human glioma cell lines, using immunohistochemical stainings with MoAb p53 (ab-2). The U87-MG cell line showed equivocal staining, and the U118-MG and A172 cell lines showed slight nuclear positivity. However, in the U251-MG, U373-MG, KMG4, and T98G cell lines, the nuclei of these malignant glioma cells were found to stain diffusely for p53 protein, with sparing of the nucleoli (Fig. 1).

We then performed biochemical analysis of p53 protein expressed in these glioma cells by immunoprecipitation with MoAb p53 (ab-1) after ^{35}S-methionine labeling. These immunoprecipitates were examined by SDS-PAGE analysis. Using this sensitive technique, the p53 protein was clearly detected in all of the human glioma cell lines except for U87-MG (Fig. 2) in which the presence of p53 protein was equivocal. There was some heterogeneity in the migration rate of p53 protein in slab gel. U251-MG and U373-MG showed a single band of p53 which had a fast migration rate and T98G and U118-MG showed slow migration bands of p53 protein. Specifically, the A172 cells showed doublet bands of p53 protein. These findings suggest that there is clear heterogeneity in p53 protein expressed in glioma cells, and that some of them may express aberrant p53 protein.

Finally, we employed pulse-chase analysis in order to determine the half-life of p53 proteins expressed in A172 and T98G cells. After 0, 30, 60, and 180 min of chase, cell lysates were immunoprecipitated and subjected to SDS-PAGE. As shown in Fig. 3, both of the p53 doublet bands in A172 cells and the single

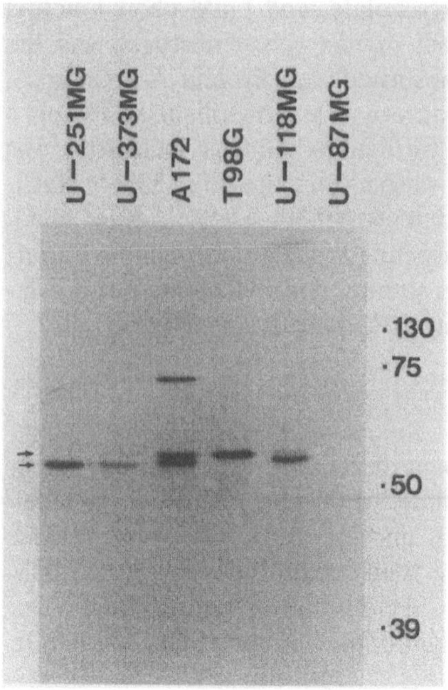

Fig. 2. SDS-PAGE analysis of p53 immunoprecipitates from human glioma cell lines. There is evident heterogeneity in the migration rate of p53 protein in slab gel (*arrows*). A172 cells in particular show a doublet band pattern

band of T98G cells continued to maintain the radioactivity even after 60 min of chase, which indicated a prolonged half-life of the p53 protein expressed in those cells, because the half-life of the wild-type p53 protein is reported to be 6–30 min [11].

Discussion

The function of p53 protein in somatic cells still remains unknown. The p53 protein was first identified as a cellular phosphoprotein that formed a complex with the large T antigen of SV40. The p53 protein also associates with the E1B protein of adenovirus and the E6 protein of human papilloma virus [12,13]. Similar behavior underlies the product of the retinoblastoma susceptibility gene (RB) which was first identified as a tumor suppressor gene. The RB protein also binds SV 40 large T antigen, adenovirus E1A and human papilloma virus E7 proteins, and inactivates those oncoproteins encoded by DNA tumor viruses. More recently, p53 protein was found to be phosphorylated in a cell cycle-dependent manner and in a substrate of cdc2 protein kinase which played a broad and key role in cell cycle control [14,15]. Thus, recent reports support the view that p53 protein plays an important role in controlling the cell cycle, particularly since it may normally act as an inhibitor of cell proliferation and as a tumor suppressor. In this study, we analyzed the p53 protein in human glioma cell lines. Our present study revealed some abnormalities regarding the expression and structure of p53 proteins expressed in human glioma cells.

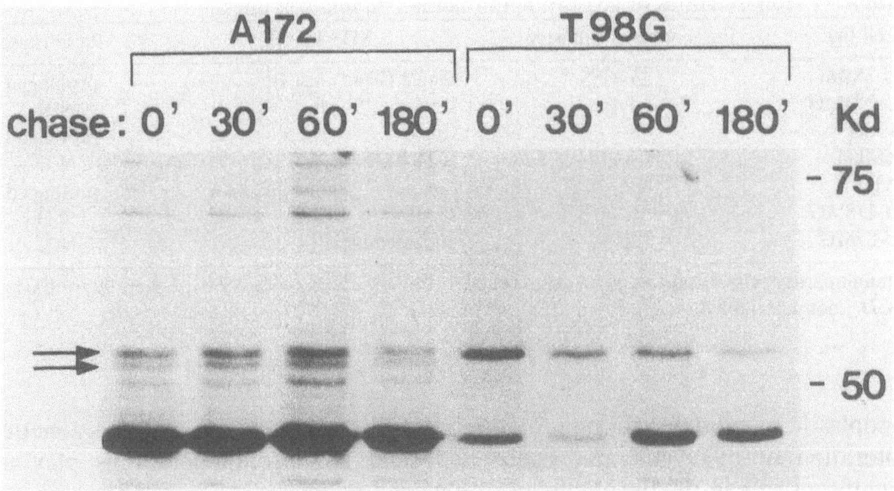

Fig. 3. Pulse-chase analysis of p53 protein in A172 and T98G cells. Both the p53 doublet band in A172 cells and the single band of T98G cells continue to maintain the radioactivity even after 60 min of chase, which indicates the prolonged half-life of p53 protein expressed in those cells

Immunohistochemical evaluation of p53 protein expression showed evident nuclear positivity in 5 out of 6 glioma cell lines. Specifically, over 90% of the cells in the U251-MG, U373-MG, KMG4, and T98G cell lines were positive for p53 protein. For the biochemical analysis of p53 protein expressed in such glioma cells, we performed SDS-PAGE and pulse-chase analyses. In the SDS-PAGE analysis, the migration rate of p53 proteins expressed in glioma cells showed unequivocal heterogeneity, and in the pulse-chase analysis, the half-life of p53 proteins expressed in both A172 and T98G cells was markedly prolonged. Previous studies on the p53 protein indicate that the mutant form may be distinguished from the wild type by abnormal migration on polyacrylamide gels [16] and by an increased half-life [17]. Indeed, a single amino acid change in the p53 protein may cause an alteration of electrophoretic mobility and a slower migration in SDS-PAGE gels. On the other hand, mutant p53 protein is reported to bind with heat shock protein and to increase its half-life.

Conclusions

The results of our present studies are summarized in Table 1. They demonstrate that several glioma cell lines have an aberrant form of p53 protein in its expression and/or in its molecular structure, and that p53 abnormalities may be a frequent event associated with the development of human glioma. The wild-type p53 protein may act as a tumor suppressor. However, over-expression of the mutant p53 protein leads to the transformation in rodent cells to a

Table 1. Abnormalities of p53 protein in human glioma cell lines

Cell line	Immunohistochemistry	SDS-PAGE		Pulse chase
U-251MG	+++	Single (band)	fast (migration)	prolonged
U-373MG	+++	single	fast	N.D.
T98G	+++	single	show	prolonged
KMG4	+++	N.D.		N.D.
A172	++	double	fast and slow	prolonged
U-118MG	++	single	slow	N.D.
U-87MG	±	undetectable		N.D.

Immunohistochemical positivity: ±, equivocal; +, 5%–49%; ++, 50%–89%; +++, 90%–100%; *N.D.*, not determined

neoplastic phenotype. In view of these data, it is concluded that the genetic alteration of p53 gene may cause abnormal p53 protein and thus play a significant role in the development of glial cell neoplasia.

References

1. El-Azouzi M, Chung RY, Farmer GE, Maltuza RL, Black PM, Rouleau GA, Hettlich C, Hedley-Whyte ET, Zervas NT, Panagopoulos K, Nakamura Y, Gusella JF, Seizinger BR (1989) Loss of distinct regions on the short arm of chromosome 17 associated with tumorigenesis of human astrocytomas. Proc Natl Acad Sci USA 86:7186–7190
2. Fujimoto M, Fults DW, Thomas GA, Nakamura Y, Heilbrun MP, White R, Story JL, Naylor SL, Kagan-Hallet KS, Sheridan PJ (1989) Loss of heterozygosity on chromosome 10 in human glioblastoma multiforme. Genomics 4:210–214
3. James CD, Carlbom E, Dumanski JP, Hansen M, Nordenskjold M, Collins VP, Cavenee WK (1988) Clonal genomic alterations in glioma malignancy stages. Cancer Res 48:5546–5551
4. Lane DP, Crawford LV (1979) T antigen is bound to a host protein in SV-40 transformed cells. Nature 278:261–263
5. Parada LF, Land H, Weinberg RA, Wolt D, Rotter V (1984) Cooperation between gene encoding p53 tumour antigen and *ras* in cellular transformation. Nature 312:649–651
6. Eliyahu D, Michalovitz D, Eliyahu S, Pinhasi-Kimhi O, Oren M (1989) Wild-type p53 can inhibit oncogene-mediated focus formation. Proc Natl Acad Sci USA 86:8763–8767
7. Baker SJ, Fearon ER, Nigro JM, Hamilton SR, Preisinger AC, Jessup JM, van-Tuinen P, Ledbetter DF, Barker DF, Nakamura Y, White R, Vogelstein B (1989) Chromosome 17 deletions and p53 gene mutations in colorectal carcinomas. Science 244:217–221
8. Masuda H, Miller C, Koeffler HP, Battifora H, Cline MJ (1987) Rearrangement of the p53 gene in human osteogenic sarcomas. Proc Natl Acad Sci USA 84:7716–7719
9. Nigro JM, Baker SJ, Preisinger AC, Jessup JM, Hostetter R, Cleary K, Bigner SH, Davidson N, Baylin S, Devilee P, Glover T, Collins FS, Weston A, Modali R,

Harris CC, Vogelstein B (1989) Mutations in the p53 gene occur in diverse human tumour types. Nature 342:705–708
10. Takahashi T, Nau MM, Chiba I, Birrer MJ, Rosenberg RK, Vinocour M, Levitte M, Pass H, Gazdar AF, Minna JD (1989) p53: A frequent target for genetic abnormalities in lung cancer. Science 246:491–494
11. Crawford LV, Pim DC, Gurney EG, Goodfellow P, Papadimitriou JT (1981) Detection of a common feature in several human tumor cell lines—53,000-dalton protein. Proc Natl Acad Sci USA 78:41–45
12. Sarnow, P, Ho YS, Williams J, Levine AJ (1982) Adenovirus E1b-58kd tumor antigen and SV40 large tumor antigen are physically associated with the same 54 kd cellular protein in transformed cells. Cell 28:387–394
13. Werness BA, Levine AJ, Howley PM (1990) Association of human papilloma virus type 16 and 18 E6 protein with p53. Science 248:76–79
14. Bischoff JR, Friedman PN, Marshak DR, Prives C, Beach D (1990) Human p53 is phosphorylated by p60-cdc2 and cyclin B-cdc2. Proc Natl Acad Sci USA 87:4766–4770
15. Milner J, Cook A, Mason J (1990) p53 is associated with $p34^{cdc2}$ in transformed cells. EMBO J 9:2885–2889
16. Matlashewski GJ, Tuck S, Pim D, Lamb P, Schneider J, Crawford LV (1987) Primary structure polymorphism at amino acid residue 72 of human p53. Mol Cell Biol 7:961–963
17. Finlay CA, Hinds PW, Tan T-H, Eliyahu D, Oren M, Levine AJ (1988) Activating mutations for transformation by p53 produce a gene product that forms an hsc70-p53 complex with an altered half-life. Mol Cell Biol 8:531–539

Detection of Retinoblastoma Gene Aberrations in Human Brain Tumor by Single-Strand Conformation Polymorphism Analysis of Polymerase Chain Reaction Products

Masako Katahira[1,2], Yoshinori Murakami[2], Kenshi Hayashi[2], Osami Kubo[1], Yasuhiko Tajika[1], Mizuo Kagawa[1], and Takao Sekiya[2]

Introduction

The gene predisposing to retinoblastoma, RB-1, has been mapped to chromosomal region 13q14 [1], and a cDNA clone has been isolated [2]. Aberrations of this gene have been found not only in retinoblastoma, but also in other human cancers, including osteosarcoma [3], small cell lung cancer [4], and bladder cancer [5]. An epidemiological study revealed that the occurrence of brain tumor in members of a family with hereditary retinoblastoma was more frequent than in normal individuals [6]. This observation suggested the involvement of aberrations of the RB gene in the genesis of brain tumor and prompted us to examine the gene in human brain tumors.

Two independent mutations, each on two copies of the RB gene, have been proposed to create null alleles and to be involved in the genesis of retinoblastoma [7,8]. Two types of mutation have been evidenced for the RB gene, one involving gross alterations including the loss of whole or part of the gene and the other involving subtle changes of the nucleotide sequence of the gene including point mutations and deletions of several nucleotides [2,5,9].

In order to detect RB gene aberrations in brain tumor, we applied single-strand conformation polymorphism (SSCP) analysis of polymerase chain reaction (PCR) products [10,11]. This method can detect subtle DNA changes and losses of the gene simultaneously [12].

Materials and Methods

Cell Lines

All 7 glioblastoma cell lines (T98G, U-638MG, U-138MG, A172, U-373MG, U-87MG, and CCF-STTG1) were obtained from the American Type Cellular Collection. These cell lines were maintained in the medium suggested by the

[1]Department of Neurosurgery, Neurological Institute, Tokyo Women's Medical College, Shinjuku-ku, Tokyo, 162 Japan
[2]Oncogene Division, National Cancer Center Research Institute, Chuo-ku, Tokyo 104 Japan

supplier. Surgical specimens were obtained at operations at the Tokyo Women's Medical College.

Northern Blot Analysis

Total cellular RNA was prepared by the method of acid guanidinium thiocyanate-phenol-chloroform extraction. About 7 μg of RNAs were subjected to electrophoresis in 1% agarose containing formamide. RNAs thus fractionated were transferred onto a nitrocellulose membrane. Hybridization with probes was performed as previously described [12].

The probe used for detection of the RB gene transcript was 3.8 kb EcoRI fragment of the 3′-region of human RB cDNA [2]. HpaII-EcoRI fragment (1.3 kb) from the 3′-region of the rat β-actin gene was used to detect the human β-actin gene transcript. The probes were labeled with [^{32}P]phosphate using a multi-prime labeling kit (Rapid Hybridization System, Multiprime, Amersham, UK) with [α-^{32}P]dCTP as a radioactive substrate.

RT-PCR-SSCP Analysis

Samples of total cellular RNA (1 μg) were annealed with synthetic deoxyoligonucleotides complementary to appropriate regions of RB mRNA and transcribed with M-MLV reverse transcriptase (RT) (Bethesda Research Laboratories) in the presence of ribonuclease inhibitor RNasin in the reaction mixture (14 μl) described previously [13]. A portion of the reaction mixture (1 μl) was used for the PCR with two appropriate oligonucleotides as primers, one of which was the same oligonucleotide used in the reverse transcriptase reaction. The 5′-ends of these primers were labeled by the polynucleotide kinase reaction with [γ-^{32}p]ATP as described previously [10,11]. An aliquot of the PCR reaction mixture (1 μl) was mixed with 0–39 μl 0.1% SDS and 20 mM EDTA. Then, 1 μl of this solution was mixed with 9 μl 90% formamide, 20 mM EDTA, and 0.05% xylene cyanol. After being heated at 80°C, samples (1 μl/lane) were analyzed by electrophoresis in a 5% polyacrylamide gel with and without 10% glycerol at 30–40 W for 2–6 h with cooling by a fan.

Results

Samples of total cellular RNA were isolated from 7 human glioblastoma cell lines and 21 surgical specimens of brain tumor. The histological types of the 21 surgical specimens are as follows: 6 glioblastomas, 3 astrocytomas, 3 mixed oligo-astrocytomas, 4 meningiomas, 2 neurinomas, 1 pituitary adenoma, 1 hemangioblastoma, 1 metastatic lung carcinoma, and 1 metastatic renal carcinoma.

RNA samples were subjected to Northern blot analysis using a 3.8 kb DNA fragment from the 3′-region of RB cDNA as a probe. The amounts of RNA were evaluated by hybridization of the same blot with the probe for β-actin mRNA as an internal control.

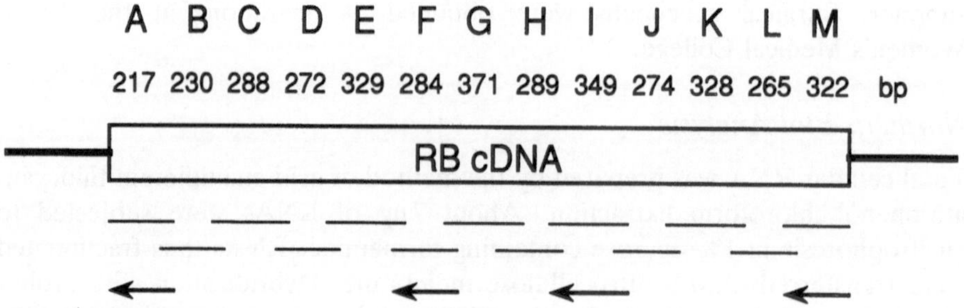

Fig. 1. Region of RB cDNA analyzed by the SSCP method. The *open box* indicates the coding region of RB cDNA. Using 13 sets of oligonucleotide primers, regions of RB cDNA were amplified into 13 fragments *A–M* by the PCR. Nucleotide lengths of fragments A–M are indicated by *numbers*. *Bars* under the open box indicate the regions amplified. *Arrows* indicate the position of primers for reverse transcriptase reaction

Since the RB gene consists of 27 exons which are located in the region of about 200 kb, analysis of genomic DNA may not be convenient for detection of aberrations. Therefore, we analyzed cDNA obtained by reverse transcriptase reaction of total cellular RNA. The reverse transcription was performed by using several primers of 20 nucleotides and was complementary to appropriate regions of RB mRNA as shown in Fig. 1. The coding sequence of RB cDNA of 2.7 kb was amplified into 13 fragments of 217–371 bp as shown in Fig. 1 A–M by the PCR using 13 sets of primers of 20 deoxynucleotides. As an example, results of the amplified fragments of M containing the nucleotide sequence of exons 24 to 27 from the cell lines are shown in Fig. 2. The results revealed that DNAs from these cell lines did not contain any mutations in the coding region (fragments A–M) of the RB gene. Although the T98G glioblastoma cell line gave a fragment with different mobility, the result was not reproducible under the following conditions; (1) electrophoresis at room temperature in 5% polyacrylamide gel containing 10% glycerol at 40 W, (2) the same condition as (1) except using gel without glycerol, (3) electrophoresis at 4°C in 5% polyacrylamide gel containing 10% glycerol at 30 W, and (4) the same condition as (3) except using gel without glycerol. DNAs from 21 surgical specimens were similarly analyzed by the PCR-SSCP method. However, the results thus far obtained did not show any aberration of the RB gene in these DNAs (data not shown).

Discussion

The PCR-SSCP analysis has been successfully applied to the detection of the loss of one of the RB alleles and of a point mutation in the remaining allele [12]. By using this simple and sensitive method, we analyzed aberrations of the RB gene in human brain tumors. Although an epidemiological observation [6,14] suggested the possible involvement of RB gene aberrations in human

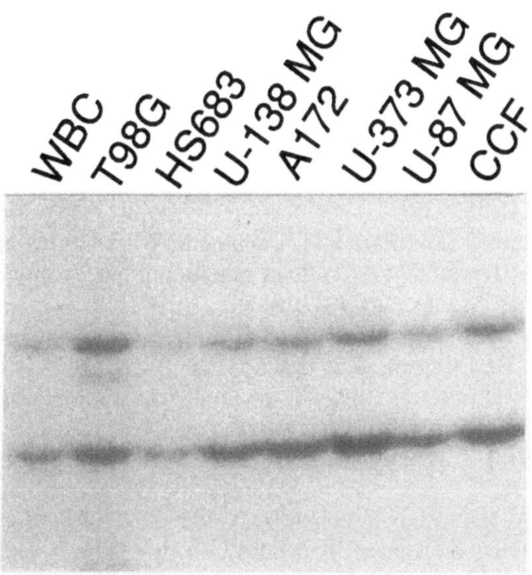

Fig. 2. SSCP analysis of fragment M (exon 24–27). Total cellular RNA isolated from the cultured cells (T98G, U-638MG, U-138MG, A172, U-373MG, U-87MG, and CCF-STTG1) were subjected to reverse transcriptase reaction. The region corresponding to fragment M was amplified by the PCR and the amplified fragments were subjected to SSCP analysis. *WBC*, RNA from normal white blood cells

brain tumors and that the aberrations were found in a variety of human cancers, we could not find any aberrations in the gene in human cell lines of glioblastoma nor in surgical specimens of brain tumors. Therefore, at present, we concluded that involvement of the aberration of the RB gene in the genesis of human brain tumor might not be of much significant, if at all.

Conclusion

We examined the RB gene transcripts in 7 cell lines and 21 surgical specimens of human brain tumor by the PCR-SSCP method. No aberration of the nucleotide sequence of the RB mRNA was observed in the brain tumors analyzed, suggesting infrequent involvement of RB gene mutations in human brain tumor.

References

1. Sparkes RS, Sparkes MC, Wilson MG, Towner JW, Benedict W, Murphree AL, Yunis JJ (1980) Regional assignment of genes for human esterase D and retinoblastoma to chromosome band 13q14. Science 208:1042–1044
2. Friend SH, Bernards R, Rogelj S, Weinberg RA, Rapaport JM, Albert DM, Dryja TP (1986) A human DNA segment with properties of the gene that predisposes to retinoblastoma and osteosarcoma. Nature 323:643–646

3. Friend SH, Horowitz JM, Gerber MR, Wang X-F, Bogenmann E, Li FP, Weinberg RA (1987) Detection of a DNA sequence in retinoblastoma and mesenchymal tumors: Organizations of the sequence and its encoded protein. Proc Natl Acad Sci USA 84:9059–9063
4. Harbour JW, Lai S-L, Whang-Peng J, Gazdar AF, Minna JD, Kaye FJ (1988) Abnormalities in structure and expression of the human retinoblastoma gene in SCLC. Science 241:353–357
5. Horowitz JM, Yandell DW, Park S-H, Canning S, Whyte P, Buchkovich K, Harlow E, Weinberg RA, Dryja TP (1989) Point mutational inactivation of the retinoblastoma antioncogene. Science 243:937–940
6. Sanders BM, Jay M, Draper GJ, Roberts EM (1989) Non-ocular cancer in retinoblastoma patients. Br J Cancer 60:358–365.
7. Knudson AG (1971) Mutation and cancer: Statistical study of retinoblastoma. Proc Nat Acad Sci USA 68:820–823
8. Comings DE (1973) A general theory of carcinogenesis. Proc Nat Acad Sci USA 70:3324–3328
9. Dunn JM, Phillips RA, Zhu X, Becker A, Gallie BL (1989) Mutations in the RB1 gene and their effects on transcription. Mol Cell Biol 9:4596–4604
10. Hayashi K, Orita M, Suzuki Y, Sekiya T (1989) Use of labeled primers in polymerase chain reaction (LP-PCR) for a rapid detection of the product. Nucleic Acids Res 17:3605
11. Orita M, Suzuki Y, Sekiya T, Kenshi H (1989) Rapid and sensitive detection of point mutations and DNA polymorphisms using the polymerase chain reaction. Genomics 5:874–879
12. Murakami Y, Katahira M, Reiko M, Hayashi K, Hirohashi S, Sekiya T (1991) Inactivation of the retinoblastoma gene in a human lung carcinoma cell line detected by single-strand conformation polymorphism analysis of the polymerase chain reaction product of cDNA. Oncogene 6:37–42
13. Kawasaki ES, Clark SS, Coyne MY, Smith SD, Champlin R, Witte ON, McCormick FP (1988) Diagnosis of chronic myeloid and acute lymphocytic leukemias by detection of leukemia-specific mRNA sequences amplified in vitro. Proc Natl Acad Sci USA 85:5698–5702
14. Abramson DH, Elisworth RM, Kitchin FD, Tung G (1984) Second nonocular tumors in retinoblastoma survivors. Ophthalmology 91:1351–1355

Oncogene Expression in Acoustic Neurinomas

Koichi Ichimura[1,3], Kimiyoshi Hirakawa[1], Atsushi Komatsuzaki[2], and Yasuhito Yuasa[3]

Introduction

Recent molecular biological studies have shown the alterations of several oncogenes in various types of primary intracranial neoplasms, such as glioblastomas [1,2], medulloblastomas [3], and meningiomas [4]. However, such studies concerning the oncogene alteration of intracranial neurinomas have not yet been reported, and it is not clear whether or not an oncogene might be involved in the oncogenesis of neurinomas. In this study, we analyzed the alterations of the c-*myc* and *sis* oncogenes in acoustic neurinomas and showed the presence of an enhanced expression of these two oncogenes.

Materials and Methods

Human Tumor Samples

Ten acoustic neurinomas were obtained at surgery. All tumors were unilateral and sporadic. Five of the patients were male and five were female, and their mean age at operation was 48.3 years, (range: 20–78 years). One recurrent tumor was included (NR13, Table 1).

Ribonucleic acid(RNA) Extraction and Northern Blotting

Messenger RNA (mRNA) was extracted from freshly frozen tumor samples by two methods. The first method was a common one described by Sambrook et al. [5], using guanidium-isothiocyanate and cesium chloride gradient. In the second method, mRNA was directly isolated from tissue samples by using the Fast Track mRNA Isolation Kit (Invitrogen, San Diego, CA). Tissues were homogenized and incubated with RNase (ribonuclease)/Protein Degrader at 45°C. Then oligo (dT) cellulose was directly applied to the homogenates after which polyadenylated RNA was eluted. The mRNA isolated by both methods

---

Departments of [1]Neurosurgery, [2]Otorhinolaryngology, and [3]Hygiene and Oncology, Tokyo Medical and Dental University School of Medicine, Bunkyo-Ku, Tokyo, 113 Japan were then electophoresed and transferred to a nylon membrane (Hybond N, Amersham) by capillary elution.

Oncogene Probes

The human c-*myc* oncogene third exon cloned at the EcoRI-Cla I site into plasmid pBR322 (pMCE2), and the viral *sis* (v-*sis*) oncogene cloned at the Pst I site into plasmid pBR322 (p-v-*sis*) were used as oncogene probes. Complementary DNA (cDNA) for mouse α-actin was cloned at the Pst I site of pBR322.

Hybridization and Quantitative Densitometry

Membranes were hybridized and washed at a high stringent condition according to the instructions supplied by the manufacturer of the membrane, and autoradiography was performed. The relative oncogene expression was quantitated by measuring the intensity of the hybridization signals of the oncogene and actin probes with Olympus-Avio Color Image Analyzer SP-500 (Olympus, Tokyo). The oncogene/actin expression ratio was compared to that of nontumorous human brain specimens.

Results

Figure 1 shows the representative results of Northern blot analysis of c-*myc* oncogene expression. The 2.4 kb c-*myc* transcripts were detected in all of the tumors examined. In control nontumorous brain, c-*myc* was also expressed at a low level. According to the densitometric data, relative expression levels of the c-*myc* oncogene were calculated and these are represented in Table 1. The enhanced expression of the c-*myc* oncogene was observed in all of the tumors compared to control brain specimens. Among them, an over fivefold expression was noted in 5 out of 10 acoustic neurinomas. In two acoustic neurinomas, NR10 and NR13, the c-*myc* oncogene was expressed at a value almost as high as HL60, a human leukemic cell line which is known to express c-*myc* oncogene at a high level [6].

The 4.2 kb *sis* transcripts were also detected in all of the samples (data not shown). The *sis* oncogene was moderately to highly expressed in most of the tumors, and 3 acoustic neurinomas showed an over fivefold expression (Table 1). There was no correlation between oncogene expression and various clinical parameters such as the patient's age and sex.

Discussion

We analyzed 10 acoustic neurinomas for alteration of two oncogenes, c-*myc* and *sis*. Our data indicate that both oncogenes were expressed at a higher level in acoustic neurinomas compared to normal brain tissue, and two showed

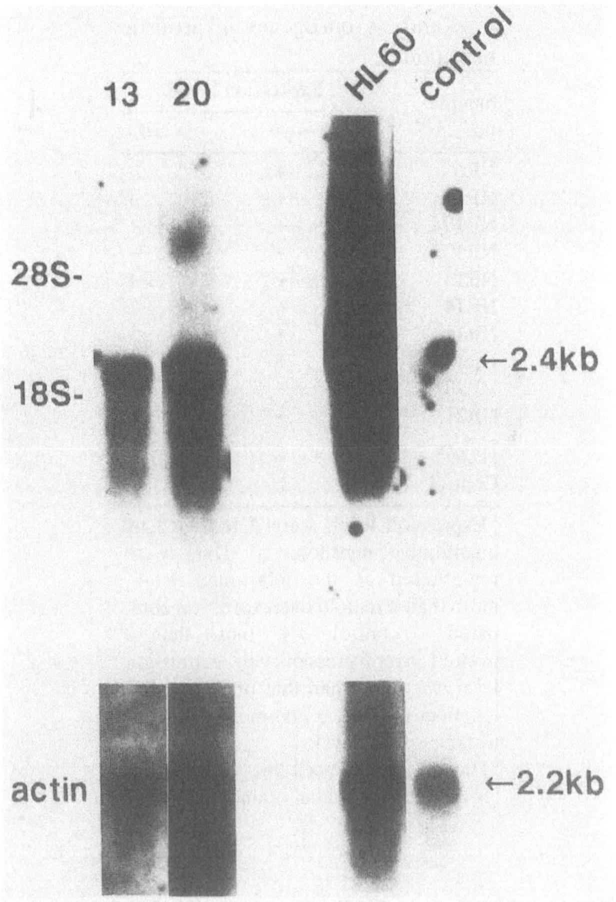

Fig. 1. Northern blot analysis of the c-*myc* oncogene expression in acoustic neurinomas (*top*). The *number* indicated at the top of each lane corresponds to the sample number shown in Table 1. The *HL60* cells are originated from human leukemic cells known to express the c-*myc* gene at a high level; *control* RNA was derived from nontumorous human brain specimen. *28S* and *18S* indicate ribosomal RNA, used as size markers. Membranes were reprobed with α-actin and used as an internal invariant standard (*bottom*)

over-expression of the c-*myc* oncogene, nearly as high as HL60. In the Southern blot analysis, no amplification nor rearrangement of the c-*myc* and *sis* oncogenes was observed in these tumors (data not shown), indicating that the enhanced expression was due to the altered regulation of transcription of these oncogenes.

The alteration of the c-*myc* oncogene has been reported in a broad spectrum of human neoplasms [7]. Although the function of c-*myc* protein has not yet been fully clarified, it is supposed to be associated with cellular DNA replica-

Table 1. Expression levels of the c-*myc* and *sis* oncogenes in acoustic neurinomas

Sample no.	Expression level[a] c-*myc*	*sis*
NR6	+	+
NR9	++	+
NR10	+++	+++
NR12	+	+
NR13	+++	++
NR14	+	++
NR16	+	+
NR17	+	+
VR20	++	+
NR21	+	+
HL60[b]	+++	±
Control[c]	±	±

[a] Expression levels were determined by quantitative densitometry. Data were represented as the following: +++, more than a tenfold overexpression compared to control; ++, more than a fivefold overexpression; +, expression level was more than that of control but less than fivefold; ±, no more than control expression level

[b] Human leukemic cell line

[c] Nontumorous human brain specimen

tion [8]. Enhanced expression of *sis* mRNA has also been observed in a variety of human tumors [9]. The c-*sis* protooncogene encodes the B chain of the platelet-derived growth factor (PDGF) [10], and the cellular transformation induced by the *sis*/PDGF-B gene product may be the result of excessive or inappropriate PDGF-mediated stimulation of growth in PDGF-responsive cell types [11]. Although the number of cases examined are too small to be conclusive, it is likely that elevated expression of the c-*myc* and *sis* oncogenes might be involved in the oncogenesis of intracranial neurinomas.

Acoustic neurinomas have a special association with meningiomas. In an extensive restriction fragments length polymorphism (RFLP) study, loss of heterozygosity on chromosome 22 was reported in both tumors [12,13]. This means that the loss of function of tumor suppressor genes on chromosome 22 might play an important role in the oncogenesis of these tumors. Meningiomas are frequently associated with neurofibromatosis type 2 (NF2) [14]. NF2 is a hereditary disorder of an autosomal dominant type, and is characterized by bilateral occurrence of acoustic neurinomas. Moreover, in a very recent study, it was reported that an enhanced expression of the c-*myc* and *sis* oncogenes without gene amplification was noted in meningiomas [4], as we showed for acoustic neurinomas in this study. Although it has not yet been determined if the neurinoma and meningioma loci are different, these data indicate that there is a kind of common oncogenic mechanism between these two closely related central nervous system tumors. Further molecular biological analyses would clarify the oncogenesis of neurinomas and the relationship between these two intracranial neoplasms.

Conclusion

We analyzed 10 acoustic neurinomas for the alteration of the c-*myc* and *sis* oncogenes. In all of the tumors, both oncogenes were expresses at a higher level compared to normal brain specimens. Among them, an over fivefold expression of the c-*myc* oncogene was noted in 5 acoustic neurinomas, and 3 showed more than a fivefold expression of the *sis* oncogene. It is suggested that the enhanced expression of the c-*myc* and *sis* oncogenes might play an important role in the oncogenesis of acoustic neurinomas.

Acknowledgements. We thank Dr. Shimotohno and the Japanese Cancer Research Resources Bank for the oncogene probes. We are also grateful to the doctors of the Otorhinolaryngology Department of the Tokyo Medical and Dental University School of Medicine for providing tumor samples.

References

1. Libermann TA, Nusbaum HR, Razon N, Kris R, Lax I, Soreq H, Whittle N, Waterfield MD, Ullrich A, Schlessinger J (1985) Amplification, enhanced expression and possible rearrangement of EGF receptor gene in primary human brain tumours of glial origin. Nature 313:144–147
2. Trent J, Meltzer P, Rosenblum M, Harsh G, Kinzler K, Mashal R, Feinberg A, Vogelstein B (1986) Evidence for rearrangement, amplification, and expression of c-*myc* in a human glioblastoma. Proc Natl Acad Sci USA 83:470–473
3. Bigner SH, Friedman HS, Vogelstein B, Oakes WJ, Bigner DD (1990) Amplification of the c-*myc* gene in human medulloblastoma cell lines and xenografts. Cancer Res 50:2347–2350
4. Kazumoto K, Tamura M, Hoshino H, Yuasa Y (1990) Enhanced expression of the *sis* and c-*myc* oncogenes in human meningiomas. J Neurosurg 72:786–791
5. Sambrook J, Fritsch EF, Maniatis T (1989) Molecular cloning, 2nd edn. Cold Spring Harbor, New York
6. Westin EH, Wong-Staal F, Gelmann EP, Favern RD, Papas TS, Lautenberger JA, Eva A, Reddy EP, Tronick SR, Aaronson SA, Gallo RC (1982) Expression of cellular homologues of retroviral *onc* genes in human hematopoietic cells. Proc Natl Acad Sci USA 79:2490–2494
7. Slamon DJ, deKernion JB, Verma IM, Clire MJ (1984) Expression of cellular oncogenes in human malignancies. Science 224:256–262

8. Ariga H, Imamura Y, Iguchi-Ariga SMM (1989) DNA replication origin and transcriptional enhancer in c-*myc* gene share the c-*myc* protein binding sequences. EMBO J 8:4273–4279
9. Eva A, Robbins KC, Andersen PR, Srinivasan A, Tronick SR, Reddy EP, Ellmore NW, Galen AT, Lautenberger JA, Papas TS, Westin EH, Wong-Staal F, Gallo RC, Aaronson SA (1982) Cellular genes analogous to retroviral *onc* genes are transcribed in human tumor cells. Nature 295:116–119
10. Doolittle RF, Hunkapiller MW, Hood LE, Devare SG, Robbins KC, Aaronson SA, Antoniades HN (1983) Simian sarcoma virus *onc* gene, v-*sis*, is derived from the gene (or genes) encoding a platetet-derived growth factor. Science 221:275–277
11. Gazit A, Igarashi H, Chiu I-M, Srinivasan A, Yaniv A, Tronick SR, Robbins KC, Aaronson SA (1984) Expression of the normal human *sis*/PDGF-2 coding sequence induces cellular transformation. Cell 39:89–97
12. Dumanski JP, Carlbom E, Collins VP, Nordenskjöld M (1987) Deletion mapping of a locus on human chromosome 22 involved in the oncogenesis of meningioma. Proc Natl Acad Sci USA 84:9275–9279
13. Seizinger BR, Martuza RL, Gusella JF (1986) Loss of genes on chromosome 22 in tumorigenesis of human acoustic neuroma. Nature 322:644–647
14. National Institutes of Health Consensus Development Conference Statement (1988) Neurofibromatosis. Meeting report. Neurofibromatosis 1:172–178

Enhanced Expression of the c-*myc* Oncogenes in Human Brain Tumors

Kiyoshi Kazumoto[1], Masahiro Matsumoto[1], Junpei Tamada[1], Ichiro Handa[1], Masaru Tamura[2], and Yasuhito Yuasa[3]

Introduction

Recent advances in molecular biology have provided evidence that the pathological expression of the oncogene is related to cell transformation in vitro and malignancy in vivo [1]. Several oncogenes are activated in different nervous system tumors, e.g., the N-*myc* gene in neuroblastomas, the c-*myc* gene [2] and others in malignant gliomas, and the *sis* and c-*myc* genes in meningiomas [3], (reviewed in [4]). Furthermore, alterations of the N-*myc* gene in neuroblastomas are correlated with disease progression and metastasis [5].

C-*myc* is an important oncogene located in cell nuclei and combined with DNA. Its effect on cellular proliferation is of great interest. Overexpression of the c-*myc* oncogene has been reported in a variety of neoplasms. In the central nervous system, the c-*myc* gene is expressed in human glioblastoma [2] and meningioma [3], and amplified in medulloblastoma cells [6].

In 1982, Hassoun et al. described central neurocytoma as a new central nervous tumor of neuronal origin [7]. The genetic foundation for this is still unknown. Therefore, we analysed c-*myc* expression in various brain tumors including central neurocytoma.

Materials and Methods

Tissue Samples

The brain tumor specimens obtained from 11 surgical patients included 5 gliomas (grades II–IV), 1 central neurocytoma, 1 metastasis from lung squamous cell cancer, and 4 meningiomas. The clinical details are summarized in Table 1. Human brain tumor cells transplanted into athymic nude mice

[1] Department of Neurosurgery, Takasaki National Hospital, Takasaki, 370 Japan
[2] Department of Neurosurgery, Gunma University School of Medicine, Maebashi, 371 Japan
[3] Department of Hygiene and Oncology, Tokyo Medical and Dental University School of Medicine, Bunkyo-ku Tokyo, 113 Japan

Table 1. Clinical summary and quantitative densitometry of the c-*myc* oncogene hybridization for brain tumors

Case no.	Sex, Age (years)	#Histopathology	Expression of c-*myc*: c-*myc*/ Actin	Expression of c-*myc*: Tumor/ control
Human brain tumors				
1	F,59	Glioma (grade III)	0.94	7.2
2	F, 4	Glioma (grade II)	0.72	5.5
3	M,62	Glioma (grade III)	0.75	5.8
4	M,50	Glioma (grade III)	0.85	6.5
5	M,35	Glioblastoma	0.80	6.2
6	M,59	Central neurocytoma	0.61	4.7
7	M,63	Metastatic tumor Squamous cell lung cancer	0.73	5.6
8	F,62	Meningioma (M)	0.79	6.1
9	F,47	Meningioma (M)	0.37	2.8
10	F,61	Meningioma (M)	0.26	2.0
11	F,54	Meningioma (P)	1.00	7.7
Tumors transplanted into athymic nude mice				
YAG	(F,66)	Glioblastoma	0.90	6.9
TYG	(F,68)	Glioblastoma	0.25	1.9
NNE	(F, 2)	Ependymoblastoma	0.53	4.1
KNM	(M,69)	Meningioma (A)	0.45	3.5
Control	M,68		0.13	1

Histopathological diagnosis of the meningiomas were classified according to the World Health Organization (1979): *M* meningotheliomatous, *P* psammomatous, *A* anaplastic

(YAG, TYG, NNE, and KNM) were also used. A control nontumorous brain specimen was obtained from a 68-year-old male with a right occipital infarction. HL60 cells, used as a positive control, originated from human promyelocytic leukemic cells with about a 10- to 30-fold amplification of c-*myc* DNA.

Recombinant DNA Probes

The human c-*myc* oncogene third exon cloned at the EcoRI-ClaI site into pBR322 and complementary DNA(cDNA) for mouse α-actin at the PstI site of pBR322 were obtained from Dr. Y. Taya and Dr. K. Shimotohno (National Cancer Center Research Institute), respectively.

RNA Isolation and Northern Blot Hybridization

Total RNA was isolated by the lithium chloride method [8]. Electrophoresis of each sample was performed on horizontal denatured formaldehyde agarose gels with subsequent transfer to nitrocellulose membranes [9]. The membranes were hybridized to ^{32}p-nick-translated DNA probes [10]. The filters were washed at high stringency and then exposed to X-ray film with intensifying screens. After exposure to the film, the filters were washed then reprobed with the actin cDNA probe to determine the amount of RNA present in each lane. The autoradiograms were analyzed by scanning densitometry with an LKB Ultrascan XL and the peaks corresponding to each hybridization signal were integrated to calculate the areas. The relative oncogene expression was quantified by comparing the hybridization peak areas for oncogene probes with those for the actin probe. The oncogene/actin expression ratio for each oncogene was then compared to that of the nontumorous brain specimen.

DNA Isolation and Southern Blot Hybridization

High molecular weight DNAs were isolated from human brain tumors, the nontumorous brain specimen, and HL60 cells [11]. Approximately 20 μg of tumor and nontumor DNAs were digested to completion with the HindIII restriction enzyme, fractionated by agarose gel electrophoresis, transferred to nitrocellulose membranes, and then hybridized to ^{32}p-nick-translated probe DNA.

Results

Expression of the c-myc Oncogene

Increased expression of the c-*myc* gene was detected as a band at 2.7 kb in all human brain tumors (Fig. 1). The increases were from 1.9- to 7.7-fold compared to the control (Table 1). The faint band of the control sample was seen clearly on the overexposed film. The transcripts were the same size as reported for c-*myc* RNA in human cells. No correlation between oncogene expression and parameters including histopathology, age, and sex of the patients was found (Table 1). Intensity differences in the hybridization bands between the lanes, using the actin probe, reflects the different amounts of RNA applied and the degradation of RNA, as demonstrated by ethidium bromide staining of the gel before transfer. No abnormal bands of RNA, e.g., due to DNA rearrangement, were observed for any sample.

Southern Blot Hybridization

A distinct band of the c-*myc* gene at 10.0 kb was observed for all of the tumors and the control sample. The fragment intensities detected by the c-*myc* probe were the same in the tumors, indicating that the tumor DNAs contained the normal number of c-*myc* gene copies. Southern blot hybridization of these brain tumor DNAs with the c-*myc* probe showed neither gene amplification nor rearrangement in any sample.

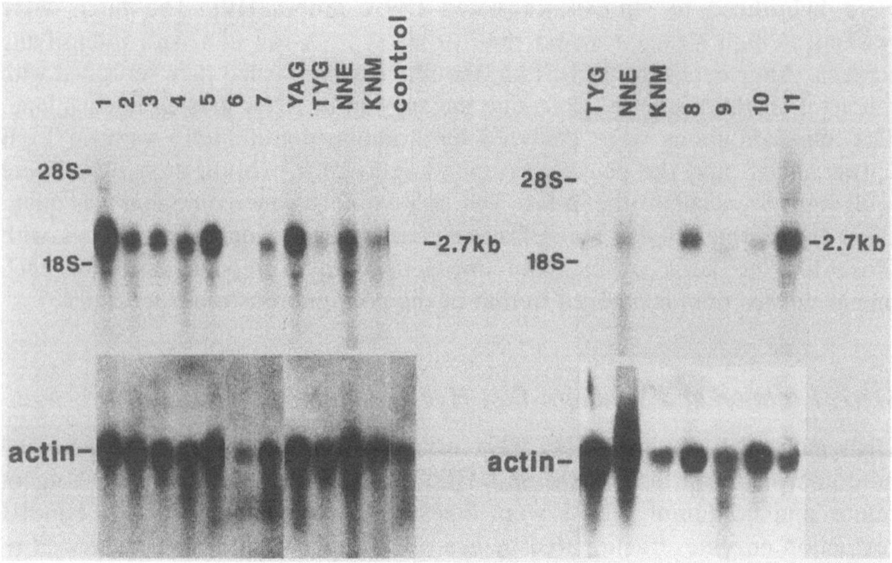

Fig. 1. Expression of the c-*myc* oncogenes in human brain tumors. The c-*myc* specific messenger RNAs were detected by hybridization and autoradiography. Ribosomal RNAs (18S and 28S) were used as markers to estimate the base size. *Numbers 1–7* represent case numbers (see Table 1), *kd* kilobase

Discussion

These results demonstrate the enhanced expression of c-*myc* oncogene in human brain tumors. The c-*myc* gene is associated with a variety of neoplasms such as lymphomas, hepatocellular carcinomas, and glial tumors [2,12]. C-*myc* gene expression was seen in all of the human brain tumors examined when compared with a nontumorous sample. The central neurocytoma sample showed a low c-*myc* gene expression. No oncogene abnormalities in central neurocytoma have previously been reported.

Neither c-*myc* gene amplification nor rearrangement was observed on Southern blot hybridization. Gene amplification is one possible reason for a high level of c-*myc* mRNA. The increased levels of c-*myc* mRNA in HL-60 cells may reflect gene amplification in these cells. However, the c-*myc* gene was not amplified in any of the brain tumors examined. Increased c-*myc* expression not associated with gene amplification was also reported in a Morris hepatoma by Hayashi et al. [12]. Recently, the instability of c-*myc* mRNA (half-time, 10 min) was demonstrated in normal and transformed cells, and a post-transcriptional regulation of the c-*myc* mRNA level by mRNA degradation was proposed [13]. Our results suggest these hypotheses may apply to brain tumors as well.

Usually, the c-*myc* gene alone is not sufficient to induce the full transformation phenotype. In the study of oncogene cooperation in mouse embryo fibroblast, oncogenes were classified into two functional groups (*myc* gene, large T of polyomavirus, etc., and *ras* gene, middle T of polyomavirus, etc.) [14]. Genes from both groups are required to induce the full transformation phenotype. In the two-step (or rather multi-step) carcinogenesis theory, the c-*myc* gene induces 'one step' in the carcinogenesis. Since various brain tumors originating from a glia, neuron, meninx, and bronchial epithelium express the c-*myc* gene, it is probably a common factor in the carcinogenesis and/or tumor proliferation of these brain tumors.

Conclusions

1. The c-*myc* oncogene is expressed in various brain tumors at different levels.
2. The post-transcriptional regulation of the c-*myc* mRNA level by mRNA degradation is likely.
3. C-*myc* expression is not associated with histological malignancy.
4. The c-*myc* oncogene is probably a common factor in the carcinogenesis and/or proliferation of brain tumors.

Acknowledgements. We wish to thank Dr. Y. Ishida for helpful histological diagnoses. This work was supported in part by a Grant-in-Aid for Cancer Reseach from the Ministry of Education, Science and Culture of Japan.

References

1. Marshall C (1985) Human oncogenes. In: Weiss R, Teich N, Varmus H, Coffin J (eds) RNA Tumor Viruses, 2nd edn. Cold Spring Harbor, New York, pp 487–558
2. Trent J, Meltzer P, Rosenblum M. Harsh G, Kinzler K, Mobert R, Feinberg A, Vogelstein B (1986) Evidence for rearrangement, amplification, and expression of c-*myc* in a human glioblastoma. Proc Natl Acad Sci USA 83:470–473
3. Kazumoto K, Tamura M, Hoshino H, Yuasa Y (1990) Enhanced expression of the *sis* and c-*myc* oncogenes in human meningiomas. J Neurosurg 72:786–791
4. Tabuchi K (1988) The cell biological characteristics of brain tumors (in Japanese). No Shinkei Geka 16:919–931
5. Brodeur GH, Seeger RC, Schwab M, Vermus HE, Bishop JM (1984) Amplification of N-*myc* in untreated human neuroblastomas correlated with advanced disease stage. Science 224:1121–1124
6. Friedman HS, Burger PC, Bigner SH, Trojanowski JQ, Brodeur GM, He X, Wikstrand CJ, Kurtzberg J, Berens ME, Halperin EC, Bigner DD (1988) Phenotypic and genotypic analysis of a human medulloblastoma cell line and transplantable xenograft (D341 Med) demonstrating amplification of c-*myc*. Am J Pathol 130:472–484
7. Hassoun J, Gambarelli D, Grisoli F, Pellet W, Salamon G, Pellissier JF, Toga M (1982) Central neurocytoma. An electron-microscopic study of two cases. Acta Neuropathol (Berl) 52:151–156

8. Auffray C, Rougeon F (1980) Purification of mouse immunoglobulin heavy chain messenger RNAs from total myeloma tumor RNA. Eur J Biochem 107:303–314
9. Southern EM (1978) Detection of specific sequences among DNA fragments separated by gel electrophoresis. J Mol Biol 98:503–517
10. Rigby PWJ, Dickmann M, Rhodes C, Berg P (1977) Labeling deoxyribonucleic acid to high specific activity in vitro by nick translation with DNA polymerase 1. J Mol Biol 113:237–251
11. Blin N, Stafford DW (1976) A general method for isolation of high molecular weight DNA from eukaryotes. Nucleic Acid Res 3:2303–2308
12. Hayashi K, Makino R, Sugimura T (1984) Amplification and overexpression of the c-*myc* gene in Morris hepatomas. Jpn J Cancer Res 75:475–478
13. Blanchard JM, Piechaczyk M, Dani C, Chambeard JC, Franchi A, Pouyssegur J, Jeanteur P (1985) C-*myc* gene is transcribed at high rate in Go-arrested fibroblasts and post-transcriptionally regulated in response to growth factors. Nature 317:443–445
14. Land H, Parada F, Weinberg RA (1983) Tumorigenic conversion of primary embryo fibroblasts requires at least two cooperating oncogenes. Nature 304:596–602

Restriction Fragment Length Polymorphism of the L-*myc* Gene and Gene Amplification in Meningiomas

Hideki Kamitani[1], Tomokatsu Hori[2], Satoshi Tanaka[2], Yasuo Hokama[1], Ichiro Okajima[2], Sachio Nomura[3], Kazuko Kawashima[3], and Susumu Nishimura[3]

Introduction

Gene amplification is a particular feature of certain human tumors. Epidermal growth factor receptor (EGFR) [1], c-*erbB2* [2], N-*myc* [3], and c-*myc* [4] are cellular oncogenes that show gene amplification of human tumor tissues of glial origin. The frequency of EGFR gene amplification is high especially in malignant glioma [1,5]. In human meningioma, however, overexpression of cellular oncogenes [6] but not gene amplification is described. In order to observe gene ampification in human meningioma, we analyzed genomic deoxyribonucleic acid (DNA) of tumor tissues with Southern blotting [7].

Restriction fragment length polymorphism (RFLP) of the L-*myc* gene is a useful marker for metastatic potential of human cancer of the lung [8] and kidney [9]. We obtained data on L-*myc* RFLP from 119 patients with brain tumors [10]. Meningioma-related data were selected, and the role of L-*myc* RFLP in human brain tumors was studied.

Material and Methods

Human Meningioma Xenografts and Surgical Specimens

We used 21 specimens which were surgically removed from patients with meningioma: 18 specimens were benign, 2 were malignant, and the remaining tumor was malignant and was propagated in an athymic Balb/3 nude mouse. Table 1 shows their properties. Tumor tissues were stored at −80°C until DNA could be isolated in the usual manner.

Human Oncogene Probe

The probes used to observe gene amplification were EGFR, c-*erbB2*, N-*myc*, and c-*myc* (Japanese Cancer Research Resources Bank, Japan). β-actin DNA (Onco Co., Japan) was used as the control probe.

---

[1] Clinic of Neurosurgery, Nojima Hospital, Kurayoshi, 682 Japan
[2] Division of Neurosurgery, Institute of Neurological Sciences, Tottori University, Faculty of Medicine, Yonago, 683 Japan
[3] Biology Division, National Cancer Center Research Institute, Chuo-ku, Tokyo, 104 Japan

Table 1. Histological subtype of meningiomas examined

Case no.	Histological subtype	Age (years)	Sex
1*	Malignant	38	Male
2	Transitional	47	Female
3	Meningotheliomatous	57	Male
4	Angiomatous	78	Female
5	Meningotheliomatous	60	Male
6	Transitional	69	Female
7	Meningotheliomatous	61	Female
8	Transitional	72	Female
9	Meningotheliomatous	59	Male
10	Malignant	51	Male
11	Fibromatous	21	Male
12	Meningotheliomatous	49	Female
13	Transitional	64	Female
14	Transitional	79	Male
15	Meningotheliomatous	54	Female
16	Unknown	64	Female
17	Fibromatous	58	Female
18	Meningotheliomatous	51	Female
19	Meningotheliomatous	47	Female
20	Malignant	78	Female
21	Psammomatous	65	Female

* Tumor propagated in a nude mouse. The case numbers are the same as in Fig. 1

Southern Blot Analysis

DNA was digested under standard conditions with restriction endonuclease *Eco*RI. An aliquot (about 10 µg) of the digested DNA was subjected to electrophoresis on 0.8% agarose gel. The fractionated DNA was transferred from the gel to a nylon membrane [7]. DNA labeling and hybridization methods followed the procedures described previously [8]. After the hybridization reaction, the filters were washed under conditions of high stringency, and autoradiographed on Kodak XAR-5 film at −80°C using an intensifier screen. The density of the band was measured with a densitometer (Fujiriken Co., Japan).

L-myc RFLP Analysis

With the polymerase chain reaction method [12], we amplified the DNA segment corresponding to the 410-base pair (bp) fragment that has L-*myc* RFLP. Genomic DNA (1 µg) was treated with the same method with 2 units of *Thermus aquaticus* DNA polymerase. The reaction mixture containing 50 pmol each of the primers was subjected to 30 cycles of amplification using a Perkins-Elmer Cetus Thermocycler: 1 min at 94°C, 1 min at 60°C, and 1.5 min at 72°C. Amplified DNA fragments were digested with *Eco*RI, and subjected to electrophoresis on 4% agarose gel.

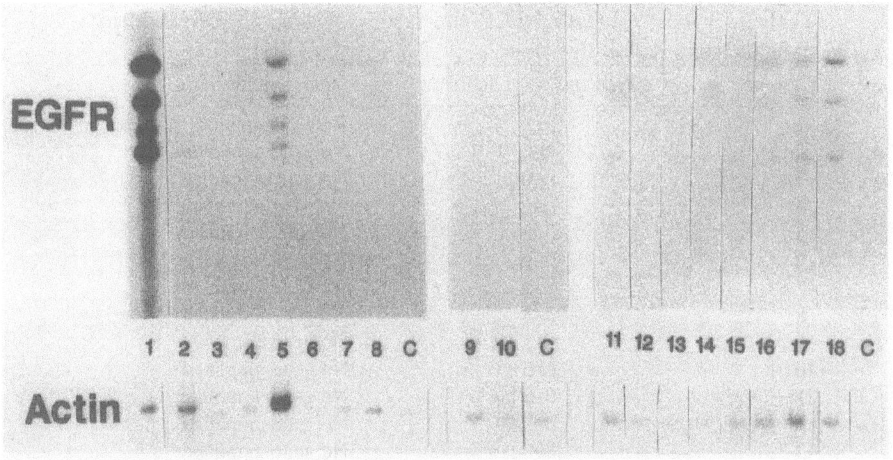

Fig. 1. Gene amplification of EGFR by Southern blot analysis. *Number* of each lane shows case described in Table 1. *C*, DNA from human placenta as a control

Results

*Eco*RI-digested DNA obtained from each patient, except for case 21, was screened by Southern blotting with the 4 above-noted probes. Of the 4 genes screened, EGFR of case 1 showed a 12-fold amplification (Fig. 1), DNA from a human placenta served as control, and c-*erbB2* of case 20 had a 2.5-fold amplification. Both meningiomas were malignant. Patients with meningioma showed typical L-*myc* RFLP patterns (Fig. 2). L-L type patients were homozygous for only the 410-bp fragment corresponding to the 10-kilobase (kb) L-*myc* fragment. S-S type patients were homozygous for 320-bp and 90-bp fragments

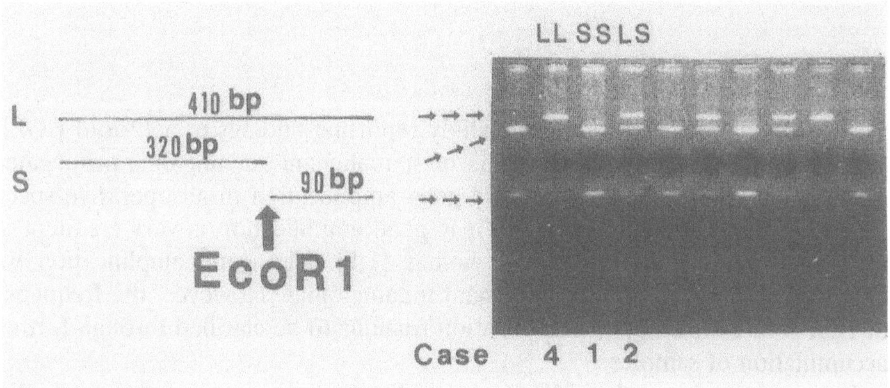

Fig. 2. L-*myc* RFLP of the patients with meningioma. The 4% agarose gel electrophoresis of PCR products after digestion by *Eco*R1 is shown. Cases 1, 2 and 4 indicate S-S, L-S, and L-L, respectively

Table 2. Types of L-*myc* RFLP and results of gene amplification in patients examined in this study

Case no.	Type of L-*myc* RFLP	Gene amplification
1	S–S	EGFR amplified, 12-fold
2	L–S	No gene amplified
3	L–S	No gene amplified
4	L–L	No gene amplified
5	L–S	No gene amplified
6	L–L	No gene amplified
7	S–S	No gene amplified
8	L–S	No gene amplified
9	L–S	No gene amplified
10	L–S	No gene amplified
11	S–S	No gene amplified
12	S–S	No gene amplified
13	S–S	No gene amplified
14	L–L	No gene amplified
15	L–L	No gene amplified
16	S–S	No gene amplified
17	L–S	No gene amplified
18	L–S	No gene amplified
19	L–S	No gene amplified
20	L–L	c-*erbB2* amplified, 2.5-fold
21	L–S	Not determined

corresponding to the 6-kb L-*myc* fragment. L-S type patients were heterozygous for 410-bp, 320-bp, and 90-bp fragments. Table 2 shows the relation between the type of L-*myc* RFLP and gene amplification in the patients examined. Malignancy was not correlated with the type of L-*myc* RFLP. In paitents older than 70 years, however, L-*myc* RFLP showed a tendency of being the L-L type (Fig. 3).

Discussion

To our knowledge, this is the first study reporting findings of a 12-fold EGFR gene amplification in tumor tissues of a malignant meningioma-propagated nude mouse, and a 2.5-fold c-*erbB2* gene amplification in an operative specimen of malignant meningioma. EGFR gene amplification is very frequent in malignant but not in low-grade gliomas [1,5]. The gene amplification we observed was also present in malignant meningiomas. However, the frequency of EGFR or c-*erbB2* gene amplification remains to be clarified through further accumulation of samples.

One study reported that 24% of surgically treated meningiomas bore malignant characteristics (25/105 patients) [12]. When a malignant meningioma relapses, mainly radiation therapy after surgery is currently recommended. A chemotherapeutic modality most valid for this tumor has been vigorously

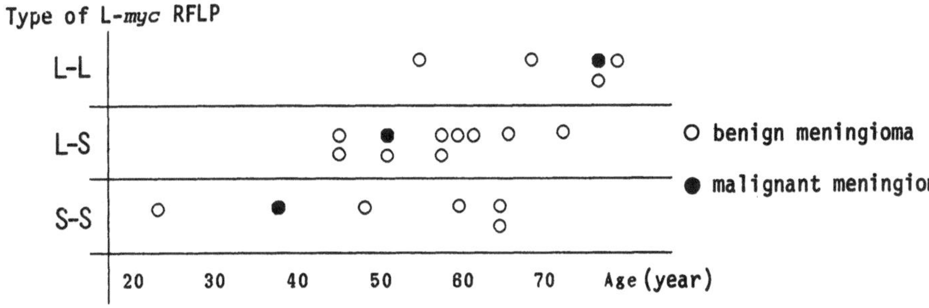

Fig. 3. Age and L-*myc* RFLP in patients with meningioma

studied. The strain of malignant meningioma that was propagated in our nude mouse and that showed EGFR gene amplification can be a good therapeutic model for chemotherapy, since EGFR kinase inhibitors are considered to be good candidates for antiproliferative agents [13].

The L-*myc* RFLP pattern was of the L-L type in 3 out of 4 patients exceeding 70 years of age, whereas many of younger patients had an S allele (Fig. 3). We suppose that persons with the L-L type are likely to have had meningioma when they were younger.

Conclusions

One of the examined 20 meningiomas showed EGFR gene amplification, and another had c-*erbB2* gene amplification. If the strain of malignant meningioma having the 12-fold EGFR amplification is propagated in nude mice, the strain can be a good therapeutical model. Aged patients with meningioma showed a tendency to have the L-L type of L-*myc* RFLP.

References

1. Libermann TA, Nusbaum HR, Razon N, Kris R, Lax I, Soreq H, Whittle N, Waterfield MD, Ullrich A, Schlessinger J (1985) Amplification, enhanced expression and possible rearrangement of EGF receptor gene in primary human brain tumors of glial origin. Nature 313:144–147
2. Yamamoto T (1988) Oncogene of brain tumor (in Japanese). No To Shinkei (Brain and Nerve) 40:817–823
3. Garson JA, McIntyre PG, Kemshead JT (1985) N-*myc* amplification in malignant astrocytoma. Lancet II:718–719
4. Trent J, Meltzer P, Rosenblum M, Harsh G, Kinzler K, Marsh R, Feinberg A, Vogelstein B (1986) Evidence for rearrangement, amplification, and expression of c-*myc* in human glioblastoma. Proc Natl Acad Sci USA 83:470–473
5. Bigner SH, Burger PC, Wong AJ, Werner MH, Hamilton SR, Muhlbaier LH, Vogelstein B, Bigner DD (1988) Gene amplification in malignant human gliomas: Clinical and histopathologic aspects. J Neuropathol Exp Neurol 47:191–205

6. Kazumoto K, Tamura M, Ohye C, Hoshino H, Yuasa Y, Igarashi H (1988) Over-expression of *sis* and c-*myc* genes and rearranged DNA sequences on chromosome 22 in human meningiomas. Proceedings of the 47th annual meeting of the Japanese Cancer Association, Tokyo, p. 217
7. Southern EM (1975) Detection of specific sequences among DNA fragments separated by gel electrophoresis. J Mol Biol 98:503–517
8. Kawashima K, Shikama H, Imoto K, Izawa M, Naruke T, Okabayashi K, Nishimura S (1988) Close correlation between restriction fragment length polymorphism of the L-*MYC* gene and metastasis of human lung cancer to the lymph nodes and other organs. Proc Natl Acad Sci USA 85:2353–2356
9. Kakehi Y, Yoshida O (1989) Restriction fragment length polymorphism of the L-*myc* gene and susceptibility to metastasis in renal cancer patients. Int J Cancer 43:391–394
10. Kamitani H, Nomura S, Hori T, Mita T, Soejima T, Kajiwara H, Kawashima K, Nishimura S (1990) RFLP of the L-*myc* gene in 119 cases of brain tumors. Proceedings of the 49th annual meeting of the Japanese Cancer Association. Tokyo, p. 281
11. Saiki RK, Gelfand DH, Stoffel S, Scharf SJ, Higuchi R, Horn GT, Mullis KB, Erlich HA (1988) Primer-directed enzymatic amplification of DNA with a thermostable DNA polymerase. Science 239:487–491
12. Kojima T, Waga S, Itoh H, Matsubara T, Kuga Y (1990) Clinical analysis of malignant meningiomas. Neurol Surg 18:939–946
13. Yaish P, Gazit A, Gilon C, Levitzki A (1988) Blocking of EGF-dependent cell proliferation by EGF receptor kinase inhibitors. Science 242:933–935

DNA Aneuploid Cells Showing Discrepancy of Expression Between c-*myc* Oncogene Products and GFAP in Malignant Glioma

Nobuyuki Sakai, Keiji Kawamoto, and Hiroshi Matsumura[1]

Introduction

There are various reports on brain tumors in the rapidly developing research on oncogenes which have been noted to be associated with human malignant tumors. We have made an analytical study of the cell growth of brain tumors using flow cytometry (FCM), and further evaluated our results by applying simultaneous double staining using anti c-*myc* or GFAP monoclonal antibodies (MoAb). In the present study we described an interesting finding in the relationship between c-*myc* oncogene products and DNA content in malignant glioma cells obtained at surgery.

Material and Methods

1. Cultured Glioma Cells

A malignant glioma cell line, U-251MG, which was kindly provided by Dr. Jun Yoshida (Nagoya University) was cultured in Dulbecco's modified Eagle's medium (DMEM) supplemented with 10% fetal bovine serum at 37°C in a humidified atmosphere of 5% CO_2. Single-cell suspension in the exponentially growing phase was obtained using 0.25% trypsin to detach adherent cells. The cells were rinsed in phosphate bufferd saline (PBS) and were fixed in 70% cold ethanol overnight.

2. Surgical Materials

Tumor specimens were obtained from 20 patients with malignant gliomas who underwent surgery in our institute from 1988 to 1990. The cells were rinsed immediately after sampling, minced in 0.25% trypsin in order to obtain a single cell suspension, and then fixed in 70% ethanol [1].

[1] Department of Neurosurgery, Kansai Medical University, Moriguchi, 570 Japan

*3. Flow Cytometric Analysis Using the Double Staining Method for the Evaluation of DNA Content and Expression of c-*myc *Oncogene Products and/or GFAP*

The specimens fixed in 70% ethanol were rinsed in PBS and centrifuged for subjection to indirect immunofluorescence staining. Antihuman-c-*myc* mouse monoclonal antibody (Cambridge Co., Ltd., USA) and antihuman-GFAP mouse monoclonal antibody (Dako Co., Ltd., Denmark) were used as the primary antibody. Normal mouse serum, instead of the primary antibody, was used as the negative control. The optimal conditions for reaction had been previously determined using a cell line as described elsewhere [2,3]. The respective concentrations of the primary antibody were 1:40 and 1:50 for c-*myc* oncogene products and GFAP, and the conditions for cultivation were 37°C for 60 min or 4°C overnight. After being rinsed in PBS and centrifuged twice, the cells were reacted with a secondary antibody, fluorescein isothiocynate (FITC)-labeled goat antimouse IgG antibody (Tago Co., Ltd., USA) at the concentration of 1:50 for 40 min in room temperature. Following rinsing in PBS and centrifugation two more times, the cells were subjected to DNA staining using 50 mg/ml propidium iodide (PI). This is the method used for simultaneous double staining which enables us to simultaneously measure the expression of c-*myc* oncogene products and/or GFAP and DNA content. A FACStar (Becton Dickinson Co., Ltd., USA) was used for flow cytometric analysis.

Results

*Double Staining of DNA and c-*myc *Oncogene Products in a Glioma Cell Line*

U-251MG, a glioma cell line, showed a two-peak pattern in the DNA-histogram (Fig. 1, top). The first peak represented the accumulation of the G_0G_1 phase and the second peak the accumulation of G_2M phase. S-phase accumulation was shown between the two peaks. FITC-labeled c-*myc* staining revealed a minor peak of negative cells and a peak of positive cells at the right (Fig. 1, lower left). Most cells were c-*myc* positive. A number of c-*myc* positive cells corresponding to the cells at the G_0G_1 phase were recognized on dot plots, and c-*myc* positive cells equivalent to the cells at the G_2M phase were also present (Fig. 1, lower right).

A Case of Malignant Glioma

1. DNA-histogram with use of PI staining. Three parts of the ridge, periphery, and center were sampled from a specimen of a glioblastoma case and were stained with PI to obtain DNA-histograms. Two peaks were shown near 2C in each histogram, showing DNA aneuploidy pattern (Fig. 2).
2. DNA/GFAP double staining. The horizontal axis represents DNA-histogram by PI staining and the vertical axis shows GFAP staining in Fig. 3. GFAP

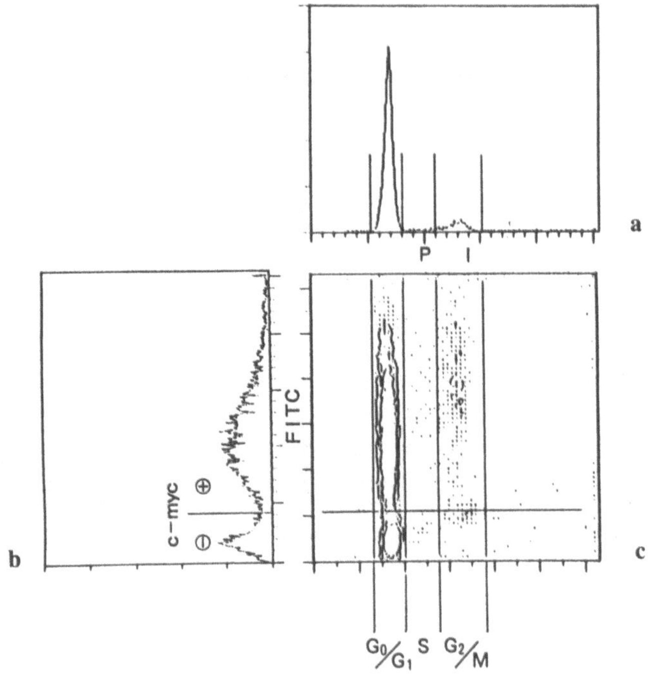

Fig. 1. Double staining of DNA/c-*myc* products in U251MG glioma cell line. **a** DNA histogram obtained by PI staining. **b** Two peaks showing accumulations of c-*myc* positive and c-*myc* negative cells were apparent on the FITC-histogram. **c** A number of c-*myc* positive cells at G_0G_1 phase were present on dot plots

positive cells had two peaks near 2C in the A region. The cells at the first peak of 2C showed a GFAP positive rate of 25.1% and a GFAP negative rate of 12.3% in all of the cells. The positive cell rate was 67.1% at the first peak. At the second peak, positive cell rate was 59.5%. The cells at the first peak were generally composed of blood cells contained in samples, but, in our present

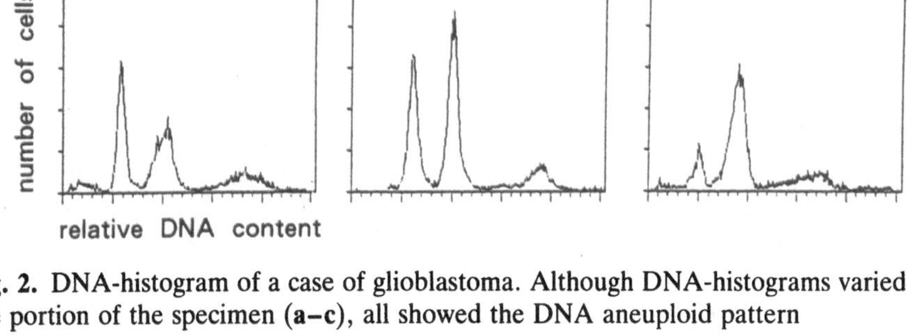

Fig. 2. DNA-histogram of a case of glioblastoma. Although DNA-histograms varied by the portion of the specimen (**a–c**), all showed the DNA aneuploid pattern

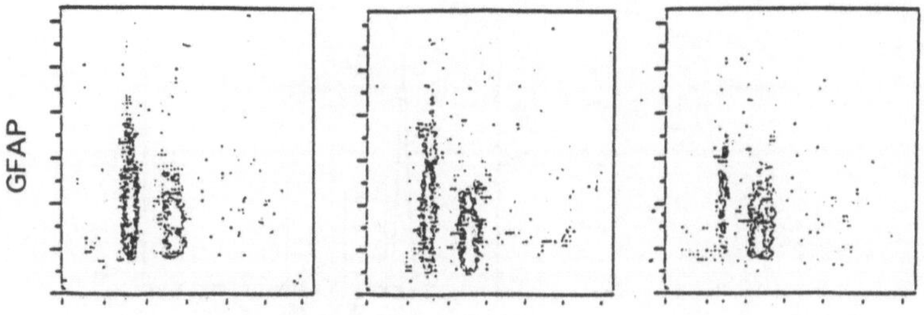

	A			B			C		
	1st peak	2nd peak	total	1st peak	2nd peak	total	1st peak	2nd peak	total
GFAP (+)	25.1	23.8	65.2	24.3	30.6	68.6	9.2	40.5	64.6
(−)	12.3	16.2	34.8	10.2	17.2	31.4	4.6	24.0	35.4
positive%	67.1	59.5	65.2	70.4	63.7	68.6	66.7	62.8	64.6

Fig. 3a–c. GFAP expression in a case of glioblastoma. The GFAP positive rate was lower in the aneuploid peak than in the diploid peak

method, these cells were considered to be glioma cells and the cells at the second peak were also considered to be another different cluster of glioma cells. The B and C regions presented similar results.

3. DNA/c-*myc* double staining. As shown in Fig. 4, c-*myc* positive cells were recognized at the first and second peaks, but the c-*myc* positive rate at the first peak of 2C was 64.6% in the A region, lower than the 71.8% percentage of the second peak of aneuploid cells. Similar results were seen in the B and C regions. Thus, the GFAP-positive rate was lower, while the c-*myc* positive rate was higher in aneuploid cells, compared with the cells of 2C.

Discussion

The number of reports on DNA-ploidy of solid tumors using FCM have been increasing. Kawamoto, et al. described a classification of DNA-ploidy, i.e., diploid, aneuploid and multimodal types using DNA/BrdU double staining [4]. The authors found heterogeneity of gliomas with two different stem lines using PI/c-*myc* double staining in our surgical cases.

With regard to the correlation between *myc* oncogenes and brain tumors, many studies have appeared since the report of N-*myc* proliferation in a 7-year-old patient with a grade III astrocytoma by Garson, et al. [5] in 1985 and others [6,7]. According to the study of m-RNA using dot hybridization by Fujimoto, et al. [8] in 1988, v-*myc* increased in malignant glioma cells and v-*sis* and v-*fos* expressions were observed in benign glioma cells. However, some studies state that c-*myc* oncogene expression increases at some stage of normal brain development [9] or during the regenerative process of liver cells [10].

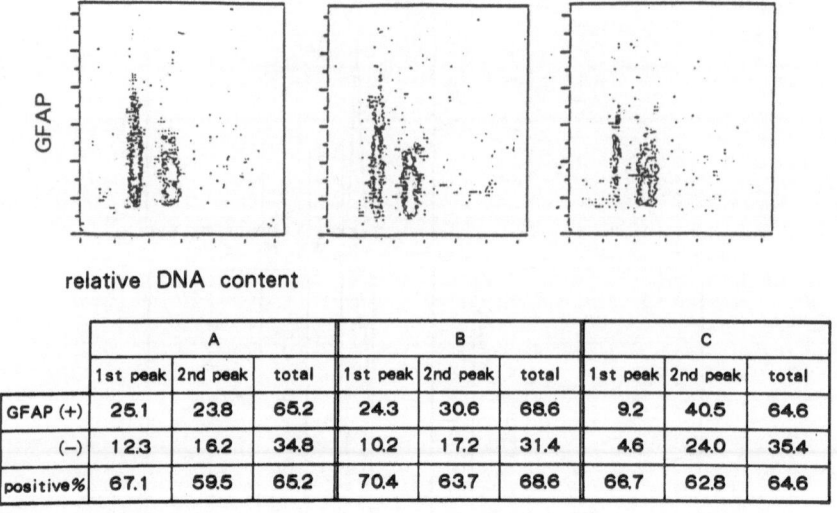

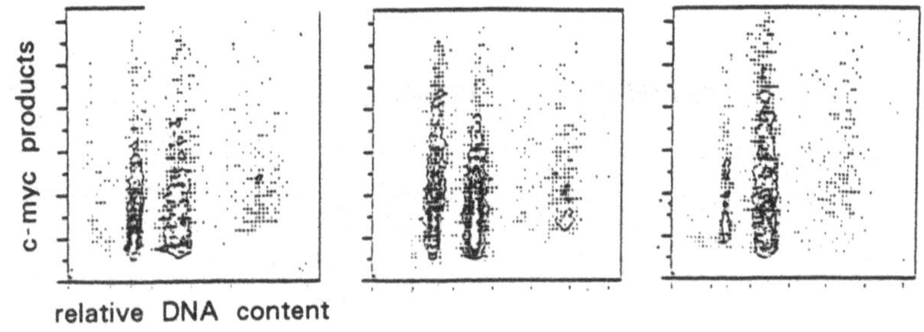

	A			B			C		
	1st peak	2nd peak	total	1st peak	2nd peak	total	1st peak	2nd peak	total
c-myc (+)	24.1	28.8	64.7	23.5	34.7	66.7	8.2	51.8	66.4
(−)	13.2	11.3	35.2	11.0	13.8	33.3	5.3	14.0	33.6
positive %	64.6	71.8	64.7	68.1	71.5	66.7	60.7	78.7	66.4

Fig. 4a–c. The expression of c-*myc* in a case of glioblastoma. The c-*myc* positive rate was higher in the aneuploid peak than in the diploid peak

Flow cytometric analysis of c-*myc* was first reported by Watson et al. [11] in 1985 in ovarian cancer. We described that the rate of c-*myc* expression was about 60% in glioma cell lines [3].

Flow cytometric measurement of the GFAP-positive rate was reported by Kawamoto, et al. [2] in glioma cells using PI-FITC-labeled GFAP double staining. Suzuki, et al. [12] performed a double staining of vimentin and GFAP to evaluate the difference by the degree of differentiation. It was reported that GFAP staining became lower in undifferentiated cells in immunological staining. We found it interesting to note that GFAP positive rate was revealed by flow cytometry to be lower in aneuploid cells than in diploid cells of 2C in glioblastoma cases. The fact that the expression of c-*myc* positive cells in aneuploid cells was higher than that in diploid cells suggested that the expression of oncogenes was higher in aneuploid cells, indicating high carcinogenesis of aneuploid cells. Discrepancy of the expression between GFAP and the c-*myc* oncogene may be a characteristic aspect of glioblastoma. This discrepancy is interesting because it suggests that aneuploid cells are undifferentiated and may potentially play an important role in the growth of tumor cell.

References

1. Sakai N, Kawamoto K, Numa Y, Shoda Y, Matsumura H (1989) Comparison of DNA aneuploidy and histological malignancy in brain tumors. Flow Cytometry 9:37–42

2. Kawamoto K, Inagaki T, Sakai N, Ohuchi M, Yasuda T, Suwa J, Seto Y, Matsumura H (1988) Correlation of the cell cycle of glioma with GFAP staining on flow cytometry, using PI-FITC-labelled GFAP double staining technique. Flow Cytometry 8:48–53
3. Sakai N, Kawamoto K, Matsumura H (1989) Flowcytometric analysis on the expression of c-*myc* products in cultured brain tumors. Neuroimmunol Res 2:183–187
4. Kawamoto K, Sakai N, Imahori T, Matsumura H (1990) Proposal for new classification of DNA-ploidy by flow cytometry. Flow Cytometry 10:124–131
5. Garson JA, McIntyre PG, Kemshed JT (1985) N-*myc* amplification in malignant astrocytoma. Lancet II:718–719
6. Bigner SH, Wong AJ, Mark J, Muhlbaier LH, Kinzler KW, Vogelstein B, Bigner DD (1987) Relationship between gene amplification and chromosomal deviations in malignant human gliomas. Cancer Genet Cytogenet 29:165–170
7. Trent J, Meltzr P, Rosenblum M, Harsh G, Kinzler K, Mashal R, Feinberg A, Vogelstein B (1986) Evidence for rearrangement, amplification, and expression of c-*myc* in a human glioblastoma. Proc Natl Acad Sci USA 83:470–473
8. Fujimoto M, Weaker FJ, Herbert DC, Sharp ZD, Sheridan PJ, Story JL (1988) Expression of three viral oncogenes (v-*sis*, v-*myc*, v-*fos*) in primary human brain tumors of neuroectodermal origin. Neurology 38:289–293
9. Zimmerman KA, Yancopoulus GD, Collum RG, Smith RK, Kohl NE, Denis KA, Nau MM, Witte ON, Toran-Allerand D, Gee CE, Minna JD, Alt FW (1986) Differential expression of c-*myc* family genes during murine development. Nature 319:780–783
10. Goyette M, Petropoonlos CJ, Shank PR, Faust N (1983) Expression of a cellular oncogene during liver regeneration. Science 219:510–517
11. Watson JV, Sikora K, Evan GI (1985) A simultaneous flow cytometric assay for c-*myc* oncoprotein and DNA in nuclei from paraffin embedded material. J Immunol Methods 83:179–192
12. Suzuki C, Nagashima C, Noritake S, Takahama M (1986) Oncobiology of the human brain tumor cells with special reference to the two-color immunofluorescence analysis of Vimentin/GFAP and BUdR labelling with use of flow cytometry. Brain Tumor Pathol 4:69–76

Oncogene Expression in High-Grade Astrocytomas: A Comparative Study of Immunogold-Silver and Peroxidase-Antiperoxidase Immunohistochemistry

SEIICHI YOSHIDA[1], RYUICHI TANAKA[1], and ANDREW H. KAYE[2]

Introduction

The expression products of many oncogenes is known to mediate cell proliferation [1–3], and much interest has been focused upon oncogene expression as a marker for neoplastic phenotypes [4]. Additionally, the level of expression of certain oncogenes in some tumors has been a significant indicator of biological behavior [5]. In this study, we examined the relative efficacy of immunogold-silver (IGS) and peroxidase-antiperoxidase (PAP) immunohistochemistry in detecting the expression product of the epidermal growth factor receptor (EGF-R), c-*myc*, *ras*, and c-*fos* in 20 high-grade astrocytomas.

Materials and Methods

Twenty high-grade astrocytomas (18 glioblastomas multiforme and 2 anaplastic astrocytomas) derived from surgical resections were fixed in 10% neutral buffered formalin, embedded in paraffin, and stained with monoclonal antisera against EGE-R, c-*myc*, *ras* (N-*ras*/c-HA-*ras*), and c-*fos* oncoproteins.

Immunogold-silver (IGS) Staining [6].

Sections of 6 µm thickness were dewaxed in xylene, immersed in Lugol's iodine for 5 min, decolorized in 2.5% sodium thiosulphate, and incubated with 5% egg albumin for 15 min. After incubation with monoclonal antisera against these oncoproteins, at dilutions of 1:400, 1:500, and 1:600 with tris-buffered saline (TBS) for 12 h at 4°C, the sections were reacted with Protein A/gold suspension diluted 1:10 with TBS at 4°C overnight. The sections were then washed in TBS and distilled water and immersed for 3 min in silver development in a dark room. After fixation in 5% sodium thiosulphate for 2 min,

[1] Department of Neurosurgery, Brain Research Institute, Niigata University, Niigata, 951 Japan
[2] Department of Surgery, Melbourne University, Victoria 3050, Australia

they were counterstained with Nuclear Fast Red B and examined by light microscopy.

Peroxidase-Antiperoxidase Staining

Sections of 6 μm thickness were treated with 5% H_2O_2 for 5 min and were then incubated with these monoclonal antisera in the same way. After incubation with unlabeled secondary antibody diluted 1:20 in TBS, they were incubated with rabbit peroxidase anti-peroxidase conjugate for 30 min and reacted with DAB and 0.001% H_20_2 until a brown reaction could be detected.

Assessment of Immunostaining

IGS staining was assessed as positive if silver grains were clearly visible above the background of negative controls and were concentrated in the appropriate cellular compartment, i.e., cell membrane for EGF-R, cell membrane and cytoplasm for *ras* and overlying nuclei for c-*myc* and c-*fos* (Fig. 1a–c). PAP staining was also assessed as positive by the presence of the brown DAB product in the appropriate cellular compartment (Fig. 2a–c).

Results

Both techniques were equivocal in detecting these four oncoproteins at a 1:400 dilution but the IGS technique was more sensitive than the PAP technique at 1:500 and 1:600 dilutions except for the detection of the c-*fos* oncoprotein (Table 1). Expression of EGF-R, c-*myc*, *ras*, and c-*fos* was found in 18, 16, 15,

Table 1. Numbers of tumors showing positive staining

	Oncoprotein 1:400	Antisera 1:500	Dilutions 1:600
EGFR			
IGS	18	17	10
PAP	17	13	7
c-*myc*			
IGS	16	13	7
PAP	16	11	4
ras (N-*ras*/c-Ha-*ras*)			
IGS	15	11	5
PAP	10	8	1
c-*fos*			
IGS	7	7	1
PAP	7	4	2

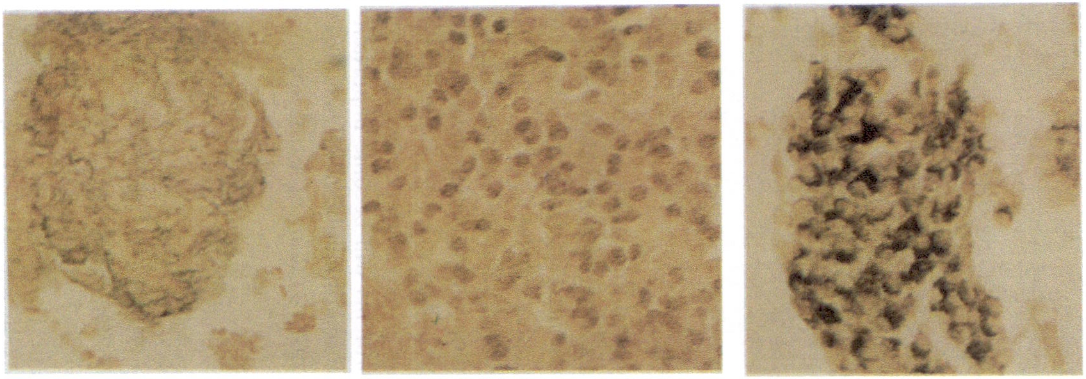

a b c

Fig. 1. **a** Immunogold-silver staining of EGF-R **b** c-*myc*, and **c** *ras* oncoproteins, × 300

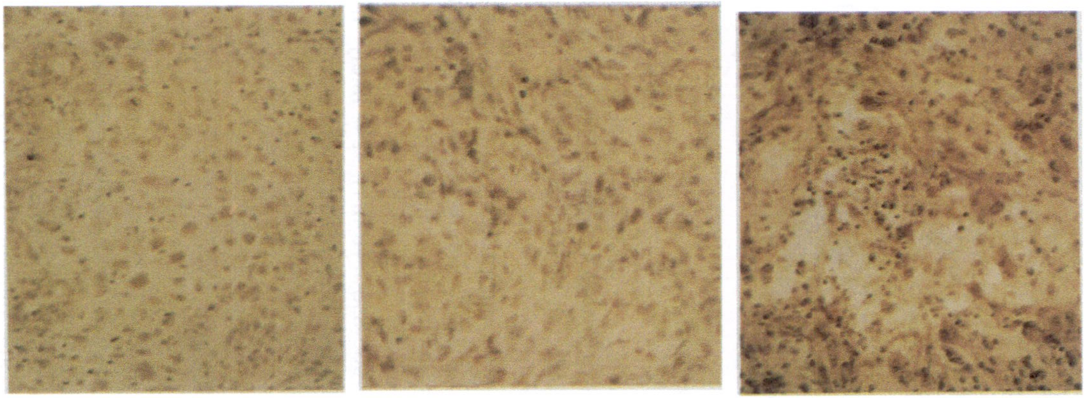

a b c

Fig. 2. **a** Peroxidase staining of EGF-R, **b** c-*myc*, and **c** *ras* oncoproteins, × 300

Table 2. Incidence of expression of each oncoprotein

Oncoprotein	No. of tumors positive by IGS or PAP	%
EGF-R	18	90
c-*myc*	16	80
ras	15	75
c-*fos*	9	35

and 9 tumors, respectively. Table 2 summarizes the patterns of co-expression. Five tumors showed positive for all four oncoproteins. Positive staining for three was seen in 11 tumors, with EGF-R/c-*myc*/*ras* the most frequently observed in four tumors. No tumor showed positive staining for only one oncoprotein.

Discussion

This study has shown that activation of oncogenes in high grade astrocytomas can be detected as immunoreactive oncoproteins in paraffin-embedded tissue by either IGS or PAP immunohisochemistry, and that IGS was more likely to detect low levels of oncoproteins. We also detected immunoreactive EGF-R and c-*myc* oncoproteins in a much greater frequency than in previous studies [7]. Our study has established a profile receptor showing cytoplasmic and nuclear oncogene overexpression in these tumors. This is in keeping with the hypotheses of multistep carcinogenesis [8] and of progression of low-grade to high-grade astrocytomas. It is likely that oncoproteins will become important as markers of neoplastic transformation and that determination of an oncoprotein profile by our methods may allow more accurate grading of astrocytomas.

Conclusions

The relative efficacy of immunogold-silver (IGS) and peroxidase-anti-peroxidase (PAP) immunohistochemistry in detecting oncogene products was compared in 20 high-grade astrocytomas. The two techniques were found to be equivocal in detecting each of the four oncoproteins (EGF-R, *ras*, c-*myc*, c-*fos*) at a 1:400 dilution. However, IGS was more sensitive at 1:500 and 1:600 dilutions. EGF-R, c-*myc*, *ras*, and c-*fos* expressions were detected by either technique at a rate of 90%, 80%, 75%, and 35%, respectively. Five tumors co-expressed all four oncoproteins, 11 tumors co-expressed three oncoproteins with EGF-R/c-*myc*/*ras*, and four tumors co-expressed two oncoproteins. We concluded that IGS is more sensitive than PAP for detecting the expression products of these oncogenes.

References

1. Hermansson M, Nister M, Betsholtz C, et al. (1988) Endothelial cell hyperplasia in human glioblastoma: Coexpression of mRNA for platelet-derived growth factor B chain and PDGF receptor suggests autocrine growth stimilation. Proc Natl Acad Sci USA 85:7748–7752
2. Libermann TA, Razon AD, Bartal Y, et al. (1984) Expression of epidermal growth factor receptors in human brain tumors. Cancer Res 44:753–760
3. Moelling KB, Heimann N, Beimling P, et al. (1984) Serine and threonine-specific protein kinase activities of purified gag-mil and gag-raf proteins. Nature 312:558–561
4. Thompson TC, Southgate J, Kitchener G, Land H (1989) Multistage carcinogenesis induced by *ras* and c-*myc* oncogenes in a reconstituted organ. Cell 56:917–930
5. Brodeur GM, Seeger RC, Shwab M, Varmus HE, et al. (1985) Amplification of the N-*myc* sequences in primary human neuroblastomas: Correlation with advanced disease stage. Prog Clin Biol Res 175:105–113
6. Holgate CS, Jackson P, Cowen PN, et al. (1983) Immunogold silver staining: A new method of immunostaining with enhanced sensitivity. J Histochem Cytochem 31:983–984
7. Filimus J, Pollak MN, Cairncross JG, et al. (1985) Amplified, overexpressed and rearranged epidermal growth factor receptor gene in a human astrocytoma cell line. Biochem Biophys Res Commun 131:207–215
8. Weinberg RA (1989) Oncogenes, antioncogenes and the molecular basis of multistep carcinogenesis. Cancer Res 49:3713–3721

Chromosomes and Clinical Features in 6 Cases of Gliomas

Takashi Houri[1], Norihiro Ibayashi[1], Masahito Fujimoto[1], Satoshi Ueda[1], Johji Inazawa[2], and Tatsuo Abe[2]

Introduction

Several characteristic and specific chromosomal changes have been observed in human solid tumors [1]. It has been assumed that these aberrations are involved in the processes of initiation and progression of the tumor. In glioblastoma, numerical and structural chromosomal abnormalities have been reported, such as gains of chromosome 7, losses of chromosome 10, structural abnormalities of chromosome 9, and double minute chromosomes (dmin) [2]. Cytogenetic analysis of the initial and recurrent tumor tissues of malignant gliomas has provided information regarding the specific and multistep chromosomal changes during initiation and progression of the lesions [3].

The following is a report on the results obtained from a cytogenetic analysis of 6 gliomas and a discussion on the correlations between chromosomal abnormalities and the development of malignant gliomas.

Materials and Methods

A chromosomal analysis was performed on 6 patients with cerebral gliomas consisting of 1 astrocytoma (case 1), 2 anaplastic astrocytomas (cases 2 and 6), and 3 glioblastomas (cases 3, 4, and 5). These patients were surgically treated at Kyoto Prefectural University Hospital between October, 1986 and September, 1989. The 2 glioblastoma cases (cases 4 and 5) were examined only in the recurrent states. Karyotypic evaluations between the initial and recurrent states were examined in case 3.

Sterile tumor tissues were obtained from the operating room and finely minced in the culture medium. The cell suspension was cultured in humidified 5% CO_2 in air at 37°C in Ham'F-10 medium supplemented with 20% fetal bovine serum. After short- or long-term tissue culture, the tumor cells were harvested for chromosomal preparations. Colcemid (0.02 μg/ml culture medium) was added for 3 h before harvesting. After hypotonic treatment for 30 min using 0.075 M KCl, the cells were fixed with 3:1 methanol/acetic acid. Air-dried

Departments of [1]Neurosurgery and [2]Hygiene, Kyoto Prefectural University of Medicine, Kyoto, 602 Japan slides were prepared for GTG and/or QFQ banding [4]. GTG-banded metaphase cells were examined and well-spread metaphase cells were photographed and analyzed. Modal numbers were determined by counting all well-spread metaphases in each preparation. In addition, specimens of chromosomes from each case were simply stained with 5% Giemsa solution, and observed for the possible presence and/or the precise number of dmin. The karyotypes were arranged according to the International System for Human Cytogenetic Nomenclature (1985) scheme [5].

Results

A summary of the clinical, histopathological, and cytogenetic data of all of the patients in this study is presented in Table 1.

Case 1 (astrocytoma) showed a normal male karyotype. The numbers of the chromosomes ranged within the near-diploid region in cases 2, 4, and in the initial state of case 3, and others, including the recurrent state of case 3, ranged within the near-triploid region. The detailed structural abnormalities of the chromosomes in all of the 6 cases are shown in Table 1. The chromosomes most frequently involved in structural rearrangements were 2, 3, 7, 9, 12, and 14. Interstitial deletion of chromosome 14, del(14)(q22q32), was observed in the recurrent state of case 3, as well as in case 6 which was not recurrent. In both the initial and recurrent glioblastoma tissues of case 3, an identical marker chromosome, t(3;15)(p21;q22), was observed, although several chromosomal aberrations were found to be increased in the recurrent tumor (Fig. 1). One case (case 4) contained homogeneously staining regions (HSR) on the long arm of chromosome 9 (Fig. 1), and 3 cases (the recurrent state of case 3 and cases 5 and 6) had dmin. There was a wide range in the size and number of dmin demonstrated among the tumors (Fig. 2).

Discussion

Previous reports on the cytogenetic analysis of gliomas have suggested that these tumors frequently show structural abnormalities involving chromosomes 1, 7, 9, 11, and 19, and numerical abnormalities involving chromosomes 1, 6, 7, 10, 22, and Y [2,6]. In our 6 cases, chromosomes 7 and 9 were also frequently involved in structural rearrangements, although each breaking point was different. Interstitial deletion of chromosome 14, del(14)(q22q32), was observed in the recurrent state of case 3, and also in case 6. Survival was extremely short in these 2 cases, suggesting that the del(14)(q22q32) may be associated with the rapid progression of these tumors. In addition, case 3 revealed common structural chromosomal abnormality of t(3;15)(p21;q22) in both initial and recurrent tumor tissues. These results suggest that the genetic alterations caused by t(3;15)(p21;q22) might have played an important role in the tumorigenesis of case 3.

Recently, cytogenetic and restriction fragment length polymorphism (RFLP) studies have shown that allelic deletions of chromosomes 10 and 17p occur in at

Table 1. Summary of the clinical, histopathological, and cytogenetic data of the 6 examined cases

Case	Age (year) and sex	Tumor location	Postop. survival (months)	Diagnosis	Type of culture (passages)	No. of Karyotypes	No. of metaphases analyzed	Modal no.	Market chromosomes	HSR	dimn
1.	38 M	R. Frontal	Alive (13)	Astrocytoma	1–3	6	29	46	(46XY)*	(−)	(−)
2.	11 M	L. Temporal	Alive (14)	Anaplastic astrocytoma	1–4	7	53	46	a. der(7)t(7;?) (p11.2;?), der(12)t(7;12) (p11.2;p11.2) der(12)t(12;?)(p13;?) b. der(12)t(9;12)(q22.3;q24.3)	(−)	(−)
3.	70 F	R. Parietal	30	Glioblastoma	0–3	9	24	43	*t(3;15)(p21;q22)*	(−)	(−)
	72 F	R. Parietal	6	Glioblastoma (recurrence)	10–15	24	58	68	del(2)(q13q37), der(2)t(2;?)(p11;?) *t(3;15)(q21;q22)*, der(9)t(2;9)(p11.2;p11) del(14)(q22q32), der(19)t(19;?)(q13.1;?)	(−)	(+)
4.	47 F	L. Temporal	12	Glioblastoma (recurrence)	1	4	10	47	der(1)t(1;?)(p36;?) der(9)t(9;HSR;?)(q11.2;HSR;?)	(+)	(−)
5.	33 F	R. Frontal	11	Glioblastoma (recurrence)	Overnight culture	8	34	80	der(3)t(3;?)(p25;?), der(4)t(4;?)(q31;?) del(4)(q31q35), der(8)t(8;?)(q24;?) del(11)(q21q23), der(12)t(12;?)(p11;?) der(13)t(13;?)(q32;?), der(15)t(15;?)(q22;?) del(X)(q22q25)	(−)	(+)
6.	37 F	L. Temporal	1	Anaplastic astrocytoma	15–20	9	21	71	a. t(2;12)(p11.1;p11.2), ins(3)t(3;?)(q21;?) *t(7;10)(q11;q11)*, der(9)t(9;?)(p12;?) der(9)t(3;9)(q21;q34), del(11)(p11.1p15.5) del(16)(q22q24) b. *t(7;10)(q11;q11)*, del(14)(q22q32) der(18)t(18;?)(q23;?)	(−)	(+)

Two clonal abnormalities indicate *a*. and *b*.
*Normal stemline; *Postop*., postoperative; *R*. right; *L*. left

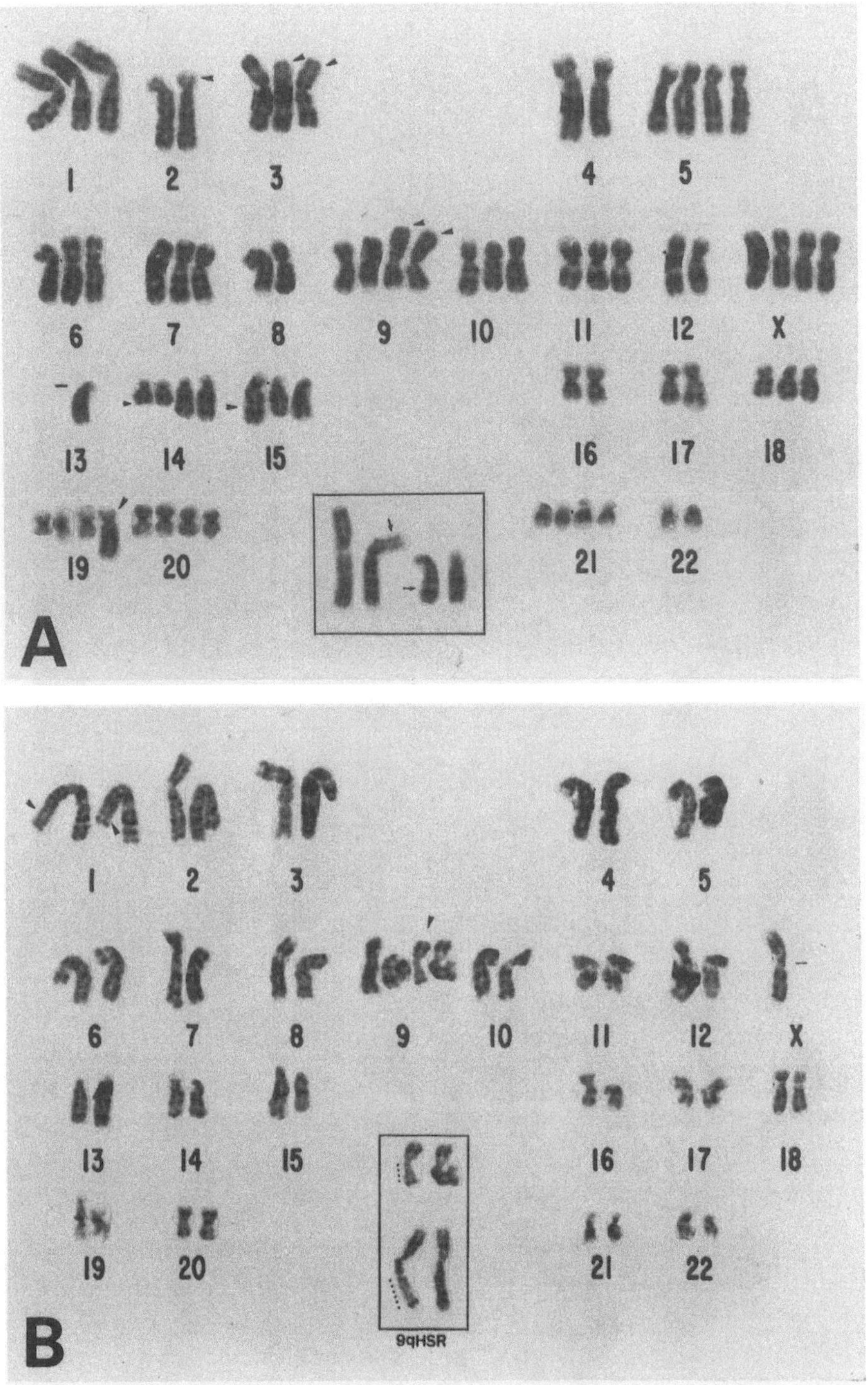

Fig. 1. A A representative karyotype in the recurrent state of case 3. *Arrowheads* indicate rearranged chromosomes. The *inset* is the partial karyotype of t(3;15)(p21;q22). **B** A representative karyotype in case 4. *Arrowheads* indicate rearrenged chromosomes. The *inset* is the homogeneously staining region (HSR) on the long arm of chromosome 9

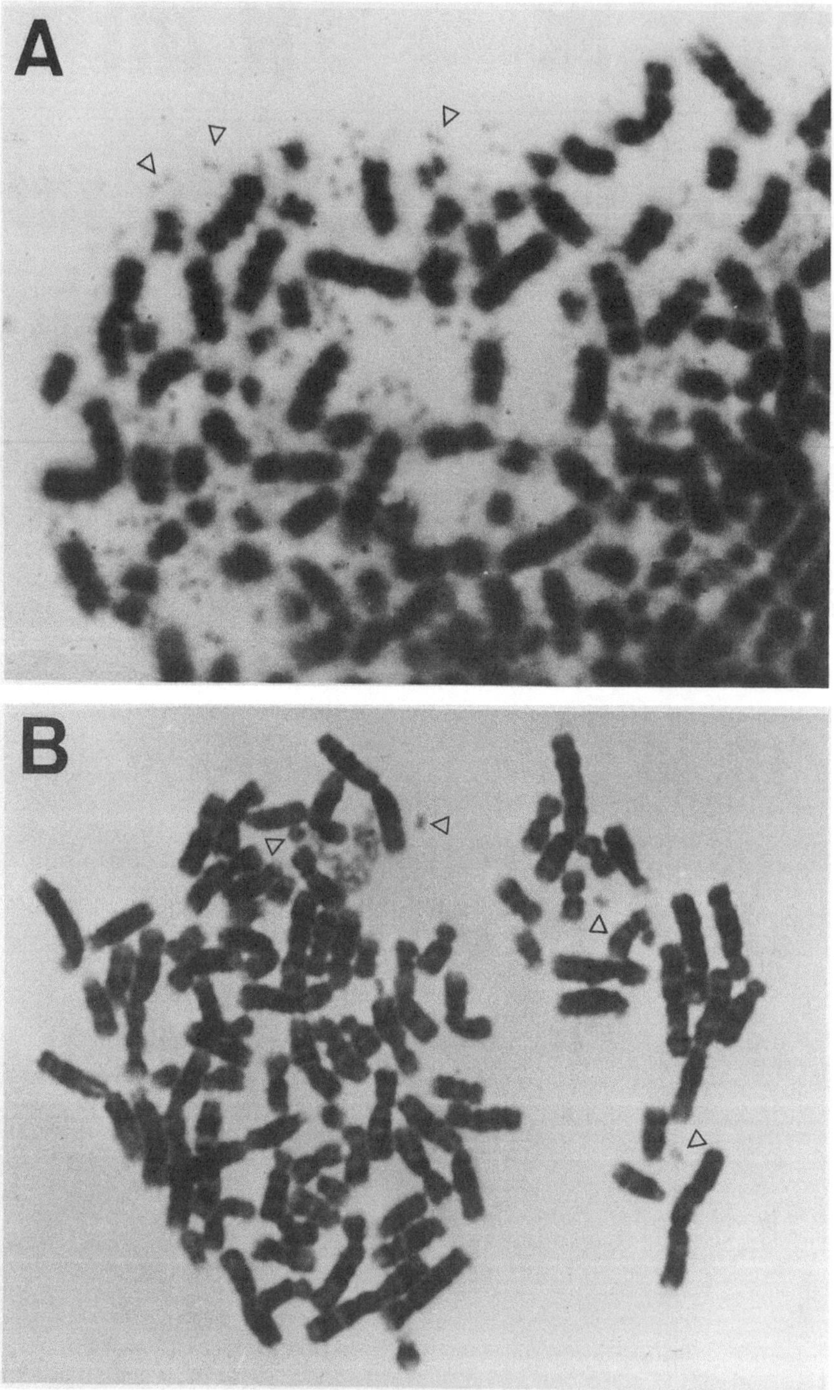

Fig. 2. **A** Partial metaphase spread in case 5 and **B** 6. The several numbers of dmin are shown (*arrowheads*). The number of dmin varied widely in each cell

least 35% of malignant human astrocytomas [7–11]. Nigro et al. reported point mutations of the p53 gene in 4 malignant gliomas with a loss of heterozygosity for chromosome 17p [12]. However, our cytogenetic studies of 6 gliomas revealed that none of the morphological deletions were detected in chromosomes 10 and 17p.

Among the 6 gliomas we examined, either dmin or HSR were observed in 4 cases (cases 3, 4, 5, and 6) with recurrent or rapidly progressive tumors. Bigner et al. reported that dmin was detected in 18 out of 32 near-diploid malignant gliomas, but HSR were not observed [2]. HSR in malignant human gliomas have not been reported thus far [3], although HSR and dmin are well known to be cytogenetic forms of gene amplification [13–15]. In malignant gliomas, specific gene amplifications have been reported, such as N-*myc*, *gli*, and the epidermal growth factor receptor (EGFR) gene [16–19]. It is suggested that the presence of these amplifications is correlated with the recurrence and rapid progression of tumors.

It would be interesting to study the possible gene amplification in our 4 gliomas showing dmin or HSR by Southern hybridization analysis and in situ hybridization.

Conclusion

1. In the 6 gliomas we examined, chromosomes 2, 3, 7, 9, 12, and 14 were frequently involved in structural chromosomal abnormalities. However, neither loss nor deletion of chromosomes 10 and 17p were observed in these cases.
2. In one glioblastoma, t(3;15)(p21;q22) was detected both in the initial and recurrent tumor cells, suggesting that the cytogenetic abnormality plays a pivotal role in the pathogeneis.
3. Four recurrent or rapidly progressive tumor cells contained either dmin or HSR, which are cytogenetic forms of gene amplification.

Acknowledgements. The authors thank Miss Yoko Yamane for technical advice. This investigation was supported in part by Grants-in-Aid for Scientific Research from the Ministry of Education, Science and Culture of Japan (No. 01480360).

References

1. Sandberg AA, Turc-Carel C, Gemmill RM (1988) Chromosomes in solid tumor and beyond. Cancer Res 48:1049–1059
2. Bigner SH, Mark J, Burger PC, Mahaley MS, Bullard DE Jr, Muhlbaier LH, Bigner DD (1988) Specific chromosomal abnormalities in malignant human gliomas. Cancer Res 88:405–411
3. Bigner SH, Wong AJ, Mark J, Muhlbaier LH, Kinzler KW, Vogelstein B, Bigner DD (1987) Relationship between gene amplification and chromosomal deviations in malignant human gliomas. Cancer Genet Cytogenet 29:165–170

4. Verma RS, Babu A (1989) Human chromosome: Manual of basic techniques. Pergamon, New York, pp 4–113
5. Harnden DG, Klinger HP (eds) (1985) ISCN. An international system for human cytogenetic nomenclature. S. Karger, Base 1
6. Jenkins RB, Kimmel DW, Moertel CA, Schultz CG, Scheithauer BW, Kelly PJ, Dewald GW (1989) A cytogenetic study of 53 human gliomas. Cancer Genet Cytogenet 39:253–279
7. Cavenee WK, Scrable HJ, James CD (1989) Molecular genetics of human cancer predisposition and progression. In: Cavenee WK, Hastie ND, Stanbridge EJ (eds) Current communications in molecular biology: Recessive oncogenes and tumor suppression. Cold Spring Harbor, New York, pp 67–72
8. James CD, Carlbom E, Dumanski JP, Hansen M, Nordenskjold M, Collins VP, Cavenee WK (1988) Clonal genomic alterations in glioma malignancy stages. Cancer Res 48:5546–5551
9. Fujimoto M, Fults DW, Thomas GA, Nakamura Y, Heilbrun MP, White R, Story JL, Naylor SL, Kagan-Hallet KS, Sheridan PJ (1989) Loss of heterozygosity on chromosome 10 in human glioblastoma multiforme. Genomics 4:210–214
10. El-Azouzi M, Chung RY, Farmer GE, Martuza RL, Black PM, Rouleau GA, Hettlich C, Hedley-Whyte ET, Zervas NT, Panagopoulos K, Nakamura Y, Gusella JF, Seizinger BR (1989) Loss of distinct regions on the short arm of chromosome 17 associated with tumorigenesis of human astrocytomas. Proc Natl Acad Sci USA 86:7186–7190
11. Fults D, Pedone CA, Thomas GA, White R (1990) Allelotype of human malignant astrocytoma. Cancer Res 50: 5784–5789
12. Nigro JM, Baker SJ, Preisinger AC, Jessup JM, Hostetter R, Cleary K, Bigner SH, Davidson N, Baylin S, Devilee P, Glover T, Collins FS, Weston A, Modali R, Harris CC, Vogelstein B (1989) Mutations in the p53 gene occur in diverse human tumor types. Nature 342:705–708
13. Schimke RT (1984) Gene amplification in cultured animal cells. Cell 37:705–713
14. Lin CC, Alitalo K, Schwab M, George D, Varmus HE, Biship JM (1985) Evolution of karyotypic abnormalities and c-*myc* oncogene amplification in human colonic carcinoma cell lines. Chromosoma 92:11–15
15. Nunberg JH, Kaufman RJ, Schimke RT, Urlaub G, Chasin LA (1978) Amplified dihydrofolate reductase genes are localized to a homogeneously staining of a single chromosomes in methotrexate-resistant Chinese hamster ovary cell line. Proc Natl Acad Sci USA 75:5553–5556
16. Libermann TA, Nusbaum HR, Rozon N, Kris R, Lax I, Soreq H, Whittle N, Waterfield MD, Ullrich A, Schlessinger J (1985) Amplification, enhanced expression and possible rearrangement of EGF receptor gene in primary human brain tumours of glial orgin. Nature 313:144–147
17. Kinzler KW, Bigner SH, Bigner DD, Trent JM, Low ML, O'Brien SJ, Wong AJ, Vogelstein B (1987) Identification of an amplified, highly expressed gene in a human glioma. Science 236:70–73
18. Wong AJ, Bigner SH, Bigner DD, Kinzler KW, Hamilton SR, Vogelstein B (1987) Increased expression of the epidermal growth factor receptor gene in malignant gliomas is invariably associated with gene amplification. Proc Natl Acad Sci USA 84:6899–6903
19. Fujimoto M, Sheridan PJ, Sharp ZD, Weaker FJ, Kagan-Hallet KS, Story JL (1989) Proto-oncogene analyses in brain tumors. J Neurosurg 70:910–915

Section 6. Basic Studies in Brain Tumor Biology and Therapy

The Influence of MHC Class I Expression on the Growth of a Glioblastoma Cell Line

NOBUAKI MOMOZAKI[1], KAZUO TABUCHI[1], MAMORU OH-UCHIDA[2], KIYONOBU IKEZAKI[1], TATSUMI HIROTSU[1], and KATSUJI HORI[2]

Introduction

MHC class I complex genes constitute a highly polymorphic gene family which encodes transmembrane glycoproteins. They consist of a 45,000 dalton integral membrane protein noncovalently associated with the 12,000 dalton polypeptide, β_2 microglobulin. MHC class I complex molecules appear to play an essential role in the presentation of tumor-specific antigens to the host's immune system (reviewed in [1]). Recently, other roles of MHC class I have been documented, such as signal transduction and glucose transport. In the present experiment, we examined the influence of MHC class I expression on the growth of human glioma cells. We constructed a dexamethasone-inducible mouse MHC class I and introduced it into a human glioblastoma cell. Using this dexamethasone-inducible MHC class I-glioblastoma cell system, the influence of the expression of mouse MHC class I on anchorage-independent cell growth was compared between MHC class I expressing and non-expressing states.

Materials and Methods

Construction of the Plasmid H-2L^d *with a MMTV Promoter*

The mouse MHC class I (*H-2L^d*) gene was obtained from plasmid pL^{d}4 [2] and the MMTV promoter was obtained from MMTV plasmid. The expression vector, pMMTV-L^d plasmid, was constructed by linking *H-2L^d* to the MMTV promoter at the 5′ non-coding sequences. The MMTV promoter is known to be inducible in the presence of dexamethasone. The pSV2-neo is the neomycin resistant gene.

Cell Culture and DNA Transfection

Human glioblastoma KMG4 cells were grown in Dulbecco's modified Eagle's medium (DMEM) with 10% fetal bovine serum (FBS) in a humidified atmos-

Departments of [1]Neurosurgery and [2]Biochemistry, Saga Medical School, Saga, 849 Japan phere of 5% CO_2 at 37°C. Fresh monolayers of KMG4 cells in 10-cm plates were transfected with 20 µg pMMTV-L^d and 1 µg of pSV2-neo by the calcium phosphate precipitation technique [3]. Transformed cells were selected as neomycin-resistant clones in a selective medium containing 400 µg/ml G418 (neomycin, GIFCO). Neomycin-resistant clones were established when they increased sufficiently in number to extract total RNA for Northern blot analysis and further experiments.

Northern Blot Analysis

Total RNA was extracted by the guanidinium/hot phenol method [4]. Twenty µg total RNA from each proliferating cells was separated by electrophoresis in 1% agarose-formaldehyde gel and transfected to a nylon membrane [5]. The filters were hybridized with a ^{32}P-labeled probe (*H-2L^d*), and the filters were washed and exposed to Kodak XAR-5 film.

Immunohistochemistry

In order to examine the expression of exogenously introduced mouse MHC class I gene expression on them, the cells were immunohistochemically examined with mouse *H-2L^d*-specific monoclonal antibody.

Anchorage-Independent Growth Analysis

The colony-forming ability in soft agar was estimated according to Carney et al. [6]. Cells were trypsinized to single-cell suspension and mixed with 0.3% agar (Bactoagar, Difco) in DMEM plus 10% FBS to a final concentration of 10^3 cells per ml. One milliliter of this suspension was layered in 10-cm culture dishes containing a base of 0.5% agar in DMEM plus 10% FBS in the presence (final concentration: 2 µM) or absence of dexamethasone. Agar plates were incubated in 5% CO_2/95% air at 37°C. Colonies were scored after 2 weeks.

Results

Transfection and Expression of H-2L^d *with MMTV Promoter in KMG4 Human Glioblastoma Cells*

The constructed expression vector of MHC class I, the plasmid pMMTV-L^d, and the pSV2-neo gene as selectable marker were cotransfected into the KMG4 cells. In addition to the parental cell line, the KMG-neo clone (KMG4 transfected with pSV2-neo only) and the KMG4-MMTV-L^d clone (KMG4 transfected with MMTV-Ld and pSV2-neo) were obtained.

Figure 1 represents the results of the Northern blot analysis in each cell line. Parental KMG4 exhibited no hybridization signal of mouse *H-2L^d* or human *HLA-B7* (data not shown) regardless of the presence or absence of dexametha-

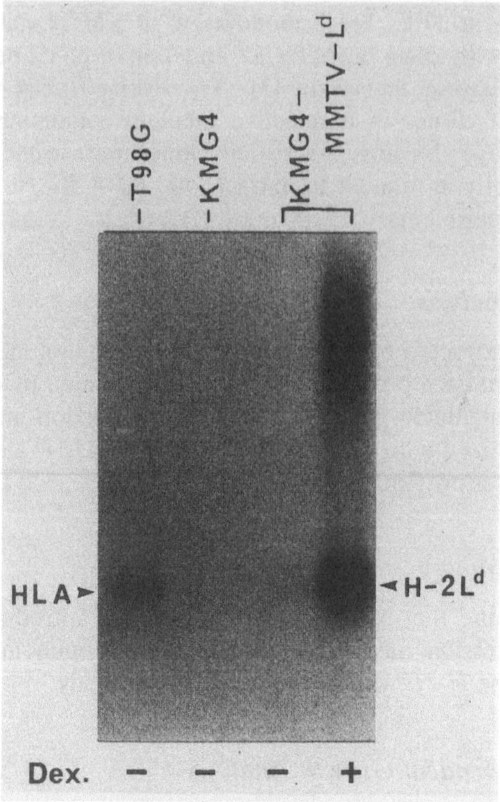

Fig. 1. Northern blot hybridization. Total RNA was extracted from proliferating cells. The denatured RNA (20 µg/lane) was electrophoresed on agarose gel, blotted to a nylon filter, hybridized with ^{32}P-labeled MHC class I probe DNA (*H-2L^d*, Bgl II fragment), and subjected to autoradiography. *Lane 1*, T98G; *Lane 2*, KMG4 (parental cell line); *Lane 3*, KMG4-MMTV-L^d, Dexamethasone (−); *Lane 4*, KMG4-MMTV-L^d, Dexamethasone (+)

sone in the culture medium. A KMG4-neo clone also showed no band (data not shown). KMG4-MMTV-L^d added with dexamethasone appeared to contain a transcript of 1.7 kb, which was not expressed at KMG4-MMTV-L^d without dexamethasone. T98G is a human glioblastoma cell line which shows the band of the MHC (HLA) class I mRNA. The expression of exogenously transfected *H-2L^d* (MHC class I gene) products on the cell surface was also examined by immunohistochemistry, and confirmed the expression of MHC class I antigen on the cell surface (data not shown).

Partial Suppression of Anchorage-Independent Growth in a Semi-Solid Medium of Mouse H-2L^d *Expressing KMG4*

KMG4-MMTV-L^d in the absence of dexamethasone, which expressed no *H-2L^d*, formed many colonies in soft agar (Fig. 2, Table 1). Contrarily, KMG4-

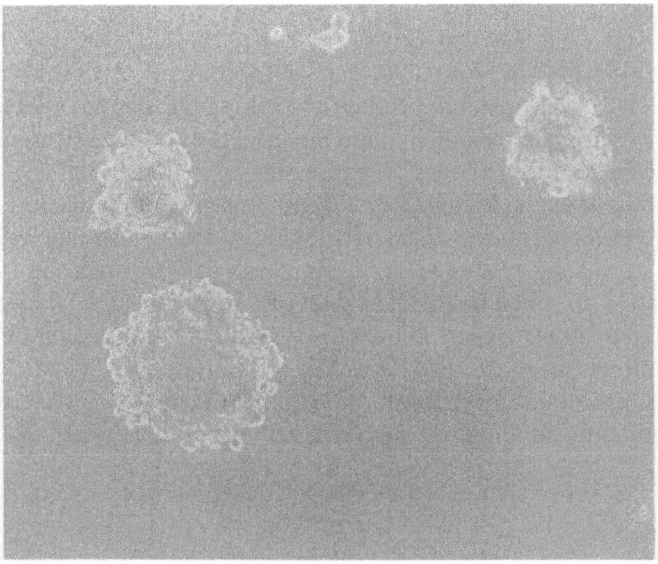

Fig. 2. Colony formation in soft agar. KMG4-MMTV-L^d, which does not express MHC class I (without dexamethasone), shows colony foramastion in soft agar, but, KMG4-MMTV-L^d, which expresses MHC class I (with dexamethasone), reveals significant reduction of colony forming ability

Table 1. The result of colony formation assays

Cell line	Efficiency of colony formation*	
Dexamethasone	−	+
KMG4-neo	++	+++
(H-2L^d expression)	(−)	(−)
KMG4-MMTV-L^d	+++	+
(H-2L^d expression)	(−)	(+)

*Results are expressed as the percentage of cells showing colony formation (> more than 50 cells). +, 1% to 10%; ++, 10% to 20%; +++, 20% to 40%; ++++, > 40%; −, no colony. KMG4-MMTV-Ld without dexamethasone formed many colonies in soft agar. Contrarily, KMG4-MMTV-L^d, which expresses *H-2L^d* by the stimulation of dexamethasone, showed partial suppression of colony formation in soft agar. As a control, KMG4-neo was also examined for its soft agar colony-forming ability. The colony-forming ability of KMG4-neo is slightly increased when dexamethasone is added into the culture medium

MMTV-L^d cells, which expressed *H-2L^d* by the stimulation of dexamethasone, showed only some microscopically identifiable colonies (Table 1). The colony-forming ability of KMG4-neo, which had only pSV2-neo (a neomycin-resistant gene), was slightly increased by the addition of dexamethasone into the culture medium compared with KMG4-neo without dexamethasone (Table 1).

Discussion

Our present results indicate that mouse MHC class I expression partially suppresses the anchorage-independent growth of the human glioblastoma cell line KMG4. Our system can eliminate the effects of the transfection procedure itself by comparing MHC class I expressing and non-expressing states of a human glioblastoma cell clone. The gene transfection procedure itself may alter the phenotype of the cells, including its colony-forming ability in soft agar. This study suggested that the MHC class I antigen might also be involved in the change of phenotypes, altering cell behavior independently of the immune system. Interferon is known to stimulate the expression of MHC class I [7], and alters the shape as well as the proliferating ability of cultured cells [8]. The suppression mechanism of tumorigenicity by interferon may be ascribed not only to immune response modification [1] but also to growth control.

Conclusions

The influence of MHC class I expression on cell growth was examined in a human glioblastoma cell line (KMG4). Parental KMG4 cells expressing from low to undetectable levels of MHC class I mRNA were introduced with the mouse MHC class I (*H-2L*^{d}) gene with a murine mammary tumor virus (MMTV)-promoter. Suppression of the colony-forming ability in soft agar was detected in MHC class I-expressing cells. Therefore, we conclude that the expression of the MHC class I gene influences the anchorage-independent cell growth and suppresses the colony formation of a human glioblastoma cell line.

Acknowledgments. We thank Dr. Junichi Miyazaki (Institute for Medical Genetics, Kumamoto University Medical School) for valuable discussions, Mr. T. Tanamachi and Mr. Y. Tateishi (Center of Medical Photography, Saga Medical School) for their photographic assistance, and Mr. K. Toukaichi for his critical reading of this manuscript.

References

1. Tanaka K, Yoshioka T, Bieberich C, Jay G (1988) Role of the major histocompatibility complex class I antigens in tumor growth and metastasis. Annu Rev Immunol 6:359–380
2. Evans GA, Margulies DH, Camerini-Otero RD, Ozato K, Seidman JG (1982) Structure and expression of a mouse major histocompatibility antigen gene, *H-2L*^{d}. 79:1994–1998
3. Gorman C, Padmanabhan R, Howard BH (1983) High efficiency DNA-mediated transformation of primate cells. Science 221:551–553
4. Maniatis, T, Fritch, EF, Sambrook, J (1982) Molecular cloning: A laboratory manual. Cold Spring Harbor, New York

5. Thomas PS (1980) Hybridization of denatured RNA and small DNA fragments transferred to nitrocellulose. Proc Natl Acad Sci USA 77:5201–5205
6. Carney DN, Gazdar AF, Minna JD (1980) Positive correlation between histological tumor involvement and generation of tumor cell colonies in agarose in specimens taken directly from patients with small cell carcinoma of the lung. Cancer Res 40:1820–1823
7. Shirayoshi Y, Burke PA, Appella E, Ozato K (1988) Interferon-induced transcription of a major histocompatibility class I gene accompanies binding of inducible nuclear factors to the interferon consensus sequence. Proc Natl Acad Sci USA 85:5884–5888
8. Kulesh DA, Greene JJ (1986) Shape-dependent regulation of proliferation in normal and malignant human cells and its alteration by interferon. Cancer Res 46:2793–2797

Association of Histocompatibility Antigen Expression with Intracerebral Tumorigenicity

Toshiki Yamasaki, Kouzo Moritake, Seiichi Nagao, Yasuhiko Akiyama, and Masako Kawahara[1]

Introduction

Although the major histocompatibility complex (MHC, H-2 in mouse) class I and class II antigens are either absent or are present only at low levels in the brain, it has been recognized that various kinds of immune reactions may take place within the brain [1–4]. With regard to the immunology of H-2 class I antigen expression, it has been reported that there is a relationship between the level of cell surface H-2 expression and cytotoxic T lymphocyte (CTL) or natural killer cell (NK) susceptibility in certain tumor systems [5]. In the central nervous system, however, little is known about natural resistance mediated by the cytotoxic cellular interaction between T cells and NK cells. Thus, in the present study, we have focused upon examining the immunosurveillance mechanism for tumor rejection selectively acting in association with MHC class I antigen expression, using a mouse lymphoma system.

Materials and Methods

Animals

All inbred mouse strains used in this study were supplied from the Department of Tumor Biology, Karolinska Institute (Stockholm, Sweden). In some experiments, thymectomized (T-depleted) and NK-depleted mice were used.

Tumor Cell Line

The Moloney virus-induced T-cell lymphoma YAC-1 and its beta-2-microglobulin (β 2 m)-deficient variant, Lym^-, were used. Lym^- was established by mutagenization and selected for its resistance to anti-H-2 antibody-complement mediated lysis. There was no difference in in vitro proliferation, as measured by doubling time and DNA synthesis between the YAC-1 and the Lym^- lines.

[1] Department of Neurosurgery, Shimane Medical University, Izumo, 693 Japan

FACS Analysis

Cell surface expression of H-2 class I antigen and β 2m was examined by fluorescence-activated cell sorter (FACS) analysis. Controls consisting of cells labeled with fluorescein-conjugated rabbit anti-mouse antibodies were included in all experiments.

Cytotoxicity Assay

For the activation of NK cells, mice were given injections of Tilorone (2 mg in 100 μl phosphate-buffered saline [PBS] orally; Sigma Chemical Co., St. Louis, Mo.) 24 h before sacrifice. The spleens were harvested aseptically and made into single cell suspensions. Anti-H-2^a- and H-2^b- (as control) specific CTL effectors were generated in a one-way mixed lymphocyte culture by using A.BY (H-2^b) anti-A/Sn (H-2^a), and A/Sn anti-A.BY spleen cells, respectively. The standard 4-h ^{51}Cr-release assay was used to measure cytotoxic activities.

Rapid Elimination Assay

Iododeoxyuridine (^{125}I-IUdR), special activity 5 Ci/mg (Amersham, Bucks, UK), was added to YAC-1 cells (usually 10^6/ml) in a tissue culture medium and incubated for 16 h at 37°C in 5% CO_2. After labeling, the cells were extensively washed at least four times in PBS. The mice were then inoculated intracerebrally with 10^5-labeled tumor cells in 10 μl PBS, intravenously with 10^6-labeled tumor cells in 0.2 ml PBS, or subcutaneously with 10^6-labeled tumor cells in 0.1 ml PBS, and subsequently sacrificed at different time periods (ranging from 6 to 24 h). Retained radioactivity (reflecting the number of surviving cells) in the heads of intracerebrally inoculated mice, in the lungs, spleen, and, liver of intravenously inoculated mice, or in the leg of subcutaneously inoculated mice was measured in an LKB gamma counter. The results were expressed as the percentage of remaining radioactivity of the total injected amount. From five to seven mice were usually used per group.

Intracerebral Tumorigenicity Assay

Tumor cells were semi-stereotactically inoculated with a microinjector into the right hemisphere of the mice in a total volume of 10 μl. From three to six mice were used in each experiment and the data from several independent experiments were pooled. In the initial experiments, the mice inoculated with tumor cells were observed daily after inoculation until they died. In subsequent experiments, the mice were sacrificed and autopsied when physiological or neurological signs indicated that they would have died within 24 h because of the tumor burden. All of the mice without any signs of tumor growth were kept alive at least 6 weeks after tumor cell inoculation. The tumor takes and survival rates were then calculated.

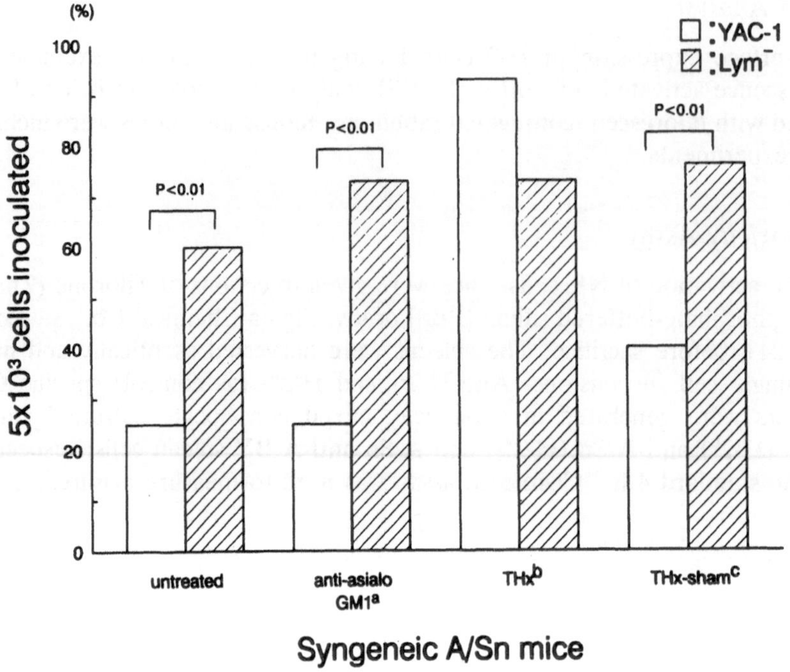

Fig. 1. Tumorigenicity after intracerebral inoculation of 5×10^3 YAC-1 (□) cells or 5×10^3 Lym⁻ (▨) cells into various kinds of syngeneic A/Sn mice. **a** NK-depleted mice were obtained by several intravenous injections of anti-asialo-GM1 antibodies. **b** T-depleted mice resulted from thymectomy, irradiation, and bone marrow reconstruction. **c** Sham control for thymectomized mice. There was no difference in tumorigenicity between YAC-1 and Lym⁻ in T-depleted groups, while YAC-1 was less tumorigenic than Lym⁻ in other groups ($P < 0.01$)

Results and Discussion

Relationship Between MHC Antigen Expression and Intracerebral Tumorigenicity

The first finding was that the highly immunogenic H-2 positive YAC-1 was less tumorigenic than H-2 negative Lym⁻ in untreated as well as NK-depleted syngeneic mice (Fig. 1). Furthermore, the variant Lym⁻ was rarely rejected in the syngeneic mice even when a smaller dose of the cells was inoculated together with YAC-1 cells into the brain. In the T cell-depleted thymectomized mice, however, YAC-1 was as tumorigenic as Lym⁻ (Fig. 1). Therefore, the intracerebral natural resistance was expressed against the highly H-2-positive YAC-1, suggesting that T cells, but not NK cells, might be involved in the YAC-1 tumor elimination, while Lym⁻ cells escaped from the natural resistance in the brain.

When a mixture of YAC-1 and Lym⁻ cells was inoculated in the brain at a cell ratio of $10^5/10^3$, even a much lower dose of Lym⁻ cells always formed

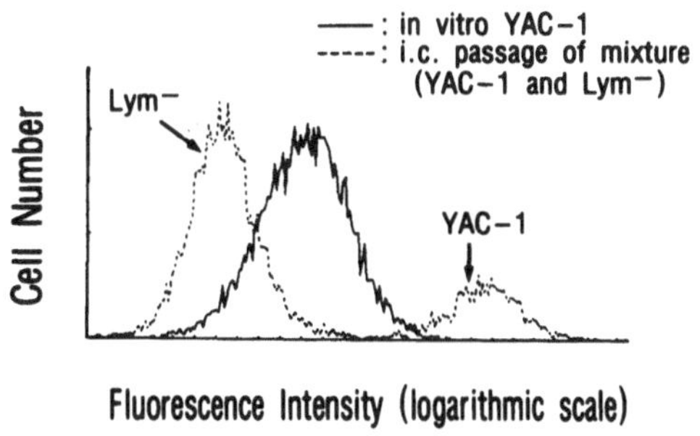

Fig. 2. FACS analysis showing a cell surface H-2 expression on in vivo passaged tumor cells after intracerebral (*i.c.*) inoculation of a mixture of YAC-1 and Lym⁻ cells at a cell ratio of 10^5–10^3

progressively growing tumors (Fig. 2). It was clearly shown that *in vivo* passaged YAC-1 cells exhibited an enhancement of H-2 class I expression (Fig. 2).

On the other hand, in vitro cytotoxicity assays showed that intracerebrally passaged YAC-1 cells decreased and increased the sensitivity to NK- and CTL-mediated lysis, respectively, in association with the enhancement of cell surface H-2 antigens (Fig. 3). In contrast, H-2 negative Lym⁻ did not alter susceptibility to either cell-mediated lysis or cell surface H-2 expression (Fig. 3).

Natural Resistance Mechanism in the Brain

As shown in Fig. 4, *in vivo* rapid elimination assays revealed that after either intravenous or subcutaneous inoculation there was a more efficient abrogation of ^{125}I-IUdR labeled YAC-1 cells in normal untreated mice compared to NK-depleted mice. Following intracerebral inoculation, however, no difference in remaining radioactivity was observed between untreated and NK-depleted

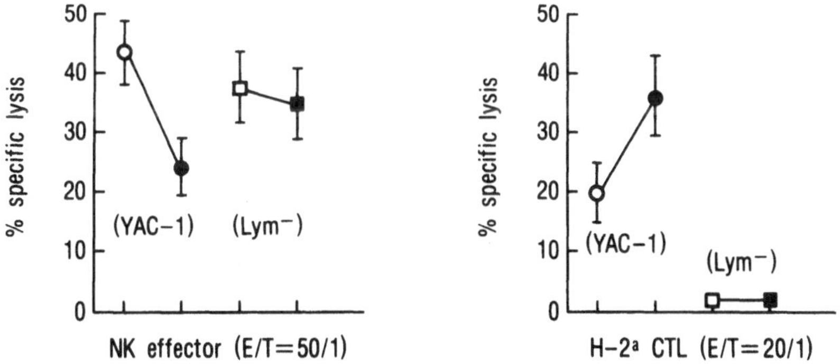

Fig. 3. In vitro cytotoxicity assay showing a significant decrease and increase in NK- and CTL-susceptibility of YAC-1 cells, respectively, after intracerebral inoculation ($P < 0.01$), but no change in Lym⁻ cells. NK cells were prepared from spleens of syngeneic mice given injection of tilorone. Anti-H-2^a CTLs were induced in a one-way mixed lymphocyte culture (see Materials and Methods). *E/T*, effector to target cell ratio

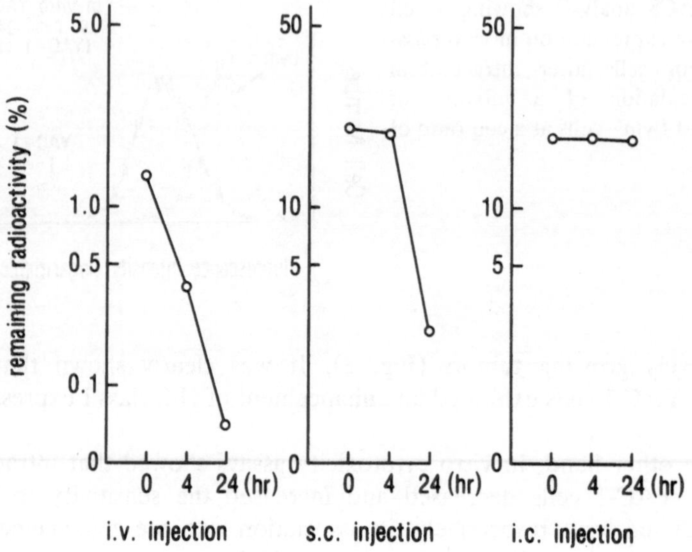

Fig. 4. Rapid elimination assay showing a survival of ^{125}I-IUdR-labeled YAC-1 cells after in vivo injection into syngeneic untreated and NK-depleted mice. Remaining radioactivity of lungs, right lower leg, and whole brain were measured 6 and 24 h after intravenous (*iv.*), subcutaneous (*s.c.*), and intracerebral (*IC*) injection of the labeled cells, respectively. A significant decline was observed at 4 and 24 h of the iv. injection group and at 24 h of the s.c. injection group in untreated mice compared to NK-depleted mice ($P < 0.01$). There was neither change nor difference in IC injection groups of untreated and NK-depleted mice

mice. This indicates that selective NK-mediated elimination of H-2 class I positive tumor cells might occur after intravenous or subcutaneous, but not intracerebral, inoculation.

Summary

The relationship between H-2 class I antigen expression and intracerebral tumorigenicity was investigated by using YAC-1 and its H-2 negative Lym$^-$. Our data suggested that the brain might be characterized by a lack of natural resistance mediated by NK cells against H-2 class I negative tumor cells, although T cell-dependent immunosurveillance can operate intracerebrally.

References

1. Lampson LA (1987) Molecular bases of the immune response to neural antigens. Trends Neurosci 10:211–216

2. Schnitzer J, Schachner M (1981) Expression of Thy-1, H-2 and NS-4 cell surface antigens and tetanus toxin receptors in early postnatal and adult mouse cerebellum. J Neuroimmunol 1:429–456
3. Morantz RA, Shain W, Cravioto H (1978) Immune surveillance and tumors of the nervous system. J Neurosurg 49:84–92
4. Yamasaki T, Handa H, Yamashita J, et al. (1983) Characteristic immunological responses to an experimental mouse brain tumor. Cancer Res 43:4610–4617
5. Kärre K, Ljunggren HG, Piontek G, et al. (1986) Selective rejection of H-2 deficient lymphoma variants suggests alternative immune defense strategy. Nature 319:675–678

Genetic Interaction Between Proto-Oncogene and Histocompatibility Antigen Gene Expressions in Cellular Differentiation of Mouse Neuroblastoma

TOSHIKI YAMASAKI[1], KOUZO MORITAKE[1], and GEORGE KLEIN[2]

Introduction

The recognition of major histocompatibility complex (MHC) class I antigens plays an important role in the function of T cells in the immune system both at the regulatory and effector levels [1]. It has been suggested that quantitative variations in target MHC class I expression would reversely influence natural killer cells (NK) compared to T cells [2], and that the MHC expression decreases as a tumor grows [3]. On the other hand, there have been reports on a relationship among N-*myc* gene expression, cellular differentiation, and tumor progression in neuroblastoma [4,5]. The aim of this study was to examine the interaction of gene regulation between proto-oncogene (N-*myc* and c-*src*) and histocompatibility antigen gene expressions, using a dimethyl sulfoxide (DMSO)-induced differentiation model of mouse neuroblastoma.

Materials and Methods

Tumor Cell Lines

A spontaneously occurring neuroblastoma of A/J Ax ($H\text{-}2^aK^kD^d$) mouse origin, MNB 85, was used. In some experiments, the Moloney leukemia virus-induced T-cell lymphoma line, YAC-1, of A/Sn ($H\text{-}2^aK^kD^d$) mouse origin and its in vivo (intraperitoneally) passaged subline, YAC ascites, were used.

Antibody

The appropriate monoclonal antibodies for H-2 antigens were used as hybridoma supernatants (H-2 K^k from 11-4.1 and H-2 D^d from 34-1-2S). Rabbit anti-mouse beta-2-microglobulin (β 2 m) antiserum was provided by Dr. Svante Paabo, Bio Medical Center, Uppsala University, Uppsala, Sweden.

[1] Department of Neurosurgery, Shimane Medical University, Izuno, 693 Japan
[2] Department of Tumor Biology, Karolinska Institute, Stockholm, Sweden

FACS Analysis

Cell surface expression of H-2 class I antigen and β 3m was examined by fluorescence-activated cell sorter (FACS) analysis. Controls consisting of cells labeled with fluorescein-conjugated rabbit anti-mouse antibodies were included in all experiments.

Isolation of DNA and RNA, and Molecular Analysis

DNA and RNA were extracted from cells under the conditions for nick translation and hybridization under high stringency. The baked filter was hybridized to various kinds of probes in a hybridization mixture containing formamide. A mixture of digests was run in a parallel slot as molecular weight markers for both Northern and Southern blots. The resulting autoradiographs were anlyzed by densitometry.

Probes

For H-2 gene analysis, a ECoRI-KpnI fragment of the cDNA clone, pH-2^d-33, corresponding to the first two and a part of the third exon of the K^d gene was used as a class I heavy chain probe. Two PstI—PstI fragments (0.3- kilobase per pair each) of the cDNA clone, pAG69, corresponding to the entire β 2m mRNA, were used as the β 2m probe. For oncogene analysis, the following cloned DNA fragments were used as hybridization probes: N-*myc* (pNbl), c-*myc* (pMC-54), v-*src* (Pvull E), actin (pAM91), and histone (pCH3-3E).

DMSO Treatment

At a 1.0%–2.0% vol dimethyl sulfoxide (DMSO), there was no change in growth rate and thymidine uptake of MNB 85 cells. Morphological examinations confirmed that DMSO treatment induced an extensive neurite outgrowth of MNB 85 cells, while untreated cells remained in their original round shapes during the *in vitro* culture. Immunohistochemical study with antibodies formed against neurofilaments showed that the neurite portion of the DMSO-treated cells was positively stained by the antibodies. Therefore, a 1.5% vol DMSO was used in all of the experiments.

Cytotoxic Cell Generation and Cytotoxicity Assay

For activation of the NK cells, mice were given injections (2 mg in 100 µl phosphate-buffered saline, per os) of Tilorone (Sigma Chemical Co., St. Louis, Mo.) 24 h before sacrifice. Anti-H-2^a and H-2^b (as control)-specific cytoxic T lymphocyte (CTL) effectors were generated in a one-way mixed lymphocyte culture by using A.BY (H-2^b), anti-A/Sn (H-2^a) and A/Sn anti-A.BY spleen cells, respectively. The standard 6 h ^{51}Cr-release assay was used to assess cytotoxicity.

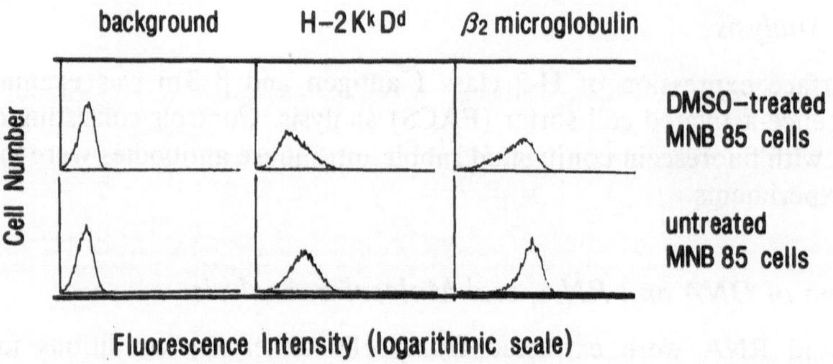

Fig. 1. FACS analysis showing a cell surface H-2 expression on dimethyl sulfoxide (DMSO)-treated and untreated mouse MNB 85 neuroblastoma cells

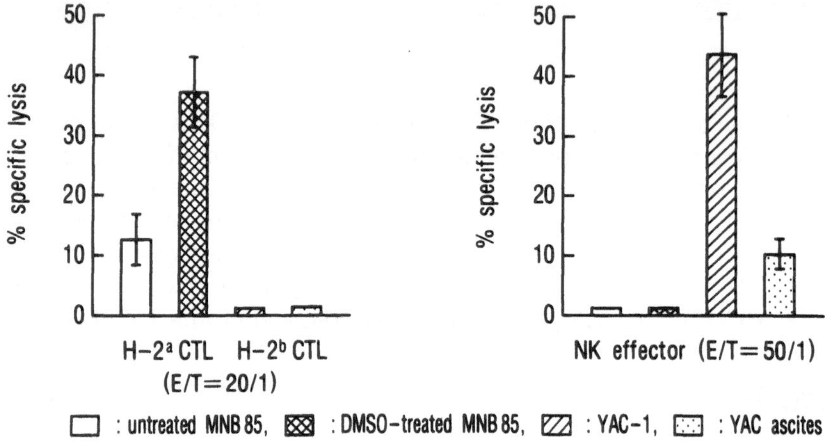

Fig. 2. *In vitro* cytotoxicity assay showing a significant increase in H-2^a CTL-susceptibility of dimethyl sulfoxide (DMSO)-treated MNB 85 neuroblastoma cells ($P < 0.01$), but no change in H-2^b CTL- and NK-susceptibility. NK cells were prepared from spleens of syngeneic mice given injections of tilorone. Anti-H-2^a and H-2^b (as control) CTLs were induced in a one-way mixed lymphocyte culture (see Materials and Methods). For an NK-mediated lysis assay, both NK-sensitive YAC-1 and NK-resistant YAC ascites cells were assessed simultaneously

Results and Discussion

Effects of DMSO Treatment on Susceptibility to CTL- and NK-Mediated Lysis in Association with Cell Surface H-2 Expression

The effects of DMSO treatment on the cell surface expression of both H-2 class I antigen and β 2m in MNB 85 cells were first investigated by FACS. Both expressions were enhanced by DMSO treatment (Fig. 1).

Fig. 3. Northern blot analysis showing a significant increase in gene transcripts of both H-2 class I antigen and beta-2-microglobulin in MNB 85 cells after dimethyl sulfoxide (DMSO) treatment

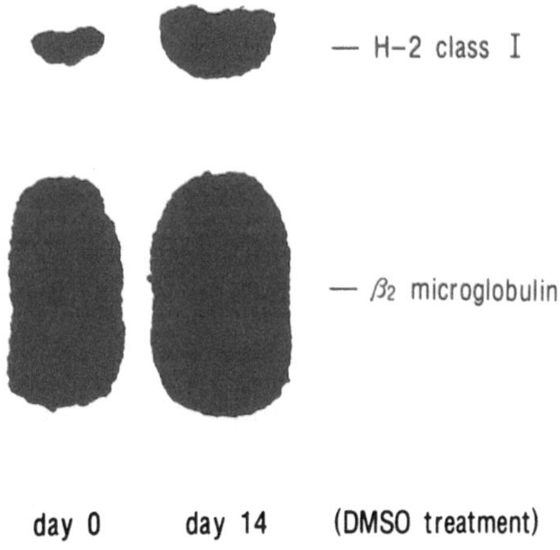

Anti-H-2[a] CTLs showed a higher killing activity against DMSO-treated MNB 85 cells than untreated cells, while anti-H-2[b] CTLs exhibited no significant cytotoxicity against either cell (Fig. 2). Furthermore, it was found that MNB 85 was far more refractory to NK-mediated lysis than relatively NK-resistant YAC ascites, and that there was no significant change in NK susceptibility of MNB 85 cells after DMSO treatment (Fig. 2).

Gene Regulation of H-2 Class I Antigen in DMSO-Induced Differentiation of Mouse Neuroblastoma

Northern blot analysis demonstrated a three- to sevenfold increase in the level of H-2 and β 2 m transcripts in DMSO-treated MNB 85 cells (Fig. 3). Thus, it was suggested that the enhancement of H-2 expression in MNB 85 cells by DMSO treatment was primarily regulated at the transcriptional level.

*Gene Control of N-*myc *and c-*src *in DMSO-Induced Differentiation of Mouse Neuroblastoma*

The N-*myc* gene transcripts of exponentially proliferating MNB 85 cells were examined before and after DMSO treatment. A decline in the level of N-*myc* transcripts was observed in DMSO-treated cells (Fig. 4), whereas there was a more than fourfold increase in the level of c-*src* transcripts. Thus, it was suggested that the N-*myc* gene was down-regulated in DMSO-induced differentiation of the mouse neuroblastoma, while primary up-regulation of c-*src* gene occurs at the transcriptional level.

Summary

The role of the MHC class I antigen gene and proto-oncogene (N-*myc* and c-*src*) expressions in DMSO-induced neuronal differentiation was examined,

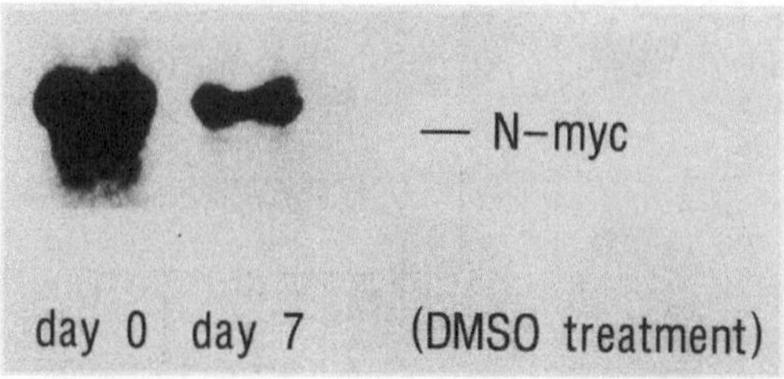

Fig. 4. Northern blot analysis showing a significant decrease in the N-*myc* gene transcripts in MNB 85 cells after dimethyl sulfoxide (DMSO) treatment

using a mouse neuroblastoma cell line. Our data suggested that protooncogene expression may be closely linked to cellular differentiation and that MHC gene expression may influence an immunogenicity of tumor cells.

References

1. Zinkernagel RM, Doherty PC (1979) MHC-restricted cytotoxic T-cells: Studies on the biological role of polymorphic major transplantation antigens determining T-cell restriction-specificity, function, and responsiveness. Adv Immunol 27:51–77
2. Kärre K, Ljunggren HG, Piontek G et al. (1986) Selective rejection of H-2 deficient lymphoma variants suggests alternative immune defense strategy. Nature 319:675–678
3. Bernards R (1987) Suppression of MHC gene expression in cancer cells. TIG 3:298–301
4. Schwab M, Ellison J, Busch M et al. (1984) Enhanced expression of the human gene N-*myc* consequent to amplification of DNA may contribute to a malignant progression of neuroblastoma. Proc Natl Acad Sci USA 81:4940–4944
5. Ramsay GM, Moscovici G, Moscovici C et al. (1990) Neoplastic transformation and tumorigenesis by the human protooncogene *MYC*. Proc Natl Acad Sci USA 87:2102–2106

Expression of Intermediate Filaments (GFAP and Vimentin) in Human Gliomas

Takashi Kokunai, Norihiko Tamaki, and Satoshi Matsumoto[1]

Introduction

Glial fibrillary acidic protein (GFAP) is expressed in developing, normal, reactive, and neoplastic glial cells [1,2]. In contrast to GFAP, vimentin, first detected in fibroblasts, characterizes the mesenchymal origin of the cells [3]. In addition to the expression of vimentin in mesenchymal cells, vimentin is thought to be a major cytoskeletal component of immature glias [3], and is expressed on some glial tumors [4].

In this paper, we describe the correlation between the expression of GFAP and vimentin, and the malignancy in astrocytoma and glioblastoma by the immunohistochemical method and the quantitative assay of GFAP and vimentin contents.

Materials and Methods

Tissue Materials

Tissues were obtained from surgical specimens of 11 cases of glioblastoma, 4 cases of anaplastic astrocytoma, 4 cases of astrocytoma, 3 cases of gliosis near the tumor tissues, and 3 cases of normal brain obtained at lobectomies for traumatic lesions.

Cytoskeletal Preparation

Triton-insoluble cytoskeletal preparations were obtained by the method reported by Starger et al. [5]. Tissues were homogenized at 4°C in a Teflon-glass homogenizer using the following Triton-extraction buffer: 1% Triton X-100, 0.6 M KCl, 10 mM $MgCl_2$, 2 mM EDTA, 1 mM EGTA, 0.15 mM PMSF, and 0.5 mg/ml p-tosyl-L-arginine methyl ester HCl in 0.1 mM phosphate-buffered saline (PBS), pH 7.1. After the homogenization, 0.1 mg/ml DNAase 1 (Sigma, type 3) was added and an additional 1 min homogenization was carried out.

[1] Department of Neurosurgery, Kobe University School of Medicine, Kobe, 650 Japan

The cytoskeletal residue was pelleted at 12,000g for 10 min and re-extracted with 10 vol. Triton-extraction buffer without DNAase 1. Following centrifugation, the cytoskeletal proteins were dissolved in 1% (w/v) sodium dodecyl sulfate (SDS) and diluted to 50 µg/ml protein in 50 mM Na_2CO_3, pH 9.6 (final SDS concentration of 0.01%).

Analysis of GFAP and Vimentin by ELISA

The 96-well microELISA plates were coated with 100 µl rabbit anti-GFAP antibody (DAKO) diluted 1:500, or rabbit anti-vimentin antibody (ICN) diluted 1:200 in 0.2 M bicarbonate buffer, pH 9.3. One day after coating, GFAP and vimentin standards (Boehringer) and diluted samples were loaded into wells and incubated overnight at 4°C. Then, anti-GFAP (× 200) or anti-vimentin (× 500) monoclonal antibodies were added to each well and incubated for 2 h at room temperature (RT). Horseradish peroxidase-conjugated rabbit anti-mouse IgG (DAKO) diluted 1:500 was added and left for 2 h at RT. Finally, 150 µl 2,2′-azino-bis(3-ethylbenzthiazoline sulfornic acid) (ABTS) (Sigma) diluted to 1 mg/ml in 0.1 M potassium phosphate pH 5.0 and 1 µl 30% peroxide were added to each well and left for 1 h. Before each of the subsequent procedures, the plates were washed three times with 0.05 M PBS. The measured optical density was 414 nm.

Immunohistochemical Staining

Deparaffinized sections were blocked with 0.3% H_2O_2 in methanol for 30 min. Before each of the subsequent procedures, the sections were washed three times with 0.05 M PBS. Sections were incubated with mouse anti-vimentin (× 100) or anti-GFAP (× 500) antibodies for 60 min at RT, after the incubation with 3% goat serum for 20 min. Then, sections were incubated with biotinylated goat anti-mouse IgG (× 500) for 30 min and incubated with peroxidase-labeled streptoavidin for 30 min. Sections were treated with 0.05% DAB and 0.01% H_2O_2 in Tris-buffered saline for 5 min and counterstained with Meyer's hematoxylin.

Results

Immunohistochemical staining of GFAP and Vimentin

Table 1 showed the results of immunohistochemical staining of GFAP and vimentin. Although GFAP was stained in all cases, including glioblastoma and normal brain, vimentin was stained in all of the 11 cases of glioblastoma, 3 out of 4 cases of anaplastic astrocytoma, none of the 4 cases of astrocytoma, none of the 3 cases of gliosis, and none of the 3 cases of normal brain. The glial and neuronal components in gliosis and normal brain were not stained, but the endothelial components were stained with anti-vimentin antibody.

Table 1. Immunohistochemical staining of GFAP and vimentin

Tissue	GFAP cases	Vimentin cases
	Positive/Total	
Glioblastoma	11/11	11/11
Anaplastic astrocytoma	4/4	3/4
Astrocytoma	4/4	0/4
Gliosis	3/3	0/3
Normal brain	3/3	0/3

Table 2. Contents of GFAP and vimentin

Tissue	Number	GFAP	Vimentin
Glioblastoma	11	12.98 ± 6.14	629.14 ± 78.43
Anaplastic astrocytoma	4	13.29 ± 7.42	243.44 ± 26.55
Astrocytoma	4	14.29 ± 3.24	13.29 ± 4.52
Gliosis	3	13.79 ± 5.21	4.47 ± 1.20
Normal brain	3	4.78 ± 1.23	6.29 ± 2.41
		μg/mg protein	ng/mg protein

Contents of GFAP and Vimentin in Various Tissues (Table 2)

There were no differences in GFAP contents between glioblastoma, anaplastic astrocytoma, astrocytoma, and gliosis. Glioblastoma showed high contents of vimentin (629.1 ± 78.43 ng/mg protein) that differed significantly from that in anaplastic astrocytoma ($P < 0.05$). The vimentin contents of anaplastic astrocytoma differed significantly from that of astrocytoma ($P < 0.05$).

Correlation Between the Survival Periods and the Contents of Vimentin in Glioblastoma

There was good correlation between the survival periods and the contents of vimentin in glioblastoma (Fig. 1). The cases with high vimentin contents had long survival periods in contrast to the cases with low vimentin contents in tumor tissues.

Discussion

There have been few reports of human brain tumors demonstrating the co-expression of GFAP and vimentin by immunohistochemistry and quantitative analysis with ELISA. In this study, GFAP was expressed in all of the astroglial tumors, both benign and malignant, but vimentin was expressed only in malignant tumors, such as glioblastoma and anaplastic astrocytoma. Moreover, from the results of the quantitative analysis, the vimentin contents were progressive-

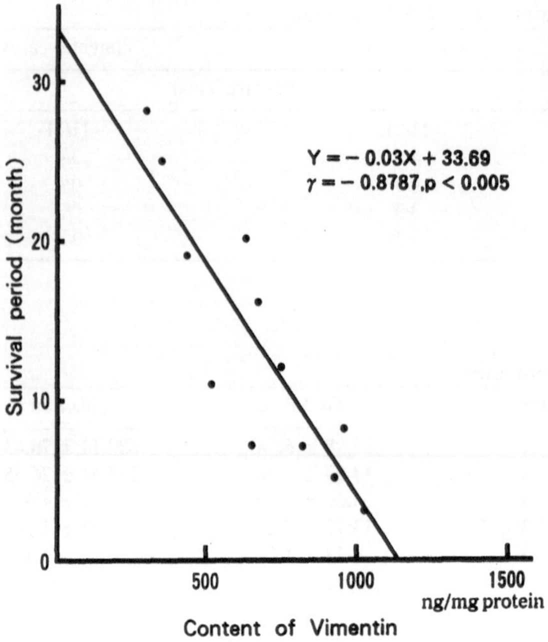

Fig. 1. Correlation between the survival periods and the contents of vimentin in 11 cases of glioblastoma

ly increased when the tumor became malignant. It was reported that an increase in the expression of vimentin of neoplastic astrocytes was observed during malignant progression [4]. Additionally, it was shown that vimentin was a major intermediate filament in immature glial cells [6]. Therefore, the presence of vimentin in astroglial tumors indicates that these tumors have characteristics of both immaturity and malignancy.

Good correlation was found between the survival periods and the vimentin contents in 11 cases of glioblastoma. Consequently, vimentin was thought to be a predictable factor in the prognosis of the patients with glioblastoma.

References

1. Eng LF (1985) Glial fibrillary acidic protein (GFAP): The major protein of glial intermediate filaments in differentiated astrocytes. J Neuroimmunol 8:203–214
2. Bonnin JM, Rubinstein LJ (1984) Immunocytochemistry of central nervous system tumors: Its contribution to neurosurgical diagnosis. J Neurosurg 60:1121–1133
3. Franke ED, Schmid E, Osborn M, Weber K (1978) Different intermediate-sized filaments distinguished by immunofluorescence microscopy. Proc Natl Acad Sci USA 75:5034–5038
4. NaKopoulou L, Kerezoudi E, Thomaides T, Litsios B (1990) An immunocytochemical comparison of glial fibrillary acidic protein, S-100p and vimentin in human glial tumors. J Neurooncol 8:33–40

5. Starger JM, Brown WE, Goldman AE, Goldman RD (1977) Biochemical and immunological analysis of rapidly purified 10 nm filaments from baby hamster kidney (BHK-21) cells. J Cell Biol 78:93–109
6. Dahl D, Rueger DC, Bignami A, Weber K, Osborn M (1981) Vimentin, the 57,000 dalton protein of fibroblast filaments is the major cytoskeletal component in immature glia. Eur J Cell Biol 124:191–196

Opposite Effects of Cyclic AMP and Cell Density on Expression of αB-Crystallin and Glial Fibrillary Acidic Protein in C-6 Glioma Cells

Akiko Iwaki[1], Toru Iwaki[2], Yoshiyuki Sakaki[1], Ronald K.H. Liem[3], and James E. Goldman[3]

Introduction

Crystallins are well known to be water-soluble proteins in the lens that can pack together efficiently to form very large aggregates. α-Crystallin is a heterogeneous aggregate produced by the products of two genes, αA and αB. Of these two genes, αA-crystallin expression seems restricted to the lens [1]. In contrast, αB-crystallin is expressed in various extra-ocular tissues such as heart, muscle, kidney, brain, nerve, and placenta [2,3]. The function of αB-crystallin in extra-ocular tissues is not yet known.

In the central nervous system, αB-crystallin is present in oligodendrocytes and in a few astrocytes [3]. The amount of αB-crystallin in normal brain is small, but it accumulates to high levels in astrocytes, especially in Rosenthal Fibers (RFs) in brains of patients with Alexander's disease [2,4]. RFs are carrot-shaped or beaded inclusions within reactive and neoplastic astrocytes, and are always associated with a marked increase of glial fibrillary acidic protein (GFAP). Immunocytochemical studies have revealed that reactive astrocytes in various disorders, such as cerebral infarction and demyelinating diseases, are also positive with an anti-αB-crystallin antibody [5]. The accumulation of GFAP is a well-known concomitant of glial scarring in the central nervous system [6]. Furthermore, it has been reported that transcripts of GFAP and αB-crystallin are expressed more in scrapie-infected brain than in normal brain [7]. These observations led us to study the regulation of αB-crystallin expression in comparison with that of GFAP. In this study we examined the effects of dibutyryl cyclic AMP (dbcAMP) and cell density on the expression of αB-crystallin and GFAP in cultured rat glioma cells.

[1] Research Laboratory for Genetic Information, Kyushu University 60, Fukuoka, 812 Japan
[2] Department of Neuropathology, Neurological Institute, Faculty of Medicine, Kyushu University 60, Fukuoka, 812 Japan
[3] Department of Pathology, Columbia University College of Physicians and Surgeons, New York, NY 10032, USA

Materials and Methods

Cell Culture

C-6, a cell line derived from a rat glioma induced by N-nitrosomethylurea [8], was obtained from the American Type Culture Collection and cultured in Ham's F-10 medium containing 10% fetal bovine serum (FBS) and penicillin-streptomycin. The C-6 cells at various cell densities were treated with 1 mM dbcAMP for 16 h before harvest.

Northern Blotting

Total RNAs from C-6 cells were isolated by the GIT method as described elsewhere [2]. RNA samples (20 μg) were electrophoresed in a 1% agarose-formaldehyde gel, transferred to a Gene Screen nylon filter, and hybridized with a GFAP probe, a 1.5 kilobase (kb) AvaI fragment obtained from a rat brain library (R.K.H. Liem, unpublished data), which was ^{32}P-labeled by random primer synthesis (Amersham). After removing the GFAP probe, the blot was hybridized with a ^{32}P-labeled αB-crystallin cDNA, a 0.4 kb insert of the RF1 clone containing the 3′ end of a human αB-crystallin cDNA [2]. Hybridization and washing conditions were described previously [6].

Results

Since rat C-6 glioma cells are homogeneous and express readily detectable amounts of αB-crystallin, we chose this cell line for study. We first examined the effect of dbcAMP on mRNA levels of αB-crystallin and GFAP in rat C-6 glioma cells. DbcAMP increases intracellular cAMP level and activates cAMP-dependent kinase. C-6 cells were treated with 1 mM dbcAMP for 16 h and then total RNAs were isolated, electrophoresed on an agarose-formaldehyde gel, and transferred to a nylon membrane. The Northern blot was hybridized with a ^{32}P-labeled rat GFAP probe (Fig. 1a). As we have already observed in primary cultures of rat astrocytes and in human astrocytoma U-373MG cell [6], GFAP mRNA levels in C-6 cells were increased by the addition of dbcAMP. The basal level of GFAP mRNA expression in C-6 was lower than those in primary astrocytes and U-373MG, but the relative induction by dbcAMP appeared to be greater in C-6 cells (data not shown). After removing the GFAP probe from the filter, the same blot was rehybridized with an αB-crystallin probe (Fig. 1b). C-6 cells mainly expressed two mRNA species for αB-crystallin, about 1.2 kb and 0.9 kb in length. The levels of both mRNA species were decreased by treatment with dbcAMP. We have recently characterized the structure of the different mRNA species in rat brain and C-6 cells. They differed in the lengths of their 5′-leader sequences and were generated by alternative initiation of transcription from a single gene [10].

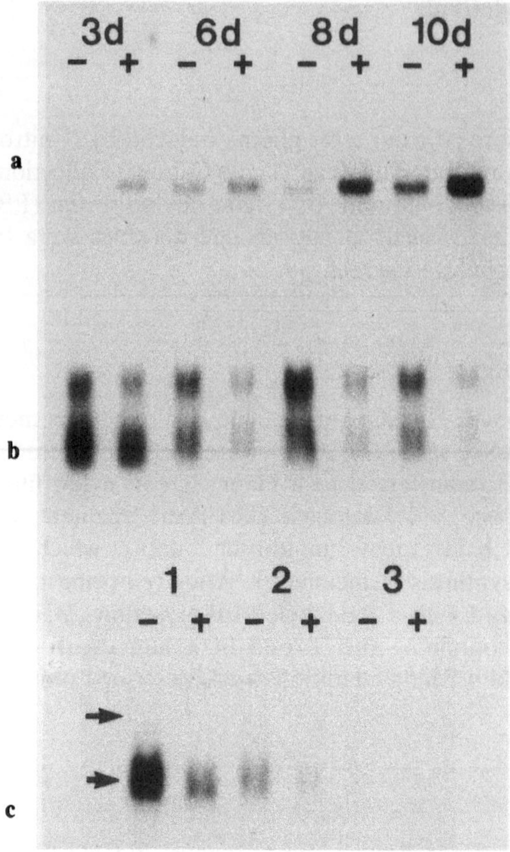

Fig. 1. GFAP and αB-crystallin mRNA expression at different cell density with or without dbcAMP. **a,b** C-6 cells were replated at 1×10^6 cells/100 mm dish and grown for 3, 6, 8, and 10 days. Fresh medium (10 ml) was supplied 1 day before the addition of dbcAMP. Cells were incubated with (+ lanes) or without (− lanes) dbcAMP for 16 h and then collected for RNA preparation on the day indicated. **c** C-6 cells were replated at the following densities: 0.5×10^6, 1×10^6, and 2.5×10^6 cells per 100 mm dish. Total RNA samples (20 μg) were separated by electrophoresis in a 1% agarose-fromaldehyde gel and transferred to a nylon membrane. **a** Northern blots were hybridized with a ^{32}P-labeled GFAP probe, and then **b,c** rehybridized with ^{32}P-labeled αB-crystallin probe. **c** The positions of the two mRNA species of αB-crystallin are marked by *arrows*.

We also examined the dependence of expression of αB-crystallin and GFAP mRNAs on the density of C-6 cells. As shown in Fig. 1a, GFAP mRNA levels increased as cells grew to higher density. The level of GFAP mRNA expression was increased by the addition of dbcAMP at all densities. In contrast, αB-crystallin mRNA levels were decreased by increasing cell density and by the addition of dbcAMP.

To examine the effect of cell density further, cells were seeded at a variety of densities and αB-crystallin mRNA levels were examined 3 days later (Fig. 1c). When the cells were seeded more sparsely than the extent shown in Fig. 1b, the ratio of the shorter mRNA to the longer one became greater. The reduction of αB-crystallin mRNA levels by dbcAMP was enhanced more at low cell density than at high cell density. The exposure time was chosen to display differences in the shorter mRNA. A longer exposure showed approximately equal signals of both mRNAs at high cell density (data not shown).

Discussion

Several observations suggest that GFAP mRNA expression may be regulated by a signal transduction pathway involving cAMP-dependent kinase. Dbc-AMP, which produces marked effects upon the morphology of normal or neoplastic astroglia in culture, increases the levels of GFAP mRNA and protein [6,9]. In the promoter region of mouse GFAP gene, there is a DNA sequence which is homologous to a consensus sequence of a cAMP-responsive element, and has been shown to be necessary for cell type specific expression of GFAP [12]. This cis-acting element and the corresponding trans-acting factors may also play an important role for up-regulation of GFAP mRNA by cAMP. The mechanism for decreasing αB-crystallin mRNA by cAMP treatment is uncertain. Negative regulatory sequences or factors for cAMP could be present in the αB-crystallin gene or in glioma cells. An analysis of promoter regions of the αB-crystallin gene may give us an answer.

Our results suggest that astrocytes regulate αB-crystallin mRNA levels in a different way from GFAP mRNA levels. This difference is also supported by our recent observation that treatment of C-6 cells with phorbol-12-myristate-13-acetate (PMA) increased αB-crystallin mRNA levels but reduced those of GFAP in C-6 cells [10]. In the 5′-flanking region of rat αB-crystallin gene, there is a PMA responsive element, a potential AP-1 binding site, suggesting regulation by protein kinase C [11].

Although both proteins often accumulate in astrocytes under pathological conditions, the effects of PMA, cAMP, and cell density on the expression of αB-crystallin were opposite to those of GFAP in cultured glioma cells. Thus, αB-crystallin mRNA is increased by PMA (involving protein kinase C) and GFAP mRNA is increased by cAMP (involving protein kinase A). We can not rule out that the two major signal transduction mechanisms cross-talk under certain pathological conditions. It is also possible that the turnover rates of those proteins may change in pathological conditions.

Summary

We have identified a major component of Rosenthal fibers as αB-crystallin and demonstrated immunocytochemical localization of αB-crystallin in glial cells of the central nervous system. In the present study, the regulation of αB-crystallin expression in a rat glioma cell line (C-6) was investigated by Northern blotting. The steady-state levels of αB-crystallin mRNA were decreased by treatment with dibutyryl cyclic AMP (dbcAMP) and by increasing the cell density. The responses to dbcAMP and cell density were opposite to those of glial fibrillary acidic protein (GFAP). Although αB-crystallin and GFAP accumulate in reactive and neoplastic glia, the expression of αB-crystallin may be regulated in a different manner from that of GFAP.

Acknowledgments. This research was supported by a Grant-in-Aid for General Scientific Research (No. 02670154) from the Ministry of Education, Science and Culture of Japan (T.I.) and by Javits Neuroscience Investigation Awards, NS 17125, USA (J.E.G.) and NS 15182 (R.K.H.L).

References

1. Dubin RA, Wawrousek EF, Piategorsky J (1989) Expression of the murine αB-crystallin gene is not restricted to the lens. Mol Cell Biol 9:1083–1091
2. Iwaki T, Kume-Iwaki A, Liem RKH, Goldman JE (1989) αB-Crystallin is expressed in non-lenticular tissues and accumulates in Alexander's disease brain. Cell 57:71–78
3. Iwaki T, Kume-Iwaki A, Goldman JE (1990) Cellular distribution of αB-crystallin in non-lenticular tissues. J Histochem Cytochem 38:31–39
4. Goldman JE, Corbin E (1988) Isolation of a major protein component of Rosenthal fibers. Am J Pathol 130:569–578
5. Iwaki T, Kume-Iwaki A, Corbin E, Goldman JE (1990) Expression of the B-chain of α-crystallin in CNS glia (abstract). J Neuropathol Exp Neurol 49:344
6. Shafit-Zagardo B, Kume-Iwaki A, Goldman JE (1988) Astrocytes regulate GFAP mRNA levels by cyclic AMP and protein kinase C-dependent mechanisms. Glia 1:346–354
7. Duguid JR, Rohwer RG, Seed B (1988) Isolation of cDNAs of scrapie-modulated RNAs by subtractive hybridization of a cDNA library. Proc Natl Acad Sci USA 85:5738–5742
8. Benda P, Lightbody J, Sato G, Levine L, Sweet W (1968) Differential rat glial cell strain in tissue culture. Science 161:370–371
9. Goldman JE, Chiu F-C (1984) Dibutyryl cyclic AMP causes intermediate filament accumulation and actin reorganization in astrocytes. Brain Res 306:85–95
10. Iwaki A, Iwaki T, Goldman JE, Liem RKH (1990) Multiple mRNAs of rat brain α-crystallin B chain result from alternative transcriptional initiation. J Biol Chem 265:22197–22203

11. Nishizuka Y (1984) The role of protein kinase C in cell surface signal transduction and tumor promotion. Nature 308:693–698
12. Miura M, Tamura T, Mikoshiba, K (1990) Cell-specific expression of the mouse glial fibrillary acidic protein gene: Identification of the cis- and trans-acting promoter elements for astrocyte-specific expression. J Neurochem 55:1180–1188

Demonstration of Microtubule-Associated Proteins in Human Gliomas

Norihiro Ibayashi, Kimirou Nakamura, Takashi Houri, and Satoshi Ueda[1]

Introduction

Microtubule-associated proteins (MAPs) are one of the major components of microtubules, and their heterogeneity appears to be a characteristic of brain tissue. Various MAPs, including MAP1, 2, 3, 4, 5 and tau, have been isolated from brain tissue. MAP1 and 2 are the major high molecular weight MAPs (Mr. 350,000 and 280,000, respectively). MAP5A (Mr. 320,000) is a subdivision of the MAP1 group which migrates between the prominent MAP1 and MAP2 bands on SDS-polyacrylamide gels. A large number of the MAPs studies have demonstrated the localization of MAPs in the central nervous system and the dynamic changes during their development in the brain [1,2]. However, previous investigations of these MAPs in brain tumors have been restricted exclusively to neuroepithelial tumors showing neuronal differentiation, such as neuroblastoma or medulloblastoma [3,4]. In the present study, we investigated MAPs in human glial tumors and tried to clarify the relationship between morphological anaplasia and the expression of these microtubule proteins in neoplastic glial cells.

Materials and Methods

Surgical specimens obtained from astrocytic gliomas (1 astrocytoma, 12 anaplastic astrocytomas, 10 glioblastomas, and 1 gliosarcoma) were used in this study. They were fixed in 10% buffered formalin or 70% ethanol and embedded in paraffin. The antibodies used were mouse anti-beta tubulin monoclonal antibody (Mabs) (BioMakor, Israel) [5], rabbit anti-glial fibrillary acidic (GFA) protein (Dako Corp., USA) [6] and three mouse anti-MAPs Mabs: (1) MAP1 (BioMakor) [7], (2) MAP2 (BioMakor) [7], and (3) MAP5 (BioMakor) [8].

After blockage of the endogenous peroxidase activity with hydrogen peroxide (0.5% in methanol), the three-step peroxidase-antiperoxidase reactions and the avidin-biotin peroxidase complex method were performed, using the polyvalent antiserum and monoclonal antibodies, respectively. Before applica-

[1] Department of Neurosurgery, Kyoto Prefectural University of Medicine, Kyoto, 602 Japan

tion of the primary antibodies, the specimens were saturated in 10% normal goat serum (Dako) (for the anti-GFA protein antiserum) or 2% normal horse serum (Vector Laboratories, USA) (for monoclonal antibodies). The sections were incubated for 1 h with anti-MAPs Mabs and anti-GFA protein antisera used at the following dilutions: (1) anti-beta tubulin Mab, 1:200, (2) anti-MAP1, 2 and 5 Mabs, 1:500, and (3) anti-GFA protein antibody, 1:100.

The immunohistochemical reactions were developed in freshly prepared 3,3′-diaminobenzidine tetrahydrochrolide. For positive controls for GFA protein and the MAPs, similarly fixed sections from adult rat brain were stained in parallel.

A double-immunostaining technique was used for the simultaneous recognition in the same sections of epitopes defined by both the anti-MAP2 antibody (applied first) and anti-GFA protein antiserum (applied second). Then, 3,3′-diaminobenzidine tetrahydrochrolide and 4-chloro-1-naphthol were used as chromogens for the first and second antibody reactions, respectively.

The details of the procedures for the immunohistochemistry have been reported previously [9,10].

Results

The immunohistochemical data on the astrocytic gliomas are summarized in Table 1. Positivity for all of the microtubule proteins in the materials fixed in 70% ethanol was higher than those fixed in 10% buffered-formalin.

1. Beta-Tubulin

In all of the samples examined, the astrocytoma, anaplastic astrocytoma, glioblastoma, and gliosarcoma tumor cells were all immunoreactive for beta-

Table 1. The results of immunohistochemistry for microtubule proteins in human gliomas

	Beta-tubulin	MAP1	MAP2	MA5
	Positive cases/total cases			
Astrocytoma				
Formalin	1/1	1/1	1/1	1/1
Ethanol				
Anaplastic astrocytoma				
Formalin	7/7	7/7	4/7	7/7
Ethanol	5/5	5/5	5/5	5/5
Glioblastoma multiforme				
Formalin	4/4	4/4	1/4	4/4
Ethanol	6/6	6/6	6/6	6/6
Gliosarcoma				
Formalin	1/1	1/1	1/1	1/1
Ethanol	1/1	1/1	1/1	1/1

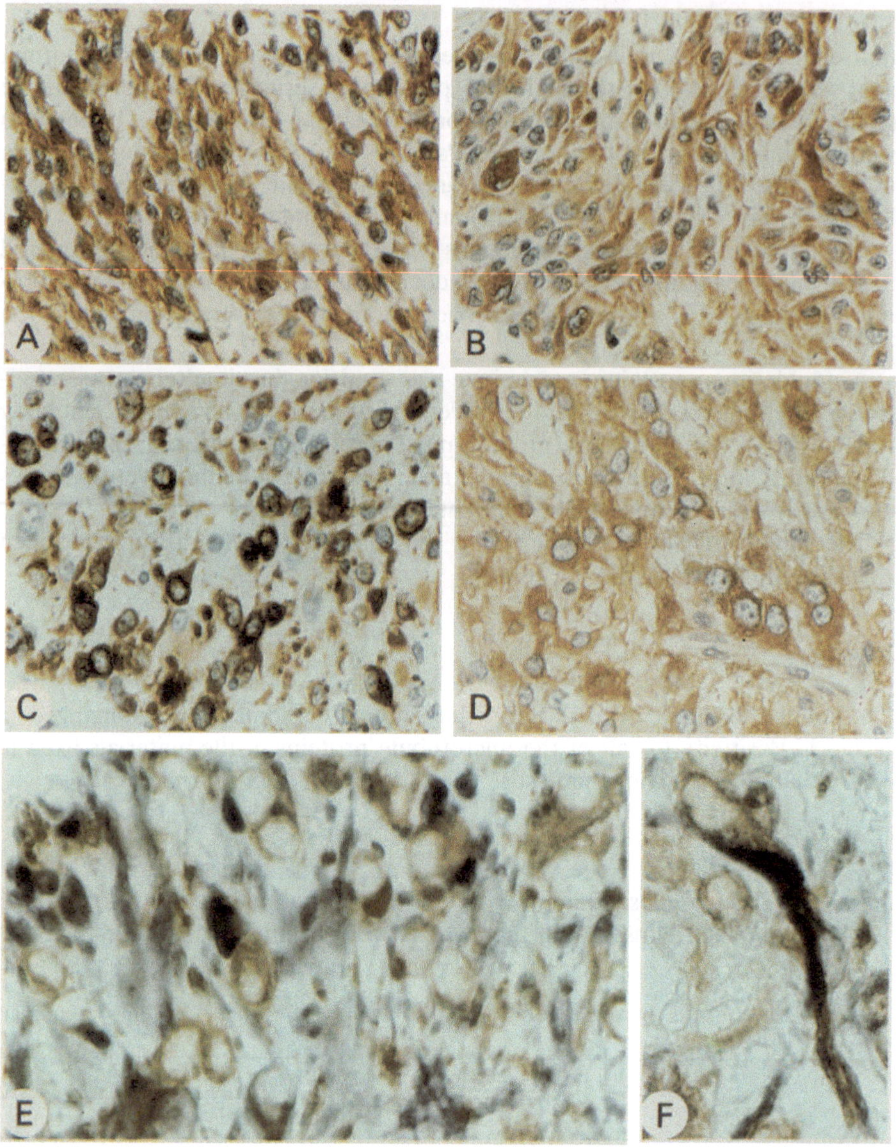

Fig. 1. Immunoperoxidase staining with **A** anti-beta-tubulin Mab, **B** anti-MAP1 Mab, **C** anti-MAP2 Mab, **D** anti-MAP5 Mab, and **E,F** double-labeling with anti-GFA protein serum and anti-MAP2 Mab. All single-labeled sections were lightly counterstained with hematoxylin. **A** Nearly all tumor cells in anaplastic astrocytoma were immunopositive for beta-tubulin, × 200. **B** Various types of tumor cells in glioblastoma were immunoreactive for MAP1, × 200. **C** Many small-sized immature cells and some plump cells in glioblastoma were immunopositive for MAP2, × 200. **D** MAP5-positive cells in glioblastoma are arranged around pseudopalisading, × 200. **E** Both MAP2-positive cells (*brown*) and GFA protein-positive cells (*dark blue*) were present in glioblastoma, × 400. **F** An anaplastic fusiform cell with a long cell process in glioblastoma was double labeled with anti-MAP2 Mab and anti-GFA protein serum, × 400

tubulin. Nearly all of the neoplastic astrocytes were positive for beta-tubulin (Fig. 1A). Sarcomatous elements in gliosarcoma were also faintly stained with anti-beta-tubulin Mab. The neuronal cell bodies, dendrites, and axons in the surrounding brain tissue of astrocytic tumors were also stained with this anti-beta-tubulin Mab.

2. *MAP1*

The fibrillary neoplastic astrocytes in 1 low-grade astrocytoma were mostly immunopositive for MAP1. The tumor cells, including giant cells and multinucleated cells in anaplastic astrocytomas and glioblastomas, also demonstrated immunoreactivity for MAP1 (Fig. 1B). There was no definitive difference in the immunoreactivity of the tumor cells when comparing low and higher-grade anaplastic astrocytomas.

3. *MAP2*

Tumor cells positive for MAP2 were found in 75% of all of the astrocytic gliomas. The percentage of MAP2-positive cells was relatively lower than those of other microtubule protein-positive cells in the astrocytic gliomas. A variety of tumor cells demonstrated immunoreactivity for MAP2 (Fig. 1C) and, most notably, giant cells or multinucleated cells were frequently stained with this monoclonal antibody.

4. *MAP5*

The immunoreactivity for MAP5 was somewhat similar to that of MAP1 in astrocytic gliomas. Most tumor cells in astrocytic gliomas were positive for MAP5 (Fig. 1D).

5. *Double-Labeled Study of MAP2 and GFA Protein*

Twelve astrocytic gliomas fixed in 70% ethanol were examined in this study. Cells positive for either MAP2 or GFA protein were present in both anaplastic astrocytomas and glioblastomas (Fig. 1E). The proportions of cells positive for each antibody were different in each case. Immunopositive cells for both MAP2 and GFA protein were also present in all of the cases, although their number was less frequent than that of the cells positive for either MAP2 or GFA protein (Fig. 1F).

Discussion

Beta-tubulin is widely present in neuronal cells, dendrites, axons, and astroglial cells in the central nervous system [2,11]. The function of beta-tubulin was closely related to axonal growth and neuronal differentiation [12], however, the significance of beta-tubulin in the astroglial cells was unclear [13]. In the present study, a strong immunopositivity for beta-tubulin was shown in the astrocytic gliomas.

Microtubule-associated proteins are a heterogenous group of molecules which promote the polymerization of tubulin [1]. MAP1, also known as MAP1a, has been shown to be widely distributed both within and outside of the nervous system [1]. MAP5, also called MAP1x or MAP1b, was present in axons, dendrites, and glial cells [8]. The study of MAPs in developing rat brain have shown that MAP5 was more abundant in brain tissue of newborn rather than that of adult rats [8], while, MAP1 was barely detectable at birth and increased steadily up to day 20. In this study, most tumor cells were positive for both MAP1 and 5, irrespective of the grade of the anaplasia.

MAP2 is the major MAP of brain tissue. Although it has been reported that some glial cells in the optic nerve demonstrate this protein, MAP2 is exclusively limited to neuronal dendrites [14]. We have shown that MAP2 was present in neoplastic astrocytes. However, we could not identify the morphological characteristics of MAP2-positive cells in astrocytic glioma, because MAP2 is present in all types of cells, such as small-sized immature cells, giant cells showing a high degree of anaplasia, multinucleated cells, as well as in fibrillary cells in astrocytic gliomas. Furthermore, the presence of double-labeled cells for MAP2 and GFA protein in astrocytic gliomas suggested that the demonstration of MAP2 was independent of astrocytic differentiation which was evaluated by GFA protein expression. GFA protein is known to be a useful marker for astrocytic differentiation, and its production is inversely correlated with the proliferating activity of glial tumors [6,9,10]. Therefore, the widespread demonstration of MAP2 and other microtubule proteins in the tumor cells may be related to the essential cytoskeletal change during neoplastic evolution.

Conclusion

The present study has shown that the presence of microtubule proteins in human astrocytic gliomas is more abundant than in normal astrocytes, and that some of these tumor cells have co-localized both microtubule proteins and GFA protein. These results suggest that the demonstration of microtubule proteins was closely related to tumorigenesis, and not to the astrocytic differentiation of the glial tumors.

Acknowledgements. This report was supported by a Grant-in Aid for Encouragement of Young Scientists from the Ministry of Education, Science and Culture of Japan (No. 02770876).

References

1. Matus A (1988) Microtubule-associated proteins: Their potential role in determining neuronal morphology. Annu Rev Neurosci 11:29–44
2. Burgoyne RD (1986) Microtubule proteins in neuronal differentiation. Comp Biochem Physiol [B] 83:1–8
3. Artlieb U, Krepler R, Wiche G (1985) Expression of microtubule-associated proteins, Map-1 and Map-2, in human neuroblastomas and differential diagnosis of immature neuroblasts. Lab Invest 53:684–691
4. Katsetos CD, Herman MM, Frankfurter A, Gass P, Collins VP, Walker CC, Rosemberg S, Barnard RO, Rubinstein LJ (1989) Cerebellar desmoplastic medulloblastomas. A further immunohistochemical characterization of the reticulin-free pale islands. Arch Pathol Lab Med 113:1019–1029
5. Gozes I, Barnstable CJ (1982) Monoclonal antibodies that recognize discrete forms of tubulin. Proc Natl Acad Sci USA 79:2579–2583
6. Eng LF, DeArmond SJ (1983) Immunohistochemistry of the glial fibrillary acidic protein. In: Zimmerman HM (ed) Progress in neuropathology, vol. 5, Raven, New York, pp 19–39
7. Huber G, Matus A (1984) Differences in the cellular distributions of two microtubule-associated proteins, MAP1 and MAP2, in rat brain. J Neurosci 4:151–160
8. Riederer B, Cohen R, Matus A (1986) MAP5: A novel brain microtubule-associated protein under strong developmental regulation. J Neurocytol 15:763–775
9. Ibayashi N, Herman MM, Boyd JC, Bigner DD, Friedman HS, Collins VP, Donoso LA, Rubinstein LJ (1989) Relationship of the demonstration of intermediate filament protein to kinetics of three human neuroepithelial tumor cell lines: Lack of neural-related proteins in most cells in S phase: A double-labeled immunohistochemical study on matrix cultures. Lab Invest 61:310–318
10. Ibayashi N, Hirakawa K, Suzuki K, Nakamura K, Houri T (1988) Immunohistochemical study of S-phase cells in human gliomas. No To Shinkei (Brain and Nerve) 40:763–769
11. Caceres A, Binder LI, Payne MR, Bender P, Rebhun L, Steward O (1984) Differential subcellular localization of tubulin and the microtubule-associated protein MAP2 in brain tissue as revealed by immunocytochemistry with monoclonal hybridoma antibodies. Neuroscience 4:394–410
12. Eddé B, de Nechaud B, Denoulet P, Gros F (1987) Control of isotubulin expression during neuronal differentiation of mouse neuroblastoma and teratocarcinoma cell lines. Dev Biol 123:549–558
13. Neto VM, Mallat M, Alliot F, Pessac B, Prochiantz A (1985) Astrocytic cerebellar cell clones synthesize the β' isoforms of the β-tubulin protein family. Neuroscience 16:333–341
14. Papasozomenos SCh, Binder LI (1986) Microtubule-associated protein 2 (MAP2) is present in astrocytes of the optic nerve but absent from astrocytes of the optic tract. J Neurosci 6:1748–1756

Human Malignant Glioma Cells Migrate to Fibronectin and Laminin: Role of Extracellular Matrix Components in Glioma Cell Invasion

Takanori Ohnishi, Norio Arita, Shoju Hiraga, Masahide Higuchi, and Toru Hayakawa[1]

Introduction

Malignant gliomas are characterized by high invasiveness, which is a major reason for the failure of treatment for these tumors with any mode. At present, the cellular and molecular mechanisms underlying glioma cell invasion are poorly understood. Tumor invasion is a process that consists of sequential events of complex interactions between tumor cells and host tissues. These include adhesion of tumor cells to the extracellular matrix (ECM), degradation of the regional ECM, and tumor cell locomotion [1]. Previous studies have shown that ECM components such as fibronectin (FN) and laminin (LN) not only play an important role in cell adhesion [2], but also promote the directed movement *in vitro* of various cells, including fibroblasts, neural crest cells, and tumor cells [3–5].

Although the characteristics of the extracellular space of the central nervous system (CNS) have not been completely clarified, immunohistochemistry has shown that several ECM glycoproteins, including FN, LN, and type IV collagen, are localized in normal brain and primary intracranial tumors [6,7]. Furthermore, our immunohistochemical studies in glioma specimens have demonstrated that FN can exist in the form of fine networks in the extracellular space, and that some tumor cells cluster at such networks of FN [8].

In the present study, we report that human malignant glioma cells can migrate to FN and LN *in vitro*. We also discuss a role of FN receptors in the glioma cell migration stimulated by the glycoprotein.

Materials and Methods

Cell Lines and Cell Culture

Four human glioblastoma cell lines, T98G, U87MG, U373MG, and A172 (all purchased from American Type Culture Collection) were grown as a monolayer in Eagle's minimum essential medium (MEM) containing 10% fetal bovine serum (FBS), 1% sodium pyruvate, and 1% non-essential amino acid

[1] Department of Neurosurgery Osaka University Medical School, Osaka, 553 Japan

for the first three cell lines, and in Dulbecco's modified Eagle's medium supplemented with 10% FBS for the last cell line.

Migration Assay

The migratory responses of cultured cells to FN and LN were assessed with a modified Boyden chamber assay method described previously [9]. Briefly, cells were harvested with 0.01% trypsin and 0.01% EDTA, washed twice with MEM, and suspended in serum-free MEM at a concentration of 5×10^5 cells/ml. These cell suspensions (50 µl) were placed in the upper wells of the chamber, and FN or LN in various concentrations were placed in the lower wells. A polycarbonate membrane filter with an 8.0 µm pore size (Nucleopore, Pleasanton, Calif.) was placed between these wells. After the chamber was incubated at 37°C for 4 h, the filter was removed, fixed, and stained with Diff-Quik (Scientific Products, Harleco). The number of cells that had migrated to the lower surface of the filter was counted in 20 random fields at $\times$ 400. The degree of migration was expressed as the number of cells per mm^2.

Haptotactic Migartion to FN and LN

In order to investigate whether glioma cells can migrate to substratum-bound FN or LN in the absence of additional soluble attractants, i.e., by haptotactic migration [10], the migration of the cells on the filter whose lower surface was precoated with FN or LN was determined.

Arg-Gly-Asp(RGD)-containing peptides

Synthetic hexapeptides, GRGDSP and GRGESP, were purchased from Iwaki Glass (Chiyoda, Tokyo). The peptides were placed in the upper wells in the indicated concentrations along with the cell suspensions. Ten µg/ml FN was used as an attractant in the lower wells, and effects of RGD peptide on the cell migration were examined.

Treatment with Cytochalasin B

Glioma cells in the upper wells of the chamber were incubated with various concentrations of cytochalasin B (Sigma) and the migration of the cells to FN or LN in the lower wells was determined.

Results

Migration of Glioma Cells to FN and LN

All glioma cell lines migrated to FN up to a concentration of 10 µg/ml in a dose-dependent manner, and the migration reached a plateau or decreased at concentrations higher than 10 µg/ml (Fig. 1a). The intensity of migratory re-

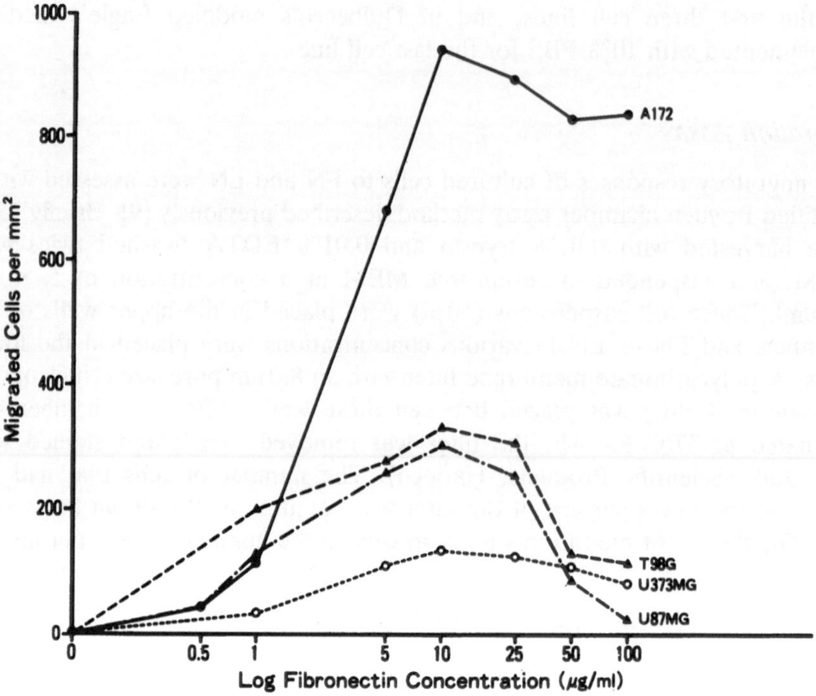

a

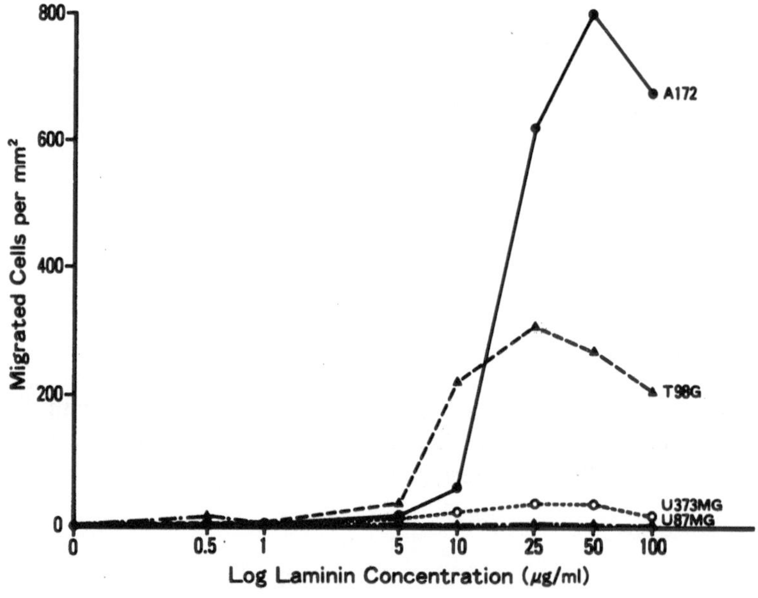

b

Fig. 1. Dose-dependent stimulation of glioma cell migration by **a** fibronectin and **b** laminin. Four human glioma cell lines, *A172, T98G, U87MG*, and *U373MG* migrated toward the attractants in soluble form to various degrees sponses to FN varied among the four glioma cell lines, i.e., A172 showed the highest migration to FN, U373MG the lowest, and T98G and U87MG had medium levels. On the other hand, the migration of these glioma cells to LN showed a different response from that to FN (Fig. 1b). A172 and T98G required 25–50 μg/ml LN to obtain a maximum migratory response. Moreover, U373MG and U87MG cells did not respond to LN at any concentration tested.

Haptotactic Migration of Glioma Cells to FN and LN

All glioma cells examined migrated to the lower surface of filters precoated with 50 μg/ml FN and two cell lines, A172 and T98G, migrated to the lower surface of filters precoated with 100 μg/ml LN (Fig. 2). U373MG cells did not migrate to the lower surface precoated with LN as in the chemotactic migration to LN.

Effects of RGD Peptide on Glioma Cell Migration to FN

T98G cell migration to FN was inhibited by synthetic peptide, GRGDSP, in response to increasing concentrations of the peptide, while the control peptide, GRGESP, had no such effect (Fig. 3). GRGDSP peptide at a concentration of more than 1 mg/ml was required for the complete inhibition of T98G cell migration to 10 μg/ml FN.

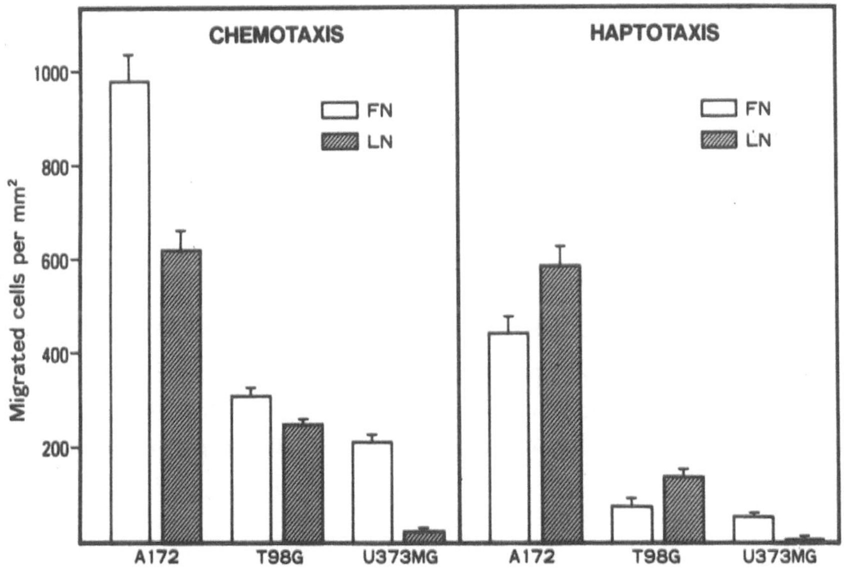

Fig. 2. Glioma cell migration to fibronectin (*FN*) and laminin (*LN*) in soluble form (chemotaxis) and in substratum-bound form (haptotaxis). For haptotaxis, filters were precoated on only the lower side with 50 μg/ml of FN or 100 μg/ml of LN. Values are means ±SD (*bars*) for triplicate experiments

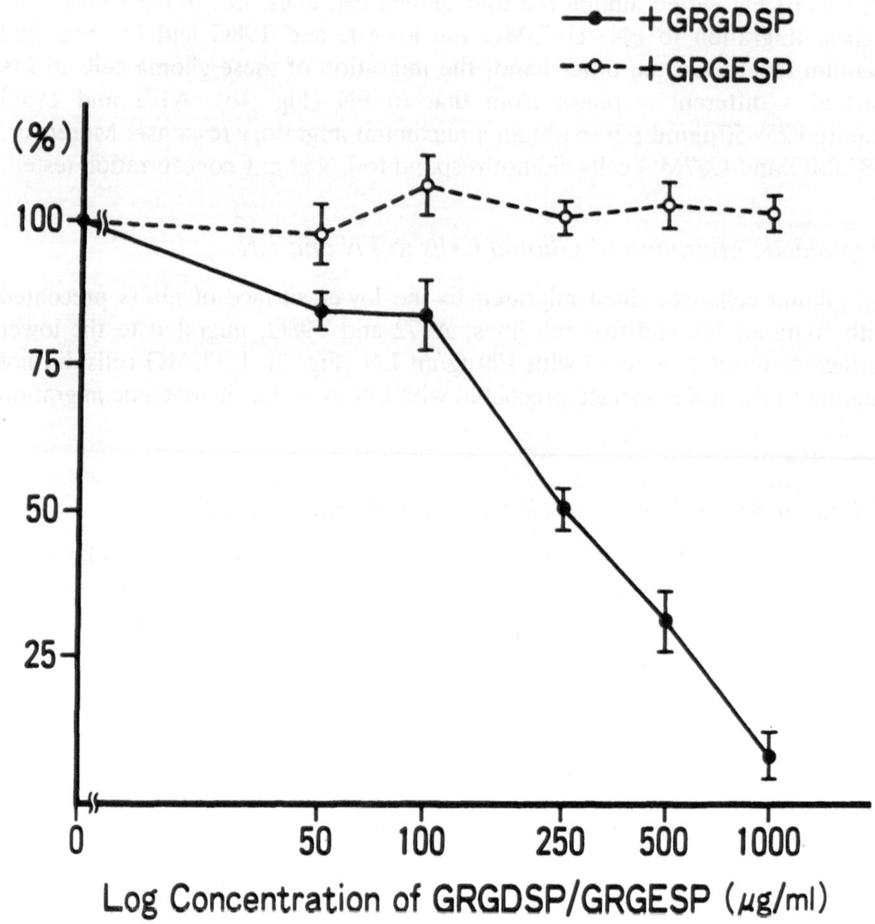

Fig. 3. The effect of Arg-Gly-Asp (*RGD*)-containing peptides on T98G cell migration stimulated by fibronectin. Ten μg/ml fibronectin was used as an attractant in lower wells. Values are means ±SD for six experiments

Effects of Cytochalasin B on Glioma Cell Migration to FN

Glioma cell migration to FN in various concentrations (5–100 μg/ml) was almost completely inhibited by treatment with 10 μg/ml cytochalasin B (Fig. 4). Glioma cell migration to LN was also inhibited by the drug (data not shown).

Discussion

In the present study, we demonstrated that human malignant glioma cells can migrate to FN and LN in various degrees. All glioma cell lines examined in this study showed highly migaratory responses to FN at the relatively low concentration of 0.5 μg/ml, whereas migration to LN required a much higher concen-

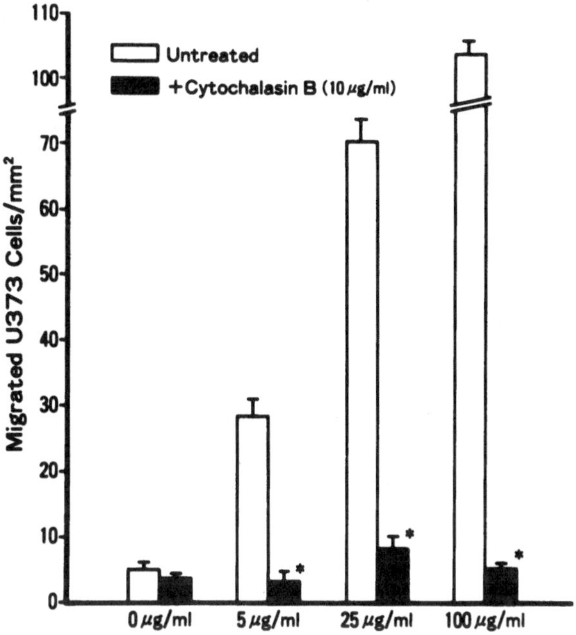

Fig. 4. The effect of cytochalasin B on U373MG cell migration stimulated by fibronectin at various concentrations. Values are means ±SD for six experiments. Significantly different from the untreated group at $^{*}P < 0.001$ (*t*-test)

tration, while two cell lines (U373MG and U87MG) did not respond to LN at any concentration tested. It has been reported that LN increases the rate and the number of tumor cells attaching to type IV collagen, thus prompting tumor metastasis [11]. In the CNS, LN has been immunolocalized in the vascular basement membrane [6–8]. These findings suggest that the lower reactivity of glioma cells to LN might relate to the low metastatic potential of these tumors.

Glioma cells showed migratory responses to FN and LN not only in soluble form (chemotaxis) but also in substratum-bound form (haptotaxis). Chemotactic migration may be involved in diffuse infiltration of tumor cells over longer distances, while haptotactic migration could be related to insoluble constituents of the ECM and promote direct invasion of tumor cells. Although FN is thought to be much more operative in the chemotactic migration of glioma cells than is LN, haptotactic migration to LN was a little stronger than that to FN in two glioma cell lines with positive responses to LN.

It has been demonstrated that FN has a specific amino acid sequence, arginine-glycine-aspartic acid (RGD), as a core structure recognized by a family of structurally related receptors (integrins), which mediates a reaction between cells and ECM components [12,13]. The fact that RGD-containing peptide inhibits the cell migration stimulated by FN may indicate that the migration of glioma cells to FN is mediated through the receptor on the cell surface. In fact, our immunohistochemical studies have demonstrated that all of these glioma cell lines express FN-receptors on their cell surfaces and that A172 cells have the most FN-receptors among these four cell lines (data not shown).

In our experiments, cytochalasin B, a disassembling agent of actin microfilaments, almost completely inhibited the cell migration stimulated by FN or LN. It has been reported that active tumor cell locomotion can occur through an alteration in cellular microfilaments such as actin [14]. These results may indicate that glioma cell migration promoted by FN or LN requires a normal organization of cytoskeletons, and that receptors for these glycoproteins play an important role in the process of tumor invasion.

Conclusion

Human malignant glioma cells showed a highly migratory response to FN. The migratory response of the cells to LN was lower than that to FN, and some cells did not respond to LN. The glioma cells migrated to these ECM glycoproteins both in soluble form (chemotaxis) and in substratum-bound form (haptotaxis). RGD peptide inhibited the glioma cell migration stimulated by FN. Furthermore, cytochalasin B almost completely inhibited the cell migration promoted by FN or LN, thus indicating a crucial role of a receptor linked to the cytoskeleton in glioma cell migration stimulated by these ECM glycoproteins.

Acknowledgement. This work was supported in part by a Grant-in-Aid 2–14 from the Ministry of Health and Welfare, Japan.

References

1. Liotta LA, Rao CN, Wewer UM (1986) Biochemical interactions of tumor cells with the basement membrane. Ann Rev Biochem 55:1037–1057
2. Terranova VP, Rohrbach DH, Martin GR (1980) Role of laminin in the attachment of PAM 212 (epithelial) cells to basement membrane collagen. Cell 22:719–726
3. Tsukamoto Y, Helsel WE, Wahl SM (1981) Macrophage production of fibronectin, a chemoattractant for fibroblasts. J Immunol 127:673–678
4. Bronner-Fraser M (1986) An antibody to a receptor for fibronectin and laminin perturbs cranial neural crest development. Dev Biol 117:528–536
5. Lacovara J, Cramer EB, Quigley JP (1984) Fibronectin enhancement of directed migration of B16 melanoma cells. Cancer Res 44:1657–1663
6. McComb RD, Bigner DD (1985) Immunolocalization of laminin in neoplasms of the central and peripheral nervous systems. J Neuropathol Exp Neurol 44:242–253
7. Rutka JT, Myatt CA, Giblin JR, Davis RL, Rosenblum ML (1987) Distribution of extracellular matrix proteins in primary human brain tumors: An immunohistochemical analysis. Can J Neurol Sci 14:25–30
8. Higuchi M, Ohnishi T, Arita N, Hiraga S, Iwasaki H, Hayakawa T (1991) Immunohistocemical localization of fibronectin, laminin and fibronectin receptor in human malignant gliomas. No To Shinkei (Brain and Nerve) 43:17–23

9. Ohnishi T, Arita N, Hayakawa T, Izumoto S, Taki T, Yamamoto H (1990) Motility factor produced by maligant glioma cells: Role in tumor invasion. J Neurosurg 73:881–888
10. Carter SB (1967) Haptotaxis and the mechanism of cell motility. Nature 213:256–260
11. Terranova VP, Liotta LA, Russo RG, Martin GR (1982) Role of laminin in the attachment and metastasis of murine tumor cells. Cancer Res 42:2265–2269
12. Hynes RO (1987) Integrins: A family of cell surface receptors. Cell 48:549–554
13. Rouslahti E, Pierschbacher MD (1987) New perspectives in cell adhesion: RGD and integrins. Science 238:491–497
14. Jokusch BM, Haemmerli G, In Albon A (1983) Cytoskeletal organization in locomoting cells of the V2 rabbit carcinoma. Exp Cell Res 144:251–263

The Effect of Matrigel on the Growth of Glioma Cells *In Vitro* and *In Vivo*

Teruaki Mori, Takamitsu Hikawa, Takashi Yoshida, Atsushi Karashima, Minoru Fujiki, and Shigeaki Hori[1]

Introduction

Extracellular matrix components, such as laminin and fibronectin, promote cellular adhesion, growth, migration, and differentiation of glioma cells [1,2]. Matrigel is a biopolymer of natural constituents containing 60% laminin, 30% type IV collagen, 5% nidogen, 3% heparin sulfate proteoglycan, and 1% entactin.

The purpose of this study was to examine the effect of Matrigel on morphological structures and growth of glioma cells in vitro and *in vivo*.

Materials and Methods

Preparation of Matrigel

Matrigel was extracted from an Engelbreth Holm Swarm (EHS) tumor using previously described methods [3].

In Vitro *Study*

Matrigel (250 µl) was used to coat the surface of 16 mm wells (Falcon #3847, 24 flat-bottom wells), and then allowed to solidify at 37°C for at least 1 h. Five kinds of cultured human glioma cells (T98G, KWN, IN301, U251, and NHG1; 55,000 cells/well) were plated to the wells.

In some cultures, Tunicamycin, an inhibitor of protein glycosylation, was also added to the culture medium. The culture plates containing the glioma cells on Matrigel were then placed overnight in an incubator, after which the cells were examined by light-microscopy.

In Vivo *Study*

Cultured human glioma cells (U251: 1×10^5 cells) were transplanted into the dorsal subcutaneous region of 6 nude mice. The U251 cells mixed with Mat-

[1] Department of Neurosurgery, Medical College of Oita, Oita, 879-56 Japan

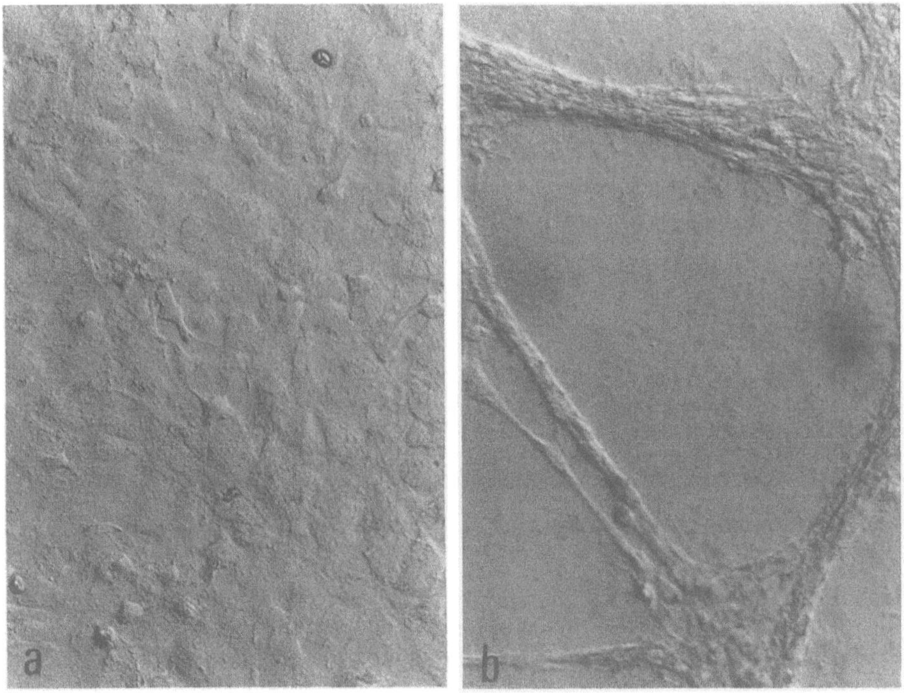

Fig. 1. Cultured human glioma cells (KWN). **a** KWN formed a normal monolayer on plastic alone and **b** network structures on Matrigel, × 40

rigel (0.01 ml) were transplanted on the right side, and the same volume of U251 mixed with Dulbecco's modified Eagle's medium (DMEM) was transplanted on the left side of the same nude mouse as control. The tumor size was measured continually, and the tumors were removed at 11 days after transplantation and examined histologically by light-microscopy.

Results

All cultured glioma cells plated on plastic alone (as control) formed a normal monolayer in culture with time. In contrast, the same glioma cells plated on Matrigel formed network structures (Fig. 1). When Tunicamycin was added to the culture medium, the glioma cells remained attached to the Matrigel, but did not form complete network structures (Fig. 2).

The subcutaneously transplanted glioma cells mixed with Matrigel grew more rapidly than those mixed with the DMEM medium: the former tumors became about 3 times heavier than the latter at 12 days after transplantation (Figs. 3, 4).

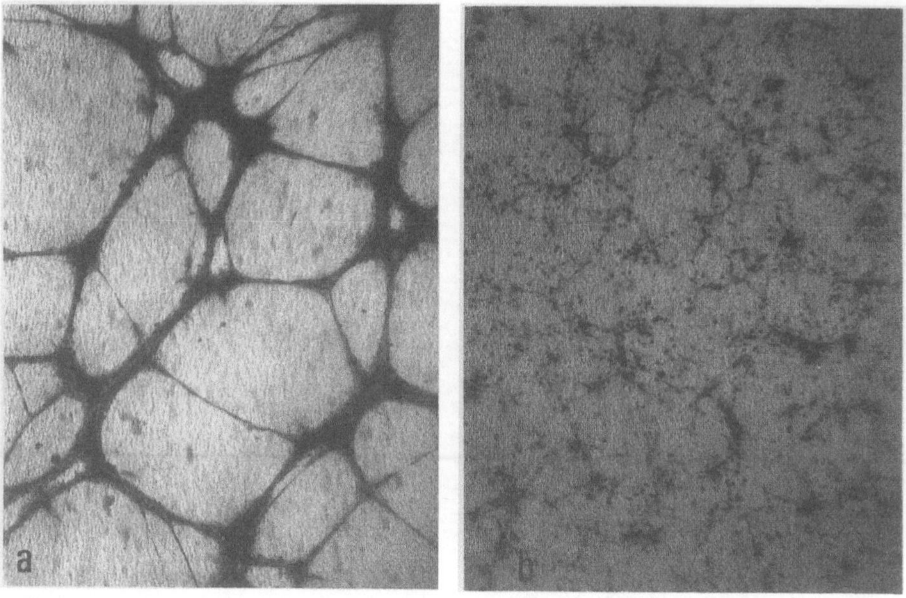

Fig. 2. Effect of Tunicamycin on network formation of KWN cultured with Matrigel. **a** Control. **b** Network structures were not formed when treated with Tunicamycin (0.5 μg/ml), × 10

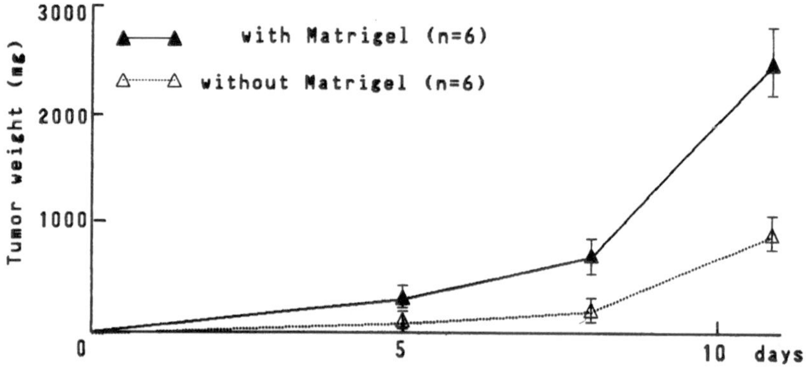

Fig. 3. Growth curves of transplanted glioma cells (U251) into nude mice. With time, the glioma cells with Matrigel produced heavier tumors than those without Matrigel

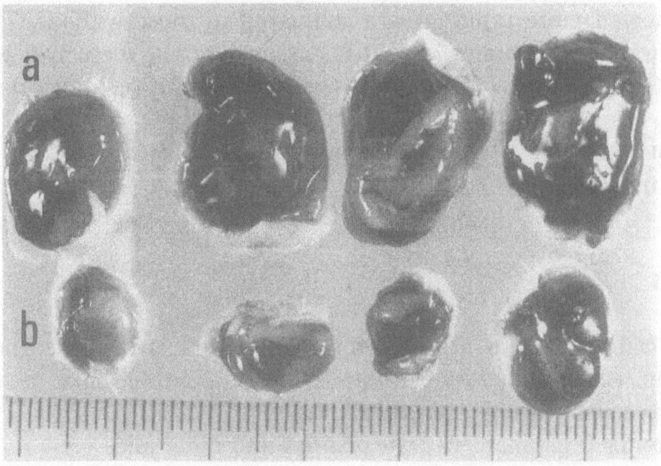

Fig. 4. Photographs of 4 tumors extirpated 11 days after transplantation of glioma cells (U251) **a** mixed with Matrigel and **b** without Matrigel

Histological examination of the extirpated tumors revealed that tumor cell population, blood vessels, collagen, and reticulin fibers were more increased in the cases with Matrigel than in those without.

Discussion

Matrigel is a biologically active substrate which induces diverse cellular responses, It was found to encourage the in vitro growth and differentiation of many cultured cells (melanoma cell, liver cell, Schwann's cell, etc.) [3]. Endothelial cells also formed capillary-like structures on Matrigel [4]. *In vivo*, it promoted peripheral nerve regeneration [5] and outgrowth of the fetal dopamine neuron [6]. However, there have been no report on the effect of Matrigel on the growth and differentiation of glioma cells.

In this study, we could observe that glioma cells formed network structures when they were cultured with Matrigel. Apparently these network structures are similar to the capillary network of endothelial cells cultured on Matrigel. Although the mechanism of the network formation is not adequately understood, it may be related to cell-to-cell and cell-to-matrix interaction and cell migration.

Tunicamycin, a blocker of protein glycosylation or monosaccharide N-acetyl-D-glucosamin, inhibited the network formation of glioma cells on Matrigel. This suggests that cell surface glycosyltransferases [7] may be related to the formation of the network structure of glioma cells.

In our *in vivo* study, the transplanted glioma cells which were mixed with Matrigel showed more rapid growth compared to those without. There were marked differences in tumor weight and size between these two glioma cell groups. Although the exact tumor-growing mechanism of Matrigel has yet to be clarified, our histological study suggested that it may promote cell growth by increasing neovascularization and the infiltrating capacity of blood vessels and connective tissues.

Conclusion

1. Glioma cells plated on Matrigel formed network structures. The network formation was inhibited by Tunicamycin treatment and may, therefore, be related to cell surface glycosyltransferases.
2. Matrigel-mixed glioma cells transplanted into nude mice grew rapidly, producing remarkably larger tumors than those in controls. Histologically, these tumors showed increases of tumor cell population, blood vessels, and connective tissue.
3. Matrigel may be useful in studying the attachment, migration, and growth of glioma cells, and the network structure of the Matrigel-mixed glioma cells may be a good three-dimensional model to study cell interaction.

References

1. Liesi P (1984) Laminin and Fibronectin in normal and malignant neuroectodermal cells. Med Biol 61:163–180
2. Rutka JT, Apodaca G, Stern R, Rosenblum M (1988) The extracellular matrix of the central and peripheral nervous systems: Structure and function. J Neurosurg 69:155–170
3. Kleinman HK, Mcgarvey ML, Hassell JR, Cannon FB, Laurie GW, Martin GR (1986) Basement membrane complexes with biological activity. Biochemistry 25:312–318
4. Grant DS, Tashiro K, Segui-Real B, Yamada Y, Martin GR, Kleinman HK (1989) Two different laminin domains mediate the differentiation of human endothelial cells into capillary-like structures *in vitro*. Cell 58:933–943
5. Madison R, da Silva CF, Dikkes P, Chiu TH, Sidman RL (1985) Increased rate of peripheral nerve regeneration using bioresorbable nerve guides and a laminin-containing gel. Exp Neurol 88:767–772
6. Haber S, Finklestein SD, Benowitz LI, Sladek JR Jr, Collier TJ (1988) Matrigel enhances survival and integration of grafted dopamine neurons into the striatum. In: Gash DM, Sladek JR Jr (eds) Progress in brain research 78. Elsevier, Netherlands, pp 427–433
7. Runyan RB, Maxwell GD, Shur BD (1986) Evidence for a novel enzymatic mechanism of neural crest cell migration on extracellular glycoconjugate matrices. J Cell Biol 102:432–441

Glycolipid in Human Glioma: Detection with Specific Antibodies and Its Application for Diagnosis of Gliomas

Osamu Nakamura[1] and Masao Iwamori[2]

Introduction

Gangliosides are acidic glycosphingolipids with sialic acid as the negative charge donor, occuring at the highest concentration in brain tissue. Their content and composition are known to change in association with malignant transformation. In general, malignant gliomas reduce the synthesizing ability of Gg4 Cer-containing molecules and contain a higher concentration of the ganglioside GD3, with the degree of malignancy appearing to correlate with the content of GD3 [1–3].

Previous studies have shown that tumor cells, such as malignant melanoma or neuroblastoma, shed gangliosides into the circulation of the blood, and suggested that gangliosides could be useful tumor markers [4,5].

In this study, we tried to clarify whether ganglioside GD3 is shed from human glioma tissues into the circulation. The results are compared with healthy controls, and the usefulness of this test in the diagnosis of malignant gliomas is assessed.

Methods

Ganglioside Extraction

Serum samples used in this study were obtained from six healthy donors, three patients with astrocytoma grade II, three with astrocytoma grade III, and nine with glioblastoma. The diagnoses of gliomas were confirmed histologically. The serum samples were frozen at −70°C until use. One milliliter of serum from each donor was lyophilized, the crude lipids were extracted successively with 2 ml chloroform-methanol-water (20:10:1), (10:20:1), (20:10:1), and (10:20:1) at 40°C, and all extracted lipids were combined. To avoid a loss of gangliosides, the lipid extracts were directly used for the analysis as follows.

[1]Department of Neurosurgery, Tokyo Metropolitan Komagome Hospital, Bunkyo-ku, Tokyo, 113 Japan
[2]Department of Biochemistry, Faculty of Medicine, Tokyo University, Bunkyo-ku, Tokyo, 113 Japan

- polygram Sil G
- develop
- dry
- + blocking buffer
  (37°C, 1hr)
- + mouse monoclonal anti-GD3 IgG antibody
  (4°C, overnight)
- wash with washing buffer
- + blocking buffer
  (37°C, 15min)
- wash with PBS
- + Peroxidase-labeled anti-mouse IgG antibody diluted with dilution buffer
  (37°C, 1hr with shaking)
- wash with washing buffer
- + 4-chloro-1-naphtol and H_2O_2
  (room temp, 15min)

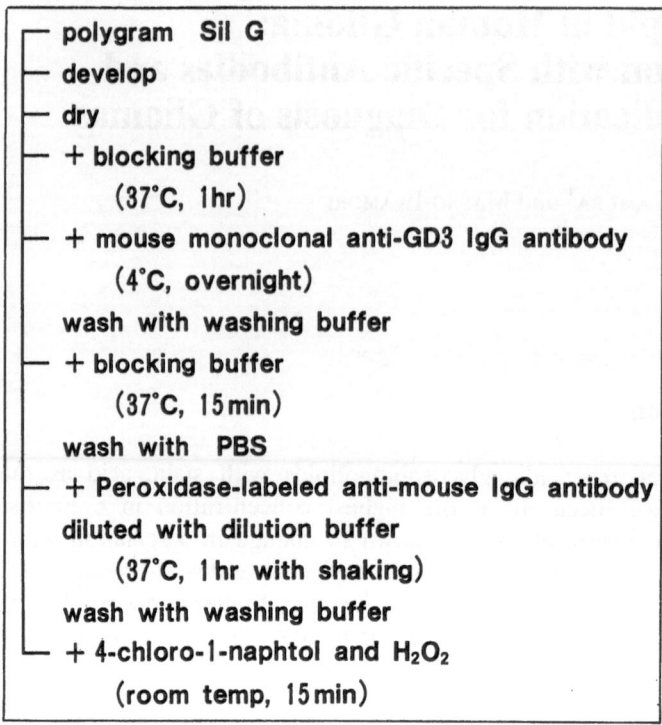

Fig. 1. Steps in TLC Immunostaining

Detection of GD3 by TLC-Immunostaining with Monoclonal Anti-GD3 Antibody

The lipid extracts corresponding to 20 µl serum were chromatographed on a thin-layer chromatogram plate (Polygram Sil), which was developed with chloroform-methanol −0.5% $CaCl_2$ (45:55:10). After blocking the plate, mouse monoclonal anti-GD3 IgG antibody, which was kindly supplied by J. Portoukalian, Center Leon Berad, Lyon, France, was allowed to react overnight at 4°C. After washing the plate, the antibody that remained on the plate was detected with peroxidase-labeled anti-mouse IgG antibody followed by 4-chloro-1-naphthol and H_2O_2. The quantitation of GD3 was made densitometrically at 420 nm with a TLC densitometer (Fig. 1).

Results

All of the results are summarized in Table 1. Ganglioside GD3 was not detected in the sera of healthy donors or in patients with astrocytoma grade II. However, serum GD3 was detected in one of the three patients with astrocyto-

Table 1. Ganglioside GD3 was not detected in the sera of healthy donors or patients with astrocytoma G2. However, serum GD3 was detected in one out of three patients with astrocytoma G3 and in seven out of nine patients with glioblastoma

Source of serum (*n*)	Positive	Negative
Control (6)	0/6	6/6
Astrocytoma G2 (3)	0/3	3/3
Astrocytoma G3 (3)	1/3	2/3
Glioblastoma (9)	7/9	2/9

Table 2. Ganglioside-sialic acid distribution (%)

Tissue	Ganglioside	GM_3	GM_2	GM_1	GD_3	GD_{1a}	GD_2	GD_{1b}	GT_{1b}
Low-grade glioma									
	N.(G-1)	2.41	2.07	8.76	5.82	73.77	tr	4.23	2.94
	O.(G-14)	7.14	1.43	74.29	7.14	2.86	tr	4.29	2.86
	A.(G-17)	9.18	8.09	29.84	14.43	14.97	tr	13.11	10.38
	S.(G-18)	11.21	7.17	38.74	7.79	15.58	ND	9.66	9.66
Malignant glioma									
	N.(G-1)	11.24	3.29	8.27	28.16	14.65	tr	13.79	20.60
	S.(G-2)	63.24	4.09	5.34	10.75	13.13	ND	1.10	2.34
	K.(G-3)	12.98	2.33	4.67	32.81	24.15	2.12	7.07	13.86
	W.(G-4)	13.57	0.01	0.01	56.42	2.67	9.40	10.19	7.73
	S.(G-5)	10.57	1.12	4.98	47.41	9.08	tr	13.21	13.63
	K.(G-12)	38.02	ND	24.79	28.93	ND	8.26	ND	ND
	A.(G-13)	27.62	3.87	14.36	37.57	ND	10.50	ND	6.08
Glioma in nude mouse		23.21	5.36	12.50	32.14	ND	5.36	ND	21.43
Metastatic tumor									
Lung	O.(M-1)	23.02	2.77	5.86	14.87	14.24	6.32	11.54	21.39
	F.(M-4)	43.78	3.97	9.13	8.06	11.64	3.22	9.46	10.75
	T.(M-14)	27.27	16.67	12.12	15.15	9.09	tr	9.09	10.61
Kidney	N.(M-3)	60.00	9.64	5.77	3.45	21.15	ND	ND	ND
	K.(M-5)	69.88	22.78	0.01	2.70	3.55	tr	tr	1.08
Colon	T.(M-2)	23.65	3.50	6.52	17.90	13.12	4.68	10.07	20.57
	T.(M-18)	28.57	23.81	14.29	14.29	9.52	ND	4.76	4.76
Malignant meningioma		10.66	10.66	27.87	13.11	13.11	ND	13.94	10.66
Reference		2.7	4.1	14.9	5.4	21.7	8.0	18.2	16.3

tr, trace; ND, not detected

ma grade III and in seven out of the nine patients with glioblastoma. These results showed that the shedding of ganglioside GD3 increases in proportion to the degree of malignancy of the gliomas. The amount of ganglioside GD3 ranged between 0.5 and 1 μg/ml.

Discussion

In a previous study we reported that the proportion of ganglioside GD3 increases in glioma tissues and that GD3 content is correlated with the malignancy of gliomas (Table 2).

In this study, we evaluated the shedding of GD3 from glioma tissues by immunochemical analysis. Serum ganglioside GD3 was detected in one of three patients with astrocytoma grade III and in seven out of nine patients with glioblastoma. It is well known that human gliomas seldom metastasize. However, this study makes it clear that gangliosides are being shed from glioma tissues. Although GD3 is a minor ganglioside in the sera, its detection may be useful in the diagnosis of gliomas. It should be noted that all of the patients with gliogblastoma in this study were at advanced stages. Considering the high reliability of radiological diagnostic techniques in the neurosurgical field, such as the CT scan and MRI, further study will be necessary to clarify the relationships between the GD3 level in serum and the properties of tumors, to enhance this technique for clinical use.

Meanwhile, gangliosides shed from tumors have been reported to show an immunosuppressive function, such as inhibition of natural killer cells or helper T cells. In other words, tumor-derived gangliosides may serve to protect tumor cells from host immune surveillance [6–9]. Further study will be necessary to clarify the functions of GD3 before anti-GD3 antibodies can be used in the diagnosis and treatment of glioblastoma.

References

1. Eto Y, Shinoda S (1982) Gangliosides and neutral glycosphinglipids in human brain tumors: Specificity and their significance. Adv Exp Med Biol 152:279–280
2. Nakamura O, Ishihara E, Iwamori M, Nagai Y, Matsutani M, Nomura K and Takakura K (1987) Lipid composition of human malignant brain tumors (in Japanese). No To Shinkei (Brain and Nerve) 39:221–226
3. Traylor TD, Hogan EL (1980) Gangliosides of human cerebral astrocytomas. J Neurochem 34:126–131
4. Bernhard H, Meyer Zum Buschenfelde KH, Dippold WG (1989) Ganglioside GD3 shedding by human malignant melanoma cells. Int J Cancer 44:155–160
5. Ladisch S, Wu Z, Frig S, Ulsh L, Schwartz E, Floutsis G, Wiley F, Lenars C, Seeger R (1987) Shedding of GD2 ganglioside by human neuroblastoma. Int J Cancer 39:73–76
6. Dippold W, Knuth A, Meyer Zum Buschenfelde KH (1984) Inhibitation of human melanoma cell growth in vitro by monoclonal anti-GD3-ganglioside antibody. Cancer Res 44:806–810
7. Hoon DB, Irie RF, Cochran AJ (1988) Gangliosides from human melanoma immunomodulate response of T cells to interleukin-2. Cell Immunol 111:410–419
8. Ladisch S, Gillard B, Wong C, Ulsh L (1983) Shedding and immunoregulatory activity of YAC-1 lymphoma cell gangliosides. Cancer Res 43:3808–3813
9. Seyfried TN, Yu RK (1985) Ganglioside GD3: Structure, cellular distribution and possible function. Mol Cell Biochem 68:3–10

Immunohistochemical Study of Protein Kinase C Isozyme in Recurrent Cases of Malignant Glioma

Osami Kubo, Yasuhiko Tajika, Masako Katahira, Yoshihiro Muragaki, Takeko Tajika, Hideaki Uchinuno, Masae Nitta, and Mizuo Kagawa[1]

Introduction

Protein kinase C (PKC) [1], an activated phorbol ester known to have a role in promoting carcinogenesis, is likely to be involved in cellular proliferation and in the process of cancer production. In their studies of gliomas, Todo et al. [2] and Reifenberger et al. [3] reported that malignant gliomas, e.g., glioblastoma, were immunohistochemically positive for the PKC-type III isozyme. The present immunohistochemical study investigated PKC isozymes in tumor tissues obtained at the first, second, or third operations from 14 cases of glioblastoma and from 4 cases of anaplastic astrocytoma.

Materials and Methods

We investigated 18 tumors, all of which were classified according to the WHO classification as human malignant glioma. The recurrent tumors were treated by surgical resection and radiochemotherapy within 1 year of the first operation in 12 cases and after 1 year after the first operation in 6 cases.

The tumor tissues were fixed by 10% formalin and embedded in paraffin, and immunohistochemical staining was performed on the paraffin sections. Monoclonal anti-rabbit brain protein kinase C (PKC) isozyme antibody (MBL Co., Japan) was used and stained by the avidin-biotin peroxidase complex (ABC) method.

Results

Anaplastic Astrocytoma

In all of the astrocytomas, we found tumor cells and vessels with PKC immunoreactivity in their cytoplasm and the walls of the vessels (Figs. 1b–d). In the glial fibrillary acidic protein (GFAP) immunostaining, only the tumor cells

[1] Department of Neurosurgery, Neurological Institute, Tokyo Women's Medical College, Shinjuku-ku Tokyo, 162 Japan

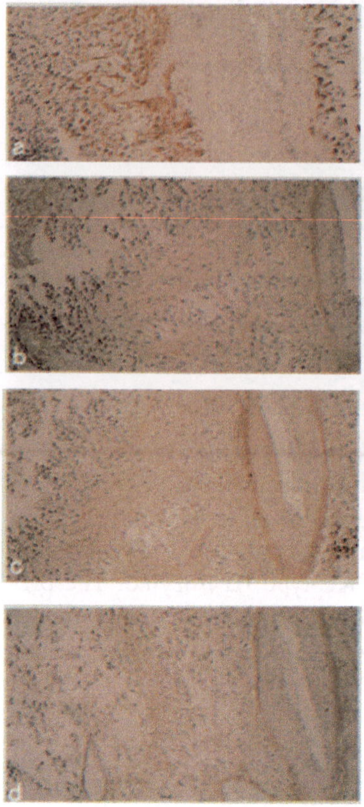

Fig. 1

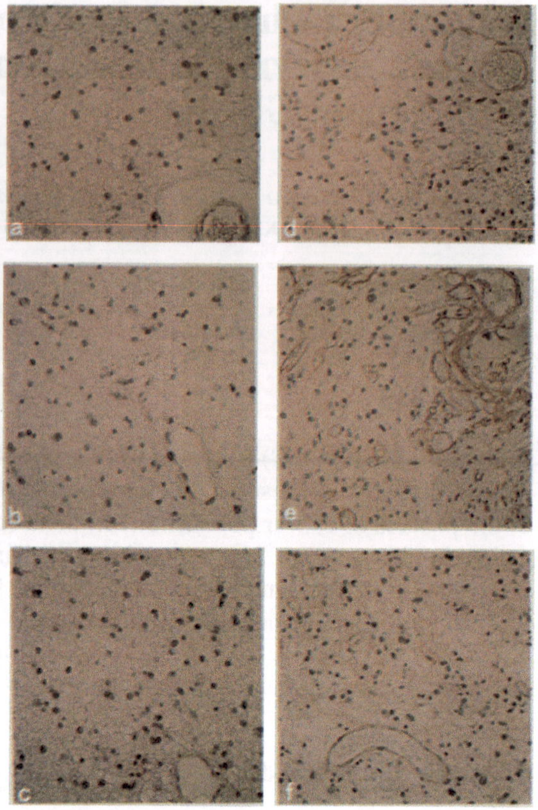

Fig. 2

Fig. 1. a GFAP immunoreactivity in tumor astrocytes around vessels in anaplastic astrocytoma. **b** PKC Type I. **c** PKC Type II. **d** PKC Type III

Fig. 2. a–c Types I, II, and III of PKC immunoreactivity in primary anaplastic astrocytoma. **d–f** Types I, II, and III of PKC immunoreactivity in recurrent anaplastic astrocytoma

were positively immunostained (Fig. 1a). PKC isozymes tended to be localized intensely in tumor vessels and cells, wherein immunoreactivity was strongest for the type II isozyme, less for type III, and least for type I.

Recurrent Astrocytoma

In all four cases of this group, the type II isozyme of PKC was more strongly positive than both types I and III (Figs. 2a–f).

Glioblastoma Multiforme

In all glioblastoma, GFAP immunoreactivity was strongly evidenced (Fig. 3a). In the isozyme of PKC, type II was more markedly immunostained than were types I and III (Figs. 3b–d).

Fig. 3

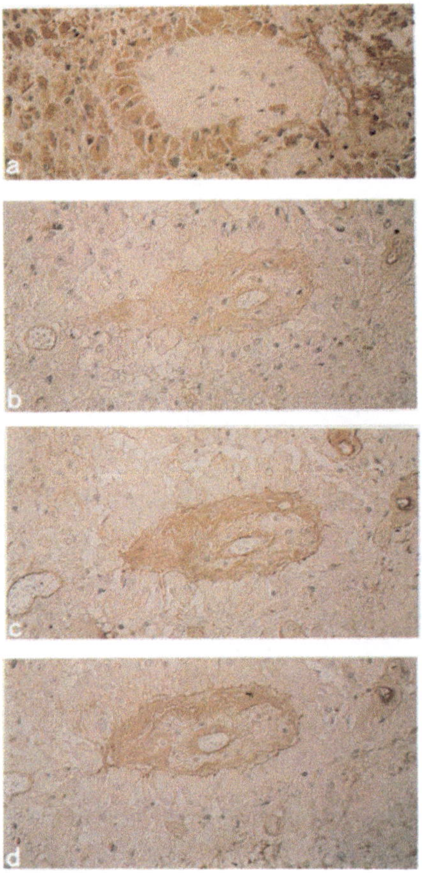

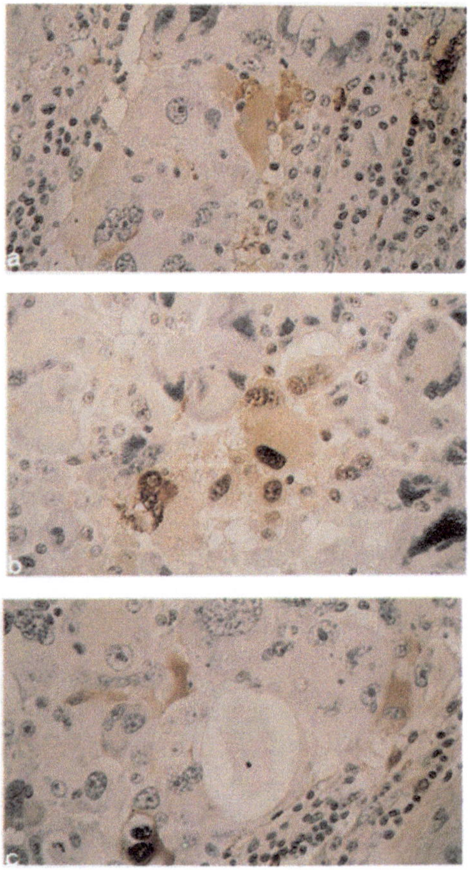

Fig. 4

Fig. 3. a GFAP immunoreactivity in tumor cells around vessels in glioblastoma. **b** PKC type I. **c** PKC type II. **d** PKC Type III

Fig. 4. a–c Types I, II, and III immunoreactivity in giant cell glioblastoma

The giant cells of the glioblastomas were also immunostained by the PKC isozyme. The immunoreactivity of type II was stronger than both types I and III (Figs. 4a–c).

Recurrent Glioblastoma

This group included 14 cases. The tumor cells and vessels were immunostained by the PKC isozyme. In all of the recurrent cases, immunoreactivity of the PKC isozyme was stronger than that in the primary tumor specimens (Figs. 5a–f). The tumor cells, both from glioblastoma and anaplastic astrocytoma, were not very strongly stained. However, in cases where the tumor cells derived from tissues which had been excised at the initial operation had been stained, the tumor cells from tissues resected at reoperation tended to be stained as well.

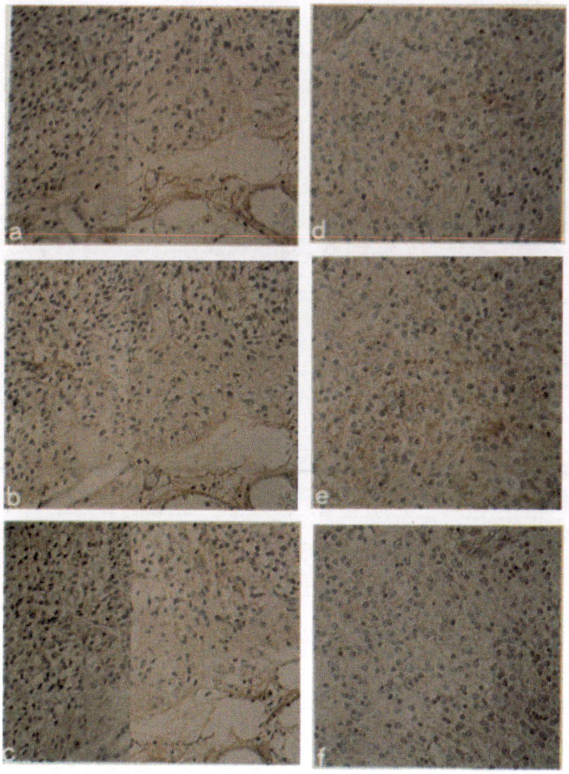

Fig. 5. a–c Types I, II, and III of PKC immunoreactivity in primary glioblastoma. **d–f** Types I, II, and III of PKC immunoreactivity in recurrent glioblastoma

Staining for the type II isozyme of PKC was stronger than that for type III, although the astrocytes adjacent to the tumor tissue were clearly stained for the type III isozyme.

Discussion

PKC is activated by tumor-promoting phorbol esters, such as TPA. It is composed of four distinct molecular types, α, βI, βII, and ψ, enclosed by three distinct genes. Isozymes of brain PKC are divided into types I (ψ), II (β), and III (α).

Our present immunohistochemical data indicate that not only tumor cells but also tumor vessels were strongly stained for PKC. The PKC isozyme was divided into three types, and the immunoreactivity of type II was shown to be stronger than types I and III.

While there are still technical problems with PKC staining in paraffin-embedded materials, the present study justifies our concluding that in each case of malignant glioma, the expression pattern of PKC isozymes was the same in primary as that in recurrent tumors.

References

1. Nishizuka Y (1984) The role of protein kinase C in cell surface signal transduction and tumour promotion. Nature 308:693–698
2. Todo T, Sidara N, Takakura K (1989) Immunohistochemical study on the expression of protein kinase C in isozymes (in Japanese). Proceedings of the 2nd annual meeting of the Society for Brain and Immunity, Tokyo, pp 178–182
3. Reifenberger G, Decker M, Wecksler W (1989) Immunohistochemical determination of protein kinase C expression and proliferation activity in human brain tumors. Acta Neuropath 78:166–175

Effects of Phorbor Esters on Cyclic AMP Accumulation in C6 Glioma Cells

HIROHIKO NAKAMURA[2], HUANG SHENG HAO[1], TETUO HARA[1], MASAO MATSUTANI[1], KINTOMO TAKAKURA[1], and NOBUYUKI SHITARA[2]

Introduction

Phorbor esters are well known tumor-promoting agents that directly activate a phospholipid- and calcium-dependent protein kinase C (PKC) [1,2]. It has recently been demonstrated that PKC can influence the β-adrenergic receptor (BAR) coupling to the cyclic AMP (cAMP)-generating system in a variety of cells and tissues, including mammalian brain. Phorbor 12-myrisate 13-acetate (PMA) enhances the cAMP response to isoproterenol or forskolin in rat brain slices [3], guinea pig cerebral cortical preparations [4], rat pinealocytes [5], and rat cerebral cortical and diencephalic neurons [6].

The C6 rat glioma cells, which respond to β-adrenergic agonists with 200-fold increases in cAMP content, have been utilized as a model for the study of β-adrenergic receptor (BAR)-coupled adenylate cyclase (AC) systems [7]. In the present study, we attempted to investigate whether such an interaction of a cAMP-generating system and PKC activation occurs in C6 glioma cells. We examined the effect of phorbor 12,13-dibutylate (PDBu) on isoproterenol- or forskolin-stimulated cAMP accumulation in rat glioma cells.

Materials and Methods

Materials

PDBu, isoproterenol, and forskolin were purchased from Sigma Chemical Co. (St. Louis, Mo., USA). The tissue culture medium, serum, and trypsin were obtained from GIBCO (Grand Island, N.Y.), and the cAMP (^{3}H) assay kit was obtained from Amersham International plc (Buckinghamshire, UK).

Cell culture

C6 glioma cells were grown in monolayer culture at 37°C in a humidified atmosphere containing 5% CO_2. The growth medium was the minimum essen-

[1] Department of Neurosurgery, University of Tokyo Hospital, Bunkyo-ku, Tokyo, 113 Japan
[2] Department of Neurosurgery, Komagome Metropolitan Hospital, Bunkyo-ku, Tokyo, 113 Japan

tial medium (MEM) supplemented with 10% fetal calf serum and 50 μg gentamycin sulfate. Confluent monolayers were removed from tissue culture flasks with 0.05% trypsin and plated at a density of 20,000 cells/cm^2 in 25 cm^2 plastic tissue culture dishes. Experiments were performed on confluent cells 5 days after plating. The medium was changed 24 h before experiments.

Assays of intracellular cAMP

After the cells were preincubated for 0, 6, and 24 h with the medium containing 500 μM PDBu, they were stimulated by 1 μM isoproterenol for 30 min or by 30 μM forskolin for 20 min. Preliminary experiments showed that isoproterenol induced cAMP maximal accumulation at 30 min and forskolin achieved this at 20 min. The reaction was terminated with the addition of ice-cold phosphate-buffered saline (PBS), and the cells were washed with 4 ml ice-cold PBS 3 times. Intracellular cAMP accumulation was extracted with 3 ml ice-cold 0.3 N perchloric acid for 10 min. The extract was neutralized with 0.3 ml 3.0 N $KHCO_3$ and kept at −80°C until the cAMP was quantified. cAMP was measured by radioimmunoassay using Amersham cAMP (^3H) assay kits.

Results

Sensitization of Intact Cell cAMP Accumulation

The effect of PDBu on cAMP accumulation in intact C6 glioma cells is shown in Fig. 1. The basal level of cAMP in C6 glioma cells was 11 pmole/mg protein. Isoproterenol (1 μM) increased the intracellular cAMP concentration by about 200-fold and forskolin (30 μM) increased it by about 230-fold, compared with the basal level. Incubation of C6 glioma cells with 500 nM PDBu alone for 30 min had no effect on cAMP content, but simultaneous incubation of C6 glioma cells with PDBu in combination with isoproterenol or forskolin significantly enhanced the effect of isoproterenol or forskolin on cAMP accumulation. In the presence of 500 nM PDBu, the isoproterenol-stimulated cAMP accumulation resulted in a 55% increase, and the forskolin-stimulated cAMP accumulation resulted in a 62% increase.

Effects of Protein Kinase C Down-Regulation on cAMP Accumulation

After C6 glioma cells were incubated with 500 μM PDBu for either 6 or 18 h, isoproterenol- or forskolin-stimulated intracellular cAMP accumulation was studied (Fig. 2). The increase of cAMP accumulation elicited by isoproterenol or forskolin was inhibited by the treatment by PDBu for more than 6 h. Pretreatment of C6 glioma cells with 500 nM PDBu for 6 h resulted in a 52% decrease of isoproterenol-stimulated cAMP production and a 48% decrease of forskolin-stimulated cAMP production. Exposure to PDBu for 24 h resulted in a 70% reduction of isoproterenol-stimulated cAMP production and a 48% reduction of forskolin-stimulated cAMP production. Pretreatment with PDBu

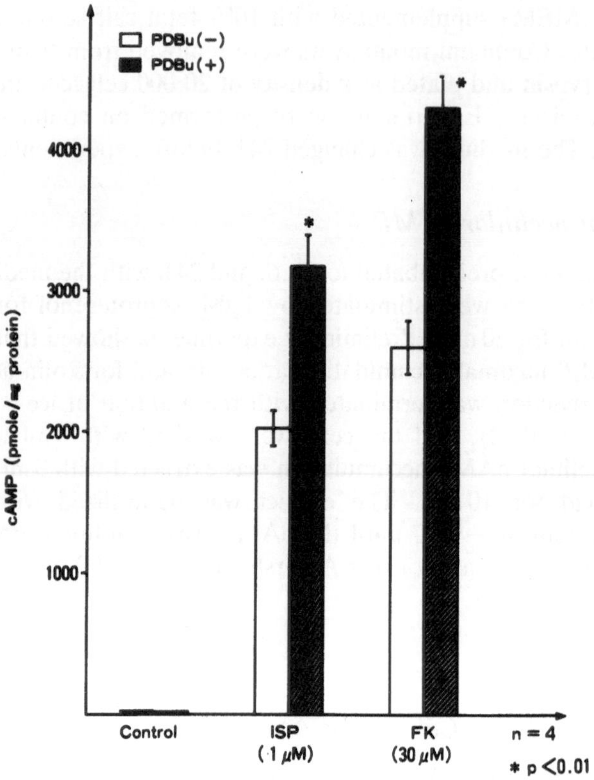

Fig. 1. Sensitization of cAMP accumulation stimulated by isoproterenol or forskolin. C6 glioma cells were exposed to MEM alone (control) or 1 μM isoproterenol for 30 min, or to 30 μM forskolin for 20 min in the absence or presence of 500 nM PDBu. PDBu significantly enhanced cAMP accumulation by isoproterenol or forskolin in C6 glioma cells, ($n = 4$, $P < 0.01$)

for more than 6 h also eliminated the enhancement of cAMP accumulation by simultaneous incubation of PDBu with isoproterenol or forskolin.

Discussion

These studies show that in C6 rat glioma cells, PDBu sensitizes isoproterenol- or forskolin-stimulated cAMP accumulation, whereas prolonged exposure to PDBu almost completely eliminates the sensitization and leads to a decrease in the ability of isoproterenol or forskolin to increase intracellular cAMP accumulation. Phorbor esters, such as PDBu and PMA, are generally recognized as activating PKC directly. Prolonged treatment of the cells with phorbor esters results in loss of PKC activity, or the so-called down-regulation [8]. Because PKC inhibitors of H7 or staurospoline inhibited PMA-induced sensitization of

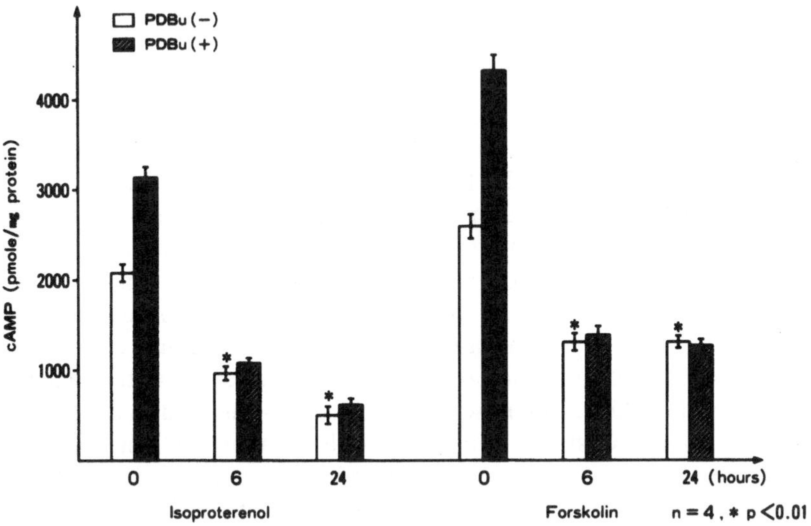

Fig. 2. Effects of PKC down-regulation on isoproterenol- or forskolin-stimulated cAMP accumulation. C6 glioma cells were preincubated with 500 nM for either 6 or 24 h. Cells were washed with PBS three times and stimulated by 1 μM isoproterenol for 30 min or by 30 μM forskolin for 20 min in the absence or presence of 500 nM PDBu. Isoproterenol- or forskolin-stimulated cAMP accumulation in C6 glioma cells preincubated with PDBu was significantly less than that in control cells ($n = 4$, $P < 0.01$). Enhancement by PDBu on cAMP accumulation was totally distinguished by preincubation of PDBu

either isoproterenol or forskolin [9], this cellular response most likely results from activation of PKC.

In previous studies, treatment of human and rat glioma cells with phorbor esters led to a decrease in BAR agonist-stimulated AC activity [10–12]. In more recent studies, however, phorbor esters have been shown to sensitize cAMP response to isoproterenol or forskolin in rat brain cells [4,5] and human glioma cells [9]. In the present study, PKC activation by phorbor esters also enhanced BAR stimulation of intracellular cAMP content in C6 glioma cells, followed by desensitization of the BAR-AC system associated with loss of PKC activity.

The mechanism of this sensitization followed by desensitization in C6 glioma cells has not yet been studied in detail. In human glioma and rat brain cells, PKC activation by the treatment of phorbor esters is assumed to cause sensitization at the post receptor site [5,6,9]. The possibility that exposure to phorbor ester reduces cAMP efflux or degradation by inactivating phosphodiesterase is eliminated [5,6,9]. It seems unlikely that the decreased inhibitory guanine nucleotide-binding protein is responsible for the observed sensitization [9]. Although multiple mechanisms appear to be involved in the overall process of sensitization and the following desensitization, modification of the activity of the catalytic unit of AC, presumably via PKC-mediated phosphorylation, seems the most likely mechanism for the sensitization of forskolin stimulation [9].

The mechanism of phorbor ester-induced desensitization is not clear either. Desensitization elicited by the treatment of PMA does not result in internalization of BAR, as assessed by sucrose density gradient centrifugation assays and by assays of competition by the hydrophilic ligand, isoproterenol, for radiological binding to intact cell receptors. PMA pretreatment does not alter the apparent affinity of the isoproterenol for intact cell BAR, nor is the potency of isoproterenol for stimulation of AC activity altered. PKC inhibitors impede the desensitization induced by PMA but not that induced by isoproterenol [12].

The findings in the present study suggest that, in glioma cells, PKC can influence BAR coupling to the cAMP-generating system, and that inactivation of PKC by prolonged treatment with phorbor esters can lead to the desensitization of the BAR-AC system. In rat as well as human glioma cells, cAMP causes a morphological change that is called "differentiation" [13,14]. Down-regulation of PKC induced by prolonged treatment of phorbor esters can block transducing information across the plasma membrane by means of the cAMP-generating system, which indicates that phorbor esters are tumor-promoting agents and cause glioma cells to be dedifferentiated.

Conclusions

The activation of PKC with PDBu sensitized isoproterenol- or forskolin-stimulated cAMP accumulation in C6 rat glioma cells, but the down-regulation of PKC caused by PDBu almost completely eliminated the sensitization and led to a decrease in the ability of isoproterenol or forskolin to increase intracellular cAMP accumulation. These findings indicate that protein kinase C is a key enzyme for regulating the BAR-AC system, and prolonged exposure to phorbor esters decreases cellular response to β-agonists, such as epinephrine or norepinephrine.

References

1. Castagna M, Takai Y, Kaibuchi K, Sano K, Kikkawa U, Nishizuka Y (1982) Direct activation of calcium-activated phospholipid-dependent protein kinase by tumor-promoting phorbor esters. J Biol Chem 257:7847–7851
2. Nishizuka Y (1984) The role of protein kinase C in cell surface signal transduction and tumour promotion. Nature 308:693–698
3. Karbon EW, Shenolikar S, Ena SJ (1986) Phorbor esters enhance neurotransmitter-stimulated cyclic AMP production in rat brain slices. J Neurochem 47:1566–1575
4. Hollingsworth EB, Sears EB, Daly JW (1985) An activator of protein kinase C (phorbor-12-myrisate-13-acetate) augments 2-chloro-adenosine-elicited accumulation of cyclic AMP in guinea pig cerebral cortical particulate preparations. FEBS Lett 184:339–342

5. Sugden O, Vanecek J, Klein DC, Thomas TP, Anderson WB (1985) Activation of protein kinase C potentiates isoprenaline-induced cyclic AMP accumulation in rat pinealocytes. Nature 314:359–361
6. Tapia-Arancibia L, Veriac S, Pares-Herbute N, Asiter H (1988) Activators of protein kinase C enhance cyclic AMP accumulation in cerebral cortical and diencephalic neurons in primary culture. J Neurosci Res 20:195–201
7. Gilman AG, Birenberg AM (1971) Effect of catecholamines on the adenosine 3′:5′-cyclic monophosphate concentrations of clonal satellite cells of neurons. Proc Nat Acad Sci USA 68:2165–2168
8. Rodriguez-Pena A, Rozengurt E (1984) Disappearance of Ca^{2+}-sensitive, phospholipid-dependent protein kinase activity in phorbor ester-treated 3T3 cells. Biochem Biophys Res Commun 120:1053–1059
9. Johnson RA, Toews ML (1989) Protein kinase C activators sensitize cyclic AMP accumulation by intact 1321N1 human astrocytoma cells. Mol Pharmacol 37:296–303
10. Mallorga P, Tallman JF, Henneberry RC, Hirata F, Strittmater WT, Axelrod J (1980) Mepacrine blocks -adrenergic agonist-induced desensitization in astrocytoma cells. Proc Natl Acad Sci USA 77:1341–1345
11. Kassis S, Zaremba T, Patel J, Fishman PH (1985) Phorbor esters and -adrenergic agonists mediate desensitization of adenylate cyclase in rat glioma C6 cells by distinct mechanisms. J Biol Chem 260:8911–8917
12. Toews ML, Liang M, Perkins JP (1987) Agonists and phorbor esters desensitize -adrenergic receptors by different mechanisms. Mol Pharmacol 32:737–742
13. Oey J (1975) Noradrenaline induces morphological alterations in nucleated and enucleated rat C6 glioma cells. Nature 257:317–319
14. Perkins JP, Macintyre EH, Riley WD, Clark RB (1971) Adenyl cyclase, phosphodiesterase, and cyclic AMP-dependent protein kinase of malignant glial cells in culture. Life Sci 10:1069–1080

Differentiation of a Medulloblastoma Cell Line Mediated by Protein Kinase A

TAKASHI KOKUNAI, NORIHIKO TAMAKI, and SATOSHI MATSUMOTO[1]

Introduction

Cyclic AMP has been implicated in the regulation of the growth and differentiation of various normal and malignant cells [1,2]. In neuroblastoma and glioma cells, it has been shown that $N^6,O^{2\prime}$-dibutyryl cyclic AMP (Bt_2-cAMP) induces morphological and biochemical differentiation in vitro [3]. It has been proposed that most, if not all, of the effects of cyclic AMP are mediated by cyclic AMP-dependent protein kinase (protein kinase A). It was also reported that the modulators of protein kinase C system might be induced by differentiation in some neuroblastoma and glioma cells [4,5].

Medulloblastomas arising from embryonal neuroectodermal tissue are the most malignant neoplasms which appear in childhood. There have been few reports analyzing the mechanisms of differentiation in medulloblastoma. The present study was undertaken to analyze the relationships between the effects of Bt_2-cAMP and 12-O-tetradecanoyl-phorbol 13-acetate (TPA) on the growth, differentiation and protein kinase activity in a human medulloblastoma cell line (MED 3).

Materials and Methods

Cell Culture

A medulloblastoma cell line (MED 3) was established in our laboratory and 2 neuroblastoma cell lines (NB-1 and GOTO) were supplied from the Japanese Cancer Research Resources Bank (JCRB). The cells were grown in an RPMI-1640 medium containing 10% fetal calf serum at 37°C in a humidified incubator with an atmosphere of 5% CO_2:95% air.

Treatment with Bt_2-cAMP and TPA

Bt_2-cAMP was dissolved in the RPMI-1640 medium and added to a regular growth medium to a final concentration of 1 mM. TPA was dissolved to a

[1] Department of Neurosurgery, Kobe University School of Medicine, Kobe, 650 Japan

10 mM concentration in dimethyl sulfoxide (DMSO) and added to a final concentration of 10 ng/ml. At these concentrations, the DMSO itself had no effect on the cells.

Assays for Inhibition of Cell Proliferation

Cells were seeded in 35-mm culture dishes and incubated at 37°C for 24 h. The medium was removed and replaced by fresh medium supplemented with 1 mM Bt_2-cAMP or 10 ng/ml TPA. The cells were detached every day and tested for viability by exclusion of 0.1% Trypan blue, using a hemacytometer.

Colony-Forming Assay in Semisolid Soft Agar

The cells (1×10^5) were suspended in 4 ml 0.33% Special Noble Agar supplemented with growth medium and plated on the growth medium containing 0.5% agar. Both soft agars contained 1 mM Bt_2-cAMP or 10 ng/ml TPA. At 14 days after cell plating, colonies consisting of over 50 cells were counted, and plating efficacy under 0.1% was defined as having no ability for colony formation.

Immunoblotting Analysis of GFAP and Neurofilament (160 K)

For immunoblotting, the cell lysates of MED 3 were fractionated by $NaDodSO_4$/7.5% polyacrylamide slab gel electrophoresis according to the discontinuous buffer system of Laemmli [6] and transferred to the nitrocellulose membrane. The membrane was incubated with mouse anti-GFAP or anti-neurofilament (160K) antibodies, and immunoreactive bands were visualized by the peroxidase-antiperoxidase method.

Cellular Content of Cyclic AMP and Protein Kinase A Activity in the Cytoplasmic Extracts

All treated and untreated cells were detached by scraping and homogenized in a buffer containing 50 mM Tris-HCl pH 7.5, 0.25 M sucrose, 3 mM $MgCl_2$, 4 mM 2-ME, 50 mM benzamide HCl, and 1 mM PMSF. After centrifugation at 12,000 g for 10 min, the supernatants were used for cellular extracts. The cellular contents of cyclic AMP were assayed by a cyclic AMP assay kit from Amersham International plc (Bucringhamshire, UK).

The protein kinase A activity was assayed under the following methods. Cellular extract proteins 20 µg were mixed with a buffer containing 50 mM sodium acetate pH 6.5, 10 mM $MgSO_4$, 10 mM dithiothreitol, 10 µM[$\gamma - {}^{32}P$]-ATP (2,000 cpm/pmol), and 1 mg/ml Histone H2B and incubated at 30°C for 10 min. Assays were conducted in the absence or presence of 10 µM cyclic AMP. The reaction mixtures were spotted on phosphocellulose membranes (p81, Whatman) which were counted for radioactivity.

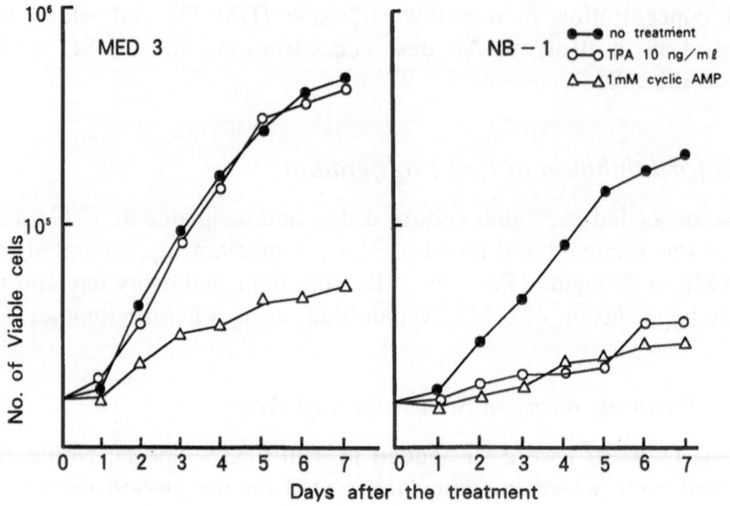

Fig. 1. Growth inhibition of 10 ng/ml TPA or 1 mM Bt_2-cAMP against MED 3 and NB-1

Table 1. Colony-forming efficacies of MED 3, NB-1, and GOTO treated with or without 1 mM Bt_2-cAMP or 10 ng/ml TPA in semisolid soft agar

	Colony-forming efficacy (%)		
Treatment	MED 3	NB-1	GOTO
None	8.53 ± 1.23	2.41 ± 0.89	6.59 ± 2.08
Bt_2-cAMP	0.18 ± 0.05	0.04 ± 0.01	1.34 ± 0.95
TPA	8.29 ± 2.07	0.02 ± 0.01	1.28 ± 0.59

Results

1. Growth Inhibition and Cell Morphology

NB-1 and GOTO inhibited cell growth by treatment with 10 ng/ml TPA or 1 mM Bt_2-cAMP. However, MED 3 inhibited cell growth only by treatment with Bt_2-cAMP (Fig. 1). Morphologically, MED 3 treated with Bt_2-cAMP developed long neurite-like processes and showed a high expression of GFAP and neurofilament (160 K) immunocytochemically (data not shown).

2. Colony-Forming Assay in Semisolid Soft Agar (Table 1)

The colony-forming efficacies of NB-1 and GOTO were 2.41 ± 0.89 and 6.59 ± 2.08, respectively, which were markedly inhibited by treatment with 10 ng/ml TPA or 1 mM Bt_2-cAMP. MED 3 showed 8.53 ± 1.23 of colony forming efficacy, which was inhibited only by treatment with Bt_2-cAMP.

Fig. 2. Immunoblotting analysis for GFAP (*top*) and neurofilament (160 K) (*bottom*). *lane 1* no treatment, *lane 2* 1 mM Bt_2-cAMP, *lane 3* 10 ng/ml TPA

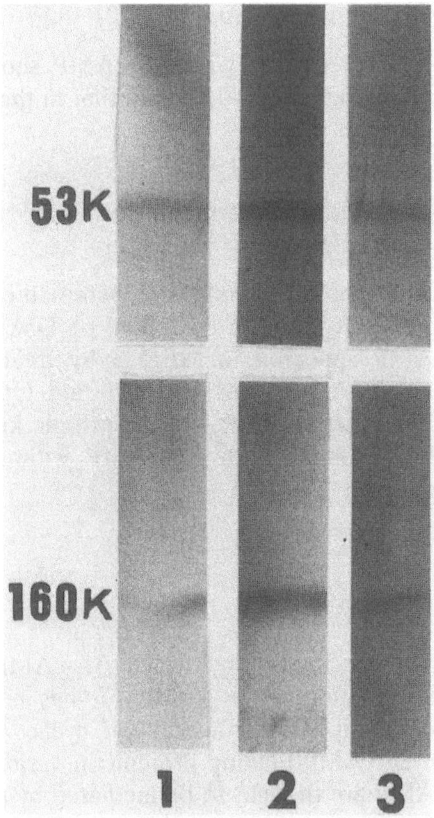

Table 2. Protein kinase activities and cyclic AMP contents in MED 3, NB-1, and GOTO treated with or without 1 mM Bt_2-cAMP or 10 ng/ml TPA

Cell	Cyclic AMP content (pmol/mg protein)	Protein kinase activity (pmol ^{32}P-incorporated/mg protein/10 min)	
		−AMP	+AMP
MED 3			
Control	14.75 ± 2.92	51.31 ± 14.92	348.29 ± 68.51
Bt_2-cAMP	18.91 ± 4.56	384.54 ± 21.81	429.55 ± 17.81
TPA	15.84 ± 3.96	57.95 ± 16.93	284.93 ± 65.84
NB-1			
Control	13.29 ± 1.84		
Bt_2-cAMP	62.84 ± 9.65	78.92 ± 7.84	282.39 ± 45.99
TPA	39.81 ± 4.56	192.54 ± 19.51	204.81 ± 32.93
		184.84 ± 12.34	264.34 ± 29.56
GOTO			
Control	14.84 ± 2.96	48.74 ± 9.91	182.34 ± 29.41
Bt_2-cAMP	48.91 ± 5.54	96.28 ± 12.33	114.57 ± 14.92
TPA	37.99 ± 5.18	86.54 ± 8.73	129.51 ± 12.32

3. *Immunoblotting (Fig. 2)*

MED 3 treated with Bt_2-cAMP showed a higher expression of GFAP and neurofilament (160 K) than that in the MED 3 treated with or without 10 ng/ml TPA.

4. *Cellular Contents of Cyclic AMP and Protein Kinase A Activities (Table 2).*

NB-1 and GOTO showed increased contents of cyclic AMP by treatment with 1 mM Bt_2-cAMP or 10 ng/ml of TPA, whereas no increased contents of cyclic AMP appeared in MED 3 by treatment with TPA or Bt_2-cAMP. Protein kinase A activities in NB-1 and GOTO were increased by treatment with Bt_2-cAMP or TPA, but the protein kinase A activity in MED 3 increased only by treatment with Bt_2-cAMP without any increase of cellular cyclic AMP content.

Discussion

The mechanism by which Bt_2-cAMP suppresses growth and promotes differentiation is not known. It has been shown that exogenously added Bt_2-cAMP increases the cellular cyclic AMP level and induces the synthesis of cyclic AMP-binding proteins in various cells [7]. Most of the effects of cyclic AMP are thought to be mediated by protein kinase A [8].

In this study, treatment with Bt_2-cAMP against neuroblastoma cells caused an increase of the cellular content of cyclic AMP and activated protein kinase A. However, in MED 3, protein kinase A was activated by treatment with Bt_2-cAMP without any increase of the cellular cyclic AMP level. It was speculated that the mechanisms involved in the activation of protein kinase A in MED 3 differed from that in neuroblastoma cells.

Furthermore, the treatment with TPA as a protein kinase c activating factor resulted in growth inhibition and differentiation in neuroblastoma cells. It was also reported that TPA caused growth inhibition and differentiation in human astrocytic glioma cells [5]. In contrast to the above results, TPA did not cause differentiation or growth inhibition in MED 3. It was suggested that the activation of protein kinase C might not be an important factor in the mechanism of differentiation in medulloblastoma.

References

1. Cohen P (1982) The role of protein phosphorylation in neural and hormonal control of cellular activity. Nature 296:613–620
2. Friedman DL (1976) Role of cyclic nucleotides in cell growth and differentiation. Physiol Rev 56:652–707

3. Prashad N, Lotan D, Lotan R (1987) Differential effect of dibutyryl cyclic adenosine monophosphate and retinoic acid on the growth, differentiation and cyclic adenosine monophosphate-binding protein on murine neuroblastoma cells. Cancer Res 47:2417–2424
4. Hama T, Huang KP, Guroff G (1986) Protein kinase C as a component of a nerve growth factor-sensitive phosphorylation system in PC 12 cells. Proc Natl Acad Sci USA 83:2353–2357
5. Couldwell WT, Antel JP, Apuzzo MLJ, Young VW (1990) Inhibition of growth of established human glioma cell lines by modulators of the protein kinase C system. J Neurosurg 73:594–600
6. Laemmli UK (1970) Cleavage of structural proteins during the assembly of the head of bacteriophage T4. Nature 227:680–685
7. Prashad N, Rosenberg RN (1978) Induction of cAMP binding protein by dibutyryl cAMP in mouse neuroblastoma cell. Biochim Biophys Acta 539:459–469
8. Greengard P (1978) Phospholylated proteins as physiological effectors. Science 199:146–152

Biological Characterization of Human Medulloblastoma (ONS-76 and ONS-81) Cell Lines

Keiji Shimizu, Masanobu Yamada, Syusuke Moriuchi, Kazuyoshi Tamura, Eiichiro Mabuchi, Yutaka Okamoto, Yasuyoshi Miyao, Kae Chang Park, and Toru Hayakawa[1]

Introduction

Medulloblastomas are the most common malignant brain tumors in children. The origins of medulloblastoma cells are controversial. Most neuropathologists believe them to have originated from immature precursor cells which have the potentiality to differentiate into either neuronal or glial cells [1]. Although it is very difficult to establish a cell line of human medulloblastoma [2,3], we have established 2 cell lines with neuronal characteristics.

The precise function of class II major histocompatibility complex (MHC) antigens is not yet completely understood. In this study, we demonstrated that class II MHC antigens were induced onto these cells by recombinant human interferon-gamma (rHuIFN-gamma). Until now, it had been reported that neuronal cells could not express class II MHC antigens, but that glial cells could be induced by these antigens under some special conditions [4–11]. These findings might suggest that the precursors of medulloblastoma differentiate into neuronal and glial cells.

Materials and Methods

Clinical History

Patient 1 was a 2-year-old female who presented with truncal ataxia in March, 1987. A computerized tomographic (CT) scan of the head showed a high density lesion (3 cm in diameter) in the midline region of the cerebellum with metastatic tumors at the right prepontine cistern. The cerebellar tumor was subtotally removed in March, 1987, and was histologically diagnosed as a medulloblastoma.

Patient 2 was a 9-year-old female with a cerebellar tumor. In February, 1984 the tumor was subtotally removed and was diagnosed as a medulloblastoma. The CT scan done in March, 1986 showed a high density area in the right lower

[1] Department of Neurosurgery, Osaka University Medical School, Osaka, 553 Japan

frontal lobe. This metastatic tumor was removed in August, 1987, and surgical specimens were submitted for cell cultures.

Primary Explant Technique for Cell Culture

The specimens were chopped as small as possible (<1 cm^3) with crossed scalpels, and were transferred to 25 cm^2 tissue culture flasks (Corning No. 25100) with 0.5–1 ml of a growth medium composed of heat-inactivated patient's serum, fetal calf serum (FCS), and RPMI 1640 (2:1:1). The flasks were incubated at 37°C in a humid 5% CO_2-in-air atmosphere. After the pieces had sufficiently adhered to the bottom of the flasks, the growth medium was gradually added for a total of 5 ml over a period of about 1 week. The first passage was carried out when the tumor cells had grown to over 1 cm^2 in diameter. The growth medium was gradually replaced with RPMI 1640 supplemented with 10% FCS, 2 mM L-glutamine, nonessential amino acids, and 1 mM sodium pyruvate. The two cell lines were designated as ONS-76 (Patient 1) and ONS-81 (Patient 2).

Immunohistochemical Studies

ONS-76 cells and ONS-81 cells were cultured in a Lab-Tek tissue culture chamber (No. 4802) for a few days and fixed with 4% paraformaldehyde at 4°C overnight. As primary antibodies, we used some polyclonal antibodies for glial fibrillary acidic protein (GFAP), S-100 protein and neuron-specific enolase (NSE) (Dakopatts), monoclonal antibodies for synaptophysin (Dakopatts), and three components of NFP (Transformation Research). As secondary antibodies, we used horseradish peroxidase (HRP)-conjugated goat anti-rabbit IgG antibody (Cappel Laboratories) and HRP-conjugated goat anti-mouse IgG antibody (Zymed).

Detection of MHC Antigens on Human Medulloblastoma Cells

The 1 to 2 × 10^6 medulloblastoma (ONS-76 and -81) cells were suspended in 10-cm-diameter Petri dishes (Corning No. 25020) with RPMI 1640 supplemented with 10% heat-inactivated FCS. These cells were harvested 48 h after cocultivation with 0.2, 2, 20, or 200 units/ml rHuIFN-gamma (Takeda Chemical Industries, Osaka, Japan). Then, the 1 × 10^6 cells were incubated with × 50 diluted monoclonal antibody for HLA-ABC antigens (Serotec) for 30 min. After washing, the cells were incubated with fluorescein isothiocyanate (FITC)-conjugated goat anti-mouse IgG (Cappel Laboratories, USA) for 30 min, and then also incubated with FITC-labeled anti-HLA-DR antibodies (Becton Dickinson Immunocytometry Systems) in order to detect the class II MHC antigen. These labeled cells were resuspended in PBS and analyzed with a fluorescence-activated cell sorter (FACS). The cells were maintained on ice at all times. Glioblastoma cells (ONS-6 and -12) and neuroblastoma cells (IMR-32 and SK-N-DZ) were also studied in the manner described above.

Table 1. Comparison of biological characteristics of medulloblastoma cell lines

Marker assayed	Cell lines				
	Daoy	D283Med	D341Med	ONS-76	ONS-81
GFAP	−	−	−	−	−
S-100 Protein	−	−	−	−	−
Neuron specific enolase	+	+	+	+	+
Neurofilament protein					
68K	−	+	−	−	−
145(160)K	−	+	+	+	+
200K	−	+	+	+	+
Synaptophysin	+	+	+	+	+

Results

1. *Biological Characteristics of Medulloblastoma Cells*

Both ONS-76 and ONS-81 cells adhered to the bottom of the tissue culture flasks, and were stellate or spindle-shaped in appearance. The population doubling time of ONS-76 and -81 cells was 18.6 and 19.2 h, respectively. These cells were passaged over 100 times in about 30 months. Immunohistochemical studies showed that both types of cells had NSE, synaptophysin, and NFP (M_r 145,000 and 200,000) without GFAP and S-100 protein (Table 1).

2. *Expression of MHC Antigens on Medulloblastoma Cells*

Glial cells could express class I and class II MHC antigens, but neurons were unable to express these antigens. We investigated class I (HLA-ABC) and class II (HLA-DR) MHC antigens on these cells. HLA-ABC antigens were expressed in 89.3% of the ONS-76 cells, while these antigens showed positive in 98.4% when IFN-gamma (200 units/ml) was added to their medium. HLA-ABC antigens were seen in 65.6% of the ONS-81 cells, and this percentage was increased to 95.3% with the addition of IFN-gamma. Class II MHC antigens were not detected on either line under ordinary culture. HLA-DR antigens were expressed on 1.9%, 17.3%, 59.4%, and 77.7% of the ONS-76 cells, when 0.2, 2, 20, and 200 units/ml IFN-gamma were added, respectively, to the cultured medium for 48 h. The corresponding percentages for the ONS-81 cells were 5.5%, 51.7%, 66.6%, and 77.3%, respectively.

Neuroblastoma (IMR-32 and SK-N-DZ) cells expressed far fewer class I MHC antigens than did glioblastoma (ONS-6 and ONS-12) and medulloblastoma (ONS-76 and ONS-81) cells. Class II MHC antigens could not be induced upon neuroblastoma cells after the addition of IFN-gamma, while they could be on medulloblastoma (ONS-76 and -81) cells with NFP (M_r 145,000 and 200,000) [12] (Table 2). The expression of MHC antigens on these medulloblastoma cells was similar to that on glioblastoma cells.

Table 2. Expression of MHC antigens on glioblastoma, medulloblastoma, and neuroblastoma cells with and without IFN-gamma

Cell lines	Medulloblastoma		Glioblastoma		Neuroblastoma	
MHC	ONS-76	ONS-81	ONS-6	ONS-12	IMR-32	SK-N-DZ
Class I (HLA-ABC)	(+)→(++)	(+)→(++)	(+)→(++)	(+)→(++)	(−)→(+)	(+)[a]→(++)
Class II (HLA-DR)	(−)→(+)	(−)→(+)	(−)→(+)	(−)→(+)	(−)→(−)	(−)→(−)

[a] The class I MHC antigen was found on 5.5% of the tumor cells

Discussion

The origins of medulloblastomas are still controversial. They have been said to originate from immature precursor cells that can differentiate into neuronal or glial cells [1]. ONS-76 and ONS-81 cells possessed NSE, synaptophysin, and NFP (M_r 145,000 and 200,000), but lacked both GFAP and S-100 protein. Therefore, these cells tended to differentiate into neuronal cells [13,14]. Cultured human glioblastoma cells could induce the HLA-DR antigen by rHuIFN-gamma, but neuroblastoma cell lines could not [12,15,16]. The medulloblastoma cells with neuronal components possessed class I antigens and rHuIFN-gamma induced class II antigens upon them. These findings might suggest that the precursor cells of medulloblastoma can differentiate into neuronal and glial cells.

References

1. Bailey P and Cushing H (1925) Medulloblastoma cerebelli: A common type of midcerebellar glioma of childhood. Arch Neurol Psychiatr 14:192–224
2. Friedman HS, Burger PC, Bigner SH, Trojanowski JQ, Wikstrand CJ, Halperin EC, Bigner DD (1985) Establishment and characterization of the human medulloblastoma cell line and transplantable xenograft D283. J Neuropathol Exp Neurol 44:592–605
3. Jacobsen PF, Jenkyn DJ, Papadimitriou JM (1985) Establishment of a human medulloblastoma cell line and its heterotransplantation into nude mice. J Neuropathol Exp Neurol 44:472–485
4. Carrel S, de Tribolet N, Gross N (1982) Expression of HLA-DR and common acute lymphoblastic leukemia antigens on glioma cells. Eur J Immunol 12:354–357
5. Hirsch MR, Wietzerbin J, Pierres M, Goridis C (1983) Expression of Ia antigens by cultured astrocytes treated with gamma-interferon. Neurosci Lett 41:199–204
6. Wong GHW, Clark-Lewis I, Harris AW, Schrader JW (1984) Effect of cloned interferon-gamma on expression of H-2 and Ia antigens on cell lines of hemopoietic, lymphoid, epithelial, fibroblastic and neuronal origin. Eur J Immunol 14:52–56
7. Wong GHW, Bartlett PF, Clark-Lewis I, Battye F, Schrader JW (1984) Inducible expression of H-2 and Ia antigens on brain cells. Nature 310:688–691

8. Wong GHW, Bartlett PF, Clark-Lewis I, McKimm-Breschkin JL, Schrader JW (1985) Interferon-gamma induces the expression of H-2 and Ia antigens on brain cells. J Neuroimmunol 7:255–278
9. Takiguchi M, Frelinger JA (1986) Induction of antigen presentation ability in purified cultures of astroglia by interferon-gamma. J Mol Cell Immunol 2:269–280
10. Massa PT, Dorries R, ter Meulen V (1986) Viral particles induce Ia antigen expression on astrocytes. Nature 320:543–546
11. Pulver M, Carrel S, Mach JP, de Tribolet N (1987) Cultured human fetal astrocytes can be induced by interferon-gamma to express HLA-DR. J Neuroimmunol 14:123–133
12. Tamura K, Shimizu K, Yamada M, Okamoto Y, Matsui Y, Park K-C, Mabuchi E, Moriuchi S, Mogami H (1989) Expression of major histocompatibility complex on human medulloblastoma cells with neuronal differentiation. Cancer Res 49:5380–5384
13. Schmechel D, Marangos PJ, Zis AP, Brightman M, Goodwin FK (1978) Brain enolase as specific markers of neuronal and glial cells. Science 199:313–314
14. Trojanowski JQ (1987) Neurofilament proteins and human nervous system tumors. J Histochem Cytochem 35:999–1003
15. Detrick B, Chader GJ, Rodrigues M, Kyritsis AP, Chan CC, Hooks JJ (1988) Coexpression of neuronal, glial, and major histocompatibility complex class II antigens on retinoblastoma cells. Cancer Res 48:1633–1641
16. Takiguchi M, Ting JPY, Buessow SC, Boyer C, Gillespie Y, Frelinger JA (1985) Response of glioma cells to interferon-gamma: Increase in class II RNA, protein and mixed lymphocyte reaction- stimulating ability. Eur J Immunol 15:809–814

Murine Models with Leptomeningeal Dissemination of Human Medulloblastoma Cells

KEIJI SHIMIZU, MASANOBU YAMADA, KAZUYOSHI TAMURA, SYUSUKE MORIUCHI, EIICHIRO MABUCHI, KAE CHANG PARK, YASUYOSHI MIYAO, and TORU HAYAKAWA[1]

Introduction

The 5-year survival rate of patients with medulloblastoma has improved as much as 70% in the past 15 years. This dramatic improvement is mainly due to advances in radiotherapy [1–3]. Although medulloblastomas are certainly radiosensitive, they are not always radiocurable because of limited irradiation dosages and adverse effects on the whole neural axis. Sooner or later, tumor regrowth takes place, and the meningeal dissemination of the tumor cells then results in the demise of most patients with medulloblastoma [4].

In order to establish further advances in the clinical treatment of medulloblastoma, we devised murine models of leptomeningeal dissemination using human medulloblastoma cells.

Materials and Methods

Human Medulloblastoma Cell Line

A human medulloblastoma (ONS-76) cell line was established from surgical specimens of a 2-year-old female patient. A computed tomography (CT) scan showed a large tumor (6 cm in diameter) at the midline of the cerebellum and a disseminated tumor in the right cerebellopontine angle. The cerebellar tumor was subtotally resected in March, 1987, and was diagnosed histologically as a medulloblastoma. The tumor specimens were mechanically minced with scissors into several fragments (<1 mm in diameter) and were then transferred to 25 cm^2 plastic culture flasks (Corning #25100) which contained about 1 ml cultured medium of a mixture of 40% patient's plasma, 40% fetal bovine serum (FBS), and 20% RPMI 1640 medium. When the outgrowths from the pieces reached about 1 cm in diameter, the outgrown cells were harvested and reinoculated with 5×10^4 cells/ml into a fresh flask. These established cells were designated as the ONS-76 cells.

---

[1] Department of Neurosurgery, Osaka University Medical School, Osaka, 553 Japan

Immunohistochemical Studies

The ONS-76 cells were cultured in a Lab-Tek tissue culture chamber (#4802, Miles Laboratories) for 2–3 days, and then were fixed overnight with 4% paraformaldehyde at 4°C. The cells were washed twice in phosphate buffer saline (PBS) and were then examined by immunoperoxidase analysis for the expression of neurofilament proteins (NFP), neuron-specific enolase (NSE), glial fibrillary acidic protein (GFAP), and S-100 protein. For primary antibodies, we used some polyclonal antibodies for anti-GFAP, S-100 protein, and NSE (Dakopatts), and monoclonal antibodies for synaptophysin (Dakopatts) and three components of NFP (Transformation Research). For secondary antibodies, we used horseradish peroxidase (HRP)-conjugated goat anti-rabbit IgG antibody (Cappel Laboratories) and HRP-conjugated goat anti-mouse IgG antibody (Zymed).

Animals

Female athymic nude mice (BALB/c, *nu/nu*, 8–12 weeks of age, Japan SLC Inc., Japan) were used for these studies.

Models of Leptomeningeal Dissemination

The ONS-76 cells were harvested and suspended in PBS at concentrations of 1×10^8, 5×10^7, and 1×10^7 cells/ml. One-hundred microliters of these cell suspensions were percutaneously transplanted into the cisterna magna of nude mice ($n = 5$) under ether anesthesia.

The general conditions and neurological signs of the models were checked daily, and their median survival time (MST) was monitored. The brains and spinal cords of the dead models were taken out together with the skulls and vertebral columns as fast as possible, and were fixed in 10% formalin. After decalcification, the coronal, transverse, and longitudinal blocks were excised and embedded in paraffin. Histological sections were prepared from each block and stained with hematoxylin and eosin.

In another experiment, 5 animals, which were inoculated with 1×10^7 tumor cells, were sacrificed to investigate the pathophysiology of disseminated medulloblastoma cells in the models every 7, 20, and 30 days after the tumor inoculation. These models were transcardially perfused with 100 ml PBS, after which the brains were removed from the skulls. Cryostat sections (8–10 µm of these fresh-frozen brains were fixed with 4% paraformaldehyde for 60 min or cold acetone for 10 min. In order to detect class I MHC antigens on the disseminated cells in models, we used monoclonal antibody for HLA-ABC (Serotec) as the primary antibody.

Results

Tumor Cell Phenotypes

The ONS-76 cells contained NSE and NFP (145,200 kd), but had no GFAP and S-100 proteins. Flow cytometry showed that 89% of the ONS-76 cells expressed class I MHC antigens, and that class II MHC antigens were absent. On the other hand, class II MHC antigens could be induced *in vitro* after cocultivation with rHuIFN-gamma (200 units/ml) for 48 h [5].

Models of Leptomeningeal Dissemination

These models began to show severe anorexia and weight loss around 30 days after tumor inoculation, and their physical activities gradually declined. They then developed paresis of the hind legs and urinary incontinence. In the terminal stage, these mice remained prone with their backs hyperflexed and hind limbs extended.

All 5 mice died within 65 days after intracisternal inoculation of 1×10^7 ONS-76 cells. Their MST was 56 days Only 1 mouse that was transplanted 5×10^6 cells died 50 days after the tumor inoculation. All of the mice which were inoculated with 1×10^6 ONS-76 cells were alive longer than 3 months after tumor inoculation.

Pathological Findings of Models

Various degrees of hydrocephalus and thickening of the leptomeninges at the cranial base were observed under macroscopic examination in all models. The tumor layers and nodules were recognized to be within the subarachnoid or epidural spaces from the cerebral hemisphere to the cauda equina. In particular, thick tumor layers were seen at the skull base (Fig. 1), and had encased major cranial nerves, such as the optic and trigeminal nerves. Many tumor cells were infiltrated into the cisterns around the brain stem, and the spinal root ganglions were also involved. The tumor cells extended into the perivascular space of the penetrating vessels (Virchow-Robin's space). Many mitotic figures were observed to be distributed in the infiltrated cells. These pathological findings were similar to those found in patients with medulloblastoma.

Immunohistochemistry of Disseminated ONS-76 cells in the Models

The transplanted ONS-76 cells possessed NFP (145,200 kd) and class I MHC antigens until 20 days after the tumor inoculation. Around 30 days after the tumor inoculation, no NFP or class I MHC antigens could be detected (Fig. 2).

Discussion

It is necessary to investigate the pathophysiology of meningeal dissemination along the pathways of the cerebrospinal fluid because tumor cell seedings are nearly always fatal in spite of improved radiotherapies. However, there have been only a few reports on animal models of meningeal dissemination using human medulloblastoma cells because of the difficulties of establishing medulloblastoma cell lines. Friedman et al. described experimental models with meningeal involvement using D341 Med cells [6]. In order to explore therapeu-

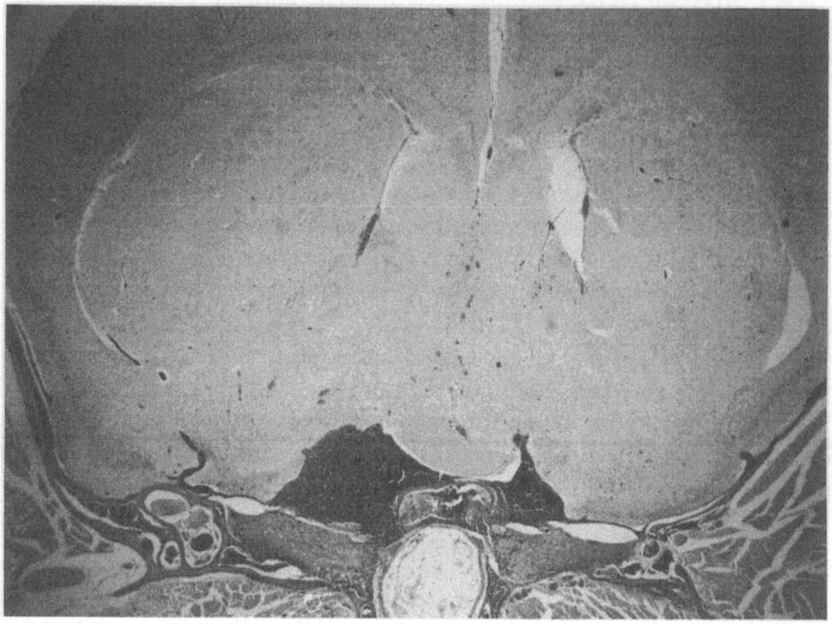

Fig. 1. Coronal section through the frontal lobe and optic chiasma

Cell markers	Days after tumor inoculation			
	7	20	30	50
NSE	+	+	±	−
NFP (200kDa)	+	+	−	−
Class I	⧺	+	±~−	N.D

Clinical states

Death

Weight loss

Neurological signs

Cell number

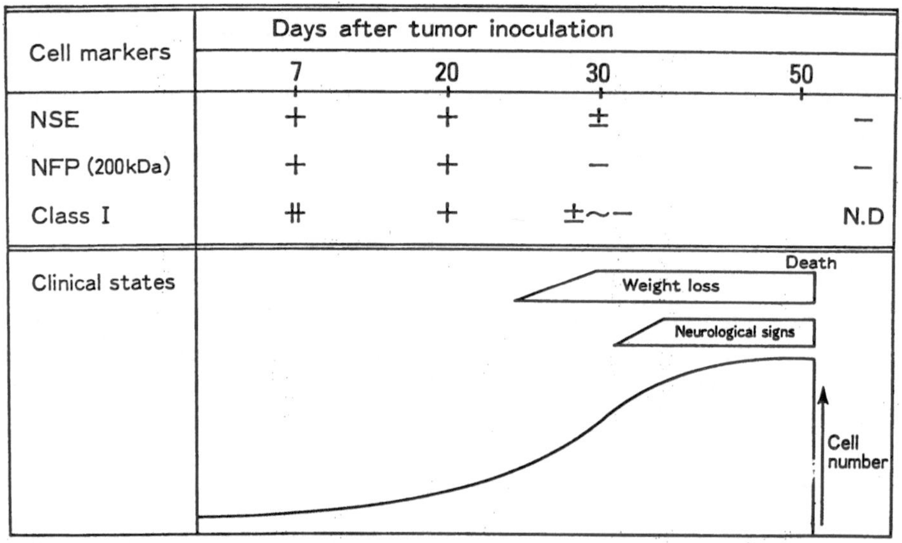

Fig. 2. Clinical signs and pathological findings of murine models with leptomeningeal dissemination. *ND*, not determined

tic strategies for their meningeal dissemination, we developed murine models with leptomeningeal dissemination using human medulloblastoma (ONS-76) cells. The neurological signs and pathological findings were closely similar to those of medulloblastoma patients.

The ONS-76 cells had class I MHC antigens on their cell surfaces, which they also expressed in the subarachnoid space. The class I MHC antigens were recognized up to the 20th day after tumor inoculation, but were markedly decreased 30 days after the inoculation (Fig. 2). At about that time, these models began to show anorexia and weight loss. This may suggest that the inoculated tumor cells began to proliferate rapidly in these models after the deleted or reduced expression of self-MHC, and that the expression of class I MHC antigens can lead to effective recognition of the disseminating tumor cells by the host immune system [7–9].

References

1. Dewit L, Van-Dam J, Rijnders A, van-de-Velde G, Ang KK, van-der-Schueren E (1984) A modified radiotherapy technique in the treatment of medulloblastoma. Int J Radiat Oncol Biol Phys 10:231–241
2. Levin VA, Vestnys PS, Edwards MS, Wara WM, Fulton D, Barger G, Seager M, Wilson CB (1983) Improvement in survival produced by sequential therapies in the treatment of recurrent medulloblastoma. Cancer 51:1364–1370
3. Park TS, Hoffman HJ, Hendrick EB, Humphreys RP, Becker LE (1983) Medulloblastoma: Clinical presentation and management. Experience at the Hospital for Sick Children, Toronto, 1950–1980. J Neurosurg 58:543–552
4. Inoya H, Takakura K, Shitara N, Manaka S (1987) Treatment of medulloblastoma. Prog Exp Tumor Res 30:91–99
5. Tamura K, Shimizu K, Yamada M, Okamoto Y, Matsui Y, Park KC, Mabuchi E, Moriuchi S, Mogami H (1989) Expression of major histocompatibility complex on human medulloblastoma cells with neuronal differentiation. Cancer Res 49:5380–5384
6. Friedman HS, Burger PC, Bigner SH, Trojanowski JQ, Brodeur GM, He XM, Wikstrand CJ, Kurtzberg J, Berens ME, Halperin EC, Bigner DD (1988) Phenotypic and genotypic analysis of a human medulloblastoma cell line and transplantable xenograft (D341 Med) demonstrating amplification of c-*myc*. Am J Pathol 130:472–484
7. Alon Y, Hammerling GJ, Segal S, Bar EM (1987) Association in the expression of Kirsten-*ras* oncogene and the major histocompatibility complex class I antigens in fibrosarcoma tumor cell variants exhibiting different metastatic capabilities. Cancer Res 47:2553–2557
8. Plaksin D, Gelber C, Feldman M, Eisenbach L (1988) Reversal of the metastatic phenotype in Lewis lung carcinoma cells after transfection with syngeneic H-2K^b gene. Proc Natl Acad Sci USA 85:4463–4467
9. Wallich R, Bulbuc N, Hammerling GJ, Katzav S, Segal S, Feldman M (1985) Abrogation of metastatic properties of tumor cells by *de novo* expression of H-2K antigens following H-2 gene transfection. Nature 315:301–305

Antitumor Effects of Human Monoclonal Antibodies on Human Malignant Glioma Xenografts and Their Clinical Application

KATSUSHI TAOMOTO[1], AKIHIRO IJICHI[1], SATOSHI MATSUMOTO[2], and HIDEAKI HAGIWARA[3]

Introduction

Human anaplastic gliomas still have a poor prognosis despite current aggressive therapies such as microsurgery, advanced radiation therapy, combined chemotherapy and/or immuno-therapy. It has been widely reported that a major limitation of these treatments is the lack of tumor specificity. Hybridoma technology has made it possible to generate large quantities of monoclonal antibodies (MAB) which are highly specific to human malignant tumors. Such tumor-associated MABs are potentially powerful tools in the diagnosis and treatment of human malignant tumors. A large number of monoclonal antibodies has been produced by hybridomas from mouse × mouse or mouse × human cells, and those antibodies were used in the diagnosis and the treatment of human cancers [1–3].

A human × human hybridoma, CLNH11, which had been produced by Hagiwara et al., was found to secrete a human immunoglobulin G(IgG) monoclonal antibody [4–6]. This monoclonal antibody, CLN-IgG was shown to react with human glioma cells as well as with autologous cervical carcinoma cells and tumor cell lines of cervical origin [7] on frozen sections of tumor tissue using immunoperoxidase staining. We studied the antitumor effect of CLN-IgG for human malignant glioma xenografts and applied CLN-IgG to patients with malignant glioma.

Materials and Methods

Cell Lines

Human glioma cell lines U-251 MG and U-87 MG were cultured in modified Eagle's essential medium (MEM) containing 10% fetal bovine serum (FBS) at 37°C in 5% CO_2: 95% air atmosphere.

[1] Department of Neurosurgery, Hyogo Prefectural Medical Center for Adults, Akashi, 673 Japan
[2] Department of Neurosurgery, Kobe University School of Medicine, Kobe, 650 Japan
[3] Department of Neurosurgery, Hagiwara Institute of Health, Hyogo, 679-01 Japan

Animals

BALB/c AJcl-nu and Jcl/AF-nu male athymic mice 5–6 weeks of age were used (10 mice in each group).

Human Tumor Xenografts

Each animal was subcutaneously inoculated in the right flank via a 26-gauge needle with 1×10^6 cells in a total volume of 0.5–0.8 ml.

Tumor Measurements

The subcutaneously growing solid tumors were measured weekly by the formula $w(mg) = (width(mm))^2 \times length(mm)/2$, using vernier calipers.

CLN-IgG Treatments

The animals were treated at 6 weeks after tumor xenografts as follows: (1) single injection of 1 mg CLN-IgG in the tumor ($n = 10$), and (2) 3 injections of 1 mg CLN-IgG at 2-weeks intervals in the tumor ($n = 10$). The mice in the control groups received single injections of 1 mg physiological saline solution in the tumor ($n = 5$).

Morphological Examinations

Light microscopic observation with hematoxylin and eosin and immunohistochemical staining of GFAP, Vimentin and S-100 protein were studied by the avidin biotin peroxidase-complex (ABC) method.

Clinical Application

The ten patients included in the study had the following tumors: 5 glioblastomas, 3 thalamic gliomas, 1 anaplastic astrocytoma, 1 pontine glioma (unknown histology), and Intra-tumoral administration (4 cases) consisted of 1 mg/ml through Ommaya's reservoir, and intravenous administrations (6 cases) consisted of 1 mg/ml once a week.

Results

Antitumor Effects of CLN-IgG

The antitumor effects of a single 1 mg intratumoral injection of CLN-IgG on the human glioma xenografts are shown in Fig. 1. At 1 or 2 weeks after the injection of CLN-IgG, the tumor growth was temporarily decreased, followed by a rapid regrowth equal to that of the control group. When 1 mg CLN-IgG was injected repeatedly, the growth rate of the human glioma xenografts was

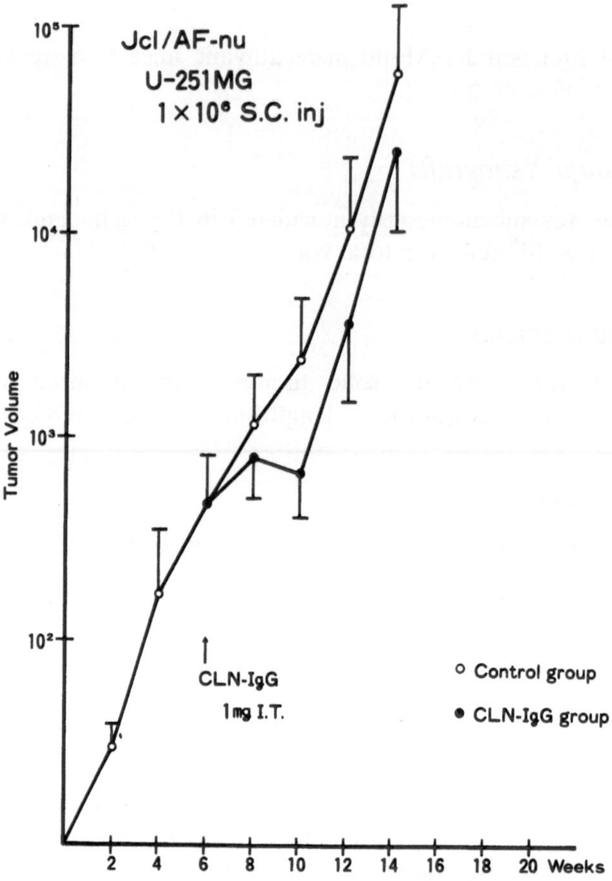

Fig. 1. Antitumoral effects of 1 mg single intratumoral (IT) injection of CLN-IgG on human glioma xenografts in athymic nude mice. *SC*, subcutaneous

decreased, and the antitumor effects were revealed gradually at around 4 weeks after intratumoral administration (Fig. 2). The group receiving six intratumoral injections of 1 mg CLN-IgG revealed definite inhibitory effects upon tumor growth (Fig. 3). However, the tumor volume was not decreased in any of the mice.

Morphology of Tumors

These subcutaneous tumors were either grossly round or lobulated masses. Macroscopically, the large tumors of the control group were generally covered with smooth cutaneous tissue but the macroscopic appearances of the CLN-IgG-treated tumors were frequently necrotic.

Microscopically, all of the tumors were well circumscribed and the growing cell nests often invaded the surrounding muscle and perineural spaces, but

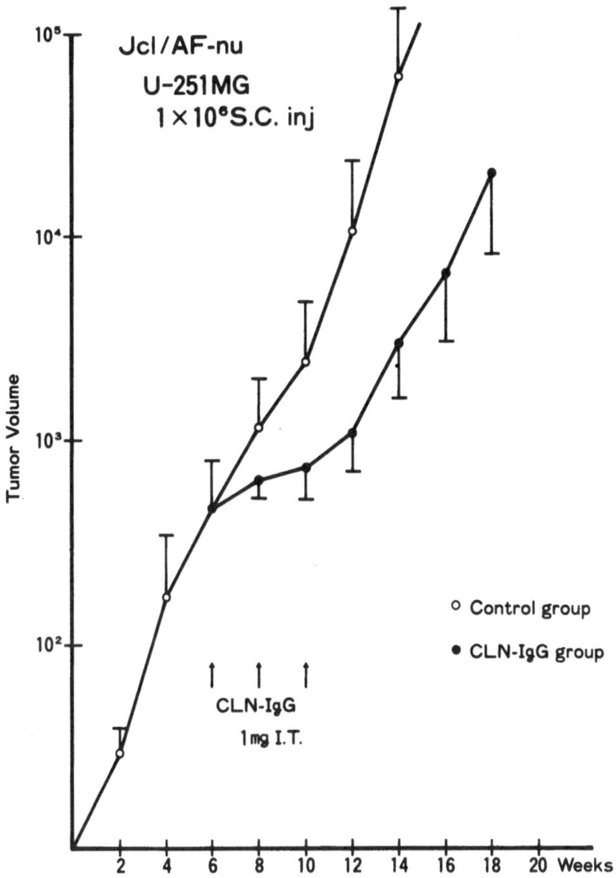

Fig. 2. Antitumoral effects of 3 injections of 1 mg CLN-IgG on human glioma xenografts in athymic nude mice. *IT*, intratumoral; *SC*, subcutaneous

there were no metastases. Tumors of the control groups were mainly composed of spindle-shaped cells punctuated by frequent large, bizarre cells and small, scattered polygonal cells. Small and scattered necroses were occasionally present in the centers of the tumors (Fig. 4a).

In the tumors receiving the 1 mg CLN-IgG treatment, some infiltrations of small round cells resembling lymphocytes were seen among tumor cells, especially at the periphery of the tumors. Tumor necroses were predominant in the centers of the tumors (Fig. 4b).

In the tumors receiving the 1 mg × 3 CLN-IgG treatment, remarkable infiltrations of small round cells were present in the forming cell groups (Fig. 4c). The most remarkable invasions of small round cells into the tumors were noted in the group of the 1 mg × 6 CLN-IgG treatment. These tumors also contained massive central necroses and abundant reticulin and collagen fibers which frequently encircled small groups of tumor cells in the peripheral active

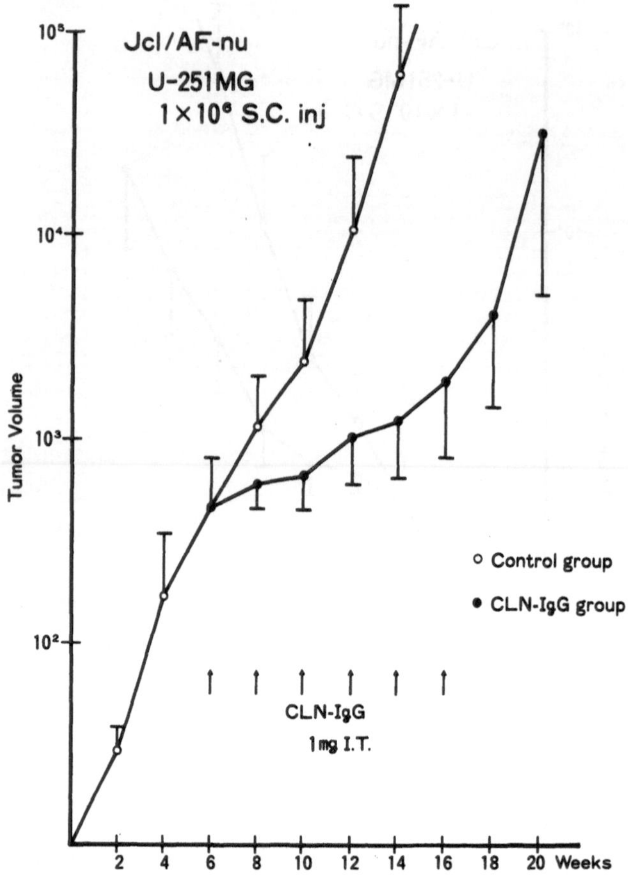

Fig. 3. Antitumoral effects of 6 intratumoral injections of 1 mg CLN-IgG on human glioma xenografts in athymic nude mice. *IT*, intratumoral; *SC*, subcutaneous

areas. These small round cells appeared to infiltrate the surrounding tumor cell nests in large numbers and this was followed by the development of tumor necroses (Fig. 4d).

Immunocytochemistry

In the subcutaneous tumors, both GFAP and Vimentin immunoperoxidase stainings were positive using the ABC procedure. Immunostaining of Vimentin was predominant compared with GFAP. Immunoperoxidase staining of frozen tissue sections for CLN-IgG in the U-251MG tumor was also weakly positive using the ABC method with a biotinylated CLN-IgG antibody.

Clinical Application

We have applied the monoclonal antibody CLN-IgG to patients with malignant glioma since January, 1989. So far, ten patients who had malignant gliomas

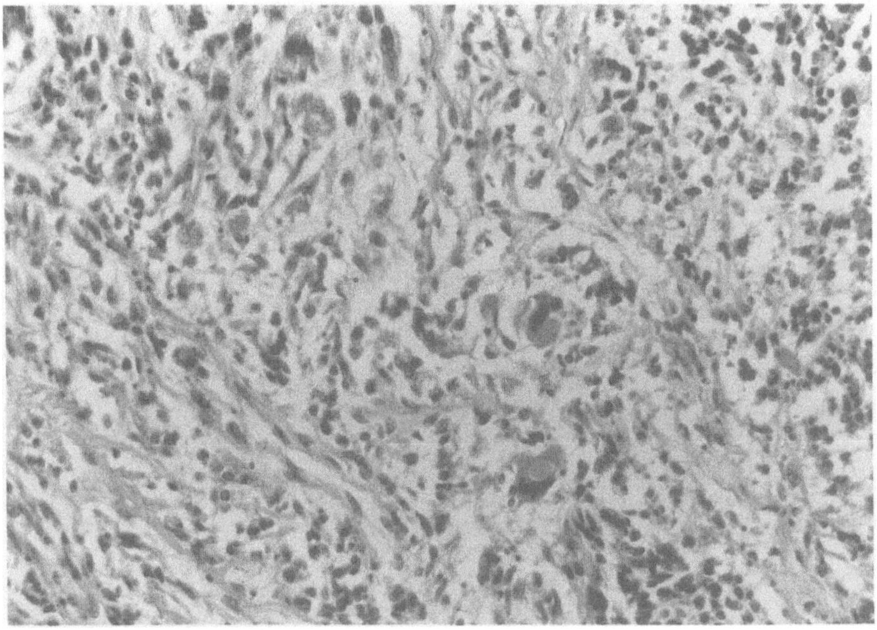

a

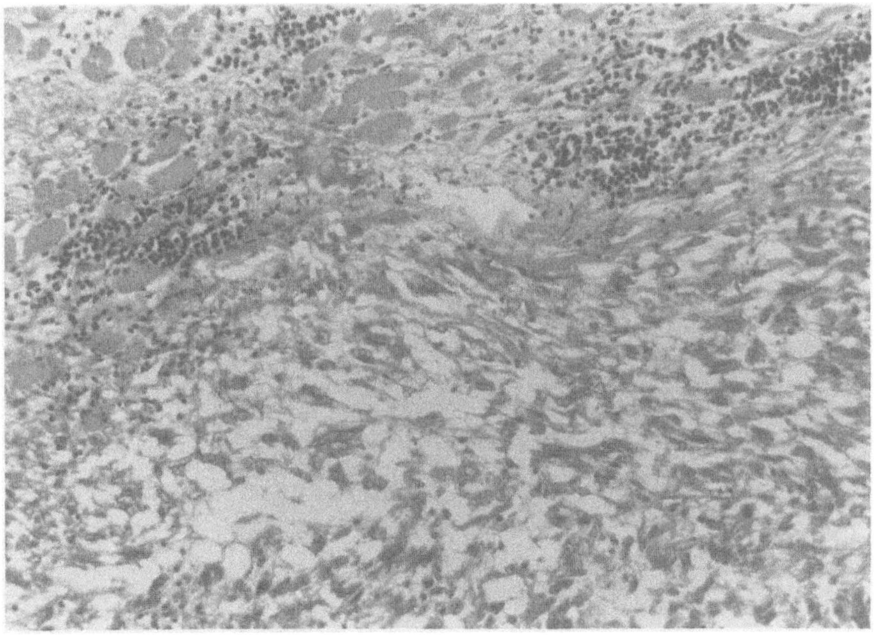

b

Fig. 4. Light microscopic findings of U-251 MG xenografts. **a** Control tumor histology, composed of spindle-shaped tumor cells punctuated by frequent bizzare large cells and scattered small round cells, × 100. **b** Some groups of small round cells which looked like lymphocytes were infiltrated at the periphery of a tumor xenograft in the case of a single intratumoral injection of 1 mg CLN-IgG, × 100. (*Continued*)

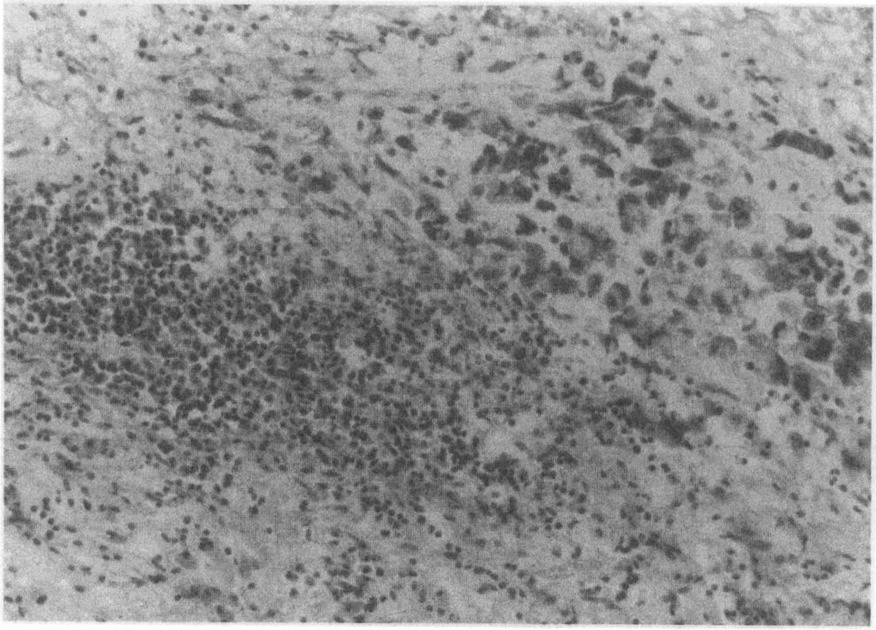

c

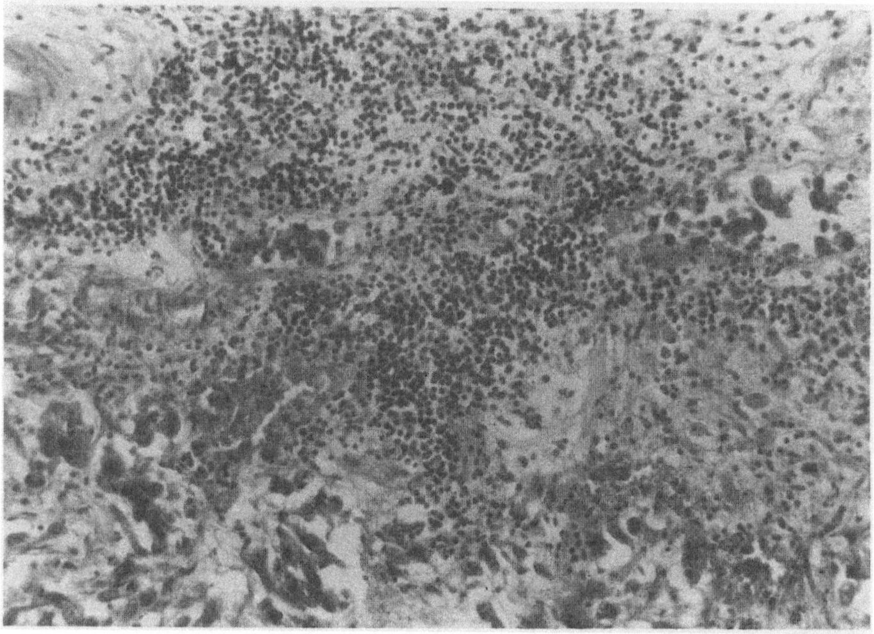

d

Fig. 4. *continued* **c** Remarkable infiltrations of small round cells were noticed in the tumor xenograft with 1 mg × 3 CLN-IgG intratumoral administration, × 100. **d** The most remarkable massive infiltrations of small round cells were seen in the case with 1 mg × 6 CLN-IgG treatment, × 100

Table 1. Clinical results of 10 cases

Case no.	Age (years)/Sex	Histology	Prior treatment	Total doses of CLN-IgG	KPS	Response (months)
1	77/F	Glioblastoma	Op. RT; 60 Gy	22 mg (IT)	40%	Dead (12)
2	68/M	Glioblastoma	Op. RT; 60 Gy MCNU	56 mg (IT, IV)	50%	Alive, *NC* (17)
3	58/M	Glioblastoma	Op. RT; 60 Gy MCNU	37 mg (IT)	50%	Dead[a] (14)
4	60/F	Glioblastoma	Op. RT; 32 Gy IFN + MCNU	4 mg (IT)	20%	Dead[b] (4)
5	60/M	Glioblastoma	Op. RT; 60 Gy	14 mg (IV)	100%	Alive, *NC* (4)
6	42/M	Thalamic glioma	Op. RT; 60 Gy	12 mg (IV)	50%	Alive, *PD* (5)
7	65/M	Thalamic glioma	Op. RT; 60 Gy	5 mg (IV)	30%	Alive *NC* (3)
8	55/M	Pontine glioma	RT; 60 Gy MCNU	20 mg (IV)	80%	Alive (9)
9	69/F	Astrocytoma	Op. RT; 50 Gy	26 mg (IV)	40%	Alive, *PD* (5)
10	42/F	Thalamic glioma	Op.	6 mg (IV)	90%	Alive, *NC* (10)

[a] CSF dissemination (ventricular and spinal subarachnoid space).
[b] Radiation encephalopathy?
KPS, Karnofsky Performance Scale; *Op.*, operation; *IT*, intratumoral injection; *IV*, intravenous injection; *NC*, no change; *PD*, progressed

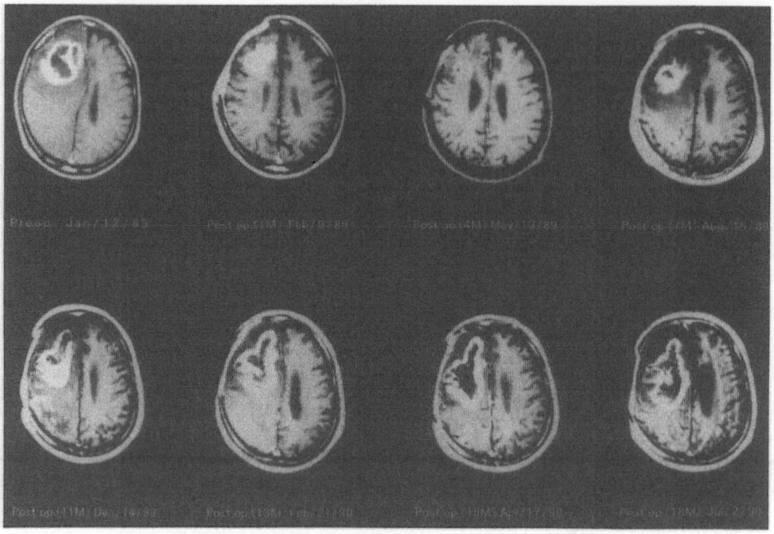

Fig. 5. Chronological changes seen in the MRI of case 2

verified by histological examination were entered into this study. Written, informed consents were obtained from each patient or from the patient's family. The 1 mg/ml purified CLN-IgG which had passed WHO criteria was injected into the tumor cavity through Ommaya's reservoir once a week in four patients. The remaining six patients were given 1 mg CLN-IgG intravenously once a week. The results of the treatment are shown in Table 1. No patient had any complications throughout the treatment due to CLN-IgG administration. Figure 5 demonstrates the chronological changes in MRI of a glioblastoma case (no. 2, a 68-year-old male).

Discussion

Since Koprowski et al. produced antibodies binding specifically to human cancer cells and applied them to the diagnosis of human cancer in 1978 [8], many monoclonal antibodies have been used to detect human cancers, including malignant gliomas, because of their relatively selective binding to tumor-associated antigens [2,9].

In addition, radio localizations of tumors have been carried out in humans using radioisotope-labeled murine and human monoclonal antibodies against brain tumors [10–12].

Approaches to the application of mice monoclonal antibodies to tumor therapy have also been carried out in experimental tumors and human tumor xenografts including gliomas [13–15]. In 1987, Lee et al. reported on radio-immuno-therapy with the ^{131}I-labeled anti-Tenascin monoclonal antibody 81C6 which has resulted in significant tumor growth delay and tumor regression [16]. However, the 81C6 monoclonal antibody itself has not shown any antitumor effects, but rather has worked as a specific carrier of human malignant gliomas.

There is only one report which demonstrated the localization of malignant glioma by a radiolabeled human monoclonal antibody, LGLI-ID6 [12]. However, we found no previously published report on malignant glioma therapy in humans using human monoclonal antibodies. In our study, the human monoclonal antibody CLN-IgG had remarkable effects of tumor growth delay, without any radioisotope or anticancer agents, when it was applied intratumorally.

Analysis of the antigen which was recognized with CLN-IgG monoclonal antibody treatment, showed it to be a protein without a sugar chain, having a molecular weight of 226 kd (non-reduced), and consisting of alpha (60 kd) and beta (53 kd) subunits [17]. The antigen was mainly located in the cytoplasm near the cell membrane and exposed its epitope on the cytoplasmic membrane; this was revealed by using high voltage immuno-electron microscopic studies of the cultured human glioma cells. In the examinations by immunoblotting and enzyme-linked immunosorbent assay (ELISA), free antigens had either not been detected or were below the threshhold of sensitivity in the serum and cerebrospinal fluid of the patient, and the supernatant of the culture medium of U-251 glioma cells (unpublished data).

These findings mean that the antigen which was recognized by CLN-IgG is not a free circulating type, which would be more convenient to use as a specific immuno-therapeutic agent than as immuno-diagnostic material. Distribution of tumor antigens on the cell surface would be essential for the therapeutic application of monoclonal antibodies against tumors, because the initial steps of an antibody-mediated cytotoxic mechanism against a tumor, such as complement-dependent cytotoxicity (CDC) and antibody-dependent cell-mediated cytotoxicity (ADCC), occur at the surface of tumor cells with exposed antigens. CLN-IgG showed ADCC against cervical carcinoma cell lines (unpublished data). The mixture of the CLN-IgG and a different human monoclonal antibody, CLN-IgG, demonstrated synergistic augmentation in CDC activity against glioblastoma cells [6].

Immunohistochemical examinations revealed that CLN-IgG had reacted markedly to the malignant gliomas, such as glioblastoma and anaplastic astrocytoma, craniopharyngioma, many cultured human glioma cell lines, and some reactive astrocytes, but had not reacted to normal adult or fetal brain tissue nor other normal extraneural tissue in frozen section (unpublished data). With the use of a tumor-specific agent, such as a monoclonal antibody, another factor that may have been involved, in addition to epitope expression in other tissues, is a specific binding to shed antigens. Two main causes of treatment failure for malignant gliomas have been proposed. One stemmed from tumor cell heterogeneity, such as clonal variations in growth potential, differential drug resistance, and antigenic heterogeneity [18]. The other cause involved the effector arm of the therapeutic approach, poor drug delivery, and lack of therapeutic agent specificity [19]. Some merits of using monoclonal antibodies for the treatment of malignant tumors are the increasing of drug delivery to the specific tumor site and the lowering of systemic toxicity. With that in mind, monoclonal antibody delivery to the tumor by intracarotid administration [16], or the use of $F(ab')_2$ fragment of the monoclonal antibody had been tried in order to increase drug delivery to malignant gliomas [20]. It is desirable to use a monoclonal antibody that has high in vivo tumor-to-normal tissue localization ratios for monoclonal antibody-targeted radiotherapy. Immunolabeling cytochemistry applying the colloidal gold techniques for electron microscopy has been recently developed.

Our experimental results with tumor localization and the inhibitory effects on tumor growth suggest that specific CLN-IgG monoclonal antibodies may play an important role not only in the diagnosis but also in immunotherapy for the primary intracranial malignant gliomas of human brain.

Conclusions

A human monoclonal antibody, CLN-IgG, which is directed against human utero-cervical carcinoma and malignant glioma has been shown to be specifically localized in U-251 MG and U-87 MG human subcutaneous xenografts in immunosupressive athymic mice using a immunohistochemical technique. This monoclonal antibody recognized the surface antigen of human malignant glioma cells by high voltage electron microscopic stereoscopic observation using gold colloid immunoreaction. Following these studies, CLN-IgG was used intratumorally to evaluate the direct antitumor effects on U-251 MG and U-87 MG human glioma. Although no remarkable inhibition of the tumor growth was noticed when 1 mg CLN-IgG was applied once at 6 weeks after the tumor implantation, apparent growth inhibition of the tumor was recognized with repeated local injections of 1 mg CLN-IgG in both U-251 MG and U-87 MG human glioma xenografts. Striking histopathological findings in CLN-IgG treated-mice included massive necrosis in the tumor and remarkable infiltration of small round cells at the periphery of the tumor. Clinically, ten patients with malignant glioma were treated with purified CLN-IgG after surgery and radiation therapy. Although the three patients with advanced stages died of malignant gliomas, five patients had neither progression of disease nor complications or side effects.

References

1. Bourdon MA, Coleman RE, Blasberg RG, et al. (1984) Monoclonal antibody localization in subcutaneous and intracranial human glioma xenografts: Paired-label and imaging analysis. Anticancer Res 4:133–140
2. Carrel S, de Tribolet N, Mach J-P (1982) Expression of neuroectodermal antigens common to melanomas, gliomas and neuroblastomas. Acta Neuropathol (Berl) 57:158–164
3. Dillman RO, Awler DL, Sobal RE, et al. (1982) Murine monoclonal antibody therapy in two patients with chronic lymphocytic leukemia. Blood 59:1036–1045

4. Glassy MC, Handley HH, Hagiwara H, et al. (1983) UC 729-6, a human lymphoblastoid B- cell line useful for generating antibody-secreting human -human hybridomas. Proc Natl Acad Sci USA 80:6327–6331
5. Hagiwara H, Sato HG (1983) Human × human hybridoma producing monoclonal antibody against autologous cervical carcinoma. Mol Biol Med 1:245–252
6. Hagiwara H, Ohtake H, Yuasa H (1985) Proliferation and antibody production of human × human hybridoma in serum-free media. In: Murakami H, Yamane I, Barnes DW, et al. (eds) Growth and differentiation of cells in defined environment. Springer Heidelberg, pp 1–6
7. Hagiwara H, Aotsuka Y (1987) Cytotoxicity of mixed human monoclonal antibodies reacting to tumor antigens (in Japanese). Acta Paediatr Jpn 29:552–556
8. Koprowski H, Steplewski Z, Herlyn D, et al. (1978) Study of antibodies against human melanoma produced by somatic cell hybrids. Proc Natl Acad Sci USA 75:3405–3409
9. Mach JP, Buchegger F, Fornai M, et al. (1981) Use of radiolabeled monoclonal anti-CEA antibodies for detection of the human carcinomas by external photoscanning and tomocintigraphy. Immunol Today 2:239–249
10. Behnke J, Mach J-P, Buchegger F, et al. (1988) In vivo localisation of radiolabeled monoclonal antibody in human gliomas. Br J Neurosurg 2:193–197
11. Blasberg RG, Nakagawa H, Bourdon MA, et al. (1987) Regional localization of a glioma-associated antigen defined by monoclonal antibody 81C6 in vivo: Kinetics and implication for diagnosis and therapy. Cancer Res 47:4432–4443
12. Phillips J, Alderson T, Sikora K, et al. (1983) Localization of malignant glioma by a radiolabeled human monoclonal antibody. J Neurol Neurosurg Psychiatry 46:388–392
13. Bullard DE, Adams CJ, Coleman RE, et al. (1986) In vivo imaging of intracranial human glioma xenografts comparing specific with nonspecific radiolabeled monoclonal antibodies. J Neurosurg 64:257–262
14. Chiou RK, Vessella RL, Limas C, et al. (1988) Monoclonal antibody-targeted radiotherapy of renal cell carcinoma using a nude mouse mode. Cancer 61:1766–1775
15. Nowak TP (1987) Monoclonal antibodies: Prospects for specific immunotherapy for gliomas. Am J Oncol 10:278–280
16. Lee Y, Bullard DE, Wikstrand CJ, et al. (1987) Comparison of monoclonal antibody delivery to intracranial glioma xenografts by intravenous and intra-carotid administration. Cancer Res 47:1941–1946
17. Aotsuka Y, Hagiwara H (1988) Identification of a malignant cell-associated antigen recognized by a human monoclonal antibody. Eur J Cancer Clin Oncol 24(5):829–838
18. Bigner DD (1981) Biology of gliomas: Potential clinical implications of glioma, cellular heterogeneity. Neurosurgery 9:320–326
19. Lee Y, Bigner DD (1985) Aspects of immunobiology and immnotherapy and uses of monoclonal antibodies and biologic immune modifiers in human gliomas. Neurol Clin 3:901–917
20. Herlyn D, Powe J, Alavi A, et al. (1983) Radioimmunodetection of human tumor xenografts by monoclonal antibodies. Cancer Res 43:2731–2735

Effects of a Human Monoclonal Antibody and Cytokines on Human Malignant Glioma Cells

Hiroshi Takahashi and Shozo Nakazawa[1]

Introduction

We have previously reported that the human monoclonal antibody (MAb) CLN-IgG, which is derived from human uterus cancer lymph node cells, binds strongly to malignant glioma cells and inhibits the tumor growth of gliomas subcutaneously transplanted into nude mice [1]. However, it may be difficult for an antibody to reach all of the tumor cells because of unequal tumor antigen expression within a large tumor mass. Some cytokines have been reported to stimulate the expression of specific membrane surface antigens [2–5]. Accordingly, we performed this study to determine whether the anti-tumor effect of CLN-IgG on glioma cells was enhanced by cytokines.

Materials and Methods

1. In Vitro *Experiment*

Human U-87MG malignant glioma cells (5×10^4 cells/well) were cultured with recombinant interferon-α(rIFN-α), human (Hu) IFN-β, HuIFN-γ, or Hu-tumor necrosis factor (TNF) for 24 h. Subsequently, the binding with CLN-IgG was determined by an enzyme immunoassay using peroxidase.

2. In Vivo *Experiment*

A cytokine which enhanced the binding of CLN-IgG in an in vitro experiment was studied with CLN-IgG. U-87MG cells (5×10^6) were transplanted subcutaneously into BALB/c nude mice aged 4–6 weeks. The mice were allocated to 4 groups, and tumor growth curves were assessed. Group 1 had CLN-IgG (1 mg) alone, group 2 had CLN-IgG (1 mg) plus IFN-β (2×10^6 IU), and group 3 had IFN-β (2×10^6 IU) alone. These agents were injected into nude mice intraperitoneally on days 0, 6, 14, and 20. Group 4 was the untreated group.

[1] Department of Neurosurgery, Nippon Medical School, Bunkyo-ku, Tokyo, 113 Japan

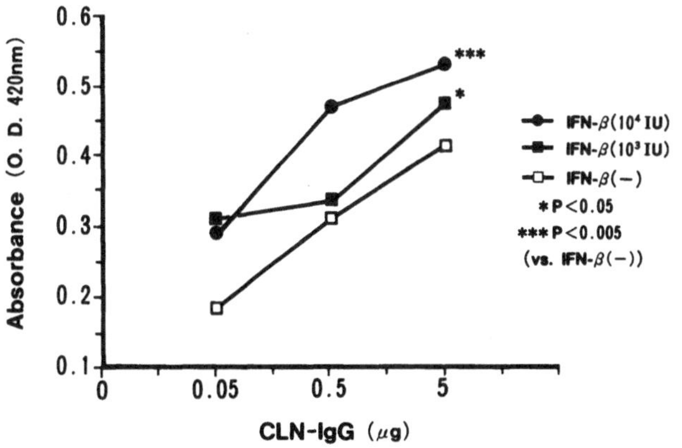

Fig. 1. Reactivity of CLN-IgG with IFN-β to U-87MG. Binding reactivity was determined by cell enzyme immunoassay. The values are the mean of triplicate data

3. *Investigation of Immunocompetent Cells*

At 3, 4 and 5 weeks after tumor inoculation, the lymphocyte subset (B cell, NK cell, and macrophage) in the peripheral blood and splenocytes were measured by flow cytometry. Measurement of B cells, NK cells, and macropahages was carried out using B220/Ly-5, anti-asialo GM 1, and anti-Mac 1 antibodies, respectively. Furthermore, splenocytes were measured for antibody-dependent cell-mediated cytotoxicity (ADCC) using an anti-chicken erythrocyte antibody and ^{51}Cr-labeled chicken erythrocytes as the target cells (effector/target ratio = 10:1).

Results

1. In Vitro *Study*

Pretreatment with HuIFN-β (10^3 and 10^4 IU) significantly increased the binding of CLN-IgG to U-87MG glioma cells compared with the untreated group ($P < 0.05$ and $P < 0.005$), and the increase was dose-dependent (Fig. 1).

HuIFN-γ (10^3 and 10^4 IU), and TNF (10^2 and 10^3 JRU) also significantly increased the binding of CLN-IgG to U-87MG cells compared with the untreated group ($P < 0.005$) in a dose-dependent manner (not shown). In addition, 10^4 IU rIFN-α increased moderately the binding of CLN-IgG to U-87MG cells in comparison with the untreated group ($P < 0.05$) (not shown).

2. In Vivo *Study*

Three weeks after the subcutaneous transplantation of malignant glioma cells, tumor growth inhibition was marked both in group 1 (CLN-IgG alone) and

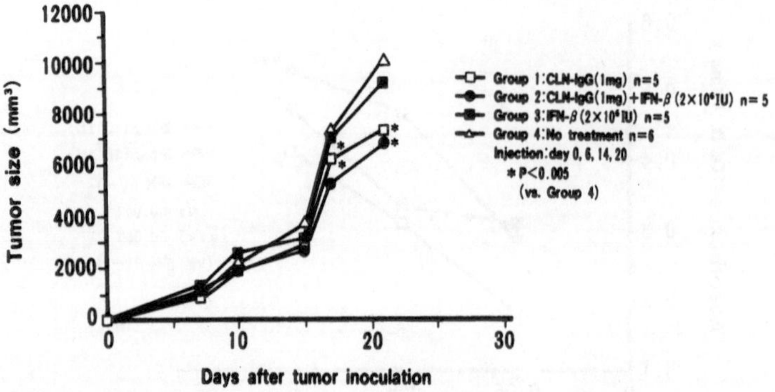

Fig. 2. Human malignant glioma xenografts treated with CLN-IgG. Groups of 5 or 6 mice with U-87MG tumor xenografts were treated with CLN-IgG and/or IFN-β. The values are mean tumor volumes of 5 or 6 mice per group

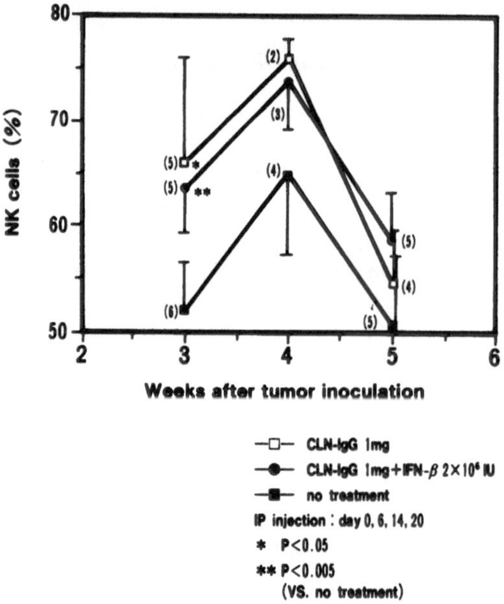

Fig. 3. Splenic NK cells of glioblastoma-bearing nude mice. Cell count was measured using anti-asialo GM1 antibody by flow cytometry. The number of mice studied is shown *in parenthesis* and *error bars* represent the standard deviation for each group

group 2 (CLN-IgG + IFNβ) compared with group 4 (untreated), with this inhibition being more prominent in group 2 (Fig. 2).

3. *Immunocompetent Cells*

Three weeks after tumor transplantation, the NK cell population among the splenocytes was significantly raised in groups 1 and 2, especially when group 2

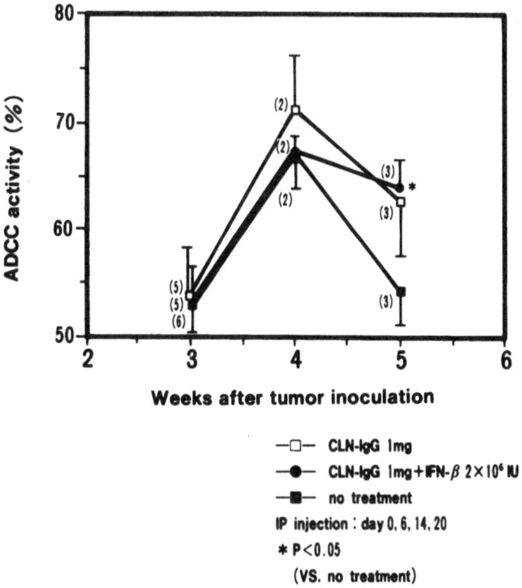

Fig. 4. Splenic ADCC activity of glioblastoma-bearing nude mice. Cytotoxicity was measured using chicken erythrocyte and anti-chicken erythrocyte antibody by ^{51}Cr release assay (effector/target ratio = 10:1). The number of mice studied is shown *in parenthesis* and *error bars* represent the standard deviation for each group

was compared with group 4 (Fig. 3). Furthermore, 5 weeks after tumor transplantation, the NK cell count of splenocytes was markedly reduced in the untreated group, while that in group 2 remained relatively unchanged.

No significant difference was noted in B cell and macrophage counts between the 4 groups at any time point, but ADCC activity was raised in group 2 at 5 weeks after transplantation compared with group 4 (Fig. 4).

Discussion

We have developed several MAbs against malignant gliomas for which no satisfactory treatment has yet been established, and have reported the results of the experimental studies aimed at their clinical application [6–8]. One of the problems was the uncertainty of the antitumor effect of the MAbs. Therefore, the stimulation of the antitumor mechanism needed to be investigated. Among the cytokines, IFN is known to have a stimulatory effect on killer cells and macrophages, as well as promoting the expression of the Ia antigen and Fc receptor. Thus, it is considered to be effective in the stimulation of a more effective MAb treatment.

The results obtained in the present study showed that concomitant use of IFN-β promoted the binding of CLN-IgG and stimulated tumor growth inhibition, compared to treatment with CLN-IgG alone, suggesting that it is necessary to consider the concomitant use of IFN-β in the future clinical application of CLN-IgG.

CLN-IgG has an ADCC activity against glioma cells and is thought to inhibit tumor growth by this mechanism. In the present study, however, enhancement of ADCC activity was observed only in the group treated with CLN-IgG with IFN-β. Flow cytometry showed that the NK cell count of splenocytes was significantly increased in the CLN-IgG treatment group, and a more marked difference was observed in the group concomitantly treated with IFN-β. These results suggest that NK cells might play an important role in the mechanism of the inhibition of CLN-IgG and IFN-β.

Conclusions

Enhancement of the accumulation of an MAb in the tumor is important in its clinical application. This study demonstrated that HuIFN enhanced the accumulation of CLN-IgG in tumors, showing a marked inhibitory effect on tumor growth. These findings may indicate some directions for the future clinical application of CLN-IgG.

References

1. Takahashi H, Nakazawa S, Herlyn D (1989) Experimental study of immunotherapy against malignant gliomas using monoclonal antibodies. Proc Jpn Cancer Assoc 48th Annu Meet, p 274
2. Gastl G, Marth C, Leiter E, Gattringer C, Mayer I, Daxenbichler G, Flener R, Huber C (1985) Effects of human recombinant α_2 arg-interferon and γ-interferon on human breast cancer cell lines: Dissociation of antiproliferative activity and induction of HLA-DR antigen expression. Cancer Res 45:2957–2961
3. Iacobelli S, Scambia G, Natoli C, Panici PB, Baiocchi G, Perrone L, Mancuso S (1988) Recombinant human leukocyte interferon-α2b stimulates the synthesis and release of a 90K tumor-associated antigen in human breast cancer cells. Int J Cancer 42:182–184
4. Real FX, Carrato A, Schuessler MH, Welt S, Oettgen HF (1988) IFN-γ-regulated expression of a differentiation antigen of human cells. J Immunol 140:1571–1576
5. Marley GM, Doyle LA, Ordonez JV, Sisk A, Hussain A, Chiu Yen R (1989) Potentiation of interferon induction of class I major histocompatibility complex antigen expression by human tumor necrosis factor in small cell lung cancer cell lines. Cancer Res 49:6232–6236
6. Takahashi H, Herlyn D, Atkinson B, Powe J, Rodeck U, Alavi A, Bruce DA, Koprowski H (1987) Radioimmunodetection of human glioma xenografts by monoclonal antibody to epidermal growth factor receptor. Cancer Res 47:3847–3850
7. Nanda A, Liwnicz B, Atkinson BF, Sela BA, Takahashi H, Belser PH, Black P, Koprowski H, Herlyn D (1989) Monoclonal antibodies with cytotoxic reactivities against human gliomas. J Neurosurg 71:892–897
8. Takahashi H, Belser PH, Atkinson BF, Sela BA, Ross AH, Biegel JB, Emanuel B, Sutton L, Koprowski H, Herlyn D (1990) Monoclonal antibody-dependent, cell-mediated cytotoxicity against human malignant gliomas. Neurosurgery 27:97–102

Antiproliferative Effect of Trapidil on a PDGF-Producing Glioma Cell Line *In Vivo*

Jun-ichi Kuratsu, Shuichi Takaki, Yosuke Mihara, Masato Kochi, and Yukitaka Ushio[1]

Introduction

Cell proliferation is regulated by growth factors which stimulate mitogenicity through binding to specific receptors on target cells. The platelet-derived growth factor (PDGF) is produced by many kinds of cells.

We previously reported that Trapidil, a PDGF antagonist, inhibits the proliferation of a PDGF-producing glioma cell (U251MG) *in vitro* [1]. The present study was undertaken to determine whether Trapidil exhibits inhibitory effects on the proliferation of PDGF-producing glioma cells *in vivo*.

Materials and Methods

Drugs

Trapidil (5-methyl-7-diethylamino-S-triazolo 1,5-a pyrimidine) was provided by Mochida Inc., Japan.

Animals

Male athymic BALB/c mice (*nu/nu* genotype, 5 weeks or older) were used for all in vivo experiments.

In Vivo *Assay*

The U251MG or U105MG tumor, which had been serially transplanted in nude mice, was removed aseptically, and a small piece of the tumor (2 mm square) was transplanted subcutaneously by trocar into the flanks of nude mice. The in vivo experiments were started on day 0 when the tumor weight reached approximately 150–200 mg. At that time, tumor-bearing mice were assigned randomly to 2 test groups consisting of 4–6 mice each. The control group

[1] Department of Neurosurgery, Kumamoto University Medical School, Kumamoto, 860 Japan

received 0.2 ml physiological saline intraperitoneally (i.p.) and the experimental group was given Trapidil, 40 mg/kg per day dissolved in 0.2 ml physiological saline, i.p. Because the U251MG tumor became cystic at about 20 days after transplantation, Trapidil was administered to U251MG tumor-bearing mice daily from day 0 to day 10. Since the U105MG tumor grows more slowly and does not become cystic, U105MG tumor-bearing mice received Trapidil daily from day 0 to day 20. The tumor was measured with sliding calipers every 5 days by the same examiner. Its width and length in mm were monitored, and the weight was calculated by the formula: $a \times b^2/2$ (a = long diameter, b = short diameter). The growth inhibition ratio was calculated as follows: $100 - Tn/T_0/Cn/C_0$, where Tn and T_0 represent tumor size on day n and day 0, respectively, in the treated group, and Cn and C_0 the tumor size on day n and day 0, respectively, in the control group. Statistical analysis was made by the Wilcoxon *t*-test.

Labeling Index Assay

At the end of the experiment, 5 mg/kg bromodeoxyuridine (BrdU) was injected i.p. and, after 60 min, the mice were sacrified under deep anesthesia. The tumors were removed, placed in chilled 70% ethanol, and embedded in paraffin. The Avidin-Biotin Peroxidase Complex method with anti-BrdU monoclonal antibody (Beckton Dickinson, Mt. View, Calif.) was performed. The ratio of BrdU-positive nuclei to total nuclei (labeling index: LI) at × 400 magnification was obtained in four fields. The average LI of the tumor was determined for each group.

Results

Antiproliferative Effect of Trapidil on Glioma Cells In Vivo

All of the mice were alive and showed no significant weight loss at the end of the experiment. The U251MG tumor-bearing control mice revealed a progressive increase in the tumor weight ratio (Table 1). At day 5, the mean tumor weight was about 3.6 and 1.2 times greater than the initial tumor weight in the

Table 1. Mean tumor weight ratios of U251MG during treatment, relative to weight on day 0

	Percentage of value on day 0		
	Day 0	Day 5	Day 10
Control (n = 4)	100	364	913
Trapidil (n = 5)	100	127*	474*

*$P < 0.05$ versus the control group

Table 2. Mean tumor weight ratios of U105MG during treatment, relative to weight on day 0

	Percentage of value on day 0				
	Day 0	Day 5	Day 10	Day 15	Day 20
Control ($n = 6$)	100	162	181	261	280
Trapidil ($n = 6$)	100	135	159	186	215

Table 3. Labeling indexes (LI) of BrdU-labeled cells of U251MG tumors in mice

	LI (%)
Control mice ($n = 6$)	17.1 ± 4.5
Trapidil-treated mice ($n = 5$)	7.3 ± 2.1

Values are means ±SD

control and Trapidil-treated mice, respectively. The growth inhibition ratio of Trapidil was about 66%, which was statistically significant ($P < 0.05$). At the end of the experiment, the mean tumor weight was about 9.1 and 4.7 times greater than the initial tumor weight in control and Trapidil-treated mice, respectively. The growth inhibition ratio of Trapidil was about 48%, which was statistically significant ($P < 0.05$). The weight of the U105MG tumor in Trapidil-treated mice at day 20 was 2.1 times greater than at day 0 (Table 2). In untreated U105MG-bearing mice, it was 2.8 times greater, resulting in a growth inhibition ratio by Trapidil of about 25%. The average LI of BrdU-labeled U251MG cells for control and Trapidil-treated mice was 17.1% and 7.3%, respectively (Table 3).

Discussion

We previously reported that a PDGF-like substance is secreted by U251MG cells but not by U105MG cells, and that there is heterogeneity among glioma cells in the production of growth factors [2]. Furthermore, the in vitro growth of U251MG cells was inhibited by anti-PDGF antibody while that of U105MG cells was not [1]. These observations suggest that the proliferation of U251MG cells is PDGF-dependent.

Trapidil is an agent capable of interfering with PDGF and can function as a competitive inhibitor, binding preferentially to PDGF receptor sites on target cells, and thus preventing PDGF from exerting its stimulating effect [3,4]. We observed that 100 μg/ml Trapidil significantly inhibited the proliferation of U251MG cells which produce the PDGF-like molecule, but did not inhibit the proliferation of U105MG cells which do not produce the PDGF-like molecule.

We now report that a daily i.p. administration of 40 mg/kg Trapidil inhibited the grwoth of xenografted U251MG tumor in nude mice. Previously, Tiell et al. [5] found that the daily administration for 17 days of 45 or 90 mg Trapidil to rats via an intragastric feeding tube markedly reduced the magnitude of arteriosclerotic smooth muscle cell plaques. Takamiya et al. [6], who studied the association of PDGF with the appearance of reactive astrocytes following brain injury, found that in rats, the appearance of reactive astrocytes in the lesion was dramatically suppressed by the administration of 40 mg/kg Trapidil.

We observed a distinct decrease in the number of BrdU-labeled cells in Trapidil-treated mice in comparison with control mice. BrdU is taken up by cells in the S phase, and the LI represents the proportion of tumor cells engaged in the S phase in preparation for mitosis [7,8]. On the other hand, the early events leading to cell proliferation are initiated by the action of PDGF [9]. Thus, because Trapidil inhibits the growth promoting action, the LI of Trapidil-treated mice was lower than that of control mice.

Our experiments demonstrated the antiproliferative effect of Trapidil, a PDGF antagonist, on a PDGF-producing glioma cell line *in vivo*, and suggested that clinical trials of this agent in patients with PDGF-producing glioma may be warranted.

Conclusions

We demonstrated that Trapidil, a specific antagonist of PDGF, inhibits the proliferation of a PDGF-producing glioma cell line. In these experiments, we investigated the inhibitory effect of Trapidil on glioma using a nude mouse xenograft system. Daily intraperitoneal administration of 40 mg/kg Trapidil significantly inhibited the growth of the PDGF-producing glioma U251MG. The labeling index, measured by BrdU intake by Trapidil-treated and untreated tumor, revealed a decrease of the growth fraction of Trapidil-treated tumors. On the other hand, the growth of PDGF-nonproducing glioma U105MG was not inhibited. These findings show that Trapidil inhibits the growth of PDGF-producing glioma *in vivo*.

References

1. Kuratsu J, Ushio Y (1990) Antiproliferative effect of Trapidil, platelet-derived growth factor antagonist, on a glioma line in vitro. J Neurosurg 73:436–440
2. Kuratsu J, Estes JE, Yokota S, Mahaley MS Jr, Gillespie GY (1989) Growth factors derived from a human malignant glioma cell line, U-251MG. J Neurooncol 7:225–236
3. Ohnishi H, Yamaguchi K, Shimada S, Suzuki Y, Kumagai A (1981) A new approach to the treatment of atherosclerosis and Trapidil as an antagonist to platelet-derived growth factor. Life Sci 28:1641–1646

4. Ohnishi H, Yamaguchi K, Shimada S, Suzuki Y, Saito Y, Kumagai A (1981) Growth-promoting activity of platelet-derived growth factor (PDGF) and effect of Trapidil. J Jpn Coll Angiol 21:409–414
5. Tiell ML, Sussman II, Gordon PB, Sanders RN (1983) Suppression of fibroblast proliferation in vitro and of myointimal hyperplasia in vivo by the triazolopyrimidine, Trapidil. Artery 12:33–50
6. Takamiya Y, Kohsaka S, Toya S, Otani M, Mikoshiba K, Tsukada Y (1986) Possible association of platelet-derived growth factor (PDGF) with the appearance of reactive astrocytes following brain injury *in situ*. Brain Res 383:305–309
7. Cho KG, Hoshino T, Nagashima T, Murovic JA, Wilson CB (1984) Prediction of tumor doubling time in recurrent meningiomas. Cell kinetics studies with bromodeoxyuridine labeling. J Neurosurg 65:790–794
8. Hoshino T, Nagashima T, Murovic JA, Edwards MSB, Gutin PH, Davis RL, DeArmond SJ (1986) In situ cell kinetics studies on human neuroectodermal tumors with bromodeoxyuridine labeling. J Neurosurg 64:453–459
9. Leof EB, Van Wyk JJ, O'Keefe EJ, Pledger WJ (1983) Epidermal growth factor (EGF) is required only during the transverse of early G1 in PDGF-stimulated density-arrested BALB/c-3T3 cells. Exp Cell Res 147:202–208

Effects of CDDP on a Monolayer Cultured 9L Glioma Cell Line—Evaluation by a FCM Study of a Cellular DNA Histogram

NOBUTOSHI RYU, SHOUBU SHIBATA, AKIRA OCHI, and KAZUO MORI[1]

Introduction

Cis-diamminedichloroplatinum (CDDP) is known to be an effective drug against many malignant tumors [1,2]. However, in brain tumors, its usefulness is limited because of the blood-brain barrier [3]. To solve this problem, we are investigating the drug delivery system with liposome [4,5]. We have already reported liposome containing CDDP (Lip-CDDP) to be more useful than free-CDDP as a targeting therapy for brain tumors when we studied organ CDDP distribution using 9L-glioma implanted rats [5].

The anti-tumoral effect of CDDP needed to be evaluated objectively, so we decided to conduct a study using flow cytometry (FCM). In this paper, we describe a basic experiment of FCM studies of cellular DNA histograms.

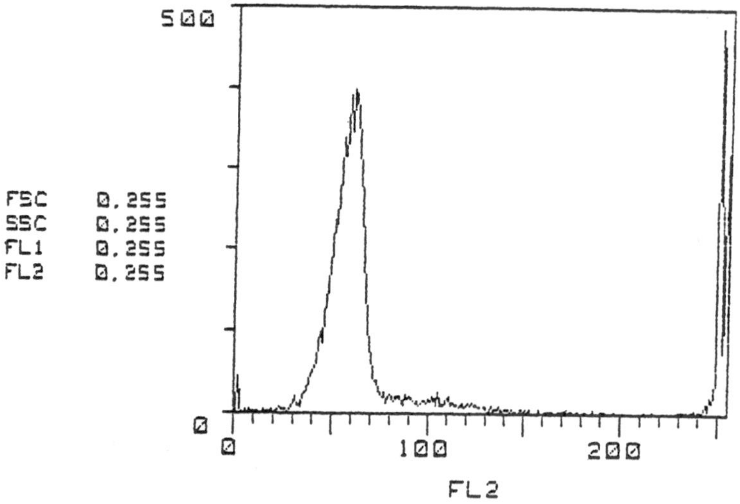

Fig. 1. DNA histogram of monolayer cultured 9L glioma cells which were not contacted with CDDP. Coefficient of variation (CV) = 9%

[1] Department of Neurosurgery, Nagasaki University School of Medicine, Nagasaki, 852 Japan

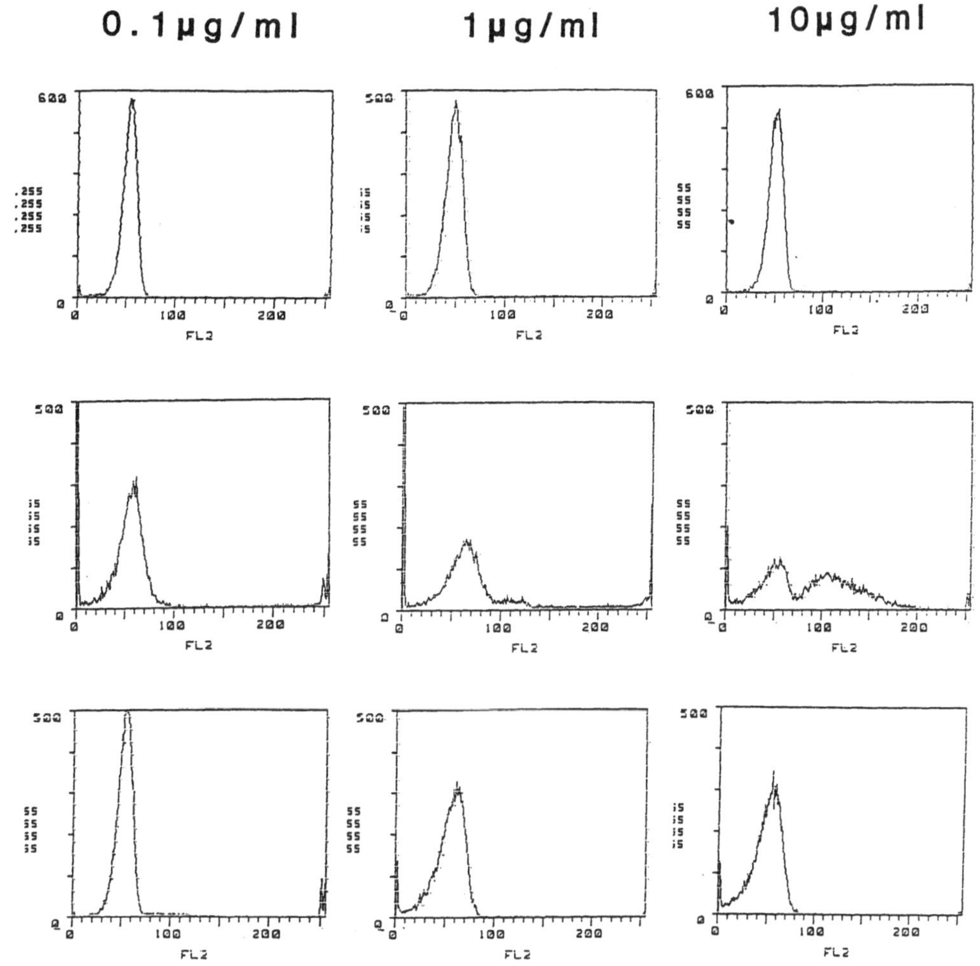

Fig. 2. DNA histograms of monolayer cultured 9L glioma cells contacted with three concentrations of free CDDP. When 9L glioma cells contacted with 1 µg/ml free CDDP, the DNA histogram showed accumulation of G2 + M phase cells at the 48 h point. At 0.1 µg/ml of CDDP, little change was seen in the DNA histogram, and at 10 µg/ml CDDP, the typical DNA histogram pattern was not seen

Materials and Methods

9L glioma cells cultured with Dulbecco's modified Eagle's medium (DMEM: Whittaker M.A. Bioproducts, Walkersville, Md.) and containing 10% fetal bovine serum (FBS: Gibco, Burlington, Ontario, Canada) were seeded into 6-well plates (1×10^5 cells/well), and incubated at 37°C. After 48 h of incubation, with the glioma cells in the exponential growth phase, the cultures were washed and refed with several test mediums and incubated. The test mediums were DMEM with 10% FBS containing concentrations of free CDDP or

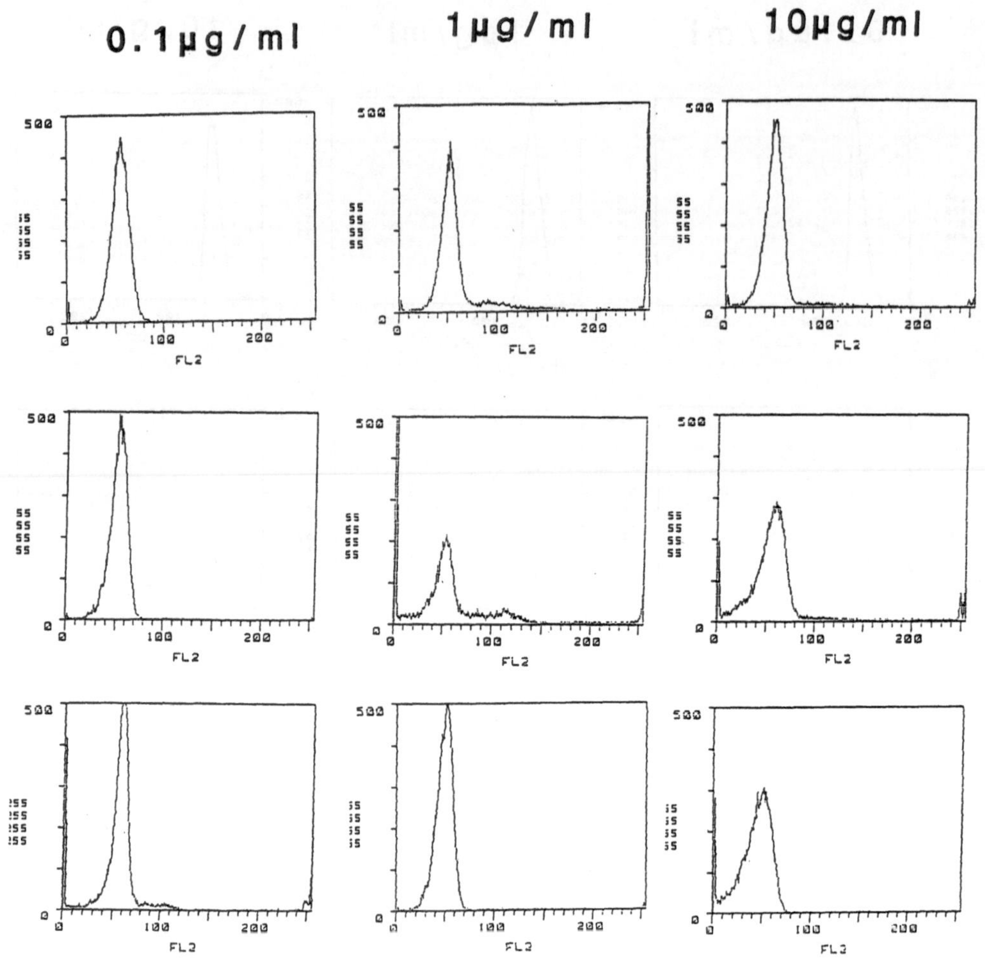

Fig. 3. DNA histograms of monolayer cultured 9 L glioma cells contacted with three concentrations of Lip-CDDP. The results were the same as those in the studies of free CDDP

Lip-CDDP of 0.1 μg/ml, 1 μg/ml, and 10 μg/ml. After 24 h of incubation, the cultures were washed and refed with DMEM containing only 10% FBS.

After 24, 48, and 72 h, the 9 L glioma cells were harvested by treatment with 0.25% trypsin and 0.02% EDTA, and prepared by single-cell suspensions for an FCM study of DNA histograms as follows:

1. Single cell suspension treated with 0.25% trypsin and 0.02% ETA
2. Fixation with 99.6% methanol for 20 min at 4°C
3. Incubation with 0.1% triton-X and 1 mg/ml RNase for 30 min at 37°C
4. Propidium Iodide (50 μg/ml) staining for 2 h at 4°C
5. Passage through a filter of 50 μm nylon mesh.

FCM studies of cellular DNA histograms were performed with FACScan (Becton Dickinson, USA).

Results

In the controls, the 9L glioma cells which were never contacted with CDDP, had DNA histograms which showed a diploid pattern (Fig. 1). The value of the coefficient of variation (CV) was about 9%. When the 9L glioma cells were contacted with a 1 μg/ml concentration of free CDDP, the DNA histogram showed an accumulation of G2 + M phase cells at 48 h. On the other hand, when the cells were contacted with 0.1 μg/ml CDDP, little change was seen in the DNA histogram, but with 10 μg/ml free CDDP, no typical DNA histogram appeared at 48 and 72 h (Fig. 2). The same results emerged from the investigations using test mediums containing Lip-CDDP (Fig. 3).

Microscopic studies of monolayer cultured 9L glioma cells with 10 μg/ml free CDDP revealed a marked decrease in the number of living cells (data not shown). Consequently, we did not agree that the DNA histogram of 9L glioma cells cultured with 10 μg/ml CDDP expressed the exact nuclear DNA content. We think that the DNA histogram was masked by cell debris and dead cells.

Discussion

We have already reported the antitumoral effect of Lip-CDDP estimated with survival rates of 9L glioma-implanted rats [5]. The survival rate, however, appeared to be influenced by nutrition, implanted tumor size, and location of the tumor in vivo. An objective indicator of the anitumoral effect of CDDP was required for these evaluations.

Many authors described the usefulness of FCM studies of DNA histograms for sensitivity tests of chemotherapeutic agents [6]. deVere White et al. [7] reported that flow cytometric analysis of the DNA histogram shape was effective in monitoring *in vivo* responses to therapy only in tumors with small G2 compartments, a large S-phase compartment, or marked aneuploid peaks. They said that the approach of short-term in vitro growth coupled with a DNA histogram analysis using FCM was useful as well. While our experimental results showed a capability of objectively estimating the antitumoral effect of CDDP in vivo, the results of the DNA histogram of 10 μg/ml CDDP seem to have been almost entirely influenced by cell debris. Additionally, the CV value of the control study seemed to be rather high. This may indicate the necessity for tests of cell viability. For a more precise evaluation of antitumoral effects with FCM, a double staining study of BrdU and Propidium Iodide (PI) would be valuable.

Conclusion

We examined the antitumoral effect of free CDDP and Lip-CDDP *in vitro* with an FCM study of cellular DNA histograms. The results of our experiment showed that there were no differences between the two drugs. BrdU and PI double staining methods in combination with FCM would probably result in more precise measurements.

References

1. Niijima H (1983) Cis-diamminedichloroplatinum: Its clinical application (in Japanese). Kyouwa-Kikaku-Tsuushin Press, pp 5–6
2. Niijima H (1982) Phase II Study of cis-diamminedichloroplatinum (in Japanese). Gan to Kagaku Ryoho 9:46–54
3. Hujita H (1983) Cis-diamminedichloroplatinum: Its clinical application (in Japanese). Kyouwa-Kikaku-Tsuushin Press, pp 11–27
4. Shibata S, Jinnouchi T, Mori K (1989) Ultrastructural study of capillary permeability of liposome-encapsulated cisplatin in an experimental rat brain tumor model. Neurol Med Chir (Tokyo) 29:696–700
5. Ochi A, Shibata S, Mori K, Satou T, Sunamoto J (1990) Targeting chemotherapy of brain tumor using liposome-encapsulated cisplatin-Part 2. Pullulan-coated liposomes to target brain tumor. Drug Del Syst 5:261–265
6. Takamoto S, Oota K (1988) Flow cytometry—technique and practical management 2nd edn (in Japanese). Kani Shobou Press, pp 450–467
7. deVere White R, Deitch AD, Olsson CA (1983) Limitation of DNA histogram analysis by flow cytometry as a method of predicting chemosensitivity in a rat renal cancer model. Cancer Res 43:604–610

Peripheral-Type Benzodiazepine Receptors in Gliomas

AKIRA TAKADA[1], YUKITAKA USHIO[1], MIRKO DIKSIC[2], and Y. LUCAS YAMAMOTO[2]

Introduction

Peripheral-type benzodiazepine receptors (PBRs) are present in high concentrations in peripheral tissues of various organs, such as lung, kidney, heart, and adrenal gland, but are sparse in the normal nervous system [1]. PBRs are thought to be located on glia rather than on neurons [2]. Moreover, PBRs have been found in rodent glial tumors [3] as well as in human glial tumors, and several studies suggested that PBRs could be useful for specific imaging of glial tumors. Black et al. [4] reported that a significant correlation was observed between the high binding of PBR ligands and the degree of malignancy in gliomas in man, but Ferrarese et al. [5] reported that the binding density of PBR ligands did not correlate with malignancy. The main purpose of this study was to try to add more light to this problem by examining the concentration (Bmax) and dissociation constant (K_d) for PBRs in human gliomas.

Materials and Methods

[3H]PK 11195 (1-(2-chlorophenyl)-N-methyl-N-(1-methylpropyl)-3-isoquinoline carboxamide) was purchased from Du-Pon-New England Nuclear (Boston, Mass.) as a ligand.

Nine pathological tissues were obtained at surgery from patients with cerebral glioma and stored at −80°C until use. Tumor samples were also examined histopathologically by two neuropathologists. The specimens were diagnosed as astrocytoma grade II (3 cases), astrocytoma grade III (1 case), and glioblastoma (5 cases). Six brain tissues (control), which were taken from patients who had undergone frontal or temporal lobectomy, were stored at −80°C.

For the binding study, 15 μM sections were cut on a cryostat and mounted onto gelatin-coated glass slides. The slides were then given three consecutive 5-min washes in buffer solution (50 mM Tris HCl, pH 7.5, 10 mM $MgCl_2$) at

[1] Department of Neurosurgery, Kumamoto University Medical School, Kumamoto, 862 Japan
[2] Cone Neurological Research Labolatory and Neuroisotope Laboratory, Montreal Neurological Institute, Montreal, Quebec, H2X 3P7 Canada

0°C, after which they were incubated in the presence of 1 nM [3 H]PK 11195 at room temperature with various concentrations of unlabeled PK 11195 as a competetive inhibitor. Non-specific binding was defined in the presence of 1 μM PK 11195. After incubation, the slides were washed twice for 5 min in the same buffer at an ice-cold temperature and then quickly rinsed in H_2O. They were rapidly and thoroughly dried under a stream of cool and dry air. In order to obtain autoradiographic images, the slides were placed in X-ray cassettes along with tissue calibrated at 3 H standards. After exposure, the sections were stained with Cresyl violet luxol fast blue and hematoxylin and easin for correlation of areas of histologically verified tumor with binding densities.

Autoradiograms were digitized and analyzed on a microcomputer-based image analysis system. Scatchard plot analysis was performed using Computer Radioligand Binding Analysis (Elsevier-Biosoft). Stastical analysis was performed using a two-trailed unpaired Student's *t*-test. $P < 0.05$ was regarded as a significant difference.

Results

There were high binding activities of periphral benzodiazepine receptor ligands in human gliomas, whereas little binding was seen in the other (normal) brain

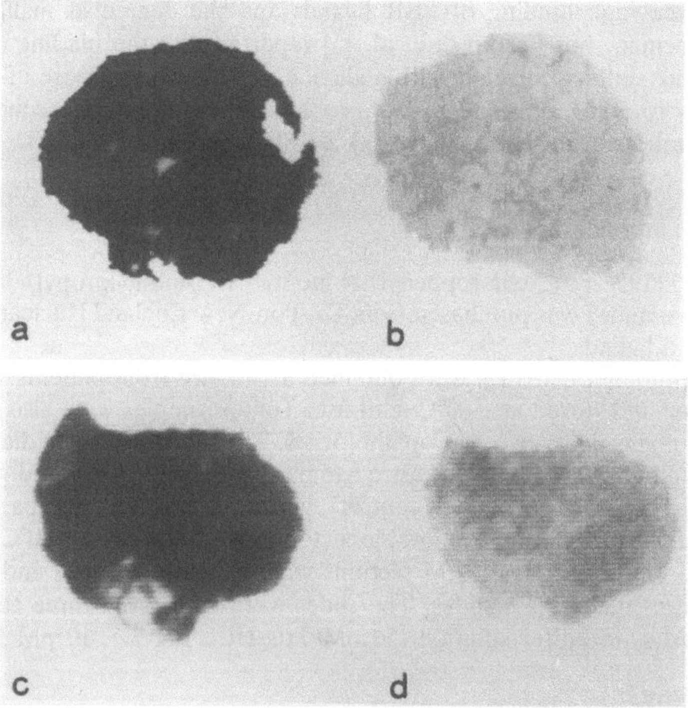

Fig. 1. [3 H]PK 11195 bindings in malignant and benign glioma. **a** Total binding and **b** non-specific binding in malignant glioma. **c** Total binding and **d** non-specific binding in benign glioma

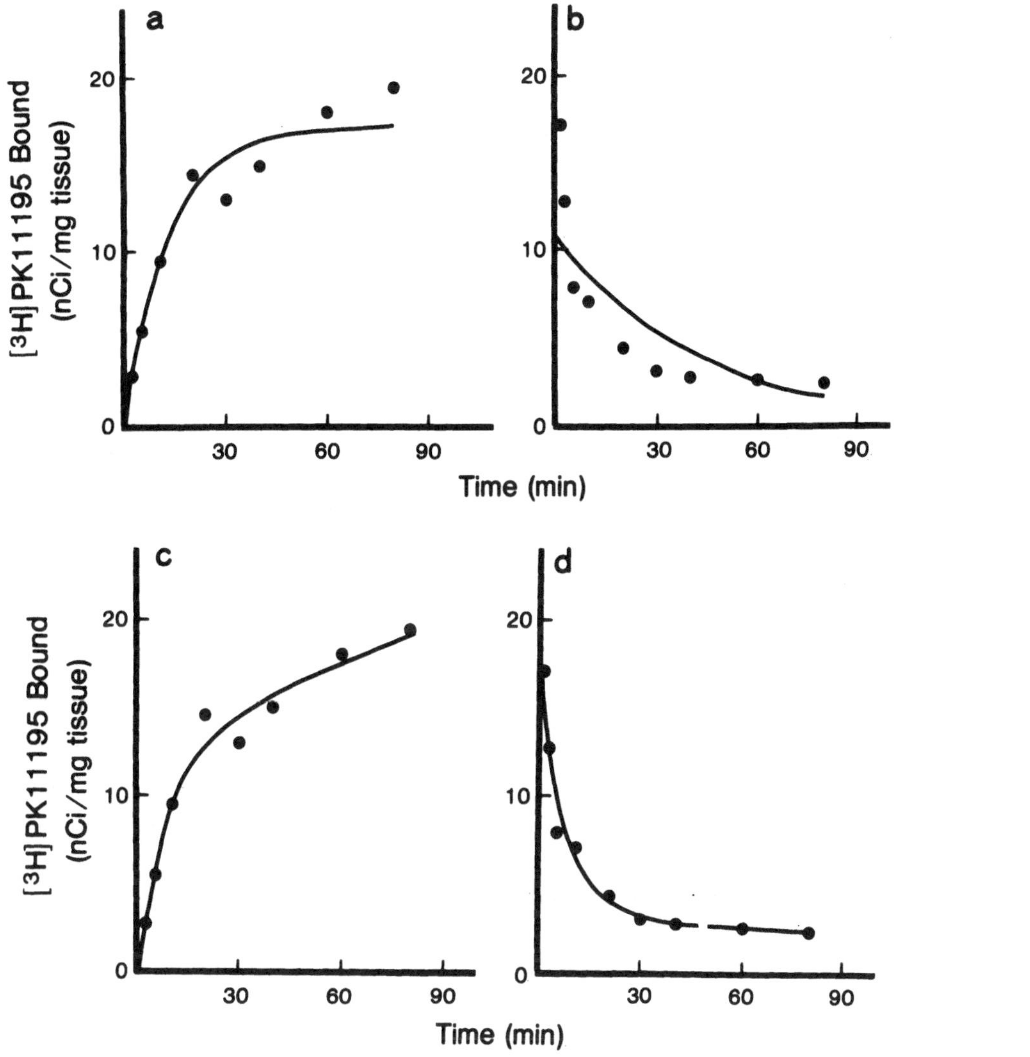

Fig. 2. Kinetics of [3H]PK 11195 binding to a benign glioma. **a,b** Association and dissociation curves fitted in a single-site model. **c,d** Association and dissociation curves fitted in a two-site model. The better fitting curve was obtained in the two-site model. Sections were incubated in the presence of 1 nM [3H]PK 11195. 1 μM PK11195 was added at zero time to measure dissociation

structures (Fig. 1). Non-specific binding of these tumors represented less than 8.4% of the total binding. There were striking correlations between high-density areas on the autoradiogram and staining for histologically determined tumors. In necrotic areas with tumor, binding was little or greatly reduced. The [3H]PK 11195 binding to human gliomas at room temperature was saturable and reversible. The data from the Scatchard analysis is shown in Table 1. The K_ds in the cortex, malignant gliomas, and benign gliomas were 3.95 ±

Table 1. [3 H]PK 11195-Binding densities and dissociation rate constants in human cortex and gliomas

Sample (n)	K_d (nM) ± SE	B_{max} (pmol/mg tissue) ± SE
Human cortex (6)	3.95 ± 0.38	0.35 ± 0.04
Malignant glioma (6)	7.24 ± 2.96[a]	1.26 ± 0.24[a]
Benign glioma (3)	5.84 ± 0.47[a]	0.64 ± 0.08[a]

[a] $P < 0.05$ when values are compared with those of human cortex. K_d dissociation constant, B_{max}, maximum binding density; *SE*, standard error

0.38 nM, 7.24 ± 2.96 nM, and 5.84 ± 0.47 nM respectively (3 cases of benign gliomas were analyzed in a single-site model). The B_{max}s in the cortex, malignant gliomas, and benign gliomas were 0.35 ± 0.04, 1.26 ± 0.24, and 0.64 ± 0.08 pmol/mg tissue, respectively. The B_{max} in malignant gliomas was 3.6 times higher than in the cortex. Both K_ds and B_{max}s in malignant and benign gliomas were significantly different when values were çompared with those of the cortex. However, there was no significant differences in K_d and B_{max} between malignant and benign gliomas.

Scatchard analysis of malignant gliomas indicated a single class of receptor site. The Hill coefficient was near the unit. Interestingly, in the Scatchard analysis of one of the benign gliomas, the better fitting curve was obtained in a two-site model than in a single-site model. Association and dissociation studies were also investigated in the same tumor, and the fitting curve in the two-site model was significantly preferrd than in a single-site model (Fig. 2). Results of the graphic analysis suggested the presence of two receptor sites in this tumor. In another case of benign gliomas, Scatchard analysis represented the better fitting line in a single-site model; however, dissociation curves in the same sample were indicative of a preference of the fitting in two-site rather than in a single site model.

Discussion

We observed increased densities in human malignant and benign gliomas in which B_{max} was 3.6–1.8 times higher than in the normal cortex. Increased densities have previously been reported in human U-87 MG gliomas, human U251 gliomas in rat, and human gliomas in humans [3–6] Our results support these findings. Recently, human gliomas have been imaged in PET and SPECT with PBR ligands [7–9], and many applications of PBR ligands for clinical investigation and diagnosis of gliomas can be expected.

We could not determine significant differences in B_{max} and K_d between malignant and benign gliomas. Black et al. [10] observed a significant correlation between density and malignancy in gliomas, while Ferrarese et al. [5] reported that density did not correlate with malignancy suggesting that PBR could be a marker of increased cellularity. Our data seems to support the latter findings, but further investigation is needed because we did not have sufficient numbers of tumors to come to definitive conclusions.

Interestingly, we found complexed receptor sites in human benign gliomas. One reason for this finding might be a heterogeneity of the tissue including adjacent gliosis and the remaining normal structure. Since malignant gliomas showed a single receptor site, it might be possible to differentiate benign from malignant gliomas with this technique.

Conclusions

The high specific binding of PBR ligands may be useful in the imaging of gliomas and in the differentiation of malignant from benign gliomas. Since necrotic lesions show little binding, it could also be possible to differentiate gliomas from radiation necrosis.

References

1. Anholt RR, De Souza EB, Oster-Granite ML, Snyder SH (1985) Peripheral-type benzodiazepine receptors: Autoradiographic localization in whole body sections of neonatal rats. J Pharmacol Exp Ther 233:517–520
2. McCarthy KD, Harden TK (1981) Indentification of two benzodiazepine biding sites on cells cultured from rat cerebral cortex. J Pharmacol Exp Ther 216:183–191
3. Starosta-Rubinstein S, Ciliax B, Penny JB, McKeever P, Young AB (1987) Imaging of a glioma using peripheral benzodiazepine receptor ligand. Proc Natl Acad Sci USA 84:891–895
4. Black KL, Ikezaki K, Toga AW (1989) Imaging of brain tumors using peripheral benzodiazepine receptor ligands. J Neurosurg 71:113–118
5. Ferrarese C, Appollonio I, Frigo M, Gaini M, Piolti R, Frattola L (1989) Benzodiazepine receptors and diazepine binding inhibitor in human cerebral tumors. Ann Neurol 26:564–568
6. Olson JMM, Junck L, Young AB, Penny JB, Mancini WR (1988) Isoquinoline and peripheral-type benzodiazepine in gliomas: Implication for diagnostic imaging. Cancer Res 48:5837–5741
7. Junck L, Olson JMM, Ciliax BJ, Koeppe RA, Watkins GL, Jewett DM, McKeever PE, Wieland DM, Kilbourn MR, Starosta-Rubinstein S, Mancini WR, Kuhl DE, Greenberg HS, Young AB (1989) PET imaging of human gliomas with ligands for the peripheral bezodiazepine binding site. Ann Neurol 26:752–758
8. Gildersleeve DL, Lin T-Y, Wieland DM, Ciliax BJ, Olson JMM, Young AB (1989) Synthesis of a high activity [125I]-labelled analog of PK 11195, a potential agent for SPECT imaging of the peripheral benzodiazepine binding site. Nucl Med Biol 16:423–429
9. Van Dort ME, Ciliax BJ, Gildersleeve DL, Sherman PS, Rosenspire KC, Young AB, Junck L, Wieland DM (1988) Radioiodinated benzodiazepines: Agents for mapping glial tumors. J Med Chem 31:2081–2086
10. Black KL, Ikezaki K, Santori E, Becher DP, Vinters HV (1990) Specific high-affinity binding of peripheral benzodiazepine receptor ligands to brain tumors in rat and man. Cancer 65:93–97

Peripheral-Type Benzodiazepine Receptors in Brain Tumors: *In Vitro* Binding Characteristics and Implication for New Image Analysis

KIYONOBU IKEZAKI[1], KEITH L. BLACK[1], and KAZUO TABUCHI[2]

Introduction

Benzodiazepines are widely used primarily as anticonvulsants, antianxiety drugs, and hypnotics in the central nervous system (CNS). Benzodiazepines bind specifically to their receptors on the plasma membrane of neurons with nanomolar affinity and exert their inhibitory effects on neurons [1,2]. This "central"-type benzodiazepine receptor has been purified, and its cDNA cloned [3]. The central-type benzodiazepine receptor is a macromolecular compex which is closely linked to gamma aminobutylic acid $(GABA)_A$ receptors and modulates the GABA-regulated chloride channel in conjunction with the recognition sites of barbiturates, picrotoxin, and bicyclophosphates [4–6].

In addition, binding sites for benzodiazepines were found to be present in several peripheral tissues, such as the kidney, and were named "peripheral"-type benzodiazepine (PBD) receptors [7–10]. These "peripheral" binding sites differ significantly from the "central"-type receptors in their pharmacological properties [11]. Although the physiological function of PBD and its receptor remains unknown, intriguing patterns of tissue distribution, an unusual subcellular localization, and a range of effects on growth, differentiation, and energy metabolism have stimulated interest in its possible biological significance.

Benzodiazepines and Receptors

Benzodiazepines are classified into three groups according to their binding affinities to specific receptors. Clonazepam and Ro15–1483 are known as central-type ligands which bind specifically to the central benzodiazepine receptor. Diazepam and flunitrazepam (mixed-type ligands) have higher affinity to the central-type receptors than to the peripheral-type receptors. In higher concentrations, they bind to PBD receptor. Synthesized Ro5–4864 [7-chloro-

[1] Division of Neurosurgery and Brain Research Institute, University of California at Los Angeles, School of Medicine, Los Angeles, CA 90024–1761, USA
[2] Department of Neurosurgery, Saga Medical School, Saga, 849 Japan

5-(4-chlorophenyl)-1,13-dihydro-1-methyl-2H-1, 4-benzodiazepine-2-one (4′-chlorodiazepam)] PK11195 [1-(2-chlorphenyl)-N-methyl-N-(1-methylpropyl)-3-isoquinoline carboxiamide [12], and PK14105 (isoquinoline carboxamide) are specific ligands for PBD receptors.

Of the two classes of benzodiazepine receptors in mammalian tissues, the "central"-type receptor is located on neuronal membranes as a macromolecular complex closely linked to $GABA_A$ receptors. The second, "peripheral", class of benzodiazepine receptor is sparse in normal nervous tissue, but prominent in many other tissues, such as the zona glomerulosa of the adrenal gland, the distal tubules and collecting ducts of the kidney, the heart muscle, the testosterone-forming Leydig cells of the testes, platelets, and lymphocytes [7,9,10,13,14]. PBD receptors have been reported to be localized on mitochondrial outer [15] or inner membrane [16]. Proteins associated with PBD receptors have been purified from rat mitochondrial preparations. Irradiation or sodium dodecyl sulfate-polyacrylamide gel electrophoresis (SDS-PAGE) analysis of the receptor with ^{3}H-flunitrazepam indicated 35 and 30 kd binding sites [17,18]. Further, photoaffinity isoquinoline carboxamide ligand ^{3}H-PK14105 labeled a single protein of approximately 17 kd, and its cDNA sequence has been determined [19,20]. Many properties of the binding of benzodiazepine and isoquinoline ligands to the receptor suggest that they interact with different sites or, perhaps, different subpopulations of receptors. Thus, potencies of isoquinolinc carboxamides are the same in various tissues and species, while relative potencies of benzodiazepines in the same tissues and species differ markedly [21].

Several compounds have been nominated as endogenous ligands for PBD receptors. Phospholipase A2 isozyme (16 kd), phospholipids, and unsaturated fatty acids do inhibit Ro5–4864 binding at micromolar concentration [22,23]. In contrast, naturally occurring porphyrins, such as heme, protoporphyrin IX, mesoporphyrin IX, and deuteroporphyrin IX have actions in the nanomolar range [24]. Ro5–4864 shows various affinities in different tissues and species. Protoporphyrins, however, have identical potencies in PBD receptors in all species and in all organs. In addition, the photosensitization of mitochondria by the tumor-localizing porphyrin dimer/poligomer fraction of hematoporphyrin derivatives was not inhibited by Ro5–4864 [25]. Thus, the nature of endogenous PBD receptor ligands is still obscure.

Localization in the CNS

There is little specific binding of PBD to normal brain structures with the exception of the olfactory bulb, the choroid plexus, ependyma cells, and the pineal gland in rats [7,9,11]. While whole rat pituitary homogenates have relatively low levels of receptors, autoradiographic analysis reveals high levels of receptors concentrated in the posterior and intermediate lobes [9]. Whole rat brain homogenates, however, have only about 2% of the adrenal gland values [26]. Unlike the rat and mouse, CNS tissue of the cat and human displays relatively high levels of PBD receptors selectively associated with gray matter, the extrapyramidal motor, vestibulo-cerebellar, visual and auditory relay, and blood pressure regulating structure [27,28]. Furthermore, experimental glial neoplasms in rats have been shown to express an elevated density of PBD receptors [29–32] compared to normal glia and to neurons [1,21]. Increased binding to PBD receptors has also been reported in human gliomas and non-glial tumors [33–36].

In Vitro Binding Characteristics of PBD Receptors in Brain Tumor

Expression of PBD receptors in brain tumor has been analyzed by Scatchard plots of radiolabeled PBD binding. There is a single class of binding sites in the rodental tumor. Although K_d values of these tumors and cortex are similar, B_{max} is maximally 20-fold higher in tumor compared to the cortex [32,33]. A comparison of Walker 256 tumors grown subcutaneously or in brain reveals no significant differences in either K_d or B_{max} [32].

Specific binding significantly increases as the histologically determined grade of malignancy increases from low- to high-grade human gliomas [33]. Relatively high specific binding is also present in normal tissue infiltrated with malignant glial cells compared to nonneoplastic tissue. ^{3}H-PK 11195 also demonstrate higher binding densities to human tumors of nonglial origin, such as meningioma, craniopharyngioma, PNET, and osteosarcoma, than nonneoplastic tissue [33]. Autoradiographical analyses display areas of increased binding of PBDs with high topographical correlation with areas of histologically verified brain tumors [32].

In Vivo Study for Imaging Brain Tumor

The mixed benzodiazepine ligand, ^{3}H-flunitrazepam, and a selective PBD ligand, ^{3}H-PK11195, could be useful *in vivo* markers to outline rat brain tumor borders. High densities of PBD binding in glial tumors by intravenous injections of ^{3}H-PK11195 or ^{3}H-flunitrazepam in combination with clonazepam have been reported [37]. These bindings are specific to PBD receptors expressed in glioma cells because ^{3}H-PBD bindings can be displaced by preadministration of excess PK11195. Topographical correlation is excellent between areas of histologically verified tumor and high densities PBD receptors [31]. The choroid plexus, the ependyma, and the pineal gland also show a moderate level of binding, but there is little binding in other normal brain structures or necrotic tissue. Binding densities are approximately three-to-five fold higher in C6 glial tumors compared to the normal cortex. Injection of mixed-type of ligands such as ^{3}H-diazepam or ^{3}H-flunitrazepam has the advantage of showing (1) normal anatomical structures, and (2) affected cortex due to tumor compression and edema with diminished binding around a larger tumor. Mixed-type ligands, however, resulted in a lower tumor/cortex ratio of radioactive densities than PBD ligands and showed neuronal inhibition at higher concentration [31].

Implication for New Image Analysis (K_d and B_{max} Images, and 3D Reconstruction)

Techniques currently utilized to image tumors in the CNS rely on differences in tissue attenuation characteristics, breakdown of the blood-brain barrier (BBB) to contrast agents, mass effect, and changes in glucose or amino acid transport [38]. The limitations of these methods are most apparent in glial and other infiltrative tumors due to their failure to identify tumor cells which reside beyond the borders of the imaging abnormality. An ability to image tumors with a ligand that (1) binds specifically to tumor cells, and (2) readily crosses the intact BBB might significantly improve tumor resolution in the brain and allow better identification of the outermost margin of tumor cells. Peripheral benzodiazepine receptor ligands appear to fulfill both criteria: they are not barred by the BBB and they have high specific binding to glial tumors.

An understanding of PBD receptor binding in brain tumors may be important to improve our ability to diagnose and manage these lesions. Positron, iodine, or ferrous particle labeled peripheral benzodiazepine ligands could, therefore, allow better delineation of tumor borders in the brain and the identification of subtle areas of tumor infiltration with positron emission tomography (PET), single photon emission computed tomography (SPECT), or magnetic resonance imaging (MRI), respectively. ^{11}C-PK11195 has been used to map heart PBD receptors *in vivo* with PET [39,40]. Even though high specific activity was essential, an ^{18}F-diazepam study revealed negative binding images of glioma in contrast with the normal cortex and reduced binding images in adjacent cortex to the tumor [41]. An *in vivo* ^{11}C-PK11195 study in glioma patients also required high specific activity to image gliomas. Gildersleeve et al. [42] reported that successively synthesized ^{125}I-labeled PK11195 did not alter the binding characteristics for the U_{251} human glioblastoma cells. *In vivo* studies using C6 glioma suggested that ^{123}I-PK11195 or a related analog as possible tools for the *in vivo* localization and characterization of glioma in humans by SPECT.

Using digital image analysis of a single saturation experiment, it is possible to produce K_d and B_{max} images of PBD binding [32]. This technique, unlike previous ligand binding methods, allows for the visual survey of specific binding, as well as of B_{max} and K_d constants obtained from an Eadie-Hofstee analysis of the saturation data for an entire tissue section [32,43]. The relationships between binding parameters and anatomic (spatial) data or histological changes can thus be more readily analyzed and quantified.

Three-dimensional images of PBD receptors in rodent brain tumor models have been generated from thionin-stained histological sections and autoradiograms [37]. It is also possible to demonstrate higher tumor/brain contrast and superior topographical correlation between anatomical and receptor mapping images of brain tumor in three dimensions. Using cut surface models, the anatomical relations can be visualized in any direction between tumor and surrounding structures. Furthermore, heterogeneities of radioactivity within the tumor might be expressing differences in the degree of distribution of the ligand itself in *in vivo* studies or differences in the degree of proliferation or metabolism of the tumor.

These new receptor mapping images may provide a more precise and biochemical image analysis of brain tumors.

Biological Roles

Although the PBD receptor was discovered 10 years ago, the cellular function of the protein(s) comprising PBD receptor remains to be elucidated. These sites could be responsible for benzodiazepine actions in cardiovascular function [44], steroidogenesis [45], and in the immune response [46]. PBD may influence epithelial regulation of electrolyte transport in the choroid plexus and ependyma of the brain [47]. Furthermore, previous studies reported the inhibitory effects of PBD on tumor growth, such as the inhibition of thymidine incorporation into the DNA of glial cells [48] and the reduction of the mitogenesis in Swiss 3T3 cells [49]. A strong positive correlation between the binding affinity of benzodiazepines for the peripheral type receptor and their antiproliferative activities was also reported in mouse thymoma cells [50], although there was no significant correlation between activities of benzodiazepines and their reported degree of affinity. Pawlikowski et al. [48] reported an antiproliferative action of PBDs on human glioma at the micromolar range (1–100 μM). Contrarily, Diwan et al. [51] reported promotion of hepatocellular carcinogenesis in B6C3F1 mice by diazepam after initiation by *N*-nitrosodiethylamine. The induction of differentiation in Friend erythroleukemia cells [49], enhancement of melanogenesis in melanoma cells [52], and the specific enhancement of *c-fos* messenger RNA induction by nerve growth factor [53] were also reported. These effects, however, were observed at micromolar concentrations while PBD receptors are saturated at concentrations in the nanomolar range. Thus, these effects of PBD might be pharmacological or toxic actions rather than biological or physiological effects, even though some of these actions were inhibited by PK11195.

Recently, Ikezaki et al. [54] reported that PBDs may be involved in the regulation of cell proliferation as a growth factor in lower concentration and as a antiproliferative agent in higher concentration. PK11195 increased the growth rate and thymidine incorporation of C6 glioma cells by 20%–30% in the nanomolar range in serum-free medium. The effect of PK11195 as a mitogenic agent was also shown by increasing DNA synthesis of Swiss 3T3 cells by 170% over control at 10 nM. Ruff et al. [55] reported that chemotaxis of human monocytes were enhanced with ED_{50} of 10^{-13} M for Ro5–4864, whereas higher concentration ($>10^{-8}$ M) resulted in a reduced chemotactic response. These findings support the results showing a biphasic effect of PBD on cell proliferation.

The possibility of a relation between PBD and the phorbol ester binding site has been proposed, because the magnitude and the persistence of down-regulation of these binding sites were similar [56]. It is interesting to note that peripheral benzodiazepines are similar to phorbol diester tumor promoters in that they exert profound effects on growth and differentiation in various kinds of cell types [56].

Although receptors for PBD are thought to exist on the mitochondrial outer membrane [15,57], it would be worthwhile to investigate further whether this receptor-ligand complex will significantly affect mitochondrial functions. As a direct effect of PBD on mitochondrial function, Hirsch et al. [58] reported that PBDs decreased respiratory control in isolated rat kidney mitochondria by increasing and decreasing the rates of respiratory state IV and III, respectively. A dose-dependent decrease of O_2 consumption has been also shown in the presence of PBDs at concentrations consistent with a receptor-mediated action [59].

There are some candidates for the protein labeled by PBD ligands on the outer membrane of the mitochondria, such as the voltage-dependent anion channel (VDAC, or porin, corresponding to the 35 kd band), the isozyme of phospholipase A2 (15–18 kd), and the membrane bound glutahione-S-transferase (15 kd) [26]. These proteins are linked to the transportation of metabolites, the cytoplasmic ADP exchange with mitochondrial ATP mediated by the bound kinase, the adenine nucleotide carrier, and phospholipid metabolism. Modulation of phospholipid metabolism is widely studied in signal transduction. Thus, it would be worthwhile to clarify whether the activated receptor transmits signals to the mitochondrial or to the nuclear DNA.

The studies of peripheral-type benzodiazepines and receptors in brain tumor may provide novel and important clues in the imaging of tumor cells and in the understanding of tumor biology.

Summary

There are two classes of benzodiazepine receptors. The central-type receptors are located on the neuronal membrane where they exert their anticonvulsant and antianxiety effects. The peripheral-type benzodiazepine receptors are found in peripheral tissues, such as the kidney, and are located on the mitochondrial membrane. Although the biological roles of PBDs have not been clarified, certain brain tumors have been shown to possess PBD receptors. PBDs have much higher affinity to brain tumors, compared to the surrounding normal brain, and easily cross the blood-brain barrier. Using these advantages of PBD, it would be promising to localize brain tumor cells with radiolabeled PBD ligands, and to characterize the biochemical behavior of brain tumors with receptor mapping images. PBDs might be deeply involved in hormonal regulation and cell proliferation in the CNS. The studies of the expression of PBD receptors in brain tumors and their biological roles in tumor cells may provide new and important clues to understand brain tumor biology.

Acknowledgements. We thank Drs. Toga, Santori, and Grafton (UCLA) for their helpful advice. This work was supported in part by grants from The California Institute for Cancer Research and American Cancer Society Institutional Grant to K.I., and the Robert Wood Johnson Foundation, the Oxnard Foundation, and NIH award 1R29NS26523-01 to K.L.B.

References

1. Tallman JF, Paul SM, Skolnick P, Gallager DW (1980) Receptors for the age of anxiety: Pharmacology of the benzodiazepines. Science 207:274–281
2. Tallman JF, Gallager DW (1985) The GABA-ergic system: A locus of benzodiazepine action. Annu Rev Neurosci 8:21–44
3. Schofield PR, Darlison MG, Fujita N, Burt DR, Stephenson FA, Rodriguez H, Rhee LM, Ramachandran J, Reale V, Glencorse TA, Seeburg PH, Barnard EA (1987) Sequence and functional expression of the GABA receptor shows a ligand-gated super-family. Nature 328:221–227
4. Tallman JF, Thomas JW, Gallager DW (1978) GABA-ergic modulation of benzodiazepine binding site sensitivity. Nature 274:383–385
5. Wastek GJ, Speth RC, Reisine TD, Yamamura HI (1978) The effect of γ-aminobutyric acid on ^{3}H-flunitrazepam binding in rat brain. Eur J Pharmacol 50:445–447
6. Olson RW (1981) GABA-benzodiazepine-barbiturate receptor interactions. J Neurochem 31:1–13
7. Braestrup C, Squires RF (1977) Benzodiazepine receptors in rat brain. Nature 266:732–734
8. Schoemaker H, Boles RB, Horst WD, Yamamura HI (1983) Specific high affinity binding sites for [^{3}H] Ro5–4864 in rat brain and kidney. J Pharmacol Exp Ther 225:61–69
9. De Souza EB, Anholt RRH, Murphy KMM, Snyder SH, Kuhar MJ (1985) Peripheral-type benzodiazepine receptors in endocrine organs: Autoradiographic localization in rat pituitary, adrenal, and testis. Endocrinology 116:567–573
10. Anholt RRH, De Souza EB, Oster-Granite ML, Snyder SH (1985) Peripheral-type benzodiazepine receptors: Autoradiographic localization in whole-body sections of neonatal rats. J Pharmacol Exp Ther 233:517–526
11. Marangos PJ, Patel J, Boulenger JP, Clark-Rosenberg R (1982) Characterization of peripheral-type benzodiazepine binding sites in brain using [^{3}H] Ro5–4864. Mol Pharmacol 22:26–32
12. Le Fur G, Perrier GM, Vaucher N, Imbault F, Flamier A, Bénavidès J, Uzan A, Renault C, Dubroeucq MC, Guérémy (1983) Peripheral benzodiazepine binding sites: Effect of PK11195, 1-(2-chlorophenyl)-N-methyl-N-(1-methylpropyl)-3-isoquinoline carboxamide. I. *In vitro* studies. Life Sci 32:1839–1847
13. Moingeon Ph, Bidart JM, Alberici GF, Bohuon C (1983) Characterization of a peripheral-type benzodiazepine binging site on human circulating lymphocytes. Eur J Pharmacol 92:147–149
14. Moingeon Ph, Dessaux JJ, Fellous R, Alberici GF, Bidart JM, Motté Ph, Bohoun C (1984) Benzodiazepine receptors on human blood plateletes. Life Sci 35:2003–2009

15. Anholt RRH, Pedersen PL, De Souza EB, Snyder SH (1986) The peripheral-type benzodiazepine receptor: Localization to the mitochondrial outer membrane. J Biol Chem 261:576–583
16. Mukherjee S, Das SK (1989) Subcellular distribution of "peripheral type" binding sites for [^{3}H] Ro5–4864 in guinea pig lung: Localization to the mitochondrial inner membrane. J Biol Chem 264:16713–16718
17. Anholt RRH, Aebi U, Pedersen PL, Snyder SH (1986) Solubilization and reassemble of the mitochondrial benzodiazepine receptor. Biochemistry 25:2120-2125
18. Paul SM, Kempner ES, Skolnick P (1981) In situ molecular weight determination of brain and peripheral benzodiazepine binding sites. Eur J Pharmacol 76:465–466
19. Antkiewicz-Michaluk L, Mukhin AG, Guidotti A, Krueger KE (1988) Purification and characterization of a protein associated with peripheral-type benzodiazepine binding sites. J Biol Chem 263:17317–17321
20. Sprengel R, Werner P, Seeburg PH, Mukhin AG, Rita Santi M, Grayson DR, Guidotti AG, Krueger KE (1989) Molecular cloning and expression of cDNA encoding a peripheral-type benzodiazepine receptor. J Biol Chem 264:20415–20421
21. Awad M, Gavish M (1987) Binding of [^{3}H]Ro5–4864 and [^{3}H]PK11195 to cerebral cortex and peripheral tissues of various species: Species differences and heterogeneity in peripheral benzodiazepine binding sites. J Neurochem 49:1407–1414
22. Mantione CR, Goldman ME, Martin B, Bolger GT, Luddens HW et al. (1988) Purification and characterization of an endogenous protein modulator of radioligand binding to "peripheral type" benzodiazepine receptor and dihydropyridine CA^{2+}-channel antagonist binding sites. Biochem Pharmacol 37:339–347
23. Beaumont K, Skowronski R, Vaughn DA, Fanestil DD (1988) Interactions of lipids with peripheral type benzodiazepine receptors. Biochem Pharmacol 37:1009–1014
24. Verma A, Snyder SH (1988) Characterization of porphyrin interactions with peripheral-type benzodiazepine receptors. Mol Pharmacol 34:800–805
25. Kessel D (1988) Interactions between porphyrins and mitochondrial benzodiazepine receptors. Cancer Lett 39:193–198
26. Verma A, Snyder SH (1989) Peripheral type benzodiazepine receptors. Ann Rev Pharmacol Toxicol 29:307–322
27. Doble A, Malgouris C, Daniel M, Daniel N, Imbault F, Basbaum A, Uzan A, Guérémy C, Le Fur G (1987) Labelling of peripheral benzodiazepine binding sites in human brain with [^{3}H]PK11195: Anatomical and subcellular distribution. Brain Res Bull 18:49–61
28. Bénavidès J, Savaki HE, Malgouris C, Laplace C, Daniel M, Begassat F, Desban M, Uzan A, Dubroeucq MC, Renault C, Guérémy C, Le Fur G (1984) Autoradiographic localization of peripheral benzodiazepine binding sites in the cat brain with [^{3}H]PK11195. Brain Res Bull 13:69–77
29. Syapin PJ, Skolnick P (1979) Characterization of benzodiazepine binding sites in cultured cells of neuronal origin. J Neurochem 32:1047–1052
30. Starosta-Rubinstein S, Ciliax BJ, Penney JB, McKeever P, Young AB (1987) Imaging of a glioma using peripheral benzodiazepine receptor ligands. Proc Natl Acad Sci USA 84:891–895
31. Black KL, Ikezaki K, Arthur WT (1989) Imaging of brain tumors using peripheral benzodiazepine receptor ligands. J Neurosurg 71:113–118
32. Ikezaki K, Black KL, Toga AW, Santori EM, Becker DP, Smith ML (1990) Imaging peripheral benzodiazepine receptors in brain tumor in rats: In vitro binding characteristics. J Cereb Blood Flow Metab 10:580–587

33. Black KL, Ikezaki K, Santori EM, Becker DP, Vinters HV (1990) Specific high-affinity binding of peripheral benzodiazepine receptor ligands to brain tumors in rat and man. Cancer 65:93–97
34. Bénavidès J, Cornu P, Dennis T, Dubois A, Hauw J-J, MacKenzie ET, Sazdovitch V, Scatton B (1988) Imaging human brain lesions with an ω_3 site radioligand. Ann Neurol 24:708–712
35. Olson JM, Junk L, Young AB, Penny JB, Mancini WR (1988) Isoquinoline and peripheral-type benzodiazepine binding in gliomas: Implications for diagnostic imaging. Cancer Res 48:5837–5841
36. Ferrarese C, Appollonio I, Frigo M, Gaini SM, Piolti R, Frattola L (1989) Benzodiazepine receptors and diazepam-binding inhibitor in human cerebral tumors. Ann Neurol 26:564–568
37. Ikezaki K, Black KL, Santori EM, Smith ML, Becker DP, Payne BA, Toga AW (1990) Three-dimensional comparison of peripheral benzodiazepine binding and histological findings in rat brain tumor. Neurosurgery 27:78–82
38. Hawkins RA, Phelps ME (1988) Applications of positron emission tomography (PET) in tumor management. In: Withers HR, Peters LJ (eds) Medical radiology. Innovations in radiation oncology. Springer Berlin, pp 209–219
39. Charbonneau P, Syrota A, Crouzel C, Valois J-M, Prenant C, Crouzel M (1986) Peripheral-type benzodiazepine receptors in the living heart characterized by positron emission tomography. Circulation 73:476–483
40. Junk L, Koeppe RA, Leonard Watkins G, Jewett DM, Wieland DM, Kilbourn MR, Greenberg HS, Ciliax BJ, Young AB (1988) Glioma imaging with a peripheral benzodiazepine ligand. Neurology 38 (Suppl 1):307
41. Grafton ST, Ikezaki K, Luxen A, Chugani D, Black KL, Mazziotta JC, Barrio JR, Phelps ME (1989) Labeling of rat C6 glioma implants with 3-[F^{18}]fluorodiazepam and [H^3]diazepam: In vitro tissue homogenate and in vivo autoradiographic results. J Cereb Blood Flow Metab 9 (Suppl 1):S18
42. Gildersleeve DL, Lin TY, Wieland DM, Ciliax BJ, Olson JM, Young AB (1989) Synthesis of a high specific activity ^{125}I-labeled analog of PK11195, potential agent for SPECT imaging of the peripheral benzodiazepine binding site. Nucl Med Biol (Int J Radiat Appl Instrum [B]) 16:423–429
43. Toga AW, Santori EM, Samaie M (1986) Regional distribution of flunitrazepam binding constants: Visualizing K_d and B_{max} by digital image analysis. J Neurosci 6:2747–2756
44. Mestre M, Carriot T, Belin C, Uzan A, Renault C, Dubroeucq MC, Guérémy C, Le Fur G (1984) Electrophysiological and pharmacological characterization of peripheral benzodiazepine receptors in a guinea pig heart preparation. Life Sci 35:953–962
45. Ritta MN, Campos MB, Calandra RS (1987) Effect of GABA and benzodiazepine on testicular androgen production. Life Sci 40:791–798
46. Zavala F, Lenfant M (1987) Peripheral benzodiazepines enhance the respiratory burst of macrophage-like P388D1 cells stimulated by arachidonic acid. Int J Immunopharmacol 9:269–274
47. Williams GL, Pollay M, Seale T, Hisey B, Robert PA (1990) Benzodiazepine receptors and cerebrospinal fluid formation. J Neurosurg 72:759–762
48. Pawlikowski M, Kunert-Radek J, Stepien H (1988) Inhibition of cell proliferation of human gliomas by benzodiazepines *in vitro*. Acta Neurol Scand 77:231–233
49. Clarke GD, Ryan PJ (1980) Tranquillizers can block mitogenesis in 3T3 cells and induce differentiation in Friend cells. Nature 287:160–161

50. Wang JKT, Morgan JI, Spector S (1984) Benzodiazepines that bind at peripheral sites inhibit cell proliferation. Proc Natl Acad Sci USA 81:753–756
51. Diwan BA, Rice JM, Ward JM (1986) Tumor-promoting activity of benzodiazepine tranquilizers, diazepam and oxazepam, in mouse liver. Carcinogenesis 7:789–794
52. Matthew E, Laskin JD, Zimmerman EA, Weinstein IB, Hsu KC, Engelhardt DL (1981) Benzodiazepines have high-affinity binding sites and induce melanogenesis in B16/C3 melanoma cells. Proc Natl Acad Sci USA 78:3935–3939
53. Curran T, Morgan JI (1985) Superinduction of c-*fos* by nerve growth factor in the presence of peripherally active benzodiazepines. Science 229:1265–1268
54. Ikezaki K, Black KL (1990) Stimulation of cell growth and DNA synthesis by peripheral benzodiazepine. Cancer Lett 49:115–120
55. Ruff MR, Pert CB, Weber RJ, Wahl SM, Paul SM (1985) Benzodiazepines receptor-mediated chemotaxis of human monocytes. Science 229:1281–1283
56. Johnson MD, Wang JKT, Morgan JI, Spector S (1986) Downregulation of [^{3}H]Ro5-4864 binding sites after exposure to peripheral-type benzodiazepines *in vitro*. J Pharmacol Exp Ther 238:855–859
57. Basile AS, Skolnick P (1986) Subcellular localization of "peripheral-type" binding sites for benzodiazepines in rat brain. J Neurochem 46:305–308
58. Hirsch JD, Beyer CF, Malkowitz L, Loullis CC, Beer B, Blume AJ (1988) Mitochondrial benzodiazepine receptors mediate inhibition of mitochondrial respiratory control. Mol Pharmacol 35:157–163
59. Larcher J-C, Vayssiere J-L, Le Marquer FJ, Cordeau LR, Keane PE, Bachy A, Gros F, Croizat BP (1989) Effects of peripheral benzodiazepines upon the O2 consumption of neuroblastoma cells. Eur J Pharmacol 161:197–202

Gadolinium Neutron Capture Therapy for Brain Tumors—Biological Aspects

MASAO TAKAGAKI[1], YOSHIFUMI ODA[1], MASATO MATSUMOTO[1], HARUHIKO KIKUCHI[1], TOORU KOBAYASHI, KEIJI KANDA, and YOWRI UJENO[2]

Introduction

The success of Boron Neutron Capture Therapy (B-NCT) has been reported for the last 25 years. [1]. This therapy requires boron to accumulate into neoplastic tissue. Gadolinium (Gd) has been proposed as an another potential nuclide for NCT [2–4] because Gd-157 has an approximately 64-fold greater thermal neutron cross-section (255,000 barns), than does Boron-10, and releases a large total kinetic energy (7.94 MeV) which it shares among prompt γ-rays, internal conversion electrons, and Auger electrons by the thermal neutron capture reaction [5]. Long ranges of high energy γ-rays and electrons deliver doses to infiltrating neoplastic satellite lesions of the main tumor [3]. Additionally, Gd-DTPA, an enhanced material for MR imaging, is clinically available as a tumor-seeking agent. In this study the tumoricidal effect of Gd-NCT was investigated using Gd-DTPA, and its killing effect was confirmed in *in vitro* and *in vivo* systems.

Materials and Methods

1. The In Vitro *System*

This work was carried out at the Deuterium Facility of the Research Reactor Institute, Kyoto University. Human glioma cells, T98G, were suspended in Teflon tubes (10 mm in diameter, 30 mm length) containing 1,500 μl Dulbecco's modified Eagle's medium supplemented with 10% fetal bovine serum and a certain amount of Gd-DTPA (Figs. 1, 2), yielding 5000 ppm Gd-n (= 780 ppm Gd-157, corresponding to the clinical standard of 50 ppm B-10) upon which thermal neutrons were exposed. After irradiation, the cells were incubated in 6-cm diameter petri dishes containing medium in a humidified atmosphere with 5% carbondioxide at 37°C. The colonies were counted after 10 days of incubation.

[1]Department of Neurosurgery, School of Medicine, Kyoto University, Kyoto, 606 Japan
[2]Research Reactor Institute of Kyoto University, Osaka, 590–04 Japan

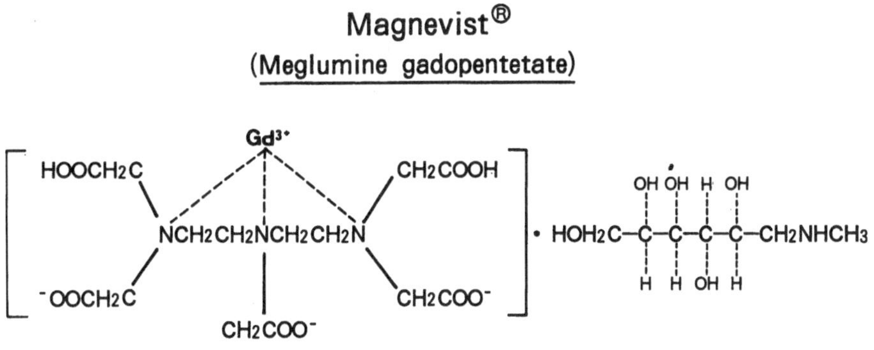

Fig. 1. Chemical structural formula of Gd-DTPA

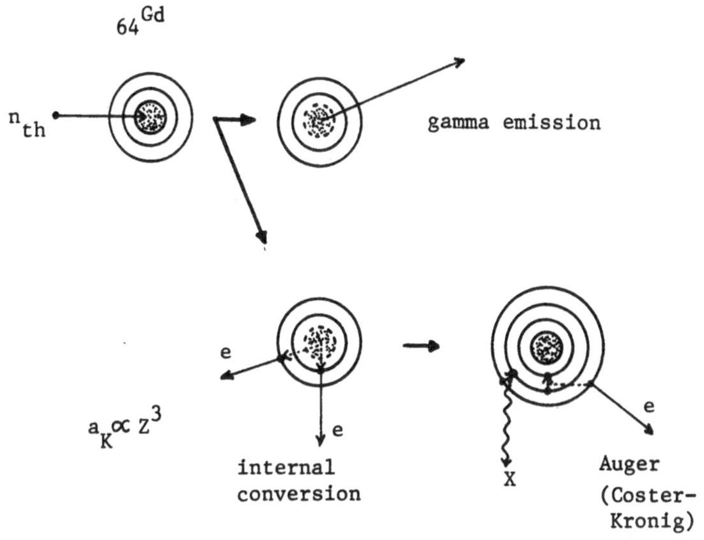

Fig. 2. Thermal neutron capture reaction of Gd-157

2. In Vivo *Study*

Fisher-344 rats (7-week-old males) bearing gliosarcoma brain tumors were prepared. 1E+5/10 μl nitrosourea-induced gliosarcoma cells (9L) were inplanted into the right parietal region by stereotactic maneuvers. The mean survival rate of the 9L-rat was approximately 2 weeks. Twelve days after implantation, which was close to their terminal stage, the 9L-rats were exposed to thermal neutrons at a fluence rate of 3E+9/s for 1 h immediately after an intravenous injection of 2 ml/kg Gd-DTPA. Thermal neutrons were vertically exposed onto the parietal scalp surface under sedation. During exposure, the animal's body was protected from neutron bombarding by an Li-6F holder. Two weeks after irradiation, the brains were removed and underwent histolo-

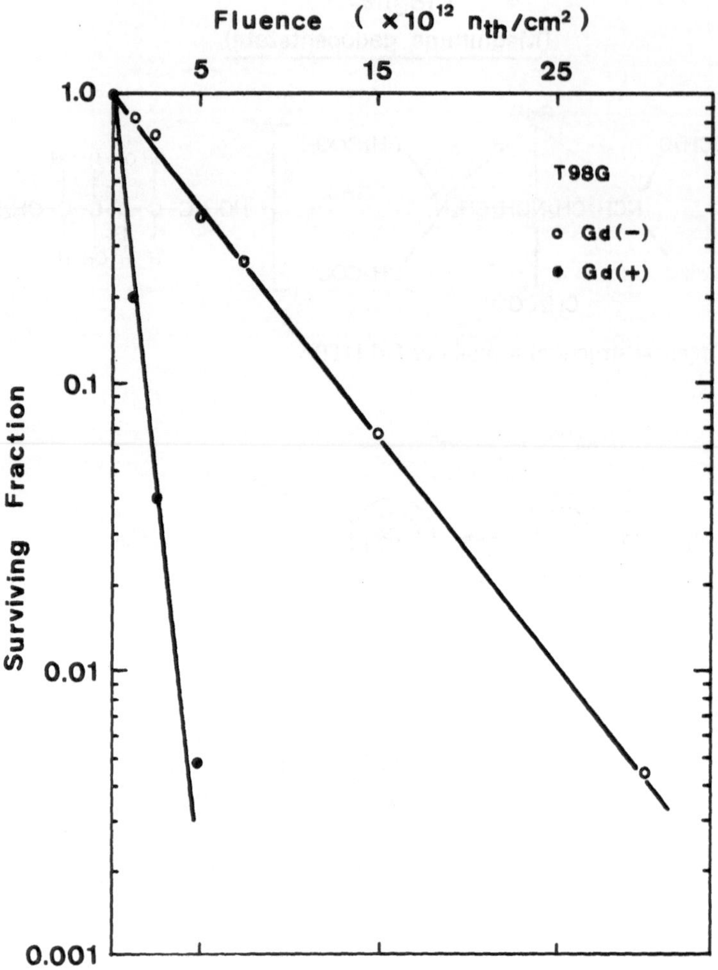

Fig. 3. Survival curve of T98G human glioma cell

gical examinations. Tumor clearance of Gd-DTPA was also measured by the prompt γ-ray spectrometry [6] from the scalp surface.

Results

1. In Vitro *Analysis*

A 1% survival level was obtained at 3.75E+12 (n/cm^2) for the Gd (+) medium and 2.50E+13 (n/cm^2) for the Gd (−) medium, obtaining an approximately 6.7-fold difference (Fig. 3).

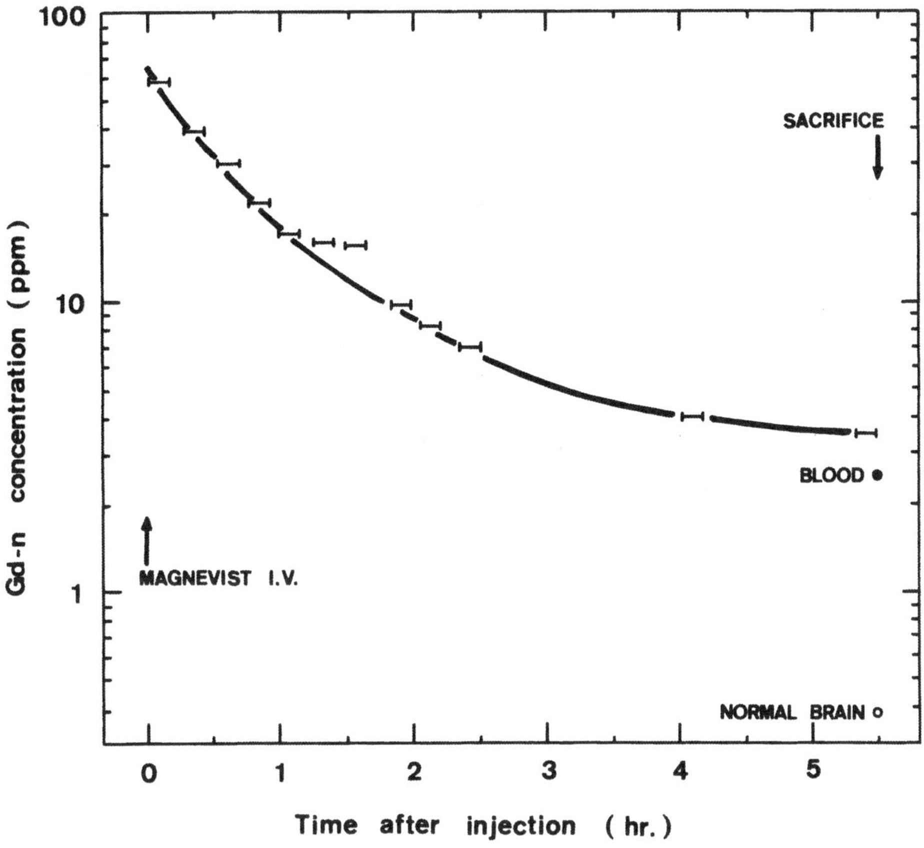

Fig. 4. Rat 9L brain tumor clearance of Gd-DTPA

2. In Vivo *Analysis*

The 9L-brain tumor cells were extensively destroyed by Gd-NCT, while almost no damage occurred to the normal brain and vessels. However, surviving viable tumor cells were also identified. Survival rates of the treated 9L-rats are now under investigation. 9L-brain tumor clearance of Gd-DTPA is shown in Fig. 4. Approximately 60 ppm Gd-n was detected immediately after iv. administration of 0.2 ml/kg Gd-DTPA. After 5.5 h from administration, only a slight difference of Gd concentration between tumor and blood levels was detected, but Gd concentration in the contralateral normal brain was under the lowest detectable limit of ca. 1 ppm. Approximately 30 min after injection, Gd concentration in tumors decreased by half.

Discussion

Gd-n concentrations in brain tumor as confirmed in this study, were less than 100 ppm. Using Gd-157-enriched DTPA, the concentration in tumor was easily elevated to sixfold of the initial value. Gd-NCT loaded with a high-dose administration of Gd-DTPA, a ten fold amount of the clinical dose, showed a tumoricidal effect in 9L-brain tumor without serious injury to normal brain and vessels after a thermal neutron exposure of 1.8E+13 (n/cm^2). If we assume the goal of Gd-n concentration in tumor to be several thousand ppm, more than a ten fold specific accumulation in tumor should be achieved. Another potential use of Gd-DTPA, intraventricular and/or intrathecal high-dose injection, can produce a supplemental killing effect in cases of subependymal or intraventricular tumor disseminations by the simultaneously combined treatment with B-NCT. In Gd-NCT, dose distribution in tumor is not uniform. Theoretically, in a spherical tumor with a radius of R, dose intensity: ϕ (r) uniformly caused by Gd (n,γ and/or e) reactions in tumor is expressed as follows:

$$d^2\phi(r)/d^2r + 2d\phi(r)/rdr + B^2\phi(r) = 0$$

$$\phi(r) = (A/r)\sin(\pi r/R)$$

$$A = \pi\phi(0)/R = \pi N\sigma\phi/R$$

where, r is the distance from the tumor center, N: Gd-157 concentration is σ: 255,000 barns, ϕ is the thermal neutron fluencey, and B is the constant depending up on the size of the spheroid. Total dose distribution is estimated as follows,

$$\gamma^* + \text{Gd-157}(n,\gamma \text{ and/or } e)\ \text{Gd-158} + \text{N-14}(n,p)\text{C-14}$$
$$= \gamma^* + [N(Gd)\ \sigma(Gd)\ RBE(\gamma \text{ and/or } e) + N(N)\ \sigma(N) RBE(p)]\phi$$

where, γ^* is caused by reactor core and structural materials, RBE is the relative biological effectiveness, and N indicates concentration of Gd-157 and/or N-14 in tissue. Dose distribution onto tumor-surrounding tissue caused by high energy γ-rays and electrons might be valid for tumors of an infiltrating type. Spacial γ^* and proton caused by N-14 are inevitably exposed, and strongly restrict the irradiation period. This frustrating situation can be lessened by Gd + B − NCT.

Conclusions

The tumoricidal effect of Gd-NCT was confirmed in an *in vitro* system suplemented with 5,000 ppm Gd-n. The concentration of Gd in 9L-rat brain tumor after intravenous injection of 0.2 mg/kg Gd-DTPA was less than 100 ppm, but Gd-NCT on 9L-rat brain tumor administrated with a ten fold dose showed a substantial killing effect on tumor without serious injury to normal brain structure. For the purpose of clinical trials, a more selective tumor affinity of Gd must be attained.

References

1. Hatanaka H (ed) (1986) Neutron capture therapy for brain tumors. Nishimura Niigata, Japan
2. Martin RF, D'cunha, G Pardee M, Allen BJ (1988) Induction of double-strand breaks following neutron capture by DNA-bound Gd-157. Int J Radiat Biol 54(2):205–208
3. Brugger RM, Shih JA (1989) Evaluation of gadolinium-157 as a neutron capture therapy agent. Strahlenther Onkol 165 (2):153–156
4. Akine Y, Tokita N, Matsumoto T, Oyama H, Egawa S, Aizawa O (to be published) Radiation effect of gadolinium neutron capture reaction and survival of Chinese hamster cells. Strahlenther Onkol
5. Greenwood RC (1978) Collective and two-quasiparticle states in Gd-158 observed through study of radiative neutron capture in Gd-157. Nucl Physiol A304:327–428
6. Kobayashi T, Kanda K (1983) Microanalysis system of ppm-order B-10 concentrations in tissue for neutron capture therapy by prompt gamma-ray spectrometry. Nucl Instr Meth 204:525–531

Index